Clinical Pediatric Anesthesiology

Clinical Pediatric Anesthesiology

Herodotos Ellinas, MD
Associate Professor
Division of Pediatric Anesthesiology
Children's Hospital of Wisconsin
Medical College of Wisconsin
Milwaukee, Wisconsin

Kai Matthes, MD, PhD
Chair, Finance Committee and Treasurer
Interisland Medical Group, Inc.
Maui, Hawaii

Walid Alrayashi, MD
Associate in Perioperative Anesthesia
Department of Anesthesiology, Critical Care and Pain Medicine
Boston Children's Hospital
Instructor of Anaesthesia
Harvard Medical School
Boston, Massachusetts

Aykut Bilge, MD, PhD
Associate in Perioperative Anesthesia
Department of Anesthesiology, Critical Care and Pain Medicine
Boston Children's Hospital
Instructor of Anaesthesia
Harvard Medical School
Boston, Massachusetts

New York   Chicago   San Francisco   Athens   London   Madrid   Mexico City
New Delhi   Milan   Singapore   Sydney   Toronto

Clinical Pediatric Anesthesiology

1 2 3 4 5 6 7 8 9 DSS 25 24 23 22 21 20

ISBN 978-1-259-58574-6
MHID 1-259-58574-3

This book was set in Minion Pro by MPS Limited.
The editors were Jason Malley and Kim J. Davis.
The production supervisor was Richard Ruzycka.
Project management was provided by Poonam Bisht, MPS Limited.
The cover designer was W2 Design.

This book is printed on acid-free paper.

Library of Congress Cataloging-in-Publication Data

Names: Ellinas, Herodotos, editor. | Matthes, Kai, editor. | Alrayashi,
    Walid, editor. | Bilge, Aykut, editor.
Title: Clinical pediatric anesthesiology / [edited by] Herodotos Ellinas,
    Kai Matthes, Walid Alrayashi, Aykut Bilge.
Description: New York : McGraw Hill, [2021] | Includes bibliographical
    references and index. | Summary: "The objective of this book is to
    provide a high-yield textbook of pediatric anesthesiology combined with
    high quality videos that can be repeatedly used to educate practitioners
    on the safest and most efficient methods. The text focuses on the unique
    aspects and considerations necessary for managing pediatric patients"—
    Provided by publisher.
Identifiers: LCCN 2020013639 (print) | LCCN 2020013640 (ebook) | ISBN
    9781259585746 (paperback ; alk. paper) | ISBN 9781259585753 (ebook)
Subjects: MESH: Anesthesia--methods | Child | Infant |
    Anesthetics--administration & dosage
Classification: LCC RD139 (print) | LCC RD139 (ebook) | NLM WO 440 | DDC
    617.9/6083--dc23
LC record available at https://lccn.loc.gov/2020013639
LC ebook record available at https://lccn.loc.gov/2020013640

This book is dedicated to my wife Libby, who has always been my pillar of support, to my children Lucas, Sophia, and Marcus who have been believers in my work, to my parents who encouraged me to dream big and aim high, and to my high school teachers Lia (English), Michalis (Math), and Nitsa (Chemistry) who taught me perseverance.

HE

To the One, who has surrounded me with a wonderful family, friends, and mentors.

WA

Contents

Contributors

Claude Abdallah, MD, MSc, FASA
Associate Professor of Anesthesiology and Pediatrics
The George Washington University Medical Center
Division of Anesthesiology
Children's National Hospital
Washington, DC
Chapter 11 Pre-procedure Medications

Gijo Alex, MD
Assistant Professor
Department of Anesthesiology and Pain Management
University of Texas Southwestern Medical Center—
    Children's Health
Dallas, Texas
Chapter 3 Monitoring, Breathing Systems, and Machines

Walid Alrayashi, MD
Associate in Perioperative Anesthesia
Department of Anesthesiology, Critical Care
    and Pain Medicine
Boston Children's Hospital
Instructor of Anaesthesia
Harvard Medical School
Boston, Massachusetts
Chapter 32 Regional Anesthesia: Truncal Blocks

Sapan Amin, MD
Assistant Professor
Division of Pediatric Anesthesiology
Children's Hospital of Wisconsin
Medical College of Wisconsin
Milwaukee, Wisconsin
Chapter 6 Hypnotics

Ingrid Fitz-James Antoine, MD
Assistant Professor, Department of Anesthesiology
Assistant Professor, Department of Pediatrics
    (Pediatric Cardiology)
Montefiore Medical Center/Albert Einstein College
    of Medicine
Bronx, New York
Chapter 33 Regional Anesthesia: Neuraxial

Adrian T. Bosenberg, MB ChB, FFA(SA)
Professor, Department Anesthesiology and Pain
    Management
Faculty Health Sciences, University Washington
Seattle Children's Hospital
Seattle, Washington
Chapter 30 Regional Anesthesia: Head and Neck Blocks

Steven Butz, MD
Professor
Division of Pediatric Anesthesiology
Children's Hospital of Wisconsin
Medical College of Wisconsin
Milwaukee, Wisconsin
*Chapter 35 Pediatric Ambulatory Anesthesia: What Is
    New and Safe?*

Veronica Carullo, MD, FAAP
New York Presbyterian Hospital / Weill Cornell Medical
    Center
Associate Professor of Clinical Anesthesiology and
    Pediatrics
Director, Pediatric Pain Management
New York, New York
Chapter 33 Regional Anesthesia: Neuraxial

Neethu Chandran, MD
Assistant Professor
Department of Anesthesiology and Pain Management
University of Texas Southwestern Medical Center—
    Children's Health
Dallas, Texas
Chapter 1 *Physiological Aspects*
Chapter 3 Monitoring, Breathing Systems, and Machines

Kallol Chaudhuri, MD, PhD, FAAP
Professor and Vice Chair (Education)
Department of Anesthesiology
Texas Tech University Health Sciences Center
Lubbock, Texas
Chapter 19 Anesthesia for Gastrointestinal Procedures

Swapna Chaudhuri, MD, PhD
Professor and Vice Chair for Administration
Associate Program Director, Curriculum and Assessment
Department of Anesthesiology
Texas Tech University Health Sciences Center
Lubbock, Texas
Chapter 21 Anesthesia for Genitourinary Procedures

Anne E. Cossu, MS, MD
Indiana University School of Medicine
Department of Anesthesia
Assistant Professor of Clinical Anesthesia
Indianapolis, Indiana
Chapter 18 Anesthesia for Thoracic Procedures

Huy Do, MD
Assistant Professor
Department of Anesthesiology and Pain Management
University of Texas Southwestern Medical Center—
    Children's Health
Dallas, Texas
Chapter 2 Anatomic Considerations

Proshad Nemati Efune, MD
Assistant Professor
Anesthesiology and Pain Management
University of Texas Southwestern Medical Center and
    Children's Health
Dallas, Texas
Chapter 38 Pediatric Critical Care Medicine

Susan E. Eklund, MD
Assistant in Perioperative Anesthesia
Boston Children's Hospital
Instructor in Anesthesia
Harvard Medical School
Boston, Massachusetts
Chapter 32 Regional Anesthesia: Truncal Blocks

Lynne R. Ferrari, MD
Associate Chair, Perioperative Anesthesia
Medical Director of Perioperative Services
Robert M. Smith Chair in Pediatric Anesthesia
Boston Children's Hospital
Associate Professor, Anesthesia
Harvard Medical School
Boston, Massachusetts
Chapter 10 Preoperative Evaluation

Doris M. Hardacker, MD
Associate Professor
Pediatric Anesthesiology
Indiana University School of Medicine
Indianapolis, Indiana
Chapter 18 Anesthesia for Thoracic Procedures

Amy Henry, MD
Pediatric Anesthesiologist
Private Practice, ANEX S.C.
Formerly from the Medical College of Wisconsin
Department of Anesthesiology, Division Pediatric
    Anesthesiology
Milwaukee, Wisconsin
Chapter 36 Anesthesia at Pediatric Offsite Locations

Jennifer Hernandez, MD
Assistant Professor
Anesthesiology and Pain Management
University of Texas Southwestern/Children's Medical Center
Dallas, Texas
Chapter 28 Intravenous Access

George M. Hoffman, MD
Professor of Anesthesiology and Pediatrics
Divisions of Pediatric Anesthesiology and Pediatric
    Critical Care
Medical College of Wisconsin
Medical Director and Chief, Pediatric Anesthesiology
Associate Medical Director, Pediatric Intensive Care Unit
Children's Hospital of Wisconsin
Milwaukee, Wisconsin
Chapter 25 Anesthesia for Liver Transplantation

Joann Hunsberger, MD
Assistant Professor, Pediatric Anesthesia
Department of Anesthesiology and CCM
Division of Pediatric Anesthesiology
Johns Hopkins Children's Center
Baltimore, Maryland
*Chapter 34 Intraoperative Complications and
    Crisis Management*

Cathie Tingey Jones, MD
Instructor, Harvard Medical School
Associate in Perioperative Anesthesia
Department of Anesthesiology, Critical Care
    and Pain Medicine
Boston Children's Hospital
Boston, Massachusetts
Chapter 23 Trauma and Special Emergencies

Nishanthi Kandiah, MD, FAAP
Assistant Professor, Department of Anesthesiology
University of Pittsburgh
Children's Hospital of Pittsburgh
University of Pittsburgh Medical Center
Pittsburgh, Pennsylvania
Chapter 30 Regional Anesthesia: Head and Neck Blocks

Asif Khan, MD
Pediatric Anesthesia Fellow
Department of Anesthesiology, Critical Care
    and Pain Medicine
Boston Children's Hospital
Harvard Medical School
Boston, Massachusetts
Chapter 27 Advanced Airway Techniques

Jeannette Kierce, MD
Assistant Professor
Pediatric Anesthesiology
VCU School of Medicine
Richmond, Virginia
Chapter 37 Post-Anesthesia Care Unit

Edgar E. Kiss, MD
Assistant Professor of Anesthesiology and Pain
 Management
University of Texas Southwestern Medical Center
Attending Anesthesiologist
Children's Health System of Texas
Dallas, Texas
Chapter 1 Physiological Aspects
Chapter 27 Advanced Airway Techniques

Benjamin Kloesel, MD, MSBS
Assistant Professor of Anesthesiology
University of Minnesota
Masonic Children's Hospital
Minneapolis, Minnesota
Chapter 29 Arterial Access

Richard F. Knox, MD
Assistant Professor
Anesthesiology and Pediatric Anesthesiology
University of South Carolina School of Medicine Upstate
Medical Director of Anesthesia Services
Shriner's Hospital for Children
Greenville, South Carolina
Chapter 22 Anesthesia for Orthopedic Procedures

Kristen L. Labovsky, MD
Assistant Professor
Division of Pediatric Anesthesiology
Children's Hospital of Wisconsin
Medical College of Wisconsin
Milwaukee, Wisconsin
Chapter 15 Anesthesia for Ophthalmic Procedures

Donna LaMonica, MD
Pediatric Anesthesiologist
Private Practice, North American Partners in Anesthesia
 of NJ LLC
St Joseph's University Medical Center
Paterson, New Jersey
Chapter 33 Regional Anesthesia: Neuraxial

Laura H. Leduc, MD
Anesthesiology and Pediatric Anesthesiology
University of South Carolina School of Medicine
Prisma Health System
Greenville, South Carolina
Chapter 22 Anesthesia for Orthopedic Procedures

Elaina E. Lin, MD
Assistant Professor
Anesthesiology and Critical Care Medicine
Children's Hospital of Philadelphia
Perelman School of Medicine at the University
 of Pennsylvania
Philadelphia, Pennsylvania
Chapter 26 Anesthesia for Fetal Surgery

Barbara J. Meinecke, MD, FASA
Assistant Professor
Division of Pediatric Anesthesiology
Children's Hospital of Wisconsin
Medical College of Wisconsin
Milwaukee, Wisconsin
Chapter 24 Anesthesia for Renal Transplantation

Shilpa Narayan, MD
Assistant Professor
Department of Pediatrics, Division of Critical Care
Children's Hospital Wisconsin
Medical College of Wisconsin
Milwaukee, Wisconsin
Chapter 39 Cardiopulmonary Resuscitation

Viviane G. Nasr, MD
Associate Professor of Anesthesia
Harvard Medical School
Department of Anesthesiology
Critical Care and Pain Medicine
Boston Children's Hospital
Boston, Massachusetts
Chapter 17 Anesthesia for Cardiovascular Procedures
Chapter 29 Arterial Access

Blake Nichols, MD
Assistant Professor
Pediatric Critical Care Medicine
University of Texas Southwestern Medical
 Center—Children's Health
Dallas, Texas
Chapter 38 Pediatric Critical Care Medicine

Patrick N. Olomu, MD, FRCA
Associate Professor of Anesthesiology and Pain Management
University of Texas Southwestern Medical Center
Attending Anesthesiologist
Children's Health System of Texas
Dallas, Texas
Chapter 27 Advanced Airway Techniques

Stacy Peterson, MD
Assistant Professor
Division of Pediatric Anesthesiology
Children's Hospital of Wisconsin
Medical College of Wisconsin
Milwaukee, Wisconsin
Chapter 8 Local Anesthetics

Sarah Reece-Stremtan, MD
Assistant Professor
Pediatrics and Anesthesiology
The George Washington University
Children's National Hospital
Washington, DC
Chapter 11 Pre-procedure Medications

Laura Rhee, MD
Assistant in Perioperative Anesthesia
Boston Children's Hospital
Instructor in Anesthesia
Harvard Medical School
Boston, Massachusetts
Chapter 40 Syndromes

Maricarmen Roche Rodriguez, MD
Instructor of Anesthesia, Harvard Medical School
Department of Anesthesiology, Critical Care and Pain
   Medicine
Boston Children's Hospital
Boston, Massachusetts
Chapter 17 Anesthesia for Cardiovascular Procedures

Iolanda Russo-Menna, MD, MEd, DABA
Associate Professor of Anesthesiology
Faculty and Attending of Pediatric Division of Anesthesia
Children Hospital of Richmond
Richmond, Virginia
Chapter 13 Pediatric Airway

Rita Saynhalath, MD
Assistant Professor
Department of Anesthesiology and Pain Management
University of Texas Southwestern Medical Center—
   Children's Health
Dallas, Texas
Chapter 12 Fluids and Acid-Base Management

John (Jake) P. Scott, MD
Associate Professor of Anesthesiology and Pediatrics
Divisions of Pediatric Anesthesiology and Pediatric
   Critical Care
Medical College of Wisconsin
Director of Pediatric Liver Transplant Anesthesia
Associate Medical Director of Pediatric Intensive Care
   Unit
Children's Hospital of Wisconsin
Milwaukee, Wisconsin
Chapter 25 Anesthesia for Pediatric Liver Transplantation

Joseph M. Sisk, MD
Assistant Professor
Department of Anesthesiology
Division of Pediatric Anesthesiology
The University of Oklahoma College of Medicine
Oklahoma City, Oklahoma
Chapter 16 Anesthesia for Otolaryngologic Procedures

Erik B. Smith, MD, JD, MS
Assistant Professor
Chief, Division of Pediatric Anesthesia
Department of Anesthesiology
Keck School of Medicine
University of Southern California
Los Angeles, California
*Chapter 34 Intraoperative Complications and
   Crisis Management*

Mary Ellen Thurman, DO
Assistant Professor, Saint Louis University
Anesthesiology and Critical Care
Division of Pediatric Anesthesiology
St. Louis, Missouri
Chapter 2 Anatomic Considerations

James A. Tolley, MD
Assistant Professor of Clinical Anesthesia
Pediatric Anesthesiology and Pain Medicine
Indiana University School of Medicine
Indianapolis, Indiana
Chapter 5 Analgesics

Kha M. Tran, MD
Associate Professor
Clinical Anesthesiology and Critical Care Medicine
Children's Hospital of Philadelphia
University of Pennsylvania Perelman School of Medicine
Philadelphia, Pennsylvania
Chapter 26 Anesthesia for Fetal Surgery

Sana Ullah, MB ChB, FRCA
Associate Professor
Department of Anesthesiology & Pain Management
University of Texas Southwestern Medical Center
Children's Health, Dallas
Dallas, Texas
Chapter 28 Intravenous Access

Galit Kastner Ungar, MD
Assistant Professor
Department of Anesthesiology and Pain Management
UT Southwestern/Children's Medical Center Dallas
Dallas, Texas
*Chapter 20 Anesthetic Considerations for Endocrine
   Disorders*

Jaya Varadarajan, MBBS
Associate Professor
Division of Pediatric Anesthesiology
Children's Hospital of Wisconsin
Medical College of Wisconsin
Milwaukee, Wisconsin
Chapter 14 Anesthesia for Neurosurgical Procedures

Tricia Vecchione, MD, MPH
Assistant Professor
Pediatric Anesthesiology and Critical Care Medicine
Johns Hopkins University School of Medicine
Baltimore, Maryland
*Chapter 31 Regional Anesthesia: Upper and Lower
    Extremity Blocks*

Barbara A. Vickers, MD, MPH
Assistant Professor of Anesthesiology and Critical Care
    Medicine
Johns Hopkins University School of Medicine
Baltimore, Maryland
Chapter 4 Neonatal Considerations

Stylianos Voulgarelis, MD
Assistant Professor
Division of Pediatric Anesthesiology
Children's Hospital of Wisconsin
Medical College of Wisconsin
Milwaukee, Wisconsin
Chapter 9 Vasoactive Medications

Cassandra Wasson, DO
Pediatric Anesthesia Fellow
Division of Pediatric Anesthesiology
Children's Hospital of Wisconsin
Medical College of Wisconsin
Milwaukee, Wisconsin
Chapter 8 Local Anesthetics

Chelsea Willie, MD
Assistant Professor of Anesthesiology
Division of Pediatric Anesthesiology
Children's Hospital of Wisconsin
Medical College of Wisconsin
Milwaukee, Wisconsin
Chapter 39 Cardiopulmonary Resuscitation

Albert C. Yeung, MD
Assistant Professor of Anesthesiology
Department of Anesthesiology
New York-Presbyterian Hospital/Weill Cornell Medical
    Center
New York, New York
Chapter 7 Muscle Relaxants

Luis M. Zabala, MD
Professor, Department of Anesthesiology and Pain
    Management
Medical Director of Pediatric Cardiac Anesthesia
UT Southwestern Medical Center
Children's Health, Dallas
Dallas, Texas
Chapter 28 Intravenous Access

Katherine L. Zaleski, MD
Instructor of Anesthesia
Harvard Medical School
Department of Anesthesiology, Critical Care and Pain
    Medicine
Boston Children's Hospital
Boston, Massachusetts
Chapter 17 Anesthesia for Cardiovascular Procedures

Preface

WHY DID WE CREATE THIS BOOK?

As a specialty, anesthesiology has two dimensions to its practice. The first is a deep fund of knowledge in human physiology, and the second is a procedural skill set needed to manipulate and treat various pathological states. Although there are a plethora of text and video sources for adult patients, there is minimal guidance for pediatric patients.

Clinical Pediatric Anesthesiology addresses this gap by providing a complete multimedia source in addition to a condensed, yet comprehensive, textbook. The text focuses on the unique aspects and considerations necessary for managing pediatric patients. For the multimedia section, found at https://accessanesthesiology.mhmedical.com/, world-renowned pediatric anesthesiologists demonstrate their techniques, selection of devices, and special considerations in an easily accessible online video format.

WHO SHOULD READ THIS BOOK?

This book is aimed at current health care providers in all specialties who deal with pediatric patients. This includes medical students, trainees, and advanced practice providers (nurse practitioners, nurse anesthetists, physician assistants, and anesthesiologist assistants). The objective is to provide a high-yield textbook of pediatric anesthesiology combined with high-quality videos that can be repeatedly used to educate practitioners on the safest and most efficient methods.

HOW IS THE BOOK ORGANIZED?

This book is divided into five major sections with 40 concise chapters written by pediatric anesthesiology leaders from multiple institutions. The goal is to have the book used as a comprehensive guide when preparing for a particular case or managing an intraoperative issue. The textbook includes text, illustrations, and graphics. However, the online multimedia source contains high-definition navigable video demonstrations that can be followed step by step. For every procedure, there is a background section and a review of the equipment, techniques, and alternatives as well as troubleshooting tips.

Each chapter features a "Focus Points" section that summarizes salient concepts guiding readers through each topic. The remainder of the chapter includes detailed topic information accompanied with tables, graphics, and references.

WHAT DO WE WANT FROM YOU?

We hope that the content of our book provides you with the necessary tools to be successful in understanding pediatric anesthesia as a subspecialty and guide you in managing pediatric anesthesia cases. That said, our book is a work in progress with always room for improvement. We welcome your comments or suggestions for future reprints. Please share them with us at UserServices@mheducation.com.

Herodotos Ellinas, MD
Kai Matthes, MD, PhD
Walid Alrayashi, MD
Aykut Bilge, MD, PhD

Basic Sciences of Pediatric Anesthesia

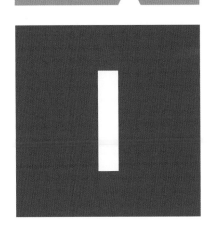

Physiological Aspects

Neethu Chandran and Edgar E. Kiss

CENTRAL AND AUTONOMIC NERVOUS SYSTEM

The brain at birth is one-tenth of the body weight. Only one-fourth of neuronal cells that exist in adults are present in the newborn. By one year of age, the cells in the cortex and brain stem are developed completely. Myelinization and synaptogenesis are not complete until the age of 3. Primitive reflexes such as Moro reflex and grasp reflex disappear with myelination. At birth, the conus medullaris is at L3, and the dural sac ends at S1. By one year of age, the conus medullaris recedes to L1 and the dural sac shortens to S1. Unlike the central nervous system, the autonomic nervous system is developed at birth, though immature. The parasympathetic system is intact and fully functional in contrast to the sympathetic component which develops by 4 to 6 months of age.[1-3]

The intracranial space has three components: brain tissue (80%), CSF (10%), and blood (10%). The Monro–Kellie hypothesis states that the sum of all intracranial components is constant (Figure 1-1). Specifically, an increase in volume of one of the components that causes an increase in intracranial pressure will result in a compensatory reduction in the other components to offset the change. The exception to this doctrine are neonates and infants since cranial sutures are open at birth.

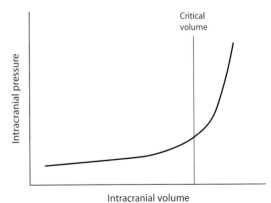

▲ **Figure 1-1.** Monro–Kellie hypothesis. An increase in volume of one of the components that causes an increase in intracranial pressure will result in a compensatory reduction in the other components to offset the change.
(Adapted with permission, from Butterworth IV JF, Mackey DC, Wasnick JD. eds. *Morgan & Mikhail's Clinical Anesthesiology,* 6e. 2018. https://accessmedicine.mhmedical.com. Copyright © McGraw Hill LLC. All rights reserved.)

The posterior fontanelle closes around 6 months of age and the anterior fontanelle around 12 to 18 months. Therefore, a slow increase in intracranial volume prior to cranial suture fusion can be compensated by an increase in head circumference. However, acute dramatic increases in ICP can still cause herniation. Children with closed fontanelles have a higher risk of herniation than adults, due to a lower intracranial compliance and smaller cranial volume.[4]

Maintaining cerebral perfusion pressure (CPP) helps prevent cerebral ischemia. CPP is dependent on mean arterial pressure (MAP), intracranial pressure (ICP), and central venous pressure (CVP). CPP is defined as MAP – ICP (or CVP if it is higher than ICP). Therefore, either an increase in ICP or a decrease in MAP can cause a decrease in CPP. Normal ICP in children and adults is less than 15 mm Hg. ICP in full-term infants is 2 to 6 mm Hg, and likely lower in premature neonates.[2] ICP can remain normal in the setting of significant intracranial pathology in infants with open fontanelles. Signs of intracranial hypertension differ in adults compared to children. Typical signs of high ICP include increased irritability, headaches, decreased feeding, and morning emesis.

Data is limited regarding normal neurophysiological values in the pediatric population. Most data is extrapolated from animal and adult data. Cerebral blood flow (CBF) varies with age (Table 1-1). CBF is coupled with cerebral metabolic rate of oxygen ($CMRO_2$). Normal $CMRO_2$ in adults is 3.5 mL/100 g/min. $CMRO_2$ in children increases to 5.2 mL/100 g/min making them more susceptible to hypoxemia, contrary to neonates who have a lower $CMRO_2$ at 3.5 mL/100 g/min making them relatively tolerant to hypoxemia.[5-8]

Cerebral autoregulation is able to keep CBF constant despite changes in CPP due to arteriolar contraction and relaxation in response to distending pressures.[5] In adults, CBF remains constant between MAP of 50 and 150 mm Hg. Beyond these limits of autoregulation, CBF is pressure dependent, which can lead to ischemia or hyperemia. Autoregulation numbers are not well known in children, although it has been shown that neonates and young children are especially vulnerable to cerebral ischemia and intraventricular hemorrhage. Attention should be given to proper blood pressure control.[9]

Cerebral spinal fluid is produced by the choroid plexus and absorbed by arachnoid villi. Adults and children synthesize about 500 mL/day, which is 0.3 to 0.4 mL/min. By the age of 5, children have the normal adult volume of CSF, which is 150 mL. Acetazolamide, furosemide, and corticosteroids all transiently decrease CSF production. Increase in ICP will cause an increase in the rate of reabsorption of CSF, unless in the setting of intracranial hemorrhage, inflammation, or obstruction in CSF flow.[1,2,4,10]

▶ Cardiovascular System

1. In fetal circulation, both the right and left ventricles provide system blood flow, and various connections allow for mixing of oxygenated blood with deoxygenated blood.

2. The three fetal connections are ductus arteriosus, ductus venosus, and foramen ovale.

3. Fetal hemoglobin has higher affinity for oxygen than adult hemoglobin helping offload oxygen to the fetus.

4. Four physiological features aid in the adequate delivery of oxygen to fetal tissues despite higher affinity for oxygen.

5. The transition from fetal to neonatal physiology begins with the neonate's first breath and involves the closure of the patent foramen ovale, patent ductus arteriosus, and ductus venosum.

6. The circulatory system undergoes a change from parallel to one in series.

7. Cardiac hemodynamic changes include decreased afterload and volume load in the right ventricle and increased afterload and volume load of the left ventricle.

8. Persistence of a patent foramen ovale occurs in up to a quarter of adults.

9. The neonate and infant myocardium is immature and is sensitive to myocardial depressive effects of various agents and anesthetics.

10. Neonates and infants have a predominance of parasympathetic autonomic innervation until the sympathetic nervous system reaches maturity in early infancy.

INTRAUTERINE ANATOMY AND PHYSIOLOGY

▶ Fetal Circulation and Anatomy

In utero, the placenta is responsible for respiratory gas exchange between the mother and the fetus. Deoxygenated blood travels through two umbilical arteries to the placenta for prenatal respiration. Blood is returned to the fetus via a single umbilical vein that carries oxygenated blood that is approximately 80% saturated, with about 30 mm Hg partial pressure of oxygen (Po_2). In comparison, the Po_2 in the umbilical arteries is approximately 16 mm Hg. Fifty percent of the blood flow bypasses the liver through the ductus venosus. The rest of the blood perfuses the left lobe

Table 1-1. CBF Variation with Age

Age	Cerebral Blood Flow (CBF)
Preterm neonate	~14–20 mL/100 g/min
Term neonate	~40 mL/100 g/min
Child	~90–100 mL/100 g/min, which is 25% of the cardiac output
Adult	~50 mL/100 g/min, which is 15% of the cardiac output

of the liver. Blood flow to the right lobe is via the portal circulation. Blood from the right and left hepatic veins combines with blood from the ductus venosus and travels to the right atrium via the inferior vena cava (IVC).[11-14]

Much of the blood that enters the right atrium is shunted to the left atrium through the *patent foramen ovale* (PFO) bypassing the right ventricle with the directional help provided by the eustachian valve located at the junction of the IVC and right atrium. The blood continues into the left ventricle and is pumped to the upper body to perfuse the brain and heart through the aorta. Oxygen saturation of the blood ejected from the left ventricle is approximately 70% due to the direct passage of flow provided by the ductus venosus. The superior vena cava carries deoxygenated blood from the upper body to the right atrium and ventricle. The high pulmonary vascular resistance (PVR) favors almost all the right ventricular output to be shunted through the *ductus arteriosus*, a connection between the pulmonary artery and aorta, to bypass the lungs and enter systemic circulation. Studies report that total pulmonary blood flow is about 25% of combined ventricular output in utero at 30 weeks of gestational age but may be as little as 13% at 20 weeks of gestational age before decreasing to 21% at 38 weeks of gestational age.[15] The lower part of the body, including the kidneys and gut, is perfused with blood that has an oxygen saturation of only 55%.[11-14]

Oxygen Delivery in Utero

The four physiological features that aid in the adequate delivery of oxygen to fetal tissues despite low oxygen saturation are (1) the presence of fetal hemoglobin (HbF), (2) low levels of 2,3-diphosphoglycerate (2,3-DPG) as well as (3) low affinity of HbF for 2,3-DPG and (4) erythropoietic environment resulting in a higher baseline hematocrit of around 17 g/dL. The P_{50}, partial pressure of oxygen at which 50% saturation of hemoglobin occurs, is lower at 19 mm Hg as opposed to that of adult hemoglobin (HbA) that has a P_{50} of 26 mm Hg. The fetal hemoglobin thus has a higher affinity for oxygen, improving the oxygen uptake from mother's blood at the placenta. In turn, the increased affinity for oxygen is offset by the slightly lower fetal pH allowing for adequate oxygen delivery to tissues.[11,16]

Perinatal Transition of Circulation

The fetal physiology undergoes dramatic changes in the first few minutes after birth to ensure survival. The once parallel circulation now changes to that in series as the pulmonary vascular resistance (PVR) significantly drops due to increased oxygen tension. Aeration of the lungs stimulates the endothelium to secrete nitric oxide and PGI_2 which are potent vasodilators. With the increased blood flow through the lungs and clamping of the umbilical vessels causing increased systemic vascular resistance (SVR), left-sided heart pressures are increased. The foramen ovale functionally closes when the left atrial pressure surpasses right atrial

pressure by exerting hydrostatic pressure on the septum primum but remains anatomically patent in most infants. Up to a quarter of adults and half of children younger than 5 years may have an anatomically patent foramen ovale.[17] The ductus arteriosus begins to close within the first hours of life due to loss of placental prostaglandins and increase oxygen tension in almost all term infants by day 4.[18] Fibrosis of the ductus arteriosus occurs within 3 weeks of birth, completing the transformation to the ligamentum arteriosum.[19,20]

Left ventricular cardiac output increases after birth due to the increased pulmonary venous return and a transient left to right shunt at the level of the ductus. There is an increase in ventricular preload, stroke volume, and heart rate to accommodate for the increased metabolic rate that is double that of an adult. The right ventricle observes a decrease in volume and pressure load due to the elimination of the umbilical vein return and decreased pulmonary vascular resistance. Flow through the ductus venosus stops after clamping of the umbilical cord and invaginates usually by week 2 of life. Hypoxia, acidosis, hypercarbia, and hypothermia have the possibility to revert neonates to a persistent fetal circulation.[11,12,15,20]

Postnatal Cardiovascular System

The neonate's immature heart has several limitations compared to that of older children and adults. Decreases in preload and heart rate are not well tolerated in neonates. The reduced number of sarcomeres and a poorly developed calcium transport system limit the heart's contractile reserve increasing its dependence on extracellular calcium for contractility. The immature myocardium, however, exhibits better tolerance to ischemia with rapid recovery of function in contrast to the adult myocardium possibly due to preference for carbohydrates and lactates as energy sources. The cardiac stroke volume is relatively fixed and cardiac output is tied to the heart rate due to a minimally compliant left ventricle, but more recent echocardiographic studies in human neonates and fetuses have demonstrated the heart's capability to increase stroke volume.[21-26]

Sympathetic system development lags behind the parasympathetic system and its activation through hypoxia, surgical stimulation, or even direct laryngoscopy can trigger bradycardia and hypotension in the neonate. The infant's vasculature is also less responsive to hypovolemia than that of older children and adults. Intravascular depletion in neonates and infants may present as hypotension without tachycardia. However, these physiological limitations usually resolve beyond infancy, if not as early as 6 months of age for a term neonate.[12,13,27-40]

Respiratory System

1. Terminal bronchioles are developed by 16 weeks of gestation, while alveolar formation begins at 36 weeks of gestation.

2. While alveoli development is completed by 18 months of age, the lungs continue to develop throughout childhood.

3. Compared to older children, the neonate lungs and chest wall both have high compliance (low elastic forces), which promotes atelectasis during inspiration.

4. Mechanisms that maintain functional residual capacity (FRC) in neonates and infants are absent under general anesthesia.

5. Apnea is common in premature and anemic patients up to 60 weeks of postmenstrual age.

6. The cricoid cartilage is the narrowest point of a child's airway.

7. Small changes in the airway diameter can lead to significant airway obstruction in children.

8. Pulmonary vascular resistance reaches adult levels by 6 months of age.

Fetal Lungs

Fetal lungs start to form in the first few weeks of life when the fetus is just 3 mm in length. The bronchial tree develops down to the terminal bronchioles by 16 weeks of gestation and the remaining distal structures develop throughout the rest of the gestation. At approximately 24 to 25 weeks of gestation during the terminal sac period, the pulmonary capillaries are formed and contact the immature alveolar epithelium. Starting at 30 weeks' gestational age, the cuboidal alveolar epithelium flattens and begins to produce pulmonary surfactant which provides alveolar stability to maintain lung inflation after birth. There is sufficient surfactant present at 34 weeks of gestation and glucocorticoid administration to the mother can hasten fetal surfactant production. A term newborn has only one-tenth of the alveoli of an adult which continue to multiply and develop significantly from birth to around 18 months of age. While in utero, the lungs remain poorly perfused and are filled with fluid that is intermittently released to form one-third of the amniotic fluid.[12,13]

Postnatal Respiratory System

The respiratory system functions primarily to maintain oxygen and carbon dioxide equilibrium in the body. With the clamping of the umbilical cord at birth, the lungs replace the placenta as the organ of gas exchange. Other components of the respiratory system include the brainstem respiratory centers; central and peripheral chemoreceptors; the phrenic, intercostal, hypoglossal, and vagal nerves; the thorax, upper and lower airways, alveoli, and lung parenchyma, as well as the pulmonary vascular system.[12,13]

The neonates' and infants' higher metabolic rates, high ventilatory requirements, and lower surface area for gas exchange of the neonate also contribute to rapid desaturations. Compared to older children, the neonate lungs and chest wall both have high compliance (low elastic forces), which promotes atelectasis during inspiration. Lung elastic fibers are poorly developed initially, but develop in the postnatal period. In neonates, there is little outward recoil of the chest wall due to the horizontal orientation of the cartilaginous rib cage poorly and developed chest wall muscles. However, FRC, the volume left in the lungs after passive exhalation, is maintained by different mechanisms than in adults. In older children and adults, the volume is maintained by the elastic forces of passive recoil of the chest balanced by the recoil of the lungs. Inspiration results largely due to the flattening of the diaphragm which is more prone to fatigue secondary to a higher proportion of type I fibers. Awake infants maintain higher end-expiratory lung volumes, therefore maintaining FRC by stiffening the chest wall with tonic contractions of the intercostal muscles and diaphragm all through the breathing cycle. In addition, they terminate their expiratory phase before lung volumes reach FRC by (1) diaphragmatic breaking and (2) glottic closure, effectively producing PEEP. However, all these mechanisms are lost while under anesthesia, resulting in atelectasis and desaturation. FRC may be only 15% of total lung capacity in young infants undergoing general anesthesia with muscle relaxation. In addition, the term neonate has only one-tenth the number terminal saccules as that of a grown child.[12,13,41–44]

Neonates and infants have a blunted response to blood carbon dioxide and oxygen concentrations. Lung inflation may result in apnea, known as the Hering-Breuer reflex. A vagal-mediated airway reflex physiologically is meant to allow for exhalation in the presence of lung hyperinflation but may lead to paradoxical apnea. Apnea is common in premature and anemic patients up to 60 weeks of postmenstrual age.[45,46] Also, breathing is independent of pulmonary arterial carbon dioxide partial pressure and hypoxia paradoxically depresses breathing.[47,48]

Compared to older children, infants have a proportionally larger head and tongue, and anterior and cephalad larynx, narrower nasal passages, and a longer omega-shaped epiglottis. The anatomic features of the neonates and infants up to 5 months of age make them obligate nasal breathers. Also, small changes in the infant airway diameter from swelling or secretions can result in significant airway obstruction.[12,13] The cricoid cartilage has been demonstrated to be the narrowest point of the airway in children less than 10 to 12 years of age, as opposed to the rima glottidis in adults.[49–56]

Regulation of Pulmonary Blood Flow

Pulmonary vascular resistance begins to decrease after birth, reaching adult levels by 6 months of age.[56] However, the neonate and infant pulmonary vasculature remains sensitive and certain conditions may increase the pulmonary vascular tone. In the neonate, these changes may result in the persistence of fetal circulation, shunting, and hypoxia even while 100% oxygen is delivered. Pulmonary disease, hypoxemia, hypercarbia, sepsis, acidosis, hypothermia, and coughing on the endotracheal tube can all increase the pulmonary vascular resistance.[57] Nitric oxide (NO), prostaglandins, histamine, and β-adrenergic catecholamines have vasodilatory effects on the pulmonary vasculature. Increases in right-sided pressures can consequently lead to right ventricular diastolic dysfunction and hypoxia from right to left shunting through the PFO.[58]

FOCUS POINTS

1. Nephrons complete formation by 36 weeks' gestation; however, the renal system is not fully mature at birth.
2. At term, GFR is only 25% of adult levels. GFR reaches adult levels at about 2 years of age.
3. All tubular transporters reliant on the sodium gradient are decreased and immature at birth. The combination of these factors decreases the newborn's ability to concentrate or dilute urine compared to adults.
4. Serum creatinine reflects maternal creatinine level at birth and then starts to decrease initially. As the child grows, creatinine clearance slowly increases and reaches adult levels at about 2 years of age due to the rapid increase in muscle mass and growth.

Renal System

Nephrons complete formation by 36 weeks' gestation; however, the renal system is not fully mature at birth. Urine output begins at 10 weeks of gestation, which helps maintain amniotic fluid balance.[59,60] The placenta helps maintain the fetus' electrolyte and fluid balance. The kidneys assume responsibility after birth. Glomerular filtration rate (GFR) and renal blood flow (RBF) are decreased in the neonate. Both increase with gestational age as renal vascular resistance decreases.[61] At term, GFR is only 25% of adult levels.[62] GFR reaches adult levels at about 2 years of age.[63,64] Similarly, tubular function also continues to increase during the first 2 years of life. All tubular transporters reliant on the sodium gradient are decreased and immature at birth. The combination of these factors decrease the newborn's ability to concentrate or dilute urine compared to adults.[65] Diluting capacity starts to mature around the fourth week of life.[66] Serum creatinine reflects maternal creatinine level at birth and then starts to decrease initially. As the child grows, creatinine clearance slowly increases and reaches adult levels at about 2 years of age due to the rapid increase in muscle mass and growth.[67]

Compared to adults, infants have lower serum bicarbonate levels and $Paco_2$. They have a greater production of endogenous acid due to calcium deposition into bone.[68] Normal bicarbonate absorption through the gastrointestinal tract helps neutralize the acid. When this process is disrupted due to gastroenteritis, starvation, or illness, infants can become extremely acidotic since they are unable to compensate for the acid load.[68] The renin–angiotensin system is present at early gestation. Serum renin activity is increased at birth and remains elevated. Renin activity decreases to adult levels by 6 to 9 years of age.[69]

REFERENCES

1. Volpe JJ. *Neurology of the Newborn*. 4th ed. Philadelphia, PA: WB Sanders; 2001:83-86.
2. Davis A, Ravussin P, Bissonnette B. Central nervous system: anatomy and physiology. In: Bissonnette B, Dalens BJ, eds. *Pediatric Anesthesia: Principles and Practice*. New York: McGraw-Hill; 2002:104-114.
3. Krass IS. Physiology and metabolism of brain and spinal cord. In: Newfield P, Cottrell JE, eds. *Handbook of Neuroanaesthesia*. Philadelphia, PA: Lippincott Williams & Wilkins; 2007:3-22.
4. Shapiro K, Marmarou A, Shulman K. Characterization of clinical CSF dynamics and neural axis compliance using the pressure-volume index: I. The normal pressure-volume index. *Ann Neurol*. 1980;7:508-514.
5. Pryds O, Edwards AD. Cerebral blood flow in the newborn infant. *Arch Dis Child Fetal Neonatal Ed*. 1996;74(1):F63-F69.
6. Chiron C, Raynaud C, Maziére B, et al. Changes in regional cerebral blood flow during brain maturation in children and adolescents. *J Nucl Med*. 1992;33:696-703.
7. Biagi L, Abbruzzese A, Bianchi MC, Alsop DC, Del Guerra A, Tosetti M. Age dependence of cerebral perfusion assessed by magnetic resonance continuous arterial spin labeling. *J Magn Reson Imaging*. 2007;25(4):696-702.
8. Kennedy L. Sokoloff: an adaptation of the nitrous oxide method to the study of the cerebral circulation in children; normal values for cerebral blood flow and cerebral metabolic rate in childhood. *J Clin Invest*. 1957;36(7):1130-1137.
9. Pryds O, Andersen GE, Friis-Hansen B. Cerebral blood flow reactivity in spontaneously breathing, preterm infants shortly after birth. *Acta Paediatr Scand*. 1990;79(4):391-396.
10. Arieff AI, Ayus JC, Fraser CL. Hyponatraemia and death or permanent brain damage in healthy children. *BMJ*. 1992;304:1218-1222.
11. Baum VC, Yuki K, de Souza DG. Cardiovascular physiology. In:Davis PJ and Cladis FP, eds. *Smith's Anesthesia for Infants and Children*, 9th ed. St. Louis, MO: Elsevier, 2017, pp. 73-107.
12. Butterworth JFIV, Mackey DC, Wasnick JD, eds. *Morgan & Mikhail's Clinical Anesthesiology*. 5th ed. New York, NY: McGraw-Hill; 2013.
13. Motoyama EK, Finder JD. Respiratory physiology. In:Davis PJ and Cladis FP, eds. *Smith's Anesthesia for Infants and Children*, 9th ed. St. Louis, MO: Elsevier, 2017, pp. 23-72.
14. Marciniak B. Growth and Development. In Coté CJ, Lerman J, and Anderson B, eds. *A Practice of anesthesia for infants and children*, 6th ed. Philadelphia, PA: Elsevier, 2019, pp. 8-24.
15. Rasanen J, Wood DC, Weiner S, Ludomirski A, Huhta JC. Role of the pulmonary circulation in the distribution of human fetal cardiac output during the second half of pregnancy. *Circulation*. 1996;94:1068-1073.

16. Carter AM. Placental oxygen transfer and the oxygen supply to the fetus. *Fetal Maternal Med Rev.* 1999;11:151-161.

17. Hagen PT, Scholz DG, Edwards WD. Incidence and size of patent foramen ovale during the first 10 decades of life: an autopsy study of 965 normal hearts. *Mayo Clin Proc.* 1984;59:17-20.

18. Reller MD, Ziegler ML, Rice MJ, et al. Duration of ductal shunting in healthy preterm infants: an echocardiographic color flow Doppler study. *J Pediatr.* 1988;112(3):441-446.

19. Fay FS, Cooke PH. Guinea pig ductus arteriosus. II. Irreversible closure after birth. *Am J Physiol.* 1972;222(4):841-849.

20. Clyman RI, Mauray F, Roman C, et al. Factors determining the loss of ductus arteriosus responsiveness to prostaglandin E. *Circulation.* 1983;68(2):433-436.

21. Rein AJ, Sanders SP, Colan SD, et al. Left ventricular mechanics in the normal newborn. *Circulation.* 1987;76:1029-1036.

22. Anderson PA. The heart and development. *Semin Perinatol.* 1996;20:482-509.

23. Baum VC, Palmisano BW. The immature heart and anesthesia. *Anesthesiology.* 1997;87(6):1529-1548.

24. Papp JG. Autonomic responses and neurohumoral control in the human early antenatal heart. *Basic Res Cardiol.* 1988;83(1):2-9.

25. Mossad EB, Farid I. Vital organ preservation during surgery for congenital heart disease. In: Lake CL, Booker PD, eds. *Pediatric Cardiac Anesthesia.* 4th ed. Philadelphia, PA: Lippincott, Williams & Wilkins; 2005:266-290.

26. DiNardo J, Zwara DA. Congenital heart disease. In: DiNardo J, Zwara DA, eds. *Anesthesia for Cardiac Surgery.* 3rd ed. Malden, MA: Blackwell Publishing; 2008:167-251.

27. Friedman WF. The intrinsic physiologic properties of the developing heart. *Prog Cardiovasc Dis.* 1972;15:87-111.

28. Gilbert JC, Glantz SA. Determinants of left ventricular filling and of the diastolic pressure-volume relation. *Circ Res.* 1989;64:827-852.

29. Hoerter J, Mazet F, Vassort G. Perinatal growth of the rabbit cardiac cell: possible implications for the mechanism of relaxation. *J Mol Cell Cardiol.* 1981;13(8):725-740.

30. Jarmakani JM, Nakanishi T, George BL, Bers D. Effect of extracellular calcium on myocardial mechanical function in the neonatal rabbit. *Dev Pharmacol Ther.* 1982;5(1-2):1-13.

31. Nayler WG, Fassold E. Calcium accumulating and ATPase activity of cardiac sarcoplasmic reticulum before and after birth. *Cardiovasc Res.* 1977;11(3):231-237.

32. Kirkpatrick SE, Pitlick PT, Naliboff J, Friedman WF. Frank–Starling relationship as an important determinant of fetal cardiac output. *Am J Physiol.* 1976;231(2):495-500.

33. Thornburg KL, Morton MJ. Filling and arterial pressures as determinants of RV stroke volume in the sheep fetus. *Am J Physiol.* 1983;244(5):H656-H663.

34. Romero T, Covell J, Friedman WF. A comparison of pressure-volume relations of the fetal, newborn, and adult heart. *Am J Physiol.* 1972;222(5):1285-1290.

35. Teitel DF, Sidi D, Chin T, et al. Developmental changes in myocardial contractile reserve in the lamb. *Pediatr Res.* 1985;19(9):948-955.

36. Winberg P, Jansson M, Marions L, Lundell BP. Left ventricular output during postnatal circulatory adaptation in healthy infants born at full term. *Arch Dis Child.* 1989;64(10 Spec No):1374-1378.

37. Kenny J, Plappert T, Doubilet P, et al. Effects of heart rate on ventricular size, stroke volume, and output in the normal human fetus: a prospective Doppler echocardiographic study. *Circulation.* 1987;76(1):52-58.

38. Papp JG. Autonomic responses and neurohumoral control in the human early antenatal heart. *Basic Res Cardiol.* 1988;83(1):2-9.

39. Sachis PN, Armstrong DL, Becker LE, Bryan AC. Myelination of the human vagus nerve from 24 weeks postconceptional age to adolescence. *J Neuropathol Exp Neurol.* 1982;41(4):466-472.

40. Burri PH. Structural aspects of postnatal lung development–alveolar formation and growth. *Biol Neonate.* 2006;89:313-322.

41. Mortola JP, Fisher JT, Smith B, Fox G, Weeks S. Dynamics of breathing in infants. *J Appl Physiol.* 1982;52(5):1209-1215.

42. Mortola JP, Hemmings G, Matsuoka T, Saiki C, Fox G. Referencing lung volume for measurements of respiratory system compliance in infants. *Pediatr Pulmonol.* 1993;16(4):248-253.

43. Kurth CD, Spitzer AR, Broennle AM, Downes JJ. Postoperative apnea in preterm infants. *Anesthesiology.* 1987;66:483-488.

44. Muller N, Volgyesi G, Becker L, et al. Diaphragmatic muscle tone. *J Appl Physiol.* 1979;47:279.

45. Gregory GA, Steward DJ. Life-threatening perioperative apnea in the ex-"premie". *Anesthesiology.* 1983;59:495-498.

46. Gao Y, Raj JU. Regulation of the pulmonary circulation in the fetus and newborn. *Physiol Rev.* 2010;90:1291-1335.

47. Thurlbeck WM. Postnatal growth and development of the lung. *Am Rev Respir Dis.* 1975;111:803-844.

48. Bayeux R. Tubage du larynx dans le Croup. *Presse Mèdicale.* 1897;6:29-33.

49. Peter K. *Handbuch der Anatomie des Kindes.* Berlin: Springer; 1936.

50. Butz RO. Length and cross-section growth patterns in the human trachea. *Pediatrics.* 1968;42:336-341.

51. Too-Chung MA, Green JR. The rate of growth of the cricoid cartilage. *J Laryngol Otol.* 1974;88:65-70.

52. Tucker GF, Tucker JA, Vidic B. Anatomy and development of the cricoid: serial-section whole organ study of perinatal larynges. *Ann Otol Rhinol Laryngol.* 1977;86:766-769.

53. Holinger LD, Green CG. Anatomy. In: Holinger LD, Lusk RP, Green CG, eds. *Pediatric Laryngology and Bronchoesophagology.* Philadelphia, PA: Lippincott-Raven; 1997:19-26.

54. Eckel HE, Koebke J, Sittel C, Sprinzl GM, Pototschnig C, Stennert E. Morphology of the human larynx during the first five years of life studied on whole organ serial sections. *Ann Otol Rhinol Laryngol.* 1999;108:232-238.

55. Wani TM, Rafiq M, Talpur S, Soualmi L, Tobias JD. Pediatric upper airway dimensions using three-dimensional computed tomography imaging. *Paediatr Anaesth.* 2017;27(6):604-608.

56. Rudolph AM. Fetal and neonatal pulmonary circulation. *Annu Rev Physiol.* 1979;41:383-395.

57. Gao Y, Raj JU. Regulation of the pulmonary circulation in the fetus and newborn. *Physiol Rev.* 2010;90:1291-1335.

58. Konduri GG, Kim UO. Advances in the diagnosis and management of persistent pulmonary hypertension of the newborn. *Pediatr Clin North Am.* 2009;56(3):579-600.

59. Jose PA, Fildes RD, Gomez RA, Chevalier RL, Robillard JE. Neonatal renal function and physiology. *Curr Opin Pediatr.* 1994;6(2):172-177.

60. Quigley R. Developmental changes in renal function. *Curr Opin Pediatr.* 2012;24(2):184-190.

61. Leake RD, Trygstad CW, Oh W. Inulin clearance in the newborn infant: relationship to gestational and postnatal age. *Pediatr Res.* 1976;10:759-762.

62. Guignard JP. Measurement of glomerular filtration rate in neonates. In: Polin RA, Fox WW, eds. *Fetal and*

Neonatal Physiology. 2nd ed. Philadelphia, PA: W.B Saunders; 2004:1593-1599.

63. Arant BSJ. Developmental patterns of renal functional maturation compared in the human neonate. *J Pediatr.* 1978;92:705-712.

64. Yared A, Ichikawa I. Postnatal development of glomerular filtration. In: Polin RA, Fox WW, eds. *Fetal and Neonatal Physiology.* 2nd ed. Philadelphia, PA: W.B Saunders; 2004:1588-1592.

65. Sulyok E, Varga F, Györy E, Jobst K, Csaba IF. On the mechanisms of renal sodium handling in newborn infants. *Biol Neonate.* 1980;37(1-2):75-79.

66. Spitzer A. The role of the kidney in sodium homeostasis during maturation. *Kidney Int.* 1982;21:539.

67. Miall LS, Henderson MJ, Turner AJ, et al. Plasma creatinine rises dramatically in the first 48 hours of life in preterm infants. *Pediatrics.* 1999;104(6):e76.

68. Malan AF, Evans A, Heese HD. Serial acid–base determinations in normal premature and full-term infants during the first 72 hours of life. *Arch Dis Child.* 1965;40(214):645-650.

69. Stalker HP, Holland NH, Kotchen JM, Kotchen TA. Plasma renin activity in healthy children. *J Pediatr.* 1976;89(2):256-258.

Anatomic Considerations

Huy Do and Mary Ellen Thurman

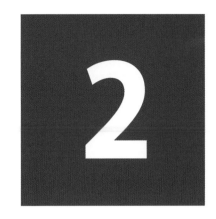

FOCUS POINTS

1. Brain growth and development occurs most rapidly in the first 5 years of life. Notable changes of the face and skull are seen in this young period. During adolescence these features approach adulthood.
2. Neonate and young infants are considered preferential nasal breathers. Any obstruction to the nares (eg, secretions) often leads to increased work in breathing.
3. A proportionately larger tongue, young epiglottic shape (long, narrow, and omega), and a cephalad larynx can affect airway management (eg, intubation). Similar to adults, the vocal cord region is the narrowest point of the airway in children.
4. The airway dimensions (short trachea, less acutely angled right main bronchi) of neonate and young children predispose them to mainstem intubation. Meticulous placement of the endotracheal tube is needed because of limited size.
5. Young pediatric patients have immature skeletal muscle and cartilaginous thorax (ie, compliant chest). These features can promote respiratory fatigue during increased demands in breathing (eg, illness).
6. The caudal level of the dura and spinal cord encompasses about two to three interspaces lowered in a neonate compared to an adult. By the first year of life, they are in the adult position.

An understanding of the anatomic changes that occur from birth through late adolescent is essential in the care for the pediatric patient. Pediatric growth may seem continuous but oftentimes occurs in sporadic stages of development (eg, infancy, childhood, adolescence) where rapid changes may be divided by a period of relatively slower or uniform pace.

SKULL

Infants and young children have a relatively large head to the size of their total body. This is attributed to the rapid growth and development of the brain. At birth, the head is one-fourth the total body length and is 25% of an adult size.[1] In the first year of life, the brain completes half its growth and by the age of 5, approximately 90% of cranial growth has occurred.[2,3] The occiput is also noted to be prominent in these early years. At birth, the anterior and posterior fontanelles are palpable. The posterior fontanel closes first, often in the first several months.[4] The anterior fontanel closes by the age of 2.[5] Except for the metopic suture, which closes completely during the first year of life, the remaining cranial sutures do not fully fuse until adulthood.[6,7] As the child matures, the body size increases relative to head size.

The face matures at a different rate compared to the head (cranium). At birth, the cranium-to-face ratio is 8:1. By the first year of life the ratio is 6:1. The facial characteristic presents as a prominent forehead and eyes in early childhood. During late adolescence, the ratio reaches adult level of 2:1. The facial complex of the nose, maxilla, and mandible increases in size with the role of development (ie, phonation and mastication). In infancy, the mandible is small with a notable oblique mandibular angle. As the child grows, the face becomes more prominent as it develops primarily downward and forward. Nasomaxillary and mandibular growths occur in parallel with dentition.[8]

Skeletal maturity of the lower face is reached during mid to late adolescence.[2] Primary (baby) teeth often occur around 6 months of age and continue in the first 2½ years of life.[9] After gradual shedding of primary teeth, permanent teeth erupt about 6 years of age and are mostly completed by age of 13.[10]

UPPER AIRWAY

Nasopharynx

Traditional teaching is that infants are obligate nasal breathers until 3 to 6 months of age.[11] It has been shown that this is not exclusively true.[12] Neonates and young infants are preferentially nasal breathers. Nonetheless, they rely upon patent nares for adequate breathing. Infant's nares are obviously small in size and rapidly increase during the first year of life. By 6 months of age the nares nearly double in dimension from birth. The nares can be quickly occluded (eg, secretions, edema) resulting in an increased work of breathing. There is linear growth of the nasopharynx during the first decade of life.[13] In early childhood, the adenoids develop and may obstruct breathing. Typically they shrink during adolescence.

Oropharynx

In proportion to the adult, the tongue of the young child is larger resulting in a decreased space inside of the oral cavity. This can compromise breathing and obstruct the airway especially when pharyngeal tone is decreased or lost. Congenital syndromes such as Down syndrome or Beckwith-Wiedemann syndrome often impede visualization of vocal cords during intubation due to the decreased amount of space due to an enlarged tongue. Similar to the adenoids, the tonsils grow rapidly in the first decade of life and often decrease in size during the teenage years. They are a common cause of airway obstruction for school-aged children.

Hypopharynx and Larynx

The epiglottis in infants differs from adults in several ways. It is proportionally longer, narrower, and omega-shaped. In addition, the epiglottis is oriented at a 45-degree angle into the lumen of the airway. In contrast, the axis of the epiglottis is parallel to the trachea in adults. These differences often impact airway management in infants especially when performing laryngoscopy (or suctioning). It is susceptible to trauma resulting in edema and obstruction around the glottic opening. In addition, in infants, the vocal cords are angled in a caudal orientation (ie, toward the feet) where the anterior location is inferior to the posterior end.[14] In adults, the vocal cord orientation is commonly at a 90-degree angle to the trachea.

During infancy, the larynx lies higher in the neck in relation to the cervical spine. In a neonate, it is at the third

and fourth cervical vertebrae (C3-C4) and descends to the adult C5 position by early adolescence (some discrepancy cited at 4–5 years). This higher position of the larynx in children results in a sharper angle between the base of tongue and the glottic opening.[15] Clinically, this is often described as being more "anterior" to an adult but in fact it is more cephalad or "superior." The cephalad location of the larynx in the young infant provides some protection against aspiration as protective reflexes (ie, swallow-breathe) develop.

Cadaveric studies from the 1950s provided the base for classical teachings of the pediatric airway.[16] For many years the pediatric larynx was taught and described as being funnel- or conical-shaped and the narrowest portion was at the level of the cricoid ring. It was believed that as the child matures between 8 and 10 years of age, the larynx transitioned into the cylindrical adult airway, in which the narrowest portion is at the rima glottis. Recent studies using advanced imaging (ie, computed tomography and magnetic resonance imaging) and direct broncho-scopic measurements have contested previous pediatric tenets.[17-19] These findings demonstrate that the pediatric larynx is similar to adult where the narrowest portion is at or immediately below (subglottic) the vocal cord. In addition, the pediatric airway is not funnel-shaped but is cylindrical in geometry. In young children, the cross-sectional area is elliptical with a greater anteroposterior (AP) to transverse dimension.[20] Despite these findings, the cricoid ring may functionally be the narrowest portion of the airway. It is completely cartilaginous and is relatively nondistensible compared to the upper glottic structures.

Lower Airway

The developmental anatomy of the respiratory system of infants and young children is another factor to take into consideration. In addition to the extrathoracic portion of the airway is the intrathoracic portion of the airway, which includes the trachea, two mainstem bronchi, bronchi, and bronchioles that conduct air to the alveoli. The pediatric population differs from adults with respect to relative length of the trachea, size difference between right and left main bronchi, the orientation of their rib cage, the compliance of their chest wall, the musculature of their diaphragm, and the incomplete alveolarization of the lung parenchyma (with regards to children less than 2 years of age).

Particularly in the neonate population, the trachea is short and measures approximately 5 cm. Therefore, precise placement and firm fixation of the endotracheal tube are essential. Table 2-1 demonstrates approximate airway dimensions (intrathoracic portion) in infants and children.

Also, regarding the main bronchi, the right main bronchus is larger than the left and is less acutely angled at its origin.[21] As discussed earlier, precision is crucial for placement of the endotracheal tube because if advancement

Table 2-1. Approximate Airway Dimensions in Infants and Children

| Age (yr) | Tracheal Length (cm) | Trachea (AP) | Diameter (mm) | |
			Right Bronchus	Left Bronchus
>0.5	5.9	5.0	4.5	3.5
0.5–1	7.2	5.5	4.8	3.7
1–2	7.5	6.3	5.1	3.9
2–4	8.0	7.5	6.4	4.9
4–6	8.6	8.0	6.7	5.3
6–8	9.5	9.2	7.9	6.1
8–10	10	9.75	8.5	6.5
10–12	11.5	10.5	9.2	6.8
12–14	13.5	11.5	9.8	7.5
14–16	14.5	13.2	11.5	8.8

AP, anteroposterior.

is too far, it almost invariably will enter the right main bronchus. It is of the utmost importance to continuously reassess the equality of bilateral breath sounds after repositioning for surgeries that require changes in position.

The anatomy of the chest wall of infants and children differs from adults in the orientation of the rib cage. At birth, ribs project at right angles from the spine. The rib cage is also more circular than in adults, thus lacking mechanical efficiency. The angle of insertion of the diaphragm in children is not oblique as in adults but almost entirely horizontal, and ventilation is mainly diaphragmatic. This leads to a decrease in contraction efficiency with a tendency of the diaphragm to pull the lower rib cage inward instead of outward.[22] The abdominal viscera are bulky and further hinder diaphragmatic excursion, especially if the gastrointestinal tract is distended.[21]

Several anatomic differences make respiration less efficient in infants. In addition to the difference in orientation, the rib cage of infants and young children is rather cartilaginous, and the thorax is too compliant to resist inward recoil of the lungs. This can allow the chest wall to retract during episodes of respiratory distress and fatigue. With the chest wall of infants being highly compliant, the ribs provide very little support for the lungs. As a result, negative intrathoracic pressure is poorly maintained, and each breath is accompanied by functional airway closure.[23] As opposed to the awake state when the chest wall maintains a relative amount of rigidity with sustained inspiratory

muscle tension, general anesthesia induces a state that affects the muscle tension by diminishing it, leading to FRC collapse and contributing to further airway closure and atelectasis.[24]

Relative to infants and smaller children, neonates' lungs are even stiffer due to greater alveolar recoil, which is offset by expression of surfactant, while the chest and abdominal walls are more compliant. As a result, the diaphragm muscle must create greater relative intrathoracic pressures to produce a given level of inspiratory airflow and tidal volume.[25]

Differences in chest wall configuration and compliance between young infants and older children can place them at a disadvantage, especially when trying to meet the increased ventilatory requirements, such as those inflicted by pulmonary disease or in the setting of increased metabolic demands. Immaturity of the respiratory muscles, combined with high chest wall compliance, can cause ventilation asynchrony and promote respiratory fatigue.[22] This is why differences in the anatomy of the microstructure of the respiratory muscular system of infants must also be taken into consideration. Skeletal muscle fibers, including those of the diaphragm, may be classified into two basic groups, type I and II, according to histochemical and electrophysiologic characteristics.[26] Type I fibers have a high capacity for oxidative phosphorylation, develop their maximal force generation slowly, also known as "slow-twitch," and are resistant to fatigue. Type II fibers rapidly develop their maximal force generation, also known as "fast-twitch," but this group is further subdivided according to additional properties. Type IIa fibers have intermediate oxidative phosphorylation and are fatigue resistant. Type IIb fibers have poor oxidative phosphorylation and fatigue easily. Type IIc fibers are found only in fetal and neonatal diaphragmatic muscle; they are highly oxidative and resistant to fatigue.

The musculature of the infant's diaphragm is characterized as immature, consisting mainly of type IIc undifferentiated fibers, which are gradually replaced by type I and type IIb fibers. Type IIc fibers co-express fetal and adult myosin heavy chains, whereas type I and type IIb fibers express only the adult myosin heavy chain isoform. The paucity of fatigue-resistant type I fibers, high proportion of fatigue-susceptible type IIC fibers, and low oxidative capacity of the neonatal diaphragm suggest that the muscle may be relatively prone to fatigue.[22]

The diaphragmatic and intercostal muscles do not achieve the adult configuration of type I muscle fibers until the child is approximately 2 years old.[23] Type I muscle fibers provide the ability to perform repeated exercise. With the lack of this type of muscle fiber in the child, any factor that increases the work of breathing will contribute to early fatigue of the respiratory muscles, thus explaining an infant's high respiratory rate, the rapidity with which hemoglobin desaturation occurs, and their propensity for fatigue and apnea. One source suggests the muscle fibers

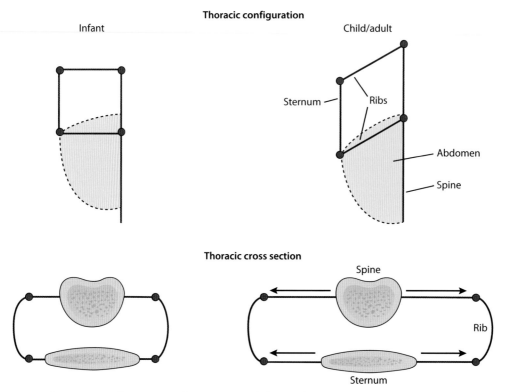

Figure 2-1. Changes in configuration and cross-sectional shape of the thorax from infancy to early childhood. (Reproduced with permission, from Taussig L, Landau L, eds. *Pediatric Respiratory Medicine.* 2nd ed. 2008. Copyright © Elsevier Health Sciences. All rights reserved.)

in the diaphragm of a preterm infant are composed of less than 10% of type I fibers, whereas the muscle fibers of a full-term infant may be 30% type I fibers, and once a child reaches his/her first year of life, the percentage of type I fibers increases to 55%, the expected adult level.[27]

Alveolarization of lung parenchyma of the infant, more specifically children under the age of 2 years, begins in late gestation. According to some sources, the number of alveoli present at birth is estimated to be less than 20% of the number in adults. Also, alveolar size of an infant is smaller than alveolar size of an adult, thus demonstrating that postnatal growth and development of the lung parenchyma increases in number as well as size of alveoli.[28]

Regarding the respiratory system, the formation of adult-type alveoli begins at 36 weeks postconception but represents only a fraction of the terminal air sacs with thick septa at full-term birth. It takes more than several years for functional and morphologic development to be complete, with a tenfold increase in the number of terminal air sacs to 400 to 500 million by 18 months of age, along with the development of rich capillary networks surrounding the alveoli, a profound difference when comparing infants and young children against adults.[24]

While multiple sources state that alveolar multiplication continues well after birth, "earlier studies suggested that postnatal alveolar multiplication might end at 8 years of age; however, more recent studies showed that alveolar multiplication was complete by 2 years of age and possibly even earlier, between 1 and 2 years of age."[22] For example, the study conducted by Thurlbeck in 1982 concludes: "The great bulk of alveoli are present by the age of 2 years and limited, or no, alveolar multiplication occurs subsequently."[29]

By 1 to 2 years of age, most septa show the adult structure characterized by a single capillary network, interwoven with connective tissue strands, that serves to stabilize the interalveolar wall. After the septal restructuring, lung development is considered complete, and the lung enters a period of normal growth that lasts until adulthood. Conclusions of postnatal human lung development consist of (a) the alveolar stage, which starts in late fetal life and lasts at about 1 to 1½ years, and (b) the stage of microvascular maturation, thought to extend from the first months after birth to the age of 2 to 3 years.[30]

It is about 2 years of age that most former studies state the number of alveoli starts to vary substantially among individuals. After the end of alveolar multiplication, the individual alveoli continue to increase in size until thoracic growth is completed.[22]

From the limited number of morphometric studies of relatively few autopsied lungs from infants and toddlers, which have used different morphometric techniques to estimate alveolar number, it remains unclear whether the process of alveolarization is complete by 6 months, 2 to 3 years, or 8 years of age.[28] It is important to realize that it is near impossible to sharply delineate the absolute completion of alveolarization. The various studies that performed quantification measures through alveolar counting procedures have their methodological inaccuracies as well. Most studies base their morphological statements on general or average structural criteria. It is safe to state, however, that the main period of alveolar formation is over before the age of 1½ years, but one cannot exclude a slower addition of further alveoli beyond that age.[30]

The end result of alveolarization and parenchymal growth produces a lung with alveolar and capillary surface areas at least 20 times that of the neonate.[31] From an anatomical standpoint, this is a concept of importance to take into consideration for the anesthetic management of an infant or child versus an adult.

BODY SIZE

Notable differences in body proportion are seen as a child ages. As noted earlier, the head changes in proportion to total length from birth (1:4) to adulthood (1:8). Similarly, a child's upper to lower segment ratio changes with maturity. This ratio is defined from the head to the symphysis pubis (SP) divided by SP to feet. At birth the ratio is approximately 1:7. At about 10 years of age, the ratio is 1. During late adolescence, the ratio is less than 1, in which the upper body is shorter than the lower body.[32]

SPINE

Age-related anatomic variations exist in the location of the caudal termination of the dural sac that can affect neuraxial anesthesia. Differential growth of the vertebrae compared to the nerves and cord accounts for a relative ascension of the cord within the canal over time.[33] By birth the dural sac ends at S3 or S4, with the conus medullaris terminating at the L3 or L4 level. It is not until approximately 1 year of age that anatomic relationships resemble that of the adult, with the spinal cord and dura mater extending to L1 and S1 to S2, respectively. The lower-lying spinal cord in young infants places them at higher risk with more vulnerability to injury for providers that choose to insert their needle at mid- to upper-lumbar levels.[34] It is possible to enter the dural sac during caudal anesthesia. If spinal anesthesia is used in this population, a low approach to entering the dural sac is warranted to avoid the cord.

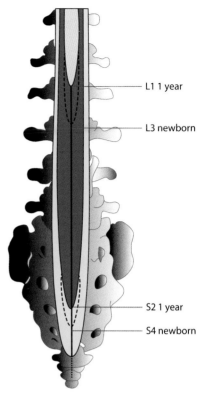

L1 1 year

L3 newborn

S2 1 year

S4 newborn

▲ **Figure 2-2.** The spinal cord terminates at a much more caudad level in neonates and in infants compared to adults. The conus medullaris ends at approximately L1 in adults and at the L2 or L3 level in neonates and infants. (Reproduced with permission, from *Pediatric Epidural and Spinal Anesthesia and Analgesia*. 2017. https://www.nysora.com. Copyright © NYSORA: New York School of Regional Anesthesia. All rights reserved.)

REFERENCES

1. Dekaban AS. Changes in brain weights during the span of human life: relation of brain weights to body heights and body weights. *Ann Neurol.* 1978;4(4):345-356.
2. Tiwana PS, Vickers A. Pediatric cranio-maxillofacial trauma: mandibular fractures. In: Khan HA, Bell RB, Bagheri SC, eds. *Current Therapy in Oral and Maxillofacial Surgery* [Internet]. Philadelphia, PA: Elsevier Saunders; 2012:841-850.
3. Marciniak B. Growth and development. In: Coté CJ, Lerman J, Anderson BJ, eds. *Coté and Lerman's A Practice of Anesthesia for Infants and Children.* 5th ed. Philadelphia, PA: Elsevier/Saunders; 2013:7-20.
4. Kiesler J, Ricer R. The abnormal fontanel. *Am Fam Physician.* 2003;67(12):2547-2552.
5. Duc G, Largo RH. Anterior fontanel: size and closure in term and preterm infants. *Pediatrics.* 1986;78(5):904-908.
6. Vu HL, Panchal J, Parker EE, Levine NS, Francel P. The timing of physiologic closure of the metopic suture: a review of 159 patients using reconstructed 3D CT scans of the craniofacial region. *J Craniofac Surg.* 2001;12(6):527-532.

7. Cohen MM Jr. Sutural biology and the correlates of craniosynostosis. *Am J Med Genet.* 1993;47(5):581-616.

8. Smartt JM Jr, Low DW, Bartlett SP. The pediatric mandible: I. A primer on growth and development. *Plast Reconstr Surg.* 2005;116(1):14e-23e.

9. Tooth eruption. *J Am Dent Assoc.* 2005;136(11):1619.

10. Tooth eruption. *J Am Dent Assoc.* 2006;137(1):127.

11. Miller MJ, Martin RJ, Carlo WA, Fanaroff AA. Oral breathing in response to nasal trauma in term infants. *J Pediatr.* 1987;111(6 pt 1):899-901.

12. Miller MJ, Carlo WA, Strohl KP, Fanaroff AA, Martin RJ. Effect of maturation on oral breathing in sleeping premature infants. *J Pediatr.* 1986;109(3):515-519.

13. Arens R, McDonough JM, Corbin AM, et al. Linear dimensions of the upper airway structure during development: assessment by magnetic resonance imaging. *Am J Respir Crit Care Med.* 2002;165(1):117-122.

14. Litman R, Fiadjoe J, Stricker P, Coté C. The pediatric airway. In: Coté CJ, Lerman J, Anderson BJ, eds. *Coté and Lerman's A Practice of Anesthesia for Infants and Children.* 5th ed. Philadelphia, PA: Elsevier/Saunders; 2013:237-276.

15. Adewale L. Anatomy and assessment of the pediatric airway. *Paediatr Anaesth.* 2009;19(suppl 1):1-8.

16. Eckenhoff JE. Some anatomic considerations of the infant larynx influencing endotracheal anesthesia. *Anesthesiology.* 1951;12(4):401-410.

17. Dalal PG, Murray D, Messner AH, Feng A, McAllister J, Molter D. Pediatric laryngeal dimensions: an age-based analysis. *Anesth Analg.* 2009;108(5):1475-1479.

18. Litman RS, Weissend EE, Shibata D, Westesson PL. Developmental changes of laryngeal dimensions in unparalyzed, sedated children. *Anesthesiology.* 2003;98(1):41-45.

19. Wani TM, Rafiq M, Talpur S, Soualmi L, Tobias JD. Pediatric upper airway dimensions using three-dimensional computed tomography imaging. *Paediatr Anaesth.* 2017;27(6):604-608.

20. Tobias JD. Pediatric airway anatomy may not be what we thought: implications for clinical practice and the use of cuffed endotracheal tubes. *Paediatr Anaesth.* 2015;25(1):9-19.

21. Lerman J, Coté CJ, Steward DJ. Anatomy and physiology. In: Lerman J, Coté CJ, Steward DJ, eds. *Manual of Pediatric Anesthesia.* 7th ed. Switzerland: Springer; 2016.

22. Gaultier C, Denjean A. Developmental anatomy and physiology of the respiratory system. In: Taussig L, Landau L, eds. *Pediatric Respiratory Medicine.* 2nd ed. Elsevier Health Sciences; 2008:15-34.

23. Coté CJ. Pediatric anesthesia. In: Miller R, Eriksson L, Fleisher L, Wiener-Kronish, Cohen N, Young W, eds. *Miller's Anesthesia.* Vol 2. 8th ed. Philadelphia, PA: Elsevier/Saunders; 2015:2757-2798.

24. Davis PJ, Motoyama EK, Cladis FP. Special characteristics of pediatric anesthesia. In: Davis PJ, Cladis FP, eds. *Smith's Anesthesia for Infants and Children.* 9th ed. Elsevier Health Sciences; 2016:2-9.

25. Mantilla CB, Fahim MA, Bradenburg JE, Sieck GC. Functional development of respiratory muscles. In: Polin RA, Abman SH, Rowitch D, Benitz WE, eds. *Fetal and Neonatal Physiology.* Vol 1. 5th ed. Elsevier Health Sciences; 2016:692-705.

26. Gutierrez JA, Duke T, Henning R, South M. Respiratory failure and acute respiratory distress syndrome. In: Taussig LM, Landau LI, eds. *Pediatric Respiratory Medicine.* 2nd ed. Elsevier Health Sciences; 2008:253-274.

27. McMurray JS. General considerations in pediatric otolaryngology. In: Lesperance MM, Flint PW, eds. *Cummings Pediatric Otolaryngology.* Philadelphia, PA: Elsevier Saunders; 2015:1-10.

28. Balinotti JE, Tiller CJ, Llapur CJ, Jones MH, Kimmel RN, Coates CE, et al. Growth of the lung parenchyma early in life. *Am J Respir Crit Care Med.* 2009;179(2):134-137.

29. Thurlbeck WM. Postnatal human lung growth. *Thorax.* 1982;37(8):564-571.

30. Zeltner TB, Burri PH. The postnatal development and growth of the human lung. II. Morphology. *Respir Physiol.* 1987;67(3):269-282.

31. Joza S, Post M. Development of the respiratory system (including the preterm infant). In: Rimensberger PC, ed. *Pediatric and Neonatal Mechanical Ventilation: From Basics to Clinical Practice.* Springer Berlin Heidelberg; 2015:3-25.

32. Nwosu BU, Lee MM. Evaluation of short and tall stature in children. *Am Fam Physician.* 2008;78(5):597-604.

33. Brull R, Macfarlane AJ, Chan VW. Spinal, epidural, and caudal anesthesia. In: Miller RD, Eriksson LI, Fleisher L, Wiener-Kronish JP, Cohen NH, Young WL, eds. *Miller's Anesthesia.* Vol 1. 8th ed. Philadelphia, PA: Elsevier/Saunders; 2015:1684-1720.

34. Birmingham PK. Pediatric postoperative pain. In: Benzon HT, Raja SN, Liu SS, Fishman SM, Cohen SP, eds. *Essentials of Pain Medicine.* 3rd ed. Elsevier/Saunders; 2011:238-242.

Monitoring, Breathing Systems, and Machines

Gijo Alex and Neethu Chandran

FOCUS POINTS

1. Serious adverse events are more common in the pediatric population, so proper understanding and implementation of monitoring tools are essential to prevent adverse outcomes.
2. The American Society of Anesthesiology recommends that during all anesthetics the patient's oxygenation, ventilation, circulation, and temperature should be continually evaluated.
3. Due to the minimal dead space and resistance, Mapleson E and F are the circuit of choice for neonates and pediatric patients.
4. Pediatric breathing systems have the same components as standard adult circuits, but are modified to decrease resistance to breathing and minimize dead space. These modifications include short and narrow tubing, valves that require reduced pressure to open and close, smaller reservoir bag, shorter Y connection, and more compact carbon dioxide absorbers.
5. The primary resistance in a pediatric circuit is determined by the internal diameter of the endotracheal tube and by the length of the tube.[1] The unidirectional valves and carbon dioxide absorber also increase breathing resistance.

MONITORING

Serious adverse events occur in the pediatric population in about 1.4 per 1000 anesthetics and the incidence of cardiac arrest is approximately 0.3 per 1000 anesthetics. This is significantly higher than in the adult population. The incidence of adverse events is inversely related to age with the highest incidence of adverse effects and cardiac arrest occurring in neonates.[2] This data suggests that children are in a high-risk population for adverse events and need to be monitored closely during anesthetic procedures. The American Society of Anesthesiology (ASA) has developed a set of commonly used standards for basic monitoring that apply to both the adult and pediatric population. Qualified anesthesia personnel must be present during the entire anesthetic encounter, continually monitoring oxygenation, electrocardiography, temperature, and the adequacy of ventilation and circulation. Instruments that quantitatively measure oxygen levels should be employed, such as pulse oximeter and an oxygen analyzer to measure oxygen concentration in the breathing system. With regards to circulation, the arterial blood pressure needs to be monitored at least every 5 minutes and the electrocardiogram needs to be displayed from the beginning of every anesthetic until departing from the anesthetizing location. Tracheal intubation or laryngeal mask airway placement needs to be confirmed by clinical assessment and by qualitative detection of carbon dioxide in the exhaled gas. Finally, every patient receiving anesthesia should have their temperature monitored when clinically significant changes in body temperature are intended, anticipated, or suspected.[2]

Pulse Oximetry

Pulse oximetry has become the standard of care in measuring arterial oxygen saturation in the operating rooms and intensive care units. The oximetry probe contains two light-emitting diodes (LEDs) which produce both red and infrared light. The LEDs and the detectors should be transversely positioned to get the best readings. In neonates, this may require placing the probe across the palm of the hand or the foot. The pulse oximeter uses two wavelengths of light, so it can only accurately detect oxyhemoglobin and deoxyhemoglobin.[3] Deoxyhemoglobin absorbs more light in the red spectrum (660 nm), whereas oxyhemoglobin absorbs more light in the infrared spectrum (940 nm).

Fetal hemoglobin has minimal effect on pulse oximetry readings, so the pulse oximetry is equally accurate in both the adult and pediatric population. Polycythemia, anemia, and sickle cell hemoglobin do not affect the accuracy of pulse oximetry.[4]

The pulse oximeter is also useful to monitor preductal and postductal oxygen saturations in neonates whenever there is a persistence of fetal circulation. A 10% decrease in postductal oxygen saturations in relation to the preductal oxygen saturation signifies significant right to left shunting as a result of pulmonary hypertension.[5,6]

The pulse oximeter is also a valuable screening tool for detection of cyanotic congenital heart disease. Neonates who have oxygen saturation values less than or approximately 95% by day 2 of life suggest a cyanotic heart disease.[7]

There are, however, certain limitations of pulse oximetry that must be taken into consideration. For example, conditions that lead to hypothermia, vasoconstriction, and hypotension make the pulse oximeter less accurate. Dyes such as methylene blue, indocynanin green, and indigo carmine may also falsely lower pulse oximeter readings by absorbing light in the red spectrum (660 nm).

Significantly elevated levels of carboxyhemoglobin or methemoglobin will also drastically alter pulse oximetry readings. Methemoglobin absorbs red and infrared light in an equal 1:1 proportion, so the pulse oximeter will read approximately 85%. Falsely high readings may occur in the presence of carboxyhemoglobin because the pulse oximeter reads carboxyhemoglobin as 90% oxyhemoglobin and only 10% deoxyhemoglobin.[8]

Electrocardiography

Electrocardiography in the pediatric population is more commonly used to detect intraoperative arrhythmias such as supraventricular tachycardias or bradyarrythmias. It is less often used to detect ischemia because ischemia rarely occurs in the pediatric population. Lead II provides the best view of atrial activity, so it is recommended for intraoperative use and the detection of arrhythmias. Bradycardia is likely to be the first indicator of hypoxia in the pediatric patient and is likely to be picked up sooner than a decrease in oxygen saturation noted by pulse oximetry. Electrolyte abnormalities can also be visualized on electrocardiography. For example, hyperkalemia will reveal peaked T waves, progressive widening of the QRS complex, and low P-wave amplitude. Hypocalcemia would reveal a prolonged QT interval.

Capnography

Capnography is the monitoring of the concentration or partial pressure of carbon dioxide (CO_2) in the respiratory gases and is an indirect monitor of CO_2 partial pressure in the arterial blood. Its main development has been as a monitoring tool for use during anesthesia and for monitoring of critically ill patients in the intensive care unit. It has become the gold standard to detect correct placement of an endotracheal tube within the trachea. According to the ASA, "When an endotracheal tube or laryngeal mask is inserted, its correct positioning must be verified by clinical assessment and by identification of carbon dioxide in the expired gas. Continual end-tidal carbon dioxide analysis, in use from the time of endotracheal tube/laryngeal mask placement, until extubation/removal or initiating transfer to a postoperative care location, shall be performed using a quantitative method such as capnography, capnometry, or mass spectroscopy. When capnography or capnometry is utilized, the end tidal CO_2 alarm shall be audible to the anesthesiologist or the anesthesia care team personnel."[3]

Changes in the shape of the capnograph can provide useful information on disease processes in an intubated patient. During ETT placement, the capnogram can readily alert the physician to endotracheal tube misplacement in the esophagus. Capnography has also long been used to determine the effectiveness of chest compressions (Figure 3-1).[9]

Near-Infrared Spectroscopy

Near-infrared spectroscopy (NIRS) is a noninvasive technique that monitors regional tissue oxygenation and perfusion status. It measures tissue oxygenation through the use of near-infrared light at wavelengths between 700 and 1000 nm.[10] It is similar to pulse oximetry in some respects. Pulse oximetry, however, depends on pulsatile blood flow and measures only the oxyhemoglobin in the arterial blood. NIRS measures the difference between oxyhemoglobin and deoxyhemoglobin in regional tissues and reflects hemoglobin saturation in arterial, venous, as well as capillary blood. This difference between oxyhemoglobin and deoxyhemoglobin reflects oxygen uptake in those areas. This measurement is reported as regional oxygen saturation (rSO_2). This is most commonly measured in the brain, renal, and splanchnic systems. In the cerebral cortex, average tissue hemoglobin is distributed in a proportion of approximately 70% venous and 30% arterial. There can be some variation between individuals with regards to cerebral arterial/venous ratios. Therefore in clinical practice, the use of NIRS as a trend monitor minimizes confounding variables.[10] Cerebral uptake of oxygen is typically higher due to higher metabolic demands, while renal and splanchnic uptakes are slightly lower. Therefore, normal cerebral readings tend to be lower (60–80), while renal and splanchnic measurements are generally higher (65–90). Lower NIRS readings indicate increased oxygen extraction at the tissue level or decreased oxygen delivery to the tissue being recorded.[11]

In the pediatric setting, NIRS is being used for pediatric cardiac surgery and neurosurgery, as well as in the neonatal intensive care units. For infants undergoing cardiac surgery,

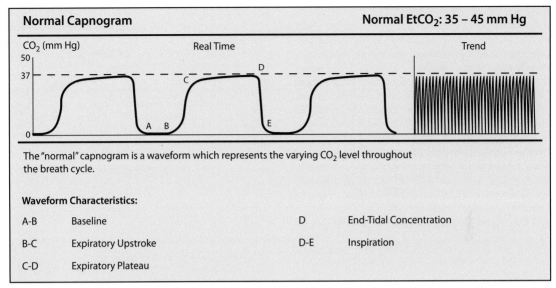

Normal Capnogram

Normal EtCO$_2$: 35 – 45 mm Hg

CO$_2$ (mm Hg) Real Time Trend

The "normal" capnogram is a waveform which represents the varying CO$_2$ level throughout the breath cycle.

Waveform Characteristics:

A-B	Baseline	D	End-Tidal Concentration
B-C	Expiratory Upstroke	D-E	Inspiration
C-D	Expiratory Plateau		

▲ **Figure 3-1.** A capnogram illustrating both the inspiratory and expiratory phases of respiration. (Reproduced with permission, from Lerman J, ed. *Neonatal Anesthesia.* 2015. https://link.springer.com. Copyright © Springer-Verlag. All rights reserved.)

perioperative cerebral and mesenteric NIRS monitoring has been shown to be beneficial in detecting changes from baseline, which represents possible hypoperfusion of tissue beds. During deep hypothermic circulatory arrest, there is little ability to monitor cerebral function, so cerebral NIRS has been used as a means of detecting cerebral ischemia.[11]

Blood Pressure Monitoring

Blood pressure can be monitored with basic noninvasive equipment such as a blood pressure cuff or through direct measurements using an arterial line.[12] The noninvasive blood pressure measurements are based on the principles of oscillometry. Systolic blood pressure is recognized by computer algorithms as the point where the rate of increase in the size of the oscillation is maximal. Diastolic blood pressure is recognized as the point of the maximal rate of decrease in the size of the oscillation. It is recommended that the blood pressure cuff width should be 40% of the circumference of the extremity.

Direct measurements of blood pressure can be used with the placement of an arterial line especially in critically ill children or in situations where noninvasive blood pressure cuff placement is not feasible. For example, in children with morbid obesity, the readings from a noninvasive blood pressure cuff may be inaccurate. In children with severe forms of osteogenesis imperfecta, the cycling of the blood pressure cuff may lead to fractures of their bones.[13]

Some common locations where arterial lines can be placed are in the radial artery, ulnar artery, brachial artery, femoral artery, posterior tibia artery, and umbilical artery. The umbilical artery is usually quite easy to access in the immediately neonatal period and is widely used in the neonatal intensive care units. Proper placement should be verified with radiographic films as improper positioning can lead to thrombotic complications which can ultimately affect organs, limbs, and even the spinal cord.[12,13]

The radial artery seems to have the lowest incidence of complications especially in the smaller pediatric patients. Axillary arterial cannulation is preferred over brachial artery cannulation as there is better collateral flow to the artery in the axillary artery. The brachial artery has poor collateral circulation, so limb ischemia is a concern with arterial line placement in this location. As with any arterial catheter, if there is evidence of impaired circulation to the extremities, the arterial catheter should be removed immediately and monitored closely.

Body Temperature Monitoring

The ASA recommends continuous temperature monitoring during anesthetic procedures. There are different sites that can be used to achieve these readings. The most commonly used sites are the axilla, rectum, bladder, skin, and esophagus. Rectal temperature is often considered the gold standard of temperature monitoring. The younger the pediatric patient, the more challenging it is to monitor and regulate their temperature in the operating theater. Neonates are especially vulnerable to heat loss and temperature regulation. They have larger surface area to body weight ratio, a thin subcutaneous fat layer, and are unable to shiver, so they depend on non-shivering thermogenesis (NST) from brown fat for heat production. NST is triggered by a surge of catecholamines, released from the sympathetic nervous system during times of cold stress.[14] With continued cold stress, the stores of brown fat become depleted and this eventually leads to hypoxia and hypoglycemia. During general anesthesia, neonates lose the ability to perform NST and so they are unable to respond effectively to even mild intraoperative hypothermia.

BREATHING SYSTEMS AND MACHINES

The breathing system is essentially an extension of the patient's lung and upper airway connecting it to the anesthesia machine.

Characteristics of an ideal breathing system include:

1. Efficient delivery of intended inspired gas mixture. This means the system should be able to deliver target concentration of gas mixture in a timely manner. Also, it should be able to adjust to rapid changes in delivery of concentration.
2. Effective elimination of CO_2 and easy removal of waste gas.
3. Minimizing dead space.
4. Minimal amount of resistance.
5. Preservation of heat and humidity in expired gases.
6. Versatility in modes of ventilation in all age groups.
7. Efficient and allows low fresh gas flow (FGF).
8. Light weight and compact while being safe and inexpensive.

Breathing systems are classified as open, semi-open, semi-closed, and closed. The classification is dependent on the presence or absence of a reservoir bag, rebreathing of exhaled gases, CO_2 absorption, and unidirectional valves (Table 3-1).

Open Breathing System

The open breathing system does not include a circuit; therefore, the patient has access to atmospheric gases. Examples of the open system include insufflation and open-drop anesthesia. Presently, insufflation is not used as a breathing system, but more as a method to administer passive oxygen during periods of apnea (eg, bronchoscopy) or as a technique for inhalational induction for pediatric patients. Similarly, open-drop anesthesia is no longer used in the United States. It consists of dripping an anesthetic (eg, ether) on a gauze, covered mask and applying it over the patient's mouth and nose. As long as flows are high there is no rebreathing of exhaled gases in the open breathing. Disadvantages of the open system include lack of conservation of humidity and heat in exhaled gases, difficult airway management, pollution of the operating room, poor control of depth of anesthesia, and inability to control ventilation.

Semi-Open Breathing System

The most common semi-open breathing system is the Mapleson system (Figure 3-2). The Mapleson system helps some of the above problems by including additional components into the breathing system. Those components include adjustable pressure limiting (APL) valves, reservoir bag, and breathing tube. Depending on the relative location of these components, Mapleson system is classified into five basic types (Mapleson A, B, C, D, and E). Mapleson F was added later, which is a Jackson-Rees modification of Mapleson E (T-piece). The Bain circuit is a modification of the Mapleson D system.

The Mapleson system lacks expiratory and inspiratory valves and carbon dioxide absorption, which reduces the resistance of the circuit; therefore, work of breathing is low. However, the lack of separation between the inspired and

Table 3-1. Breathing System Classification

Breathing Systems	Types	Reservoir Bag	CO₂ Absorption	Rebreathing of Gases	Unidirectional Valves
Open	Insufflation, open-drop anesthesia	–	–	–	–
Semi-open	Mapleson circuits	+	–	–	1 valve
Semi-closed	Circle system (FGF < MV)	+	+	Partial	3 valves
Closed	Circle system where FGF equals patient's basal oxygen requirements (FGF = uptake)	+	+	Total	3 valves

FGF, fresh gas flow; MV, minute ventilation.

high. Monitoring end-tidal CO_2 is the best way to determine the ideal amount of FGF.[15]

Historically, pediatric patients less than 10 kg were anesthetized with either the Mapleson D or F breathing system. Mapleson circuits are infrequently used because most hospitals have converted to the circle system due to cost containment and cost of newer anesthetic agents. Currently, the most commonly used Mapleson systems are the Jackson-Rees and Bain circuit. The B and C systems are rarely used today. For adults, Mapleson A is the circuit of choice for spontaneous respiration because there is no rebreathing during spontaneous ventilation when the FGF is greater than 75% of the minute ventilation.[16] Although Mapleson D and its Bain modification require a little more FGF during spontaneous ventilation to eliminate rebreathing, it is the most efficient circuit for controlled ventilation for adults.[1]

Due to the minimal dead space and resistance, Mapleson E and F are the circuit of choice for neonates and pediatric patients.[15] They both allow for observation of ventilation during spontaneous breathing, as well as positive pressure ventilation by applying pressure to the bag. Hence, Mapleson F is commonly used to transport a child post-anesthesia to the recovery room or other parts of the hospital.

An important clinical consideration of the Mapleson system is that any anesthetic concentration changes made to the vaporizer will have immediate effects on the concentration reaching the patient. This can be advantageous for a more rapid induction; however, it also increases the risk of possible anesthetic overdose compared to the circle system. Although the Mapleson system is able to address some of the problematic issues with the open system, it shares others.[17] This includes the need for high gas flow to prevent rebreathing which causes more operating room pollution, loss of conservation of humidity and heat in exhaled gases, and waste of anesthetic gases increasing cost.

Circle System

The circle absorber may be used as a closed or semi-closed system. A semi-closed circle absorber is the most commonly used breathing system. In a semi-closed system, the pressure relief valve is opened, allowing excess gas to escape. This allows higher FGF rates to be used to reduce rebreathing of gases. This system is more stable since excess gas can escape if the system fills up to capacity.[15] High FGF also allows the ability to rapidly change concentration of anesthetic gases delivered. Disadvantages of the semi-open circle system are increased anesthetic and oxygen usage and atmospheric pollution.

In a closed system, the pressure-relief valve is closed so that no gas escapes. The FGF equals the patient's basal oxygen requirements. This system is less stable because if inflow gas does not exactly match oxygen consumption,

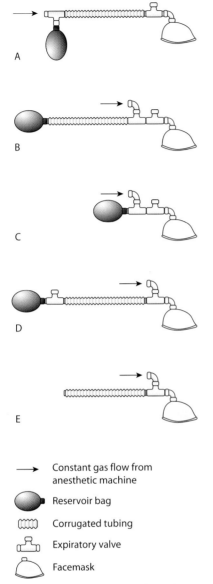

A

B

C

D

E

→ Constant gas flow from anesthetic machine

Reservoir bag

Corrugated tubing

Expiratory valve

Facemask

▲ **Figure 3-2.** Depending on the relative location of expiratory valve, reservoir bag, and corrugated tubing, Mapleson system is classified into five basic types (Mapleson A, B, C, D, and E). (Adapted with permission, from Mapleson WW. The elimination of rebreathing in various semi-closed anaesthetic systems. *Br J Anaesth.* 1954;26(5):323–332. https://bjanaesthesia.org.)

expired gases causes rebreathing to occur when inspiratory flow exceeds FGF. Therefore, the amount of rebreathing is highly dependent on FGF. Rebreathing can help conserve heat, humidity, and anesthetic gases. However, if CO_2 is not monitored correctly, the risk of hypercarbia and acidosis is the patient will have difficulty breathing.[15] Also, low FGF prevents rapid changes in concentration of anesthetic gases. The advantage of the closed system is that anesthetic and oxygen usage is optimized and atmospheric pollution is minimized.

Components of the circle include a gas inlet, unidirectional inspiratory and expiratory valves, corrugated tubing, CO_2 absorber canister, adjustable pressure-limiting (APL) valve, reservoir bag, and a Y piece connector. The most efficient configuration of the components diagrammed in Figure 3-3 includes a unidirectional valve on either side of the reservoir bag, the APL valve should be positioned before the absorber in the expiratory limb, FGF should enter between the absorber and inspiratory valves, and the reservoir bag is located in the expiratory limb.[15]

Dead space in the circuit is located distal to where inspiratory gases mix with exhaled gases located at the Y piece. The goal for pediatric patients is to reduce dead space as much as possible especially for younger patients. Unlike the Mapleson system, the tubing length does not affect dead space.[18] The primary resistance in a pediatric circuit is determined by the internal diameter of the endotracheal tube and by the length of the tube.[1] The unidirectional valves and carbon dioxide absorber also increase breathing resistance.

Pediatric breathing systems have the same components as standard adult circuits, but are modified to decrease resistance to breathing and minimize dead space. These modifications include short and narrow tubing, valves that require reduced pressure to open and close, smaller reservoir bag, shorter Y connection, and more compact carbon dioxide absorbers.[17] This helps decrease compliance of the circuit and allows rapid changes in concentration of anesthetic gases.

Most of the issues associated with the Mapleson system are solved with the circle system. Some disadvantages include bulkiness and less portability, increased resistance to breathing due to the addition of valves and CO_2 absorbent, and increased possibility for disconnection and failure due to different components.

Anesthesia Machines

Currently, there are no anesthesia machines designed only for pediatric use. Standard adult breathing machines can be used as long as the user understands how to

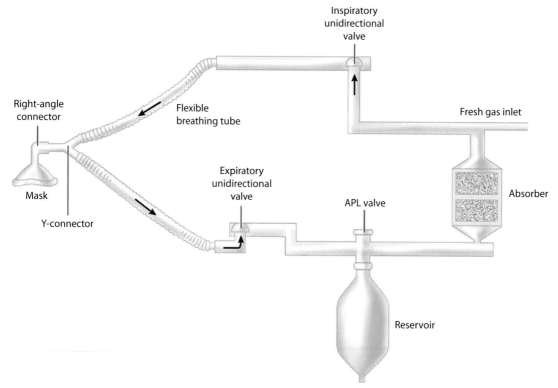

▲ **Figure 3-3.** The most efficient configuration of circle system. (Reproduced with permission, from Butterworth IV JF, Mackey DC, Wasnick JD. eds. *Morgan & Mikhail's Clinical Anesthesiology,* 6th ed. 2013. Copyright © McGraw Hil LLC. All rights reserved.)

compensate for their limitations. Advanced ventilators are the biggest difference between newer and older anesthesia machines.[19] In the past, anesthesia ventilators were unable to accurately deliver small tidal volumes for neonates, accommodate the high respiratory rate required for neonatal ventilation, and offer other modes of ventilation other than volume control.[20] Anesthesiologists resorted to using the ICU ventilators in the operating room. Newer anesthesia machines are able to provide different modes of ventilation and also estimate and compensate for circuit compliance. This feature is called circuit compliance compensation.[19] The compensation consists of delivering slightly more than the set tidal volume to compensate for volume lost to the circuit. Low compliance is desirable to minimize the amount of volume lost to expanding and contracting the circuit during ventilation. Ideally the circuit should be stiff and not distensible. Newer machines also have FGF decoupling, which means there is no change in tidal volume regardless of changes in fresh gas flow. Fresh gas flow decoupling and compliance compensation have increased the safety profile of ventilators and anesthesia machines in the pediatric population.

REFERENCES

1. Waters DJ, Mapleson WW. Rebreathing during controlled respiration with various semiclosed anesthetic systems. *Br J Anaesth*. 1961;33:374-381.
2. Kurth CD, Tyler D, Heitmiller E, Tosone SR, Martin L, Deshpande JK. National pediatric anesthesia safety quality improvement program in the United States. *Anesth Analg*. 2014;119(1):112-121.
3. The American Society of Anesthesiology. Standards for basic anesthesia monitoring. October 2015.
4. Jubran A. Pulse oximetry. *Critical Care*. 2015;19:272.
5. Patino M, Kurth D, McAuliffe J. *Monitoring the Neonate: Basic Science, Neonatal Anesthesia*. New York: Springer; 2015.
6. Steward D. *Monitoring the Neonate: Practical Considerations, Neonatal Anesthesia*. New York: Springer; 2015.
7. Arlettaz R, Bauschatz AS, Monkhoff M, Essers B, Bauersfeld U. The contribution of pulse oximetry to the early detection of congenital heart disease in newborns. *Eur J. Pediatr*. 2006;165:94-98.
8. Webb RK, Ralston AC, Runciman WB. Potential errors in pulse oximetry, II. Effect of changes in saturation and signal quality. *Anaesthesia*. 1991;46:207-212.
9. Thompson J, Jaffe M. Capnographic waveforms in the mechanically ventilated patient. *Respir Care*. 2005;50(1):100-108; discussion 108-109.
10. Murkin J, Arango M. Near-infrared spectroscopy as an index of brain and tissue oxygenation. *Br J Anaesth*. 2009;103(suppl 1): i3-i13.
11. Marin T, Moore J. Understanding near-infrared spectroscopy. *Adv Neonatal Care*. 2011;11(6):382-388.
12. Steward D. Monitoring the Neonate: Practical Considerations. In: Lerman J, ed. *Neonatal Anesthesia*. New York: Springer; 2015:191-196.
13. Lockman J, Alex G. *Monitors in Pediatric Anesthesia. Pediatric Anesthesiology Review Topics*. Montgomery, AL: Naerthwyn Press; 2013.
14. Waldron S, MacKinnon R. Neonatal thermoregulation. *Infant*. 2007;3(3):101-104.
15. Mackey DC, Butterworth JF, Mikhail MS, Morgan GE, Wasnick JD. *Morgan & Mikhail's Clinical Anesthesiology*. 5th ed. New York: McGraw-Hill Education; 2013.
16. Kaul TK, Mittal G. Mapleson's breathing systems. *Indian J Anaesth*. 2013;57:507-515.
17. Coté CJ. Pediatric breathing circuits and anesthesia machines. *Int Anesthesiol Clin*. 1992;30:51-61.
18. Brown ES, Hustead RF. Resistance of pediatric breathing systems. *Anesth Analg*. 1969;48(5):842.
19. Rothschiller JL, Uejima T, Dsida RM, Coté CJ. Evaluation of a new operating room ventilator with volume-controlled ventilation: the Ohmeda 7900. *Anesth Analg*. 1999;88:39-42.
20. Moynihan R, Coté CJ. Fresh gas flow changes during controlled mechanical ventilation with the circle system have significantly greater effects on the ventilatory parameters of toddlers compared with children. *Paediatr Anaesth*. 1992;2:211-215.

Pharmacology

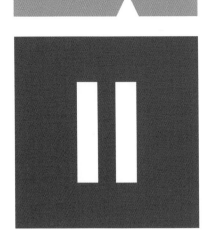

Neonatal Considerations

Barbara A. Vickers

As one considers the anesthetic to be delivered to a neonatal patient, it is prudent to give special attention to the ontogeny that will affect this plan. Neonates are children typically defined as age birth to 1 month. However, if born prematurely, as early as 24 weeks, this "neonatal" period is extended. Since neonates are not simply small adults, one must review the developmental aspects of pharmacokinetics and pharmacodynamics prior to administering anesthesia.

The emphasis on a neonatal tailored anesthetic originates from the very basic facts. Start with growth and maturation. Compared with adults, neonates have larger heads, shorter extremities, and larger torsos. Their skin as a vital organ accounts for a much larger percentage of body weight playing a significant role in pharmacokinetics. The rest of their organs are immature in function affecting a drug's ultimate action. With advances in neonatal critical care, infants are born at birth weight of 500 g and gestational age of 24 weeks creating a different physiologic state than previously seen.

PHARMACOKINETICS

When caring for a premature infant, a clinician must respect developmental nuances that make essential a thorough review of neonatal pharmacology prior to anesthetic administration.

All infants, but especially premature ones, undergo rapid developmental changes in the postnatal period, which affect each aspect of pharmacokinetics. Pharmacokinetics refers to the disposition of a drug in the body and the processes that affect its course. These processes include drug absorption, distribution, metabolism, and elimination. We will review each process through the neonatal perspective. Fundamental parameters common among these processes include volume of distribution (V_d), clearance, and **half-life**.[1]

a. V_d is a concept used to define the volume required to contain the total amount of a drug at a concentration equal to that in plasma. This "volume" is affected by hydrophilicity and lipophilicity. When a drug is highly water-soluble, it will have a small V_d because it must remain in the intravascular space only. Conversely, when a drug is lipophilic, it is distributed to the entire body and its V_d is much larger. Neonates are considered to have a much larger volume of distribution for hydrophilic drugs compared to a smaller volume of distribution for lipophilic drugs.

b. Clearance is the organ's ability to clear or eliminate a drug from an amount of fluid (blood or plasma). This is a concept that will be further elaborated in the section on elimination. This capability is also affected by the eliminating organ's maturity, whether it will be the liver or the kidney.

c. Half-life is the time required for half the amount of a drug in the blood to be removed from the body[2]

Absorption

The first process in the pathway of pharmacokinetics is absorption, that is, the transfer of a drug from the site of administration into the circulation.[3] There are many factors that can affect the rate of absorption just like there are many modes of medication administration to consider. Possible routes for a neonate include oral (or via a feeding tube), rectal, intramuscular, subcutaneous, and topical. There is a great variability in drug absorption into a neonate's circulation, as their fat, muscle, fluid, and skin compartments are all underdeveloped and not taken into consideration when the initial drug studies are designed. While in the operating room, absorption is not commonly a concern as most of our medications are administered intravenously. However, anesthesia providers must consider alternative modes of administration should the need arise.

Enteral absorption is not reliable in a neonate for two main reasons. Neonates are susceptible to delayed gastric emptying and venous congestion. Delayed gastric emptying and poor intestinal absorption are multifactorial related to gastroesophageal reflux, poor perfusion due to illness, disease of the intestines (short-gut syndrome), irregular peristalsis, and the composition of breast milk or formula consumed.[2] Gastric emptying will reach adult rates by 6 to 8 months of life. Drugs administered via the rectum will also be affected by similar factors though the mechanism proposed is passive diffusion. If the drug is placed in the superior aspect of the rectum it will enter the portal circulation and undergo hepatic first-pass metabolism as compared to a lower rectal placement that will initially bypass the liver.[2]

Intramuscular (IM) absorption depends primarily on blood flow which can be compromised in states of low perfusion such as respiratory distress and hypoxemia, cardiac dysfunction, and sepsis all more frequently seen in premature neonates. Absorption also depends on skeletal mass which is less in neonates than in adults; medication contact time is decreased resulting in reduced absorption. Lack of muscle movement/activity from illness or a muscle relaxant agent may also affect absorption and thus peak serum concentration. Higher density of skeletal muscle capillaries has a theoretical increase in absorption after IM injection in neonates.[1] Medications commonly used intramuscularly in the operating room include atropine, glycopyrrolate, opioids, ketamine, and succinylcholine.

Percutaneous absorption has clinical significance but is often overlooked. It is related to skin hydration and surface area, but inversely related to the thickness of the stratum corneum.[2] A neonate has a larger ratio of surface area to body weight and a thinner stratum corneum, and when combined with better perfusion as seen in full-term infants,[1] topical medication bioavailability may be increased. It is estimated that when a medication is applied topically, neonates are *exposed* to 2.7 times the amount intended as compared to a similar application to an adult or child.[4] For example, in the operating room when cleansing solutions are used before a peripheral nerve block or an epidural catheter is placed, and prior to venous or arterial catheterization, toxic exposure can be a real risk. Similarly, when topical local anesthetics (EMLA, LTA, lidocaine gel) of various concentrations are used prior to procedures (ENT procedures, orogastric tube placement, nasotracheal intubation) clinicians need to be cognizant of their potency to prevent toxicity.

Other risk factors associated with toxicity include damaged skin due to trauma, burn, or infection and prematurity due to immature barrier.

Distribution

Distribution is the next step in the process of pharmacokinetics and involves medication distribution into compartments of the body. A key factor in this process is the age of the patient and its related physiologic changes—circulating binding proteins, compartment sizes, and membrane permeability. Other factors include affinity to circulating proteins, available binding sites, disease states, hemodynamics and presence of endogenous compounds such as bilirubin.

Protein binding becomes significant because it limits the amount of active drug available in circulation. Total drug in the body is the sum of bound drug (drug + protein) and unbound drug. The "bound" drug molecules are not active and not capable of crossing membranes or binding to receptors to trigger pharmacologic action, metabolism, and excretion. Binding to serum proteins is a rapidly reversible process that creates a dynamic system of drug availability to transfer across membranes.[1] The amount of unbound drug is much larger in neonates who have an altered ratio and affinity of proteins. Plasma proteins that most commonly bind to medications include albumin and alpha-1-acid glycoprotein. Albumin binds acidic medications and the affinity between the two is not at adult levels at birth, nor are total plasma protein levels. Albumin levels at birth are approximately 75% to 80% of adult levels which they reach at about a year of age.[1,2] Alpha-1-acid glycoprotein is at 50% of adult levels at birth.[1] Although the total amount of drug concentration appears to be in the therapeutic range for adults and older children, the free-drug concentration may in fact lay in a toxic range for the premature patient.

When cord blood has been studied and tested for protein binding, it is shown that there is a significant reduction in binding medications such as lidocaine and propranolol as compared to the serum of an adult.[2]

Aside from protein availability to determine distribution, total body water also makes a significant contribution. Composition of body compartments, such as total water and total fat varies with gestational age (Table 4-1), alter the volume of distribution for each drug and will theoretically influence medication concentration available for distribution and effect.

Hydrophilic drugs such as acetaminophen or vancomycin have a larger volume of distribution in a newborn per kilogram of body weight compared with an adult. Theoretically, neonates and infants could require larger doses per weight to reach therapeutic serum concentrations. Conversely, for a full-term healthy baby, his or her fat content is large enough to make the assertion that lipophilic drugs will have a large volume of distribution, similar to hydrophilic medications. The low-fat content of the extremely premature infants' brain may affect distribution of centrally acting

Table 4-1. Percentage Fat Based on Gestational Age[3]

Gestational Age	% Body Weight	% Fat
24 wks	89	0.1–0.5
40 wks	75	15
6 mos	60	30
Adult	65	20

Table 4-2. Pharmacology of Intravenous Anesthetic Agents in Extremely Premature Infants[5]

Medications	Dose (mg/kg)	V_d (L/kg)	Elimination Half-Life (h)
Propofol	2.5	9.5	
Phenobarbital	2 PO TID	0.8–1.2	60–180
Fentanyl	0.001–0.005	1.0	4.2
Morphine	0.05–0.1		6.8
Acetaminophen	10–15 PO (60 mg/d max)	1.0	4.8
Rocuronium	0.6–1.2		
Midazolam	0.1	1.15	14.1

Source: Data from Khan KS, Hayes I, Buggy DJ. Pharmacology of anaesthetic agents I: intravenous anaesthetic agents. *Cont Ed Anaesth Crit Care Pain*. 2014;14:3. https://www.journals.elsevier.com/british-journal-of-anaesthesia

Table 4-3. Pharmacology of Intravenous Anesthetic Agents in Adults[5]

Medications	Dose (mg/kg)	V_d (L/kg)	Elimination Half-Life (h)
Propofol	1–2	4.6	4–7
Phenobarbital	30–120 PO TID	0.5–0.6	53–118
Fentanyl	—	4.0	3.7
Morphine	0.05–0.1		
Acetaminophen	12.5	0.9	2
Rocuronium	0.6–1.2		
Midazolam	—	1.1	1.9

Source: Data from Khan KS, Hayes I, Buggy DJ. Pharmacology of anaesthetic agents I: intravenous anaesthetic agents. *Cont Ed Anaesth Crit Care Pain*. 2014;14:3. https://www.journals.elsevier.com/british-journal-of-anaesthesia.

medications as outlined in Table 4-2 as compared to their adult counterpart in Table 4-3. For example, propofol is a lipophilic drug routinely administered in the pediatric operating room. Neonates have lower total body fat compared to an adult, which allows propofol to have a smaller volume of distribution in the central compartment and higher plasma concentrations. This scenario places the neonate at risk for toxicity that is unique to their population.

Membrane permeability of the newborn blood-brain barrier (with incomplete myelinization) is increased, thus creating a higher drug concentration in the central nervous system with possible perioperative effects.[4]

Increased presence of unconjugated bilirubin and free fatty acids can compete with medications that are protein bound, displacing those drugs and creating an increase in free drug concentration. Hyperbilirubinemia as seen in the jaundiced neonate can reduce protein binding of penicillin, ampicillin, and phenobarbital necessitating dose adjustments. In combination with an increase in unbound drug, by nature of immature plasma proteins, hyperbilirubinemia

creates a scenario in which the amount of drug now free for distribution to the tissues may place the infant at risk of toxic exposure. Presence of certain medications such as diazepam and phenytoin can displace bilirubin from albumin binding sites, increasing the risk of kernicterus.[6] Otherwise known as bilirubin encephalopathy, kernicterus results from deposition of bilirubin in the brain potentially leading to cerebral palsy, hearing loss, vision problems, or mental retardation. The binding affinity of albumin for bilirubin increases with age and does not reach adult levels until approximately 5 months of age. If a neonate is on one of these bilirubin-displacing medications, preoperative discussion should ensue to avoid perioperative morbidity.

Metabolism

Metabolism encompasses bioactivities by which a drug may get activated, inactivated (for elimination), or converted into a toxic metabolite. These reactions are identified as phase I, oxidation, reduction, or hydrolysis; or phase II, conjugation reactions which are glucuronidation, sulfation, and acetylation.[3] Phase I reactions modify the structure of the drug, altering a functional group and causing it to become polar(water-soluble). This results in activation or inactivation of the parent drug. Phase II reactions add an endogenous molecule to the drug or its metabolite. This process makes the product further water-soluble allowing it to be eliminated via bile or urine.[1] These transformations occur primarily in the liver. Other sites of metabolism include the kidneys, red blood cells, intestines, lungs, and skin. Phase I reactions in the liver are supported by the cytochrome P-enzymes (CYP). Many of the medications administered in the operating room during a general anesthetic are metabolized by these two reactions. Each site of metabolism plays a role and it is important to remember that during compromised perfusion states in the operating room the overall ability of the body to activate and eliminate medications may be altered. Specifically for newborns, hepatic blood flow is increased at birth as the ductus venosus is eliminated. This change occurs during the first week of life. However, it is not fully mature until age three.

Phase I Enzymes

Newborns have a reduced total quantity of cytochrome P450 microsomes and at term will only reach 50% of adult values.[3] It can be assumed that a reduced enzyme concentration in neonates will dictate prolonged half-lives of medications such as caffeine, phenytoin, and phenobarbital. However, due to the complexities of the developmental patterns of cytochrome enzymes, one cannot make broad generalizations regarding a neonate's metabolizing capabilities. CPY3A, an important such enzyme associated with many substrates such as acetaminophen, alfentanil, diazepam, lidocaine, midazolam, verapamil, and R-warfarin, is functionally active in the fetus mainly as CYP3A7 with activity reaching 75% of adult levels by 30 weeks' gestation. Postnatal activity has been found to be low but is near adult level by 6 to 12 months. It is also induced by dexamethasone, phenobarbital, and phenytoin requiring adjustment of substrate medication dosing.[3]

Phase II Reactions

The purpose of phase II reactions is to change the substrate to make it easier to be eliminated through the kidneys. The enzymes associated with phase II conjugation reactions include glucuronosyltransferase, sulfotransferase, N-acetyltransferase, glutathione S-transferase, and methyl transferase. There isn't as much known of these reactions, but there are some developmental changes that will affect drug clearance.

Morphine is metabolized via glucuronidation to morphine-3-glucuronide and morphine-6-glucuronide. Its metabolism takes place in the liver and kidney, while its elimination is dependent on urine and bile. It is the M6G metabolite that competes for the mu receptor and potentially contributes to the overall analgesic effect of morphine, whereas M3G does not appear to compete for opioid receptor binding. A neonate's ability to glucuronidate morphine is limited and thus its clearance may be limited[7] necessitating a dose adjustment to avoid complications with respiratory depression. Maturation of function of this enzymatic process may not be complete until 6 to 18 months of age.

Acetaminophen appears to be preferentially metabolized in neonates and children. It is metabolized by three phase II reactions: sulfation, glucuronidation, and through cytochrome P450-2E1. The sulfotransferase system is mature in the neonate as compared to the glucuronosyltransferase system previously discussed in the context of morphine. The excretion of acetaminophen is not significantly prolonged in an infant likely due to the formation of the acetaminophen-sulfate conjugate which compensates for the other immature enzyme system. This will become the nondominant product as the liver matures and glucuronidation takes over in the adult. Toxicity is a risk with acetaminophen administration in all humans when glutathione stores cannot compete with frequent dosing. The mechanism of this relates to the P450 pathway which produces N-acetyl-p-benzoquinone imine (NAPQI), a toxic metabolite. NAPQI is then metabolized via glutathione to nontoxic cysteine and mercapturic acid. If NAPQI is not metabolized, hepatocyte damage and necrosis of the liver can occur. Acetaminophen's elimination half-life is prolonged in infants from approximately 2 hours in adults to 3.5 hours. While this may not be of concern after a single dose in the operating room, repeated dosing at shorter intervals may lead to potential toxicity in this patient population.[8]

▶ Pharmacokinetics: Elimination

Elimination is the final step in the life of a drug in the human body and refers to processes that remove a drug from the body. Metabolism via biotransformation, as discussed in the section above, with inactivation of the end-product, facilitates elimination. Routes available for excretion and elimination include biliary tract, lungs, and kidneys. Renal elimination plays the largest role in the body's ability to eliminate medications. Drug elimination half-life describes medication removal from the blood and is the time required for half the amount to be removed.[2] Renal clearance is described as the volume of plasma that is cleared of a drug per unit of time through the kidneys.[4] Glomerular filtration, tubular secretion and tubular reabsorption collectively are responsible for renal clearance. If a drug is nonvolatile, water soluble, and has a low molecular weight it will most likely be eliminated by the kidney.

Each of these processes may mature at different times and with a different pattern. Renal function maturation is complete in early childhood. Nephrogenesis is complete after 34 weeks' gestation, which means a premature patient will have difficulty concentrating his or her urine. Any insult to the development of the fetus will affect renal function, for example, growth retardation and nephrotoxic drugs administered to the mother. Similarly, any insult in the postnatal period such as hypoxemia, hypoperfusion, or nephrotoxic drugs will cause renal injury and alter rates of drug elimination for the newborn. Regarding glomerular filtration, this function is not fully developed until 8 to 12 months of age. In a premature infant it can be as low as 0.6 to 0.8 mL/min. Postnatal decrease in renal vascular resistance coupled with an increase in renal blood flow allow for a dramatic increase in GFR within the first 2 weeks of life. Tubular secretion is an active process that is also immature at birth and reaches adult values similarly to the GFR, at 7 to 12 months of age. This activity will alter the course of medications such as antibiotics (penicillins and cephalosporins) which are frequently administered in the operating room. Lastly, tubular reabsorption is a passive process that depends on the characteristics of the drug and fluids present within the proximal and distal tubule.[4] The maturation of this last eliminating process is continual with a peak occurring between 1 and 3 years of age.

Upon conclusion of a review of the principles of pharmacokinetics it should be clear to the reader that when assuming care of a neonate who is either premature or fullterm, the practitioner should bear in mind anatomic and developmental differences that may alter the anesthetic plan. Preoperative assessment should include discussion with the neonatologist and pediatric pharmacist for proper dosing strategies in light of renal and hepatic limitations.

PHARMACODYNAMICS

Pharmacokinetics takes into consideration how the body processes a drug, whereas pharmacodynamics (PD) encompasses what actions that drug has on the human body. It is the relationship between the drug's concentration at the receptor and the response evoked. It is that concentration which is dependent on the pharmacokinetic processes that determine if the result will be therapeutic or toxic. Therefore, the concepts to understand when reviewing pharmacodynamics include receptor binding, post-receptor effects, and chemical interactions.[4] With the interaction between these two systems, proper management of medications for the newborn and premature patient can be established. Unfortunately, pharmacodynamics of neonates is not something that has been well studied to the extent of pharmacokinetics. What has been explained is that the PD response should be different in a neonate due to immature receptors and has been studied with a focus on specific medications. An increased sensitivity and risk for toxicity is the overall outcome associated with a neonate's receptors.[9]

An explanation as to the effect of ontogeny on the drug-response dynamic can be extrapolated by examples from the literature. Mu opioid receptors have been shown to have an increased expression in neonates as compared to adults. This would then place the patient at increased risk of narcotics commonly administered in the pediatric operating room, such as morphine or fentanyl.[10] Similarly, a neonate's dose-response to calcium channel blockers is more profound compared to an adult's response with regard to bradycardia and hypotension. Alternatively, a neonatal heart has reduced calcium stores and their myocardium is sensitive to administration of calcium, causing an enhanced contractility response.[11]

DRUG-SPECIFIC CONSIDERATIONS

This section focuses on commonly administered anesthetics and effects seen in the neonatal population. The first is *inhaled anesthetics* which have effects on several biologic systems including the cardiovascular, respiratory, and central nervous systems. The PD response observed in the neonatal cohort frequently in the operating room is a dose-dependent decrease in mean arterial pressure and systemic vascular resistance due to direct myocardial depression and depression of baroreceptor reflex, respectively. Other attributes are shared with adults, such as an increase in the respiratory rate and reduction in tidal volume and functional residual capacity. Dose-dependent increases in cerebral blood flow is coupled with a decrease in cerebral metabolic oxygen consumption.[12]

Morphine is considered the gold standard of narcotics by which other *opioids* are compared. Concerns arise due to an infant's risk of increased sensitivity, specifically to the respiratory depressant properties, as described in the pharmacodynamics section. From a cardiovascular point of view, there is a wide margin of safety for narcotics when used as an anesthetic though depressant effects are observed when used in combination with other medications such as volatile anesthetics and benzodiazepines. Of additional concern is the prolonged elimination half-life of opioids which is significant in a neonate and compounded by changes in hepatic blood flow.[12] An exception is with remifentanil which when studied was found to have a more rapid clearance with a comparable half-life to adults.[13] The most likely explanation for this phenomenon is remifentanil's degradation by red blood cell and tissue esterases which quickly render it inactive.

Benzodiazepines are used routinely in the perioperative period. Their function is multifold: alleviating preoperative anxiety and providing perioperative amnesia, as an adjunct to a balanced anesthetic, as well as for reduction in pain caused by muscle spasm associated with surgical procedures. Their cardiovascular effects are minimal when used alone. The receptors for this class of medications, gamma-aminobutyric acid (GABA), are located in the cerebral cortex, hypothalamus, cerebellum, corpus striatum, and medulla oblongata. These medications have been safely used in the neonatal population; however, studies have shown a prolonged elimination half-life of diazepam and its active metabolites.[14]

Sedative-hypnotic agents such as ketamine have a long history in anesthesiology providing reliable effects for general anesthesia as well as for sedation. Ketamine is an amnestic and holds analgesic properties but is associated with dysphoria and increased secretions. It is also emetogenic, discouraging practitioners from using it more frequently. Ketamine's cardiopulmonary profile is relatively safe as it does not cause the significant respiratory depression and hypotension as predictably as does propofol. The caveat to this is that its effects on the myocardium are indirect via the central nervous system causing increased sympathetic tone. The result is an increased heart rate, systemic blood pressure, and cardiac output. It is important to remember that ketamine directly stimulates the myocardium with a negative inotropic effect. In the chronically ill patient who cannot mount a sympathetic surge, its direct negative effects on the heart will be revealed. Focusing on the neonates, its half-life is significantly prolonged as compared to older children and adults, thus cautious administration at longer intervals should be considered.[15]

Lastly, added in the armamentarium for anesthesiology, sugammadex is now used at hospitals across the United States for the purpose of rapid reversal of nondepolarizing muscle relaxants such as rocuronium and vecuronium. Its reported use in the neonatal and pediatric population is in its infancy at this point. Sugammadex works as a selective relaxant binding agent and its chemical structure is a ring formation. It forms a complex with aminosteroid muscle relaxants such as rocuronium and vecuronium. By binding these drugs at the neuromuscular junction the amount available for action at the receptor is reduced. Metabolism of sugammadex is limited and it is excreted via the kidneys unchanged. The paralytic–sugammadex complex is eliminated via the urine. This process is rapid with approximately 70% of the dose administered excreted in 6 hours. Due to the dependence on the renal elimination, it should not be used in patients with significantly reduced renal function. One study demonstrating its use in neonates dosed sugammadex at 4 mg/kg ($N = 23$) with residual neuromuscular blockade following surgery. Time to recovery of TOF to 0.9 ranged from 1.2 to 1.4 minutes. Recurarization was not observed in this study.[16] Similar rapid results were reported in a premature infant with residual weakness after a vecuronium infusion. In this infant though, reoccurrence of weakness was seen but was attributed to the infant's chronic illness.[17]

REFERENCES

1. Tofovic S. Developmental pharmacology. In: Davis PJ, Cladis FP, eds. *Smith's Anesthesia for Infants and Children.* Elsevier; 2016:168-175.

2. Blumer J, Reed MD. Principles of neonatal pharmacology. In: Yaffe SJ, Aranda JV, eds. *Neonatal and Pediatric Pharmacology.* Philadelphia, PA: Lippincott Williams & Wilkins; 2011:179.

3. Ward RM, Lugo RA. Drug therapy in the newborn. In: MacDonald MG, Seshia MMK, Mullette MD, eds. *Avery's Neonatology.* 6th ed. Philadelphia, PA: Lippincott Williams & Wilkins; 2005:1508-1557.

4. Tayman C. Neonatal pharmacology: extensive interindividual variability despite limited size. *J Pediatr Pharmacology.* 2011;16(3):170-184.

5. Kahn K, et al. Pharmacology of anaesthetic agents I: intravenous anaesthetic agents. *Br J Anesthes.* 2014;14(3):100-105.

6. Volpe JJ. Bilirubin-induced brain injury. In: Volpe JJ, ed. *Neurology of the Newborn.* 5th ed. Philadelphia, PA: Elsevier Saunders; 2008, pp. 619-649.

7. Christrup LL. Morphine metabolites. *Acta Anaesth Scand.* 1997;41(1 pt 2):116-122.

8. Baker CF. Acetaminophen-induced hepatic failure with encephalopathy in a newborn. *J Perinatol.* 2007;27:133-135.

9. Ku L. Dosing in neonates: special considerations in physiology and trial design. *Pediatr Res.* 2015;77:2-9.

10. Mulla H. Understanding developmental pharmacodynamics: importance for drug development and clinical practice. *Paediatr Drugs.* 2010;12:223-233.

11. Anderson BJ. Pharmacology in the very young: anesthetic implications. *Eur J Anaesth.* 2012;29:261-270.

12. Vitali SH, Camerota AJ, Arnold JH. Anesthesia and analgesia in the neonate. In: MacDonald MG, Seshia MMK, Mullette MD, eds. *Avery's Neonatology.* 6th ed. Philadelphia, PA: Lippincott Williams & Wilkins; 2005:1558-1572.

13. Ross AK. Pharmacokinetics of remifentanil in anesthetized pediatric patients undergoing elective surgery or diagnostic procedures. *Anesth Analg.* 2001;93:1393-1401.

14. Morselli PL. Diazepam elimination in premature and full-term infants, and children. *J Perinat Med.* 1973;1:133-141.

15. Grant IS. Ketamine disposition in children and adults. *Br J Anaesthesiology.* 1983;55:1107-1111.

16. Alonso A. Reversal of rocuronium-induced neuromuscular block by sugammadex in neonates. *Anesthesiology.* 2009;110(2):284-294.

17. Oduro-Dominah L. Sugammadex for the reversal of prolonged neuromuscular blockage in a preterm neonate. Case Report. *Pediatr Anesth Crit Care J.* 2015;3(1):49-52.

Analgesics

James A. Tolley

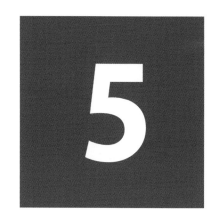

5

One of the primary roles of the anesthesiologist as perioperative physician is to provide adequate analgesia both during and after a painful procedure. It is therefore imperative to have a good working knowledge of the various analgesics that can be used to accomplish this goal. The purpose of this chapter is to provide that working knowledge.

Pharmacology can be divided into two broad areas, pharmacokinetics and pharmacodynamics. Pharmacokinetics (PK) can be thought of as "what a body does to a drug" and includes such topics as drug absorption, distribution, metabolism, and elimination. Pharmacodynamics (PD) can be thought of as "what the drug does to the body" in terms of interacting with a target and eliciting a clinical response, and its potential side effects and toxicities.[1,2] Much more is known about pharmacokinetics in pediatric patients than is known about pharmacodynamics.[3]

The chapter begins with the basic pharmacokinetic differences of the pediatric patient compared to the adult before discussing the pharmacology of acetaminophen and other NSAIDs, multiple opioids used both intraoperatively and postoperatively, and an assortment of other drugs that are used in the perioperative setting for pain modulation and treatment. The pharmacology of local anesthetics is covered in a separate chapter.

MATURATIONAL PHARMACOKINETICS

Pediatric patients, especially neonates and infants, are not simply small adults. There are many rapidly maturing biological systems which can have an influence on the absorption, distribution, metabolism, and elimination of drugs. As a result, drug dosing and dosing schedules, accumulation of active, inactive, and toxic metabolites, and pathways of biotransformation and elimination can differ significantly from older patients. In this rapidly changing environment, it is essential for the pediatric anesthesiologist to understand the basic pharmacokinetic differences that occur during the first weeks and months of life.

Absorption

Since most analgesics utilized by the pediatric anesthesiologist are given via the intravenous route, absorption plays a little role in the pharmacokinetics of those drugs. However, some developmental changes occur which the anesthesiologist should be aware of.

Generally, gastric pH is elevated in the neonate, which can affect drug stability and absorption, and does not reach adult levels until 2 years of age. In addition, neonates have prolonged gastric emptying time which may lead to a slower overall rate of absorption,[4–6] not reaching adult levels until 6 to 8 months of age.[7,8] Intestinal motility is also reduced in the neonate.[7,9] These differences may or may not ultimately impact the bioavailability, maximum concentration (C_{max}), or time to maximum concentration (T_{max}) of a particular drug.

Ontogenetic changes in intestinal enzymes can also affect the overall absorption of various drugs. Drug metabolizing enzymes (DMEs), such as CYP3A4, are located in the small intestine. Its activity is very low at birth but increases to about 50% of adult levels by 6 to 12 months of age, meaning that less intestinal metabolism occurs at younger ages.[7,10] An active drug transporter, P-glycoprotein (P-gp), can be detected in the intestine at 1 month of age, but does possess large interindividual variability.[7,11] Rectal absorption can also be highly variable depending upon the characteristics of the drug and its residence time in the rectum.[7]

Percutaneous absorption of drugs in the neonate and infant is often elevated due to a greater surface area to body mass ratio, greater hydration of the skin, and increased blood flow.[7,12] Furthermore, preterm neonates have enhanced absorption for the first 3 weeks postnatally as the epidermis rapidly matures.[13] Intramuscular absorption of drugs can also be enhanced in younger patients due to the increased capillary density surrounding muscle that occurs at this young age.[14]

Distribution

Once absorbed, a drug is distributed to the various tissues of the body based upon its physicochemical properties and can be described by its volume of distribution (V_d). Body composition and protein binding can have a large impact upon the V_d of a drug. Because a newborn's body weight is composed of a greater percentage of water than an adult, hydrophilic drugs will have a greater apparent V_d requiring a larger initial dose to achieve therapeutic plasma concentrations.[6,7] The total body water content approaches adult levels by 4 months of age.

Neonates and infants also have decreased levels of circulating proteins, such as albumin and alpha-1-acid glycoprotein, that bind drugs in the plasma. The result is a larger apparent V_d as the resulting free fraction of drug distributes throughout the body tissues.[7,15] Circulating levels of plasma proteins reach adult levels by 3 years of age, but the impact upon the free fraction can vary depending on the drug.[16]

Metabolism

The liver serves as the primary organ for biotransformation of drugs into more water-soluble compounds for elimination. Phase I reactions create a more polar compound through reduction, oxidation, or hydrolysis. The cytochrome P450 (CYP) enzymes are primarily responsible for phase I reactions and with the exception of CYP3A7 are not very active at birth. Some, such as CYP2D6, will develop fairly rapidly while others will take several months to reach adult levels.[2,7,17,18]

Phase II reactions involve conjugation of small chemical groups to a drug or to its phase I metabolite. These enzymes will also demonstrate variable expression during different stages of development. Sulfation is fully present at birth, whereas glucuronidation will develop more slowly with some isoenzymes reaching adult levels in the first few years of life and others not reaching adult levels until sometime after age 10.[2,7,19]

The variable expression of metabolizing enzymes at different stages of development can lead to interesting clinical implications when a drug is forced down a particular metabolic pathway. Furthermore, the presence of genetic polymorphisms can have profound effects on the efficacy or toxicity of several analgesics, which will be discussed when reviewing the pharmacology of the individual drugs later in the chapter.

Excretion

The kidney is the primary organ of excretion for the body. The glomerular filtration rate (GFR) is low at birth but rapidly increases, doubling in the first week of life. Adult GFR is reached by the first birthday and will exceed adult values by 20% to 30% until the age of 5, perhaps requiring larger weight-based dosing in this age group.[7,20] In addition to passive filtration of a drug and its metabolites, the kidney may actively secrete these compounds, although little is known about the development of the processes involved. This is an area where additional research is needed.[20]

Acetaminophen (Paracetamol)

Acetaminophen is one of the most widely used analgesics in the world. It is available in oral, rectal, and intravenous forms. When administered via the gastrointestinal tract, it is absorbed by passive nonionic diffusion primarily in the proximal portion of the small intestine.[21] It has an oral bioavailability of approximately 80%,[22] and while some experts suggest a bioavailability of close to 70% when given rectally,[23] there have been reports of great variability including significant differences in male vs female neonatal absorption.[24]

Protein binding of acetaminophen is relatively low (10–25%), leading to a V_d of approximately 1 L/kg.[22] Acetaminophen has no known pharmacologically active metabolites.[22] Its primary means of metabolism is glucuronidation via UGT1A6, with sulfation playing a greater role in the neonate due to the ontogeny of the hepatic enzymes.[22,25] A small amount of acetaminophen is oxidized via CYP2E1 to form N-acetyl-p-benzoquinone imine (NAPQI), the compound responsible for the hepatic toxicity of acetaminophen in the event of an overdose.[1,22,26] Since CYP2E1 activity is reduced in neonates, this group of patients seems to be somewhat resistant to the hepatotoxic effects of acetaminophen as demonstrated by several reports of neonatal overdose without long-term sequelae.[22,27-30]

Acetaminophen and its metabolites are primarily excreted in the urine with acetaminophen sulfate representing approximately 50% of renal clearance in infants.[22,31] Acetaminophen sulfate is highly protein bound (>50%), and in the presence of unconjugated hyperbilirubinemia, clearance is reduced by 40%. It has been recommended to reduce the dose of acetaminophen if this condition exists.[32,33]

The true mechanism of action of acetaminophen is unknown but is postulated to involve centrally mediated cyclooxygenase (COX) inhibition. It seems to have little clinical effect on peripheral inflammation, edema, and platelet aggregation.[34] Acetaminophen crosses the blood-brain barrier via passive diffusion, requiring a sufficient gradient between serum and CSF concentrations.[23] The existence of a central mechanism of action is suggested by a delay of approximately 1 hour between maximal effectiveness and peak plasma concentrations.[35]

The actual serum concentration associated with analgesia is unknown but is presumed to be 10 to 20 mcg/mL[23,35] with some suggestion that an analgesic ceiling effect exists.[36] When equal doses of acetaminophen are utilized, intravenous administration results in greater plasma and CSF concentrations with an earlier peak than either oral or rectal administration.[35]

Acetaminophen has been shown to have an opioid-sparing effect following major noncardiac thoracic or abdominal surgery in neonates and infants less than 1 year of age.[37] It also has been shown to benefit patients following tonsillectomy with or without adenoidectomy[38] and cleft palate repair.[38] The reduction in rescue opiate requirements was approximately 40% to 50%[37,39] when the IV form was used. Conversely, rectal acetaminophen was *not* effective in reducing postoperative narcotic requirements

in young infants up to 2 months of age following major noncardiac thoracic or abdominal surgery,[40] nor was it effective in patients up to 24 months of age in cleft palate repair despite a maximum plasma concentration of 21 mcg/mL in the 40 mg/kg group.[41]

When oral elixir was compared to rectal paracetamol in children undergoing tonsillectomy, the oral form yielded significantly higher plasma concentrations and superior pain relief.[42] In pediatric outpatient surgery, rectal acetaminophen doses of 40 mg/kg were required to produce a morphine-sparing effect.[43] In contrast, for pediatric ophthalmic surgery, even 20 mg/kg was more effective than placebo.[44] Thus, analgesic efficacy may be determined by the proper combination of drug delivery method and case selection.

The current IV acetaminophen product in the United States is approved for mild to moderate pain in patients 2 years of age and older.[45] Dosing recommendations are as noted in Tables 5-1 and 5-2.

Table 5-1. Acetaminophen IV Dosing Based on PMS*

Age	Weight	Dosage	Max
Any	<50 kg	15mg/kg q6h	75 mg/kg/day
PMA 32–34 wks		20 mg/kg load, 10 mg/kg q6h maintenance	
PMA 28–31 wks		20 mg/kg load, 10 mg/kg q12h maintenance	

*Postmenstrual age is defined as gestational age plus chronological age in weeks.[46]

Table 5-2. Acetaminophen Dosing[47]

Administration	Dosage	Max
IV	15mg/kg q6h	75 mg/kg/day
Oral	15mg/kg q4–6h	60 mg/kg/day
Rectal	40 mg/kg load, 20 mg/kg q6h	?

Recommended rectal doses in children aged 2 to 12 years showed large interindividual variability in pharmacokinetics with only 48% of observed plasma concentrations within the target range of 10 to 20 mcg/mL.[48]

Source: Data from de Martino M, Chiarugi A. Recent advances in pediatric use of oral paracetamol in fever and pain management. *Pain Ther.* 2015;4:149-168. https://www.springer.com/journal/40122.

Nonsteroidal Anti-Inflammatory Drugs (NSAIDS)

NSAIDs as a group contain such drugs as acetylsalicylic acid (aspirin), ibuprofen, ketoprofen, naproxen, indomethacin, ketorolac, celecoxib, parecoxib, and others. Many of these drugs are available in oral, rectal, and IV formulations. Rarely will the anesthesiologist be using rectal NSAIDs, so the discussion will be limited to oral and IV preparations. Furthermore, given the association of aspirin with Reye syndrome and the decreased usage in pediatric patients,[49] this drug will not be addressed.

Ibuprofen, ketoprofen, and *naproxen* are propionic acid derivatives and possess several similar pharmacokinetic characteristics but also some unique differences. These drugs are all weak acids with pK_a values of 5.38, 5.94, and 4.15, respectively.[50-52] They all have oral bioavailability approaching 100%, and a rate of absorption that depends upon the precise formulation.[51,53-55] In premature neonates, oral ibuprofen also has excellent bioavailability with drug being detectable in plasma within 1 hour of administration.[56,57] Usage of ketoprofen and naproxen in neonates has not been reported. Cystic fibrosis can significantly impact the oral absorption of ibuprofen resulting in a decrease in peak serum concentration that is almost 30% lower than healthy individuals.[58]

Because these drugs are highly protein bound at 98% to 99%, the V_d approximates plasma volume.[51,53,59] Ibuprofen and ketoprofen are commonly administered as racemic drugs that undergo unidirectional inversion by hepatic enzymes from the inactive (R)-enantiomer to the biologically active (S)-enantiomer, whereas (R)-naproxen is known to be hepatotoxic necessitating the clinical use of the pure (S)-naproxen enantiomer.[60,61]

Ibuprofen is oxidized primarily by CYP2C9, and to a lesser extent CYP2C8, to inactive metabolites.[53,62,63] Genetic polymorphisms for CYP2C9 have been identified, but the clinical impact is unknown.[63] In neonates, the half-life of ibuprofen decreases rapidly from a mean of 43 hours on the third day of life to a mean of 27 hours on the fifth day of life. This is due to the rapidly increasing activity of CYP2C9 and CYP2C8 in the first week of life.[64] Ketoprofen undergoes glucuronidation, although the precise enzymes involved have not been completely elucidated.[63,65] About 60% of a dose of naproxen is metabolized by glucuronidation; oxidation via CYP2C8 and CYP1A2 also occurs.[63] These drugs and their metabolites are primarily excreted in the urine.[51,53,66]

The mechanism of action for NSAIDs, which explains their anti-inflammatory and analgesic properties, is the ability to block the production of prostaglandin via inhibition of the COX-1 and COX-2 enzymes. COX-1 is present in nearly all human tissues, while COX-2 is primarily found in the renal and central nervous systems (CNS).[67] COX-2 is also expressed in injured tissues[67] but may also play a significant role in the organogenesis of the small intestine, lungs, and kidneys.[68]

The serum level of ibuprofen that is required for analgesia is 5 to 10 mcg/mL.[69] Intravenous ibuprofen (10 mg/kg) given preoperatively to children undergoing tonsillectomy had a significant opioid sparing effect compared to placebo with no increase in serious adverse events, including surgical and postoperative blood loss.[70] A meta-analysis that looked at 18 studies of pediatric pain comparing ibuprofen and acetaminophen found that ibuprofen was at least as effective as, if not superior to, acetaminophen with no significant difference in adverse events.[71]

In neonates, ibuprofen is most often utilized as an alternative to indomethacin for closure of a patent ductus arteriosus (PDA). An intravenous dose of 10 mg/kg followed by two additional doses of 5 mg/kg every 24 hours is just one of the many dosing regimens. Alternatively, 10 mg/kg orally every 24 hours for 3 days can also be used.[67] Adverse side effects associated with ibuprofen in neonates include the rare possibility of severe nephrotoxicity and acute renal failure, pulmonary hypertension,[72] and intestinal perforation.[73]

Ketoprofen has also been studied in the perioperative setting. Intravenous doses of 1 to 2 mg/kg have been used effectively in tonsillectomy and adenoidectomy, ocular surgery, and orthopedic or soft tissue surgery. For major noncardiac surgeries, a loading dose of 1 mg/kg followed by a 4 mg/kg infusion over a 24-hour period for 1 to 3 days postoperatively provided superior analgesia compared to placebo as an adjunct to epidural sufentanil.[74]

Intravenous naproxen is not commercially available, so perioperative usage is limited in its scope.

Indomethacin and *ketorolac* are both acetic acid derivatives and like the other NSAIDs are weak acids that have an oral bioavailability of nearly 100% with peak plasma concentrations occurring approximately 1 to 1.5 hours after an oral dose.[75,76] Even in premature neonates as young as 27 weeks' gestation and 1 kg, the bioavailability of oral indomethacin is over 98%.[77] Oral ketorolac usage in neonates has not been reported. Both drugs are highly protein bound with indomethacin being at least 90% bound,[75,78] and ketorolac even more so at greater than 99%[76] resulting in a small V_d. Indomethacin is metabolized in the liver by CYP2C9 and UGT2B7.[78] The metabolites of indomethacin are inactive and excreted in the urine. About one-third are also excreted in feces.[75] Not surprisingly, in premature neonates there is a greater interindividual variability in both V_d and clearance due to the immaturity of the hepatic and renal systems.[78] These values reach adult levels by 1 year of age.[79]

The majority of ketorolac is excreted unchanged in the urine with the remainder undergoing various degrees of glucuronidation and hydroxylation in the liver.[80] There are enantiomeric differences that exist with ketorolac. The (S)-enantiomer is active, but there is no chiral inversion from (R)-ketorolac to (S)-ketorolac in the body. Furthermore, the clearance of (S)-ketorolac is four to five times higher leading to a half-life that is about 30% to 40% that of (*R*)-ketorolac. The half-life of (*S*)-ketorolac is about 1 hour in infants and 1.5 hours in children, as infants demonstrated a greater plasma clearance.[80,81]

Indomethacin is a nonselective inhibitor of COX-1 and COX-2. It is currently the drug of choice for prophylactic treatment of PDA in premature neonates due to lower incidence of pulmonary hemorrhage and severe intraventricular hemorrhage versus ibuprofen, which is the drug of choice for symptomatic treatment because of a decreased association with necrotizing enterocolitis and renal effects.[82] Indomethacin is unique among NSAIDs in that it is a known vasoconstrictor and decreases cerebral blood flow.[75] It has not, however, been extensively used in the perioperative period as ketorolac.

Ketorolac is also a nonselective inhibitor of COX-1 and COX-2. Because of its effectiveness in mitigating postoperative pain, it has been investigated following a wide range of surgical procedures and is available for use in oral, IV, IM, rectal, and intranasal formulations. In pediatric patients, ketorolac has been shown to be as effective as morphine for procedures causing moderate to severe pain, such as tonsillectomy, orthopedic surgery, or plastic surgery. In addition, patients had less postoperative nausea and vomiting.[83] Ketorolac infusion compared favorably to fentanyl infusion in patients undergoing ureteroneocystostomy, resulting in less rescue analgesia and frequency of bladder spasms.[84] Ketorolac has been used safely in neonates and infants following cardiac surgery without adverse hematologic or renal sequelae.[85]

The main concerns regarding side effects of ketorolac relate to the role that prostaglandins play in body homeostasis. Prostaglandins play a vital role in renal vascular tone and inhibition of COX-2 by NSAIDs leading to decreased renal blood flow and glomerular filtration rate.[86] The risk of acute renal failure was found to double in patients receiving more than 5 days of therapy.[87]

Prostaglandins are important in regulation of osteoclastic and osteoblastic activity, so concern has been raised regarding the use of NSAIDs during bone healing;[88] however, a retrospective review of 327 children undergoing 682 lower extremity osteotomies showed no difference in delayed union, wound complications, or bleeding in patients receiving ketorolac versus those that did not.[89] Nor was there any difference in pseudoarthrosis formation following posterior spinal fusion for idiopathic scoliosis in adolescents between those that received ketorolac postoperatively and those that did not.[90]

Ketorolac has been shown to increase bleeding time in healthy volunteers.[91] A meta-analysis revealed that its use in tonsillectomy patients led to a fivefold increased bleeding risk in adults, but not in children under 18.[92] The precise explanation for this difference is unclear. A retrospective review of 1451 pediatric neurosurgical patients did not show any association between clinically significant bleeding events and ketorolac use.[93] Thus, it would appear that short-term perioperative usage of ketorolac for pain management is acceptable in most pediatric patients for the majority of surgical procedures.

COX-2 selective inhibitors, such as **celecoxib** and *parecoxib*, were developed with the hope of minimizing the gastrointestinal and renal side effects associated with nonselective inhibition since COX-2 is preferentially induced during inflammation. Unfortunately, these drugs have shown an increased risk of thrombotic events such as myocardial infarction, stroke, and unexplained death, leading to withdrawal of some of them from the market.[94] Celecoxib is only available in oral form and parecoxib is not currently approved in the United States.

Opioids

As experts in analgesia, anesthesiologists are expected to be especially knowledgeable about opioids since this class of drugs is typically on the top of the list when it comes to pain medications due to their long history of use and effectiveness at managing pain. Anesthesiologists should also be keenly aware of the adverse effects, including the potential for addiction. Opioids can be classified into those that occur naturally, those that are semi-synthetic, and the synthetic opioids.[95] Morphine and codeine are the naturally occurring opioids that have therapeutic uses. Codeine is a prodrug that is converted to morphine for its analgesic effects,[96] so these drugs will be discussed together.

Both **codeine** and **morphine** are commonly used in oral and injectable formulations. Oral absorption is extensive with both drugs, but due to first-pass hepatic metabolism, the bioavailability is 60% to 70% for codeine and only about 24% to 40% for morphine, and somewhat variable.[97–99] The drug transporter, P-glycoprotein, may also help limit the bioavailability of morphine by pumping drug back into the intestinal lumen.[100]

Codeine is about 30% bound to plasma proteins, although it has been found to be about twice that value in patients with sickle cell anemia. This can be partially explained by the increased levels of gamma-globulin in the plasma of sickle cell patients.[101] Morphine binding ranges from 20% to 40%, and it has a V_d of 2.1 to 4.0 L/kg.[98]

In order to manifest its analgesic effects, codeine is metabolized in the liver by CYP2D6 to the active metabolite, morphine.[102] Over 100 different alleles of CYP2D6 have been identified. This degree of polymorphism has led to a great deal of interindividual variation in the ability to metabolize codeine into morphine. Patients have been separated into several phenotypes as a result. Poor metabolizers (PM) possess 2 of 15 possible inactive genes. Intermediate metabolizers (IM) have two copies of reduced activity genes or one reduced and one inactive gene. Extensive metabolizers (EM) have one or both copies of genes encoding for normal enzymatic activity, while ultra-rapid metabolizers (UM) have more than two copies of the wild-type allele because of gene duplication.[103]

These differences can have profound clinical implications ranging from little analgesic effect of codeine in PM to morphine overdose in UM due to a 30-fold or greater plasma concentration difference in morphine between the two extremes.[104] Pharmacokinetic modeling suggests that 10% of a codeine dose is converted to morphine in PM, compared to 40% in EM, and 51% in UM[105] with the remainder metabolized to norcodeine via CYP3A4 or via conjugation to codeine-6-glucuronide, which itself has analgesic activity.[106,107] These compounds are then excreted in the urine.[104]

Numerous deaths in children following adenotonsillectomy have prompted the reevaluation of using codeine in the pediatric population.[108,109] A review from 1984 to 2010 found 17 post-tonsillectomy deaths related to opioid toxicity.[110] These complications of codeine usage led the United States Food and Drug Administration (US FDA) to issue a warning contraindicating codeine use for pain or cough in children younger than 12 years in April 2017.[111] Furthermore, the report of a death in a breastfed infant whose mother was taking codeine for postpartum pain[112] has led to an additional warning.[111]

Morphine is likewise metabolized in the liver with the primary pathway being glucuronidation into morphine-3-glucuronide (45–55%) and morphine-6-glucuronide (10–15%), which are then excreted in the urine.[98] The primary enzyme responsible for these reactions is UGT2B7, although other isoforms may contribute to the formation of morphine-3-glucuronide (M3G).[113] Genetic polymorphisms of UGT2B7 are also being discovered, although the clinical significance is unclear at this time with one study showing no ability to predict postoperative morphine requirements[114] and another showing a significant difference in postoperative morphine requirements.[115] A small pilot study in preterm neonates showed that one of the UGT2B7 polymorphisms significantly influenced the pharmacokinetics of morphine metabolism in addition to postnatal age.[116]

As a metabolite, M3G is devoid of analgesic activity and is a mild opioid antagonist. On the other hand, morphine-6-glucuronide (M6G) is an opioid agonist more potent than the parent compound.[98,117] Thus, the ratio of M3G to M6G may be an important factor in a particular patient's response to morphine analgesia.

In general, opioids produce their therapeutic and adverse effects through binding with three main types of opioid receptors (mu, delta, and kappa) which are located in the central and peripheral nervous systems and in the neuroendocrine, gastrointestinal, and immune systems. Opioid receptors are G protein–coupled receptors that, when activated, ultimately influence the transmembrane gradients of calcium, sodium, and potassium ions or influence the release of neuropeptide transmitters such that the transmission of painful impulses is reduced.[118] The complete intracellular mechanism is beyond the scope of this chapter, but two excellent reviews on opioid receptors[118] and the molecular mechanism[119] of the pain pathway have been published.

All three opioid receptors play a role in analgesia both centrally and in the periphery but differ as to their adverse effects. The most serious adverse effect, respiratory depression, is mediated by centrally acting mu-receptors. These receptors are also responsible for the euphoria that is associated with opioid use, while central kappa-receptors are associated with dysphoria. Both mu- and delta-receptors contribute to constipation.[118] Neonates are especially sensitive to the central depressant effects of opioids partially due to the decreased levels of P-gp, which functions as an active drug transporter, present in the blood-brain barrier. Adult levels of P-gp are not reached until 3 to 6 months of age.[120]

The presence of polymorphisms at the mu-receptor may play a role not only in the analgesic efficacy of morphine but also in the development of adverse effects. The OPRM1 gene codes for the mu-receptor and a single nucleotide polymorphism exist at base pair 118 in which adenine is substituted with guanine such that patients homozygous for 118GG have been found to have increased postoperative morphine requirements by several multiples.[117,121,122] A more recent study in adolescents undergoing spinal fusion demonstrated higher pain scores in patients with the presence of the G allele suggesting decreased sensitivity to morphine with less respiratory depression.[123] The G allele may also offer protection from other opioid-related side effects including pruritus from epidural morphine.[124]

Despite the potential for adverse effects in neonates, opioids have become an integral part of pain management in this population both in the perioperative period as well as in the neonatal intensive care unit based on a landmark study which showed a decreased sympathetic response and decreased mortality in neonates undergoing cardiac surgery.[125] Subsequently, morphine was shown to reduce circulating norepinephrine[126] and adrenaline[127] levels in ventilated preterm neonates leading to the inclusion of opioids, especially morphine and fentanyl, as part of the latest recommendations for managing procedural pain in the neonate.[128] However, information concerning the long-term effects is conflicting: one study has shown a negative impact on a short-term memory task and more social problems compared to placebo,[129] while another study has shown that morphine may even have beneficial effect on executive functions at 8 to 9 year follow-up.[130]

Morphine is available in oral, rectal, and injectable preparations and serves as the gold standard in perioperative pain management against which other analgesic compounds and techniques are measured. When given intravenously, morphine has been shown to be superior to placebo at reducing postoperative pain in children as well as reducing the need for rescue analgesia, albeit with a significantly higher incidence of nausea, vomiting, and sedation.[131] Epidural and intrathecal morphine has also been shown to be more effective at relieving pain than no intervention but with significantly more nausea, vomiting, pruritus, and respiratory depression when used epidurally.[131] Intraarticular morphine has also been shown to be more effective than placebo following arthroscopic knee surgery,[132] although little pediatric data exists.

Hydrocodone, oxycodone, and *hydromorphone* are semisynthetic opioids derived from naturally occurring opiates.[95] The first two drugs are mainly used for acute, postoperative, or chronic pain as there is no currently available injectable product in the United States, unlike hydromorphone. The oral bioavailability of hydrocodone has not been well studied in humans but is estimated to be between 38% and 60% but with interindividual variability.[133,134] Oxycodone has a bioavailability ranging from 60% to 87% due to less first-pass metabolism compared to some of the other opioids.[135]

Volume of distribution estimates for hydrocodone would suggest lower levels of plasma protein binding[133] when compared to oxycodone, which is 45% bound to albumin and has a V_d of approximately 2.5 L/kg.[135] Hydromorphone shows a similar V_d to that of oxycodone at roughly 2 to 3 L/kg, suggesting a similar degree of serum protein binding.[136,137]

Hydrocodone is metabolized in the liver primarily by *N*-demethylation via the enzyme CYP3A4 to norhydrocodone which is a less potent, active metabolite when compared to the parent drug,[138,139] but which may also accumulate during chronic administration due to its longer half-life.[139] Norhydrocodone has been shown to have central neuroexcitatory effects.[139] Hydrocodone is also metabolized via CYP2D6 to hydromorphone, which has a much stronger affinity for the opioid receptor than the parent compound. Due to the polymorphisms of CYP2D6, it has been suggested that the probability of hydrocodone acting as a pro-drug is 44% in the UM phenotype, 22% in EM, and 5% in PM.[140] The relative contribution of each metabolic pathway depends upon an individual's phenotype.[141,142]

Oxycodone is also metabolized in the liver via the two major pathways mentioned above with the major metabolite being the weakly active noroxycodone formed by CYP3A4. Oxymorphone is an active metabolite produced by *O*-demethylation via CYP2D6[135,143] which again raises the issue of the clinical impact of genetic polymorphisms.[141,144,145]

Hydromorphone is structurally like morphine and undergoes conjugation in the liver to hydromorphone-3-glucuronide via UGT2B7.[135,146] It also undergoes reduction reactions which serve as minor pathways yielding small amounts of active metabolites that may only become clinically important in renal failure.[136] The metabolites of all three of these drugs are excreted in the urine.[135,136,138]

In the United States, hydrocodone and oxycodone are only available in oral formulations so usage is limited to acute medical or postsurgical pain or chronic pain with hydrocodone being the most commonly prescribed opioid for pediatric emergency department patients in the decade ending in 2010.[147] Hydrocodone in combination with acetaminophen was prescribed to over 2% of pediatric hospitalized patients in 2008.[148] In a recent review of over 34,000 outpatient opioid prescriptions, the majority (73%) were for oxycodone.[149] Concerns have been raised about the risk of opioid-related deaths in pediatric patients given the role of CYP2D6 in the metabolism of both hydrocodone and oxycodone and whether patients would benefit from preoperative genotyping.[150]

Given hydromorphone's structural similarity to morphine, it should not be surprising that it would also be available in rectal, oral, and injectable formulations and used in a similar manner clinically to morphine. In pediatric patients, hydromorphone has been used as a continuous infusion in mechanically ventilated infants and children.[151] It has been used as an epidural infusion alone[152] or in combination with bupivacaine for posterior spinal fusion.[153] When compared to epidural morphine and fentanyl, epidural hydromorphone showed fewer side effects and similar analgesia for pediatric patients undergoing orthopedic procedures.[154]

Fentanyl is a synthetic opioid available in many types of formulations. It is highly lipid soluble, and, although not commonly ingested, has an oral bioavailability of about 30% due to a high degree of first-pass metabolism in the liver.[155] Oral transmucosal fentanyl has a bioavailability of approximately 50% and buccal tablets are higher at 65%.[156] Intranasal fentanyl, with a bioavailability of 89%, may even be able to enter the cerebrospinal fluid directly through the olfactory mucosa without having to cross the blood-brain barrier.[157] Finally, transdermal fentanyl has the highest bioavailability at 92%,[158] although there is some individual variation in all of these values.

Fentanyl is about 80% to 85% protein bound, primarily to albumin,[159] and has a V_d of approximately 1 to 4 L/kg.[155] It is metabolized in the liver by *N*-dealkylation to the inactive metabolite, norfentanyl, via the phase I enzyme CYP3A4 with additional contributions from CYP3A5 and CYP3A7.[155] This means that fentanyl seems less likely to be impacted by polymorphisms of the cytochrome P450 system; however, polymorphisms in CYP3A5 have led to increased serum concentrations of fentanyl[160] and alterations in the *ABCB1* gene encoding for P-gp can result in more CNS adverse effects in individuals with decreased function of P-gp.[155,161] Ultimately, the metabolic products of fentanyl are excreted in the urine.[155]

As a mu-receptor agonist, fentanyl is about 100 times more potent than morphine despite similar binding affinity in vitro. This is felt to be due to the lipophilicity of fentanyl and its ability to easily cross the blood-brain barrier.[162] Fentanyl's lipophilicity and ability to cross biologic membranes have permitted numerous formulations and applications for sedation and acute and chronic pain.

Fentanyl is one of the 10 most commonly used drugs in the NICU worldwide.[163] When used in combination with propofol for lumbar puncture in children with acute leukemia, it is associated with fewer adverse events and more rapid recovery than when propofol is used alone.[164] Fentanyl has been nebulized along with lidocaine as premedication for bronchoscopy in pediatric patients and was found to result in more stable hemodynamics and fewer intraprocedural respiratory difficulties, albeit with prolonged time to emerge compared to lidocaine alone or placebo.[165] Oral fentanyl has been suggested as a safe alternative to preoperative oral midazolam in children,[166] whereas oral *transmucosal* fentanyl caused mild pruritus, sedation, and preoperative emesis with no benefit in terms of separation,[167] although the episodes of emesis may have been a result of the amount of time between premedication and induction of anesthesia.[168]

In terms of pediatric pain management, fentanyl has found extensive applications from minor procedures to cardiac surgery and acute to chronic pain. Intranasal fentanyl has been shown to be more effective than placebo following bilateral myringotomy tube placement without an increase in adverse effects.[169] In the emergency department, it is effective in reducing pain from traumatic fracture within 10 minutes of administration allowing for more rapid analgesia despite lack of intravenous access.[170] At 25 mcg/kg intravenously, fentanyl is effective at reducing the stress response of open-heart surgery in infants and children.[171]

Transdermal fentanyl has been used to manage the pain of acute sickle cell crisis[172] and oral mucositis in pediatric patients undergoing stem cell transplant.[173] It has also been used as a convenient and well-tolerated alternative to oral morphine in patients with severe chronic pain from both malignant and nonmalignant diseases.[174,175]

One of the most concerning adverse effects of opioids is muscle rigidity, especially of the chest and respiratory muscles. There have been several reports of this phenomenon occurring in infants and children,[176] including an unusual report that occurred intraoperatively during maintenance of general anesthesia.[177] It has also been reported in neonates at delivery following administration to the mother during cesarean section[178] and in a parturient requiring mechanical ventilation.[179] These varied episodes may resolve in a self-limited fashion or require supportive treatment with muscle relaxation and intubation or antagonism with naloxone.[176–179] Rarely, epinephrine has been required to treat severe bradycardia or asystole.[176]

Both *alfentanil* and *sufentanil* are synthetic derivatives of fentanyl[180] and are not commonly ingested, although alfentanil has been used orally in research as a probe for CYP3A activity[181] with a suggested oral bioavailability of 20% to 30% due to a combination of hepatic first-pass metabolism and intestinal activity of CYP3A4.[182] Nasal alfentanil has a reported average bioavailability of 65%.[183] These values compare to an oral bioavailability for sufentanil of 9%[184] and nasal bioavailability of 78%.[185] Sublingual and buccal bioavailability rates of sufentanil have also been investigated and found to be 59% and 78%, respectively.[184]

Alfentanil is bound to alpha-1-acid glycoprotein at a rate of approximately 92% leading to a smaller V_d than fentanyl.[186] Sufentanil is also highly protein bound with ranges of 88% to 92% in adults.[187,188] This value was more strongly correlated with alpha-1-acid glycoprotein levels across age groups likely explaining the observed protein binding in neonates of only 80%.[188] The V_d for sufentanil in pediatric patients has been reported to range from 1.3 to 4.1 L/kg.[189]

Alfentanil is metabolized in the liver via N-dealkylation at two different locations in its structure to form the inactive metabolites, noralfentanil and N-phenylpropionamide. These reactions are mediated by CYP3A4; however, there is considerable structural similarity between CYP3A4 and CYP3A5 such that CYP3A5 has been shown to be as active in alfentanil metabolism[190] leading to suggestions that the polymorphisms seen in CYP3A5 may help explain the interindividual variability in alfentanil clearance. However, when this question was examined, no difference in pharmacokinetic parameters based upon genotype was found[181] to the surprise of investigators.

Sufentanil is also metabolized into inactive metabolites primarily by CYP3A4, although the involvement of other cytochrome enzymes may be a possibility.[191] The metabolic byproducts of both drugs are excreted in the urine.[192,193]

Alfentanil is four times less potent than fentanyl but has a more rapid onset and shorter duration of action which is likely due to the fact that it is less ionized than fentanyl at physiologic pH.[180] These characteristics would suggest that it might have a role in procedures where rapid awakening would be beneficial. In cardiac bypass surgery, alfentanil allowed earlier tracheal extubation than fentanyl or sufentanil.[194] Alfentanil has been shown to be an effective sedative alone or in combination with midazolam for bone marrow aspiration in children.[195] When combined with propofol, alfentanil led to a greater incidence of respiratory depression compared to propofol and ketamine combined.[196]

Alfentanil has also been found to be effective in decreasing the pain upon injection of propofol,[197] reducing the movement associated with injection of rocuronium,[198,199] and decreasing the incidence of emergence agitation following sevoflurane anesthesia in children.[200] Its use in neonates without concomitant use of muscle relaxants is not recommended due to the high incidence of muscle rigidity impacting ventilation in this population.[201,202]

Sufentanil is 5 to 10 times more potent than fentanyl.[189] It has been used in pediatric cardiac surgery and is comparable to fentanyl in terms of hemodynamic effects[203] but should not be used as the sole anesthetic agent as a one-time bolus.[204] Sufentanil has been used intranasally alone[189] and in combination with ketamine[205] for premedication and for painful procedures in children. When added to caudal levobupivacaine, it is more effective in reducing the hemodynamic response to spermatic cord traction in orchidopexy than levobupivacaine alone,[206] and epidural sufentanil provides better postoperative analgesia after 24 hours than epidural fentanyl in pediatric urologic surgery.[207] When epidural ropivacaine and sufentanil infusion are used in infants, the plasma concentration of sufentanil increases throughout the duration of the infusion and continues to increase after the infusion is stopped, necessitating continued monitoring of vital signs for several hours following its cessation.[208]

Remifentanil is another synthetic opioid that has some unique properties. It is only available in injectable form and so does not possess a defined bioavailability, and although there has been one study utilizing nasal remifentanil to facilitate intubation in pediatric patients, the nasal bioavailability was not reported.[209] In that study, peak plasma concentrations were found to occur at 3 minutes and 47 seconds. Remifentanil is 92% protein bound, primarily to alpha-1-acid glycoprotein[210,211] and has a V_d that ranges from approximately 450 mL/kg in neonates to approximately 250 mL/kg in older children and adolescents.[212]

The main factor that contributes to remifentanil's uniqueness among opioids is its chemical structure which contains an ester linkage allowing it to be metabolized by non-specific blood and tissue esterases.[213] Its metabolism is not impacted by pseudocholinesterase deficiency.[214] Over 80% of remifentanil undergoes ester hydrolysis to remifentanil acid (RA) which is excreted in the urine.[213,215] RA has been determined to be 4600 times less potent in dogs than the parent compound[216] and does not appear to alter the clinical effect of remifentanil infusion of up to 72 hours duration in patients with severe renal impairment.[215] Likewise, the pharmacokinetics of remifentanil and RA are not impacted in patients with severe hepatic impairment awaiting liver transplantation.[211]

Clinically, remifentanil has found broad application in pediatric anesthesia both in neonates and older children and adolescents. It has been used as an infusion for sedation in preterm neonates intubated for respiratory distress syndrome allowing for more rapid awakening and extubation compared to morphine infusion[217] or for laser surgery in neonates with retinopathy of prematurity.[218] It has also been used effectively for neurosurgical, thoracic, cardiovascular, and intraabdominal surgeries in neonates as well as to mitigate the stress response of endotracheal intubation in this population.[218] The simple fact that remifentanil possesses similar pharmacokinetics with rapid, non-organ dependent metabolism and a non-active metabolite across the age spectrum has allowed for its diversity of clinical uses.

Complicating the use of remifentanil in the perioperative period is the concern for the development of acute tolerance or opioid-induced hyperalgesia. While the exact mechanisms are unknown, these phenomena appear to be dose-related and may contribute to the development of persistent postsurgical pain.[219,220] Furthermore, concerns regarding tolerance and hyperalgesia may not be limited solely to remifentanil as demonstrated by a retrospective review comparing remifentanil and fentanyl for pediatric scoliosis surgery in which the fentanyl group had significantly higher pain scores and opioid usage in the immediate postoperative period.[221]

Meperidine, also known as pethidine, was the first synthetic opioid developed in 1939 as an anticholinergic[222,223] but was soon found to possess analgesic properties becoming widely used for pain for many years. It is available in oral and injectable forms, possessing an oral bioavailability of approximately 50% to 60%[224,225] which increases to 70% to 80% when given rectally[224] or in the presence of cirrhosis[225] due to the high first-pass metabolism. Meperidine is about 65% to 75% protein bound and has a volume of distribution of about 3.5 L/kg.[226]

Meperidine undergoes two main routes of metabolism in the liver. The primary route is via hydrolysis to meperidinic acid, an inactive metabolite.[223,226] It also undergoes N-demethylation to normeperidine, a reaction catalyzed by CYP2B6, CYP3A4, and CYP2C19.[222] Normeperidine is an active metabolite that possesses about half the analgesic effect of the parent drug but also has central excitatory and neurotoxic effects that can lead to anxiety, hyperreflexia, myoclonus, and seizures[223] as it accumulates due to its half-life being about seven times that of meperidine.[222] These metabolites are then excreted in the urine.[226]

Historically, meperidine was felt to cause fewer effects on smooth muscle, specifically the sphincter of Oddi, leading to its widespread use for pain associated with biliary colic and pancreatitis. Compared to other opioids at equianalgesic doses, this supposition has not proven to be true.[223] Meperidine has also been used extensively in sickle cell patients, for the treatment of migraines, and for rigors and shivering associated with certain drugs or following anesthesia; however, suitable and safer alternatives exist for all of these indications.[227]

Because of the ready availability of safer, more effective alternatives and the presence of serious neurotoxic effects of meperidine use, pediatric hospitals have begun to restrict its use,[228] and meperidine can no longer be recommended for use in the treatment of acute or chronic pain in pediatric patients.[229]

Methadone is a synthetic opioid with complex pharmacokinetics that shows a high degree of variability between individuals and within an individual over time. It is a chiral molecule administered as a racemic mixture with (R)-methadone being the active enantiomer.[230] It is available in oral and injectable formulations and has also been administered rectally, nasally, intramuscularly, subcutaneously, and epidurally.[230-232] An excellent review lists an oral bioavailability of 70% to 80% with a range in the literature of 36% to 100%,[230] while two studies comparing methods of administration found oral bioavailability of 85% to 86% with a rectal bioavailability of 76%[231] and a nasal bioavailability of 86%.[232] Methadone is highly bound to plasma proteins, primarily alpha-1-acid glycoprotein (AAG), at 87% with a V_d of 4.0 L/kg.[230]

Methadone is metabolized in the liver into two main inactive metabolites which are excreted in the urine. It undergoes N-demethylation to 2-ethylidene-1,5-dimethyl-3,3-diphenylpyrrolidine (EDDP) and is also metabolized to 2-ethyl-5-methyl-3,3-diphenyl-1-pyrroline (EMDP) by enzymes of the cytochrome P450 system.[230] There is some debate in the literature as to the role that each isoenzyme plays in the metabolism of methadone, but there are suggestions that CYP3A4, CYP3A7, CYP2B6, CYP2C9, CYP2C19, CYP2D6, and CYP2D8 may be involved[230,233–235] leading to enantiomeric differences in metabolism. Furthermore, polymorphisms of the various cytochromes can add to the pharmacokinetic complexity of methadone.[236]

(R)-methadone is the enantiomer responsible for the typical opioid effects by acting on the mu-opioid receptor[236] with (S)-methadone being implicated in prolongation of the QT interval and the risk of sudden death from torsade de pointes.[237] Methadone also acts as a non-competitive antagonist of the N-methyl-D-aspartate (NMDA) receptor, much like ketamine, and may have a role in the management of chronic neuropathic pain and opioid-induced hyperalgesia.[238–241]

In pediatric patients, methadone serves as first-line treatment for neonatal abstinence syndrome which results from in utero exposure to opioids.[242] When compared to morphine, methadone has been found to result in lower pain scores and reduced supplemental opioid requirements for 36 hours following major surgery in 3- to 7-year-old children without adverse events.[243] It has been studied in adolescents undergoing posterior spinal fusion for scoliosis, but a single intraoperative dose was rapidly redistributed and did not maintain a therapeutic serum concentration into the postoperative period,[244] nor did it result in lower postoperative pain scores or lower opioid consumption.[245] However, when a single dose of methadone was added to a multimodal analgesia regimen for the Nuss procedure, it was found to be superior with lower postoperative opioid consumption and shorter length of stay compared to all other regimens including general anesthesia with epidural analgesia.[246] Methadone is also used in pediatric patients with malignant pain.[247]

Tramadol is a synthetic analogue of codeine that has two chiral centers and is available as a racemic mixture for oral, injectable, and rectal use.[248,249] Oral bioavailability has been reported at 65% to 70% due to first-pass metabolism.[249] Rectal bioavailability is reported at 77%.[250] Tramadol shows little protein binding at 20%[251] and has a V_d of 3.4 to 3.8 L/kg in pediatric patients.[252]

Tramadol can be considered a prodrug since one of its primary metabolites, (+)-O-desmethyltramadol (M1), is the major contributor to tramadol's pharmacologic mu-agonist effect. This reaction is catalyzed by CYP2D6[253] which, like codeine, is affected by the abundance of polymorphisms that exist impacting side-effect profile.

M1 is ultimately inactivated by glucuronidation via UGT2B7.[253] CYP2B6 and CYP3A4 form inactive metabolites through N-demethylation,[251] all of which are excreted in the urine. Tramadol has also been shown to inhibit serotonin and norepinephrine reuptake, possibly contributing to its analgesic effect.[249]

In pediatric patients, tramadol has been evaluated in multiple perioperative settings including neurosurgery, major abdominal surgery, and adenotonsillectomy.[254] It has been used as an adjunct in epidural blocks[255,256] for postoperative analgesia. Other applications have been peritonsillar infiltration for adenotonsillectomy,[257] prevention of pain from propofol injection,[258] sublingual usage for orthopedic trauma,[259] as well as an infusion for the treatment of sickle cell crisis.[260] It had been suggested that tramadol might fill the void in treating moderate pain that was created when codeine usage became restricted, but the experts rightly pointed out the similar pharmacokinetics between the two drugs and urged caution.[261] This caution was well founded in April 2017, the US FDA added a contraindication to the drug labels of codeine and tramadol stating that these two drugs should not be used for treating pain in children younger than 12 years of age and that tramadol should not be used to treat pain following adenotonsillectomy in any patient younger than 18.[111]

Butorphanol is a synthetic analogue of morphine that has mixed agonist-antagonist activity at the mu-receptor and agonist activity at the kappa-opioid receptor.[262] It undergoes extensive first-pass hepatic metabolism resulting in an oral bioavailability of 5% to 17%,[263] which increases to 70% when given transnasally. The serum protein binding is about 80%.[264] The V_d ranges from 466 to 637 L in adult humans.[265] Butorphanol is metabolized into the inactive hydroxybutorphanol and norbutorphanol, which are then conjugated with glucuronide along with the parent drug prior to excretion in the urine.[266]

One of the potential benefits of butorphanol for use in moderate pain is the lack of dose-related respiratory depression.[266] Due to its effects on the kappa-receptor, sedation is also a prominent pharmacodynamic response.[262] In pediatric patients, butorphanol has compared favorably with midazolam for preoperative sedative effect with more sedation at the time of induction with less need for intraoperative and postoperative rescue analgesia.[267] It has been used intranasally for postoperative pain associated with myringotomy tube placement.[268,269] Butorphanol has been used as an adjunct in caudal analgesia and was found to prolong the duration of caudal bupivacaine[270] by almost 6 hours without an increase in side effects.[271] It has also been added to epidural morphine infusion to relieve pruritus.[272]

Ketamine

Ketamine is a derivative of phencyclidine, commonly known as PCP. It is a chiral molecule and is often utilized as a racemic mixture[273] that can be given orally, rectally, intranasally, and injected intravenously, intramuscularly, and into the epidural space. S(+) ketamine has four times the analgesic potency, but a shorter duration of action than the R(−) isomer.[273]

Due to extensive first-pass hepatic metabolism, oral and rectal bioavailability are only 17–20% and 25%, respectively.[273,274] Bioavailability by the nasal route is 50%, whereas IM administration results in a high bioavailability of 93%.[274] There is a range of values (10–60%) reported for protein binding of ketamine depending upon the patient group studied. Since ketamine has a much greater affinity for AAG, which is increased under physiologically stressful conditions, this may explain the disparity of results.[275] The V_d of ketamine is 2.3 L/kg.[274]

In the liver, most ketamine undergoes N-demethylation to norketamine, which has about 20% to 30% of the analgesic activity of the parent compound.[274] There is some disagreement in the literature as to whether this occurs primarily via CYP2B6, CYP3A4, or one of the other isoenzymes;[273] however, a recent study found no changes in single-dose ketamine pharmacokinetics associated with CYP2B6 polymorphisms,[276] which would suggest the potential involvement of several enzymes for its metabolism. A small amount of ketamine is hydroxylated in other tissues, such as the intestine, kidney, and lungs. These metabolites are then conjugated with glucuronide and excreted in the urine.[274]

Ketamine exerts its pharmacodynamic effects primarily via noncompetitive antagonism at the NMDA receptor in the CNS. It likely exerts some influence on opioid receptors, either directly or indirectly via the release of endogenous substances.[273] Ketamine's unique qualities result in "dissociative anesthesia," during which the eyes remain open, often with nystagmus, and laryngeal and corneal reflexes remain intact.[274] Patients often maintain spontaneous respirations, although apnea can occur if ketamine is given rapidly intravenously.[277] Ketamine increases systemic vascular resistance and cardiac output.[278] It is a strong bronchodilator and has been efficacious in the treatment of status asthmaticus.[273] Adverse effects include emergence delirium and hallucinations, the incidence of which may be decreased by concomitant use of midazolam.[273] It is also a sialagogue and is emetogenic especially when given intramuscularly.[277]

In pediatric patients, ketamine has found a wide range of applications across all age groups because it can provide for amnesia as well as analgesia. It has been used for induction of anesthesia in congenital cardiac surgery and as the sole anesthetic agent in burns.[278] It is also used for procedural sedation in the emergency department and other intrahospital settings.[277] Ketamine has been used alone or as an adjunct with local anesthetics in caudal analgesia.[278]

Recently, concern has been raised regarding the use of ketamine in pediatric patients, especially in neonates, since ketamine has been shown to have a role in apoptosis in developing brains in various animal models.[279,280] However, ketamine has also been shown to reduce cell death in an experimental inflammatory pain model in the neonatal rat.[281] An excellent summary of this research has been published and is left for the reader to review.[280]

CONCLUSION

The pendulum has swung from a time when neonates were not believed to experience pain to an understanding that pain can have profound physiologic consequences and developmental sequelae. However, the many analgesics that are currently being used in pediatric patients can have their own distinct pharmacokinetics in preterm neonates, infants, children, and adolescents as the various organ systems undergo the maturational process. Furthermore, genetic influences can produce profound differences in the pharmacology of the drugs that pediatric anesthesiologists use daily, making the pharmacology of analgesics a rapidly changing topic requiring further research and investigation.

REFERENCES

1. Allagaert K, van de Velde M, van den Anker J. Neonatal clinical pharmacology. *Pediatr Anesth.* 2014;24:30-38.
2. Anderson BJ, Allagaert K. The pharmacology of anaesthetics in the neonate. *Best Pract Res Clin Anaesthesiol.* 2010;24:419-431.
3. Kearns GL, Artman M. Functional biomarkers: an approach to bridge pharmacokinetics and pharmacodynamics in pediatric clinical trials. *Curr Pharmaceut Des.* 2015;21:5636-5642.
4. Anderson GD. Developmental pharmacokinetics. *Sem Pediatr Neurol.* 2010;17:208-213.
5. van den Anker JN. Developmental pharmacology. *Develop Disab Res Rev.* 2010;16:233-238.
6. Anderson GD, Lynn AM. Optimizing pediatric dosing: a developmental pharmacologic approach. *Pharmacotherapy.* 2009;29:680-690.
7. Funk RS, Brown JT, Abdel-Rahman SM. Pediatric pharmacokinetics: human development and drug disposition. *Pediatr Clin N Am.* 2012;59:1001-1016.
8. Heimann G. Enteral absorption and bioavailability in children in relation to age. *Eur J Clin Pharmacol.* 1980;18:43-50.
9. Berseth CL. Gestational evolution of small intestine motility in preterm and term infants. *J Pediatr.* 1989;115:646-651.
10. de Wildt SN, Kearns GL, Leeder JS, et al. Cytochrome P450 3A: ontogeny and drug disposition. *Clin Pharmacokinet.* 1999;37:485-505.
11. Fakhoury M, Litalien C, Medard Y, et al. Localization and mRNA expression of CYP3A and P-glycoprotein in human duodenum as a function of age. *Drug Metab Dispos.* 2005;33:1603-1607.
12. Wester RC, Maibach HI. Cutaneous pharmacokinetics: 10 steps to percutaneous absorption. *Drug Metab Rev.* 1983;14:169-205.
13. West DP, Halket JM, Harvey DR, et al. Percutaneous absorption in preterm infants. *Pediatr Dermatol.* 1987;4:234-237.
14. Carry MR, Ringel SP, Starcevich JM. Distribution of capillaries in normal and diseased human skeletal muscle. *Muscle Nerve.* 1986;9:445-454.
15. Wood M, Wood AJJ. Changes in plasma drug binding and alpha-1-acid glycoprotein in mother and newborn infant. *Clin Pharmacol Therapeut.* 1981;29:522-526.

16. Sethi PK, White CA, Cummings BS, et al. Ontogeny of plasma proteins, albumin and binding of diazepam, cyclosporine, and deltamethrin. *Pediatr Res*. 2016;79:409-415.

17. Starkey ES, Sammons HM. Practical pharmacokinetics: what do you really need to know? *Arch Dis Childhood-E*. 2015;100:37-43.

18. Hines RN, McCarver DG. The ontogeny of human drug-metabolizing enzymes: phase I oxidative enzymes. *J Pharmacol Exp Ther*. 2002;300:355-360.

19. McCarver DG, Hines RN. The ontogeny of human drug-metabolizing enzymes: phase II conjugation enzymes and regulatory mechanisms. *J Pharmacol Exp Ther*. 2002;300:361-366.

20. Chen N, Aleksa K, Woodland C, et al. Ontogeny of drug elimination by the human kidney. *Pediatr Nephrol*. 2006;21:160-168.

21. Raffa RB, Pergolizzi JV Jr, Taylor R Jr, et al. Acetaminophen (paracetamol) oral absorption and clinical influences. *Pain Pract*. 2014;14:668-677.

22. Ji P, Wang Y, Li Z, et al. Regulatory review of acetaminophen clinical pharmacology in young pediatric patients. *J Pharmaceut Sci*. 2012;101:4383-4389.

23. Singla NK, Parulan C, Samson R, et al. Plasma and cerebrospinal fluid pharmacokinetic parameters after single-dose administration of intravenous, oral, or rectal acetaminophen. *Pain Pract*. 2012;12:523-532.

24. van Lingen RA, Deinum HT, Quak CME, et al. Multiple-dose pharmacokinetics of rectally administered acetaminophen in term infants. *Clin Pharmacol Therap*. 1999;66:509-515.

25. Allegaert K, Vanhaesebrouck S, Verbesselt R, et al. In vivo glucuronidation activity of drugs in neonates: extensive interindividual variability despite their young age. *Therap Drug Monitor*. 2009;31:411-415.

26. Martin LD, Jimenez N, Lynn AM. A review of perioperative anesthesia and analgesia for infants: updates and trends to watch. *F1000Research*. 2017;6:120.

27. Porta R, Sanchez L, Nicolas M, et al. Lack of toxicity after paracetamol overdose in an extremely preterm neonate. *Eur J Clin Pharmacol*. 2012;68:901-902.

28. Nevin DG, Shung J. Intravenous paracetamol overdose in a preterm infant during anesthesia. *Pediatr Anesth*. 2009;20:105-114.

29. Isbister GK, Bucens IK, Whyte IM. Paracetamol overdose in a preterm neonate. *Arch Dis Childhood-F*. 2001;85:70-72.

30. de la Pintiere A, Betremieux PE. Intravenous paracetamol overdose in a term newborn. *Arch Dis Childhood-F*. 2003;88:351-352.

31. van der Marel CD, Anderson BJ, van Lingen RA, et al. Paracetamol and metabolite pharmacokinetics in infants. *Eur J Clin Pharmacol*. 2003;59:243-251.

32. Morris ME, Levy G. Renal clearance and serum protein binding of acetaminophen and its major conjugates in humans. *J Pharmaceut Sci*. 1984;73:1038-1041.

33. Palmer GM, Atkins M, Anderson BJ, et al. I.V. acetaminophen pharmacokinetics in neonates after multiple doses. *Br J Anaesth*. 2008;101:523-530.

34. Toussaint K, Yang XC, Zielinski MA, et al. What do we (not) know about how paracetamol (acetaminophen) works? *J Clin Pharm Therapeut*. 2010;35:617-638.

35. Gibb IA, Anderson BJ. Paracetamol (acetaminophen) pharmacodynamics: interpreting the plasma concentration. *Arch Dis Childhood*. 2008;93:241-247.

36. Hahn TW, Mogensen T, Lund C, et al. Analgesic effect of iv paracetamol: possible ceiling effect of paracetamol in postoperative pain. *Acta Anaesthesiol Scand*. 2003;47:138-145.

37. Ceelie I, de Wildt SN, van Dijk M, et al. Effect of intravenous paracetamol on postoperative morphine requirements in neonates and infants undergoing major noncardiac surgery. *J Am Med Assoc*. 2013;309:149-154.

38. Subramanyam R, Varughese A, Kurth CD, et al. Cost-effectiveness of intravenous acetaminophen for pediatric tonsillectomy. *Pediatr Anesth*. 2014;24:467-475.

39. Nour C, Ratsiu J, Singh N, et al. Analgesic effectiveness of acetaminophen for primary cleft palate repair in young children: a randomized placebo-controlled trial. *Pediatr Anesth*. 2014;24:574-581.

40. van der Marel CD, Peters JWB, Bouwmeester NJ, et al. Rectal acetaminophen does not reduce morphine consumption after major surgery in young infants. *Br J Anaesth*. 2007;98:372-379.

41. Bremerich DH, Neidhart G, Heimann K, et al. Prophylactically-administered rectal acetaminophen does not reduce postoperative opioid requirements in infants and small children undergoing elective cleft palate repair. *Anesth Analg*. 2001;92:907-912.

42. Anderson B, Kanagasundarum S, Woollard G. Analgesic efficacy of paracetamol in children using tonsillectomy as a pain model. *Anaesth Intensive Care*. 1996;24:669-673.

43. Korpela R, Korvenoja P, Meretoja OA. Morphine-sparing effect of acetaminophen in pediatric day-case surgery. *Anesthesiology*. 1999;91:442-447.

44. Gandhi R, Sunder R. Postoperative analgesic efficacy of single high dose and low dose rectal acetaminophen in pediatric ophthalmic surgery. *J Anaesthesiol Clin Pharmacol*. 2012;28:460-464.

45. OFIRMEV [package insert]. Hazelwood, MO: Mallinckrodt Hospital Products; 2017.

46. Veyckemans F, Anderson BJ, Wolf AR, et al. Intravenous paracetamol dosage in the neonate and small infant [Letter to the Editor]. *Br J Anaesth*. 2014;112:380-381.

47. de Martino M, Chiarugi A. Recent advances in pediatric use of oral paracetamol in fever and pain management. *Pain Ther*. 2015;4:149-168.

48. Birmingham PK, Tobin MJ, Fisher DM, et al. Initial and subsequent dosing of rectal acetaminophen in children: a 24-hour pharmacokinetic study of new dose recommendations. *Anesthesiology*. 2001;94:385-389.

49. Hall SM. Reye's syndrome and aspirin: a review. *J R Soc Med*. 1986;79:596-598.

50. Domanska U, Pobudkowska A, Pelczarska A, et al. pK_a and solubility of drugs in water, ethanol, and 1-octanol. *J Phys Chem B*. 2009;113:8941-8947.

51. Rencber S, Karavana SY, Ozyazici M. Bioavailability file: ketoprofen. *FABAD J Pharmaceut Sci*. 2009;34:203-216.

52. Li X, Cooper MA. Measurement of drug lipophilicity and pK_a using acoustics. *Analyt Chem*. 2012;84:2609-2613.

53. Davies NM. Clinical pharmacokinetics of ibuprofen: the first 30 years. *Clin Pharmacokinet*. 1998;34:101-154.

54. Leung GJ, Rainsford KD, Kean WF. Osteoarthritis of the hand II: chemistry, pharmacokinetics and pharmacodynamics of naproxen, and clinical outcome studies. *J Pharm Pharmacol*. 2013;66:347-357.

55. Dewland PM, Reader S, Berry P. Bioavailability of ibuprofen following oral administration of standard ibuprofen, sodium ibuprofen or ibuprofen acid incorporating poloxamer in healthy volunteers. *BMC Clin Pharmacol*. 2009;9:19-28.

56. Barzilay B, Youngster I, Batash D, et al. Pharmacokinetics of oral ibuprofen for patent ductus arteriosus closure in preterm infants. *Arch Dis Childhood-F*. 2012;97:F116-F119.

57. Sharma PK, Garg SK, Narang A. Pharmacokinetics of oral ibuprofen in premature infants. *J Clin Pharmacol.* 2003;43:968-973.

58. Han EE, Beringer PM, Louie SG, et al. Pharmacokinetics of ibuprofen in children with cystic fibrosis. *Clin Pharmacokinet.* 2004;43:145-156.

59. Valitalo P, Kumpulainen E, Manner M, et al. Plasma and cerebrospinal fluid pharmacokinetics of naproxen in children. *J Clin Pharmacol.* 2012;52:1516-1526.

60. Nguyen LA, He H, Pham-Huy C. Chiral drugs: an overview. *Int J Biomed Sci.* 2006;2:85-100.

61. Khan SJ, Wang L, Hashim NH, et al. Distinct enantiomeric signals of ibuprofen and naproxen in treated wastewater and sewer overflow. *Chirality.* 2014;26:739-746.

62. Gregoire N, Gualano V, Geneteau A, et al. Population pharmacokinetics of ibuprofen enantiomers in very premature neonates. *J Clin Pharmacol.* 2004;44:1114-1124.

63. Rodrigues AD. Impact of *CYP2C9* genotype on pharmacokinetics: are all cyclooxygenase inhibitors the same? *Drug Metab Dispos.* 2005;33:1567-1575.

64. Pacifici GM. Clinical pharmacology of ibuprofen in preterm infants: a meta-analysis of published data. *Med Exp.* 2014;1:55-61.

65. Kuehl GE, Lampe JW, Potter JD, et al. Glucuronidation of nonsteroidal anti-inflammatory drugs: identifying the enzymes responsible in human liver microsomes. *Drug Metab Dispos.* 2005;33:1027-1035.

66. Vree TB, van den Biggelaar-Martea M, Verwey-van Wissen CPWGM, et al. The pharmacokinetics of naproxen, its metabolite *O*-desmethylnaproxen, and their acyl glucuronides in humans. Effect of cimetidine. *Br J Clin Pharmacol.* 1993;35:467-472.

67. Morris JL, Rosen DA, Rosen KR. Nonsteroidal anti-inflammatory agents in neonates. *Pediatric Drugs.* 2003;5:385-405.

68. Olson DM, Mijovic JE, Zaragoza DB, et al. Prostaglandin endoperoxide H synthase type 1 and type 2 messenger ribonucleic acid in human fetal tissues throughout gestation and in the newborn infant. *Am J Obstetr Gynecol.* 2001;184:169-174.

69. Mehlisch DR, Sykes J. Ibuprofen blood plasma levels and onset of analgesia. *Int J Clin Pract.* 2013;67(suppl 178):3-8.

70. Moss JR, Watcha MF, Bendel LP, et al. A multicenter, randomized, double-blind placebo-controlled, single dose trial of the safety and efficacy of intravenous ibuprofen for treatment of pain in pediatric patients undergoing tonsillectomy. *Pediatr Anesth.* 2014;24:483-489.

71. Pierce CA, Voss B. Efficacy and safety of ibuprofen and acetaminophen in children and adults: a meta-analysis and qualitative review. *Ann Pharmacother.* 2010;44:489-506.

72. Erdeve O, Sarici SU, Sari E, et al. Oral-ibuprofen-induced acute renal failure in a preterm infant. *Pediatr Nephrol.* 2008;23:1565-1567.

73. Tatli MM, Kumral A, Duman N, et al. Spontaneous intestinal perforation after oral ibuprofen treatment of patent ductus arteriosus in two very-low-birthweight infants. *Acta Paediatr.* 2004;93:999-1001.

74. Kokki H. Ketoprofen pharmacokinetics, efficacy, and tolerability in pediatric patients. *Pediatr Drugs.* 2010;12:313-329.

75. Lucas S. The pharmacology of indomethacin. *Headache.* 2016;56:436-446.

76. Jung D, Mroszczak E, Bynum L. Pharmacokinetics of ketorolac tromethamine in humans after intravenous, intramuscular and oral administration. *Eur J Clin Pharmacol.* 1988;35:423-425.

77. Al Za'abi M, Donovan T, Tudehope D, et al. Orogastric and intravenous indomethacin administration to very premature neonates with patent ductus arteriosus: population pharmacokinetics, absolute bioavailability, and treatment outcome. *Therapeut Drug Monitor.* 2007;29:807-814.

78. Alqahtani S, Kaddoumi A. Development of physiologically based pharmacokinetic/pharmacodynamic model for indomethacin disposition in pregnancy. *PLOS One.* 2015;10:e0139762.

79. Olkkola KT, Maunuksela EL, Korpela R. Pharmacokinetics of postoperative intravenous indomethacin in children. *Pharmacol Toxicol.* 1989;65:157-160.

80. Kauffman RE, Lieh-Lai MW, Uy HG, et al. Enantiomer-selective pharmacokinetics and metabolism of ketorolac in children. *Clin Pharmacol Therapeut.* 1999;65:382-388.

81. Lynn AM, Bradford H, Kantor ED, et al. Ketorolac tromethamine: stereo-specific pharmacokinetics and single-dose use in postoperative infants aged 2-6 months. *Pediatr Anesth.* 2011;21:325-334.

82. Sallmon H, Keohne P, Hansmann G. Recent advances in the treatment of preterm newborn infants with patent ductus arteriosus. *Clin Perinatol.* 2016;43:113-129.

83. Watcha MF, Jones MB, Lagueruela RG, et al. Comparison of ketorolac and morphine as adjuvants during pediatric surgery. *Anesthesiology.* 1992;76:368-372.

84. Jo YY, Hong JY, Choi EK, et al. Ketorolac or fentanyl continuous infusion for post-operative analgesia in children undergoing ureteroneocystostomy. *Acta Anaesthesiol Scand.* 2011;55:54-59.

85. Moffett BS, Wann TI, Carberry KE, et al. Safety of ketorolac in neonates and infants after cardiac surgery. *Pediatr Anesthes.* 2006;16:424-428.

86. Cheng HF, Harris RC. Renal effects of non-steroidal anti-inflammatory drugs and selective cyclooxygenase-2 inhibitors. *Curr Pharmaceut Design.* 2005;11:1795-1804.

87. Feldman HI, Kinman JL, Berlin JA, et al. Parenteral ketorolac: the risk for acute renal failure. *Ann Intern Med.* 1997;126:193-199.

88. Vuolteenaho K, Moilanen T, Moilanen E. Non-steroidal anti-inflammatory drugs, cyclooxygenase-2 and the bone healing process. *Basic Clin Pharmacol.* 2007;102:10-14.

89. Kay RM, Leathers M, Directo MP, et al. Perioperative ketorolac use in children undergoing lower extremity osteotomies. *J Pediatr Orthopaed.* 2011;31:783-786.

90. Sucato DJ, Lovejoy JF, Agrawal S, et al. Postoperative ketorolac does not predispose to pseudoarthrosis following posterior spinal fusion and instrumentation for adolescent idiopathic scoliosis. *Spine.* 2008;33:1119-1124.

91. Singer AJ, Mynster CJ, McMahon BJ. The effect of IM ketorolac tromethamine on bleeding time: a prospective, interventional, controlled study. *Am J Emerg Med.* 2003;21:441-443.

92. Chan DK, Parikh SR. Perioperative ketorolac increases post-tonsillectomy hemorrhage in adults but not children. *Laryngoscope.* 2014;124:1789-1793.

93. Richardson MD, Palmeri NO, Williams SA, et al. Routine perioperative ketorolac administration is not associated with hemorrhage in pediatric neurosurgery patients. *J Neuros-Pediatr.* 2016;17:107-115.

94. Shi S, Klotz U. Clinical use and pharmacological properties of selective COX-2 inhibitors. *Eur J Clin Pharmacol.* 2008;64:233-252.

95. Rudd RA, Seth P, David F, et al. Increases in drug and opioid-involved overdose deaths—United States, 2010–2015. *Morbid Mortal W.* 2016;65:1445-1452.

96. Wilcox RA, Owen H. Variable cytochrome P450 2D6 expression and metabolism of codeine and other opioid prodrugs: implications for the Australian anaesthetist. *Anaesth Intensive Care.* 2000;28:611-619.

97. Tobias JD. Weak analgesics and nonsteroidal anti-inflammatory agents in the management of children with acute pain. *Pediatr Clin N Am.* 2000;47:527-543.

98. Lugo RA, Kern SE. Clinical pharmacokinetics of morphine. *J Pain Palliat Care Pharmacother.* 2002;16:5-18.

99. Masood AR, Thomas SHL. Systemic absorption of nebulized morphine compared with oral morphine in healthy subjects. *Br J Clin Pharmacol.* 1996;41:250-252.

100. Kharasch ED, Hoffer C, Whittington D. Role of P-glycoprotein in the intestinal absorption and clinical effects of morphine. *Clin Pharmacol Therapeut.* 2003;74:543-554.

101. Mohammed SS, Christopher MM, Mehta P, et al. Increased erythrocyte and protein binding of codeine in patients with sickle cell disease. *J Pharmaceut Sci.* 1993;82:1112-1117.

102. Poulsen L, Brosen K, Arendt-Nielsen L, et al. Codeine and morphine in extensive and poor metabolizers of sparteine: pharmacokinetics, analgesic effect and side effects. *Eur J Clin Pharmacol.* 1996;51:289-295.

103. Zahari Z, Ismail R. Influence of cytochrome P450, family 2, subfamily D, polypeptide 6 (CYP2D6) polymorphisms on pain sensitivity and clinical response to weak opioid analgesics. *Drug Metab Pharmacokinet.* 2014;29:29-43.

104. Kirchheiner J, Schmidt H, Tzvetkov M, et al. Pharmacokinetics of codeine and its metabolite morphine in ultra-rapid metabolizers due to CYP2D6 duplication. *Pharmacogenom J.* 2007;7:257-265.

105. Linares OA, Fudin J, Schiesser WE, et al. CYP2D6 phenotype-specific codeine population pharmacokinetics. *J Pain Palliat Care Pharmacother.* 2015;29:4-15.

106. Leppert W. CYP2D6 in the metabolism of opioids for mild to moderate pain. *Pharmacology.* 2011;87:274-285.

107. Vree TB, van Dongen RTM, Koopman-Kimenai PM. Codeine analgesia is due to codeine-6-glucuronide, not morphine. *Int J Clin Pract.* 2000;54:395-398.

108. Ciszkowski C, Madadi P. Codeine, ultrarapid-metabolism genotype, and postoperative death [Letter to the Editor]. *New Engl J Med.* 2009;361:827-828.

109. Kelly LE, Rieder M, van den Anker J, et al. More codeine fatalities after tonsillectomy in North American children. *Pediatrics.* 2012;129:e1343-e1347.

110. Subramanyam R, Varughese A, Willging JP, et al. Future of pediatric tonsillectomy and perioperative outcomes. *Int J Pediatr Otorhinolaryngol.* 2013;77:194-199.

111. FDA Drug Safety Communication: FDA restricts use of prescription codeine pain and cough medicines and tramadol pain medicines in children; recommends against use in breastfeeding women. Available at https://www.fda.gov/Drugs/DrugSafety/ucm549679.htm. Accessed February 5, 2017.

112. Koren G, Cairns J, Chitayat D, et al. Pharmacogenetics of morphine poisoning in a breastfed neonate of a codeine-prescribed mother. *Lancet.* 2006;368:704.

113. Stone AN, Mackenzie PI, Galetin A, et al. Isoform selectivity and kinetics of morphine 3- and 6-glucuronidation by human UDP-glucuronosyltransferases: evidence for atypical glucuronidation kinetics by UGT2B7. *Drug Metab Dispos.* 2003;31:1086-1089.

114. De Gregori M, Garbin G, De Gregori S, et al. Genetic variability at *COMT* but not at *OPRM1* and *UGT2B7* loci modulates morphine analgesic response in acute postoperative pain. *Eur J Clin Pharmacol.* 2013;69:1651-1658.

115. Bastami S, Gupta A, Zackrisson AL, et al. Influence of *UGT2B7, OPRM1* and *ABCB1* gene polymorphisms on postoperative morphine consumption. *Basic Clin Pharmacol.* 2014;115:423-431.

116. Matic M, Norman E, Rane A, et al. Effect of UGT2B7 -900G>A (-842G>A; rs7438135) on morphine glucuronidation in preterm newborns: results from a pilot cohort. *Pharmacogenomics.* 2014;15:1589-1597.

117. Mazoit JX, Butscher K, Samii K. Morphine in postoperative patients: pharmacokinetics and pharmacodynamics of metabolites. *Anesth Analg.* 2007;105:70-78.

118. Stein C. Opioid receptors. *Ann Rev Med.* 2016;67:433-451.

119. Basbaum AI, Bautista DM, Scherrer G, et al. Cellular and molecular mechanisms of pain. *Cell.* 2009;139:267-284.

120. Lam J, Baello S, Iqbal M, et al. The ontogeny of P-glycoprotein in the developing human blood-brain barrier: implication for opioid toxicity in neonates. *Pediatr Res.* 2015;78:417-421.

121. Sadhasivam S, Chidambaran V. Pharmacogenomics of opioids and perioperative pain management. *Pharmacogenomics.* 2012;13:1719-1740.

122. Janicki PK, Schuler G, Francis D, et al. A genetic association study of the functional A118G polymorphism of the human mu-opioid receptor gene in patients with acute and chronic pain. *Anesth Analg.* 2006;103:1011-1017.

123. Chidambaran V, Mavi J, Esslinger H, et al. Association of *OPRM1* A118G variant with risk of morphine-induced respiratory depression following spine fusion in adolescents. *Pharmacogenom J.* 2015;15:255-262.

124. Tsai FF, Fan SZ, Yang YM, et al. Human opioid mu-receptor A118G polymorphism may protect against central pruritus by epidural morphine for post-cesarean analgesia. *Acta Anaesthesiol Scand.* 2010;54:1265-1269.

125. Anand KJS, Phil D, Hickey PR. Halothane-morphine compared with high-dose sufentanil for anesthesia and postoperative analgesia in neonatal cardiac surgery. *New Engl J Med.* 1992;326:1-9.

126. Quinn MW, Otoo F, Rushforth JA, et al. Effect of morphine and pancuronium on the stress response in ventilated preterm infants. *Early Hum Dev.* 1992;30:241-248.

127. Quinn MW, Wild J, Dean HG, et al. Randomized double-blind controlled trial of effect of morphine on catecholamine concentrations in ventilated pre-term babies. *Lancet.* 1993;342:324-327.

128. AAP Committee on Fetus and Newborn and Section on Anesthesiology and Pain Medicine. Prevention and management of procedural pain in the neonate: an update. *Pediatrics.* 2016;137:e20154271.

129. Ferguson SA, Ward WL, Paule MG, et al. A pilot study of preemptive morphine analgesia in preterm neonates: effects on head circumference, social behavior, and response latencies in early childhood. *Neurotoxicol Teratol.* 2012;34:47-55.

130. de Graf J, van Lingen RA, Valkenburg AJ, et al. Does neonatal morphine use affect neuropsychological outcomes at 8 to 9 years of age? *Pain.* 2013;154:449-458.

131. Duedahl TH, Hansen EH. A qualitative systematic review of morphine treatment in children with postoperative pain. *Pediatr Anesth.* 2007;17:756-774.

132. Joshi GP, McCarroll SM, O'Brien TM, et al. Intraarticular analgesia following knee arthroscopy. *Anesthes Analg.* 1993;76:333-336.

133. Melhem MR, Rubino CM, Farr SJ, et al. Population pharmacokinetic analysis for hydrocodone following the administration of hydrocodone bitartrate extended-release capsules. *Clin Pharmacokinet.* 2013;52:907-917.

134. Liu W, Dutta S, Kearns G, et al. Pharmacokinetics of hydrocodone/acetaminophen combination product in children ages 6-17 with moderate to moderately severe postoperative pain. *J Clin Pharmacol.* 2015;55:204-211.

135. Lugo RA, Kern SE. The pharmacokinetics of oxycodone. *J Pain Palliat Care Pharmacother.* 2004;18:17-30.

136. Sarhill N, Walsh D, Nelson KA. Hydromorphone: pharmacology and clinical applications in cancer patients. *Supp Care Canc.* 2001;9:84-96.

137. Jeleazcov C, Saari TI, Ihmsen H, et al. Population pharmacokinetic modeling of hydromorphone in cardiac surgery patients during postoperative pain therapy. *Anesthesiology.* 2014;120:378-391.

138. Cone EJ, Heltsley R, Black DL, et al. Prescription opioids. II. Metabolism and excretion patterns of hydrocodone in urine following controlled single-dose administration. *J Analyt Toxicol.* 2013;37:486-494.

139. Navani DM, Yoburn BC. In vivo activity of norhydrocodone: an active metabolite of hydrocodone. *J Pharmacol Exp Therapeut.* 2013;347:497-505.

140. Linares OA, Fudin J, Daly AL, et al. Individualized hydrocodone therapy based on phenotype, pharmacogenetics, and pharmacokinetic dosing. *Clin J Pain.* 2015;31:1026-1035.

141. de Leon J, Dinsmore L, Wedlund P. Adverse drug reactions to oxycodone and hydrocodone in CYP2D6 ultrarapid metabolizers [Letter to the Editor]. *J Clin Psychopharmacol.* 2003;23:420-421.

142. Madadi P, Hildebrandt D, Gong IY, et al. Fatal hydrocodone overdose in a child: pharmacogenetics and drug interactions. *Pediatrics.* 2010;126:e986-e989.

143. Poyhia R, Vainio A, Kalso E. A review of oxycodone's clinical pharmacokinetics and pharmacodynamics. *J Pain Sympt Manag.* 1993;8:63-67.

144. Zwisler ST, Enggaard TP, Mikkelsen S, et al. Impact of the CYP2D6 genotype on post-operative intravenous oxycodone analgesia. *Acta Anaesthesiol Scand.* 2010;54:232-240.

145. Andreassen TN, Eftedal I, Klepstad P, et al. Do *CYP2D6* genotypes reflect oxycodone requirements for cancer patients treated for cancer pain? A cross-sectional multicentre study. *Eur J Clin Pharmacol.* 2012;68:55-64.

146. Toyama K, Uchida N, Ishizuka H, et al. Single-dose evaluation of safety, tolerability and pharmacokinetics of newly formulated hydromorphone immediate-release and hydrophilic matrix extended-release tablets in healthy Japanese subjects without co-administration of an opioid antagonist. *J Clin Pharmacol.* 2015;55:975-984.

147. Mazer-Amirshahi M, Mullins PM, Rasooly IR, et al. Trends in prescription opioid use in pediatric emergency department patients. *Pediatr Emerg Care.* 2014;30:230-235.

148. Lasky T, Ernst FR, Greenspan J. Use of analgesic, anesthetic, and sedative medications during pediatric hospitalizations in the United States 2008. *Anesth Analg.* 2012;115:1155-1161.

149. George JA, Park PS, Hunsberger J, et al. An analysis of 34,218 pediatric outpatient controlled substance prescriptions. *Anesth Analg.* 2016;122:807-813.

150. Sadhasivam S, Myer CM III. Preventing opioid-related deaths in children undergoing surgery [Letter to the Editor]. *Pain Med.* 2012;13:982-983.

151. Reiter PD, Ng J, Dobyns EL. Continuous hydromorphone for pain and sedation in mechanically ventilated infants and children. *J Op Manag.* 2012;8:99-104.

152. Hong R, Gauger V, Caird MS, et al. Narcotic-only epidural infusion for posterior spinal fusion patients: a single-center, retrospective review. *J Pediatr Orthopaed.* 2016;36:526-529.

153. Gauger VT, Voepel-Lewis TD, Burke CN, et al. Epidural analgesia compared with intravenous analgesia after pediatric posterior spinal fusion. *J Pediatr Orthopaed.* 2009;29:588-593.

154. Goodarzi M. Comparison of epidural morphine, hydromorphone and fentanyl for postoperative pain control in children undergoing orthopaedic surgery. *Paediatr Anaesth.* 1999;9:419-422.

155. Lotsch J, Walter C, Parnham MJ, et al. Pharmacokinetics of non-intravenous formulations of fentanyl. *Clin Pharmacokinet.* 2013;52:23-36.

156. Darwish M, Kirby M, Robertson P Jr, et al. Absolute and relative bioavailability of fentanyl buccal tablet and oral transmucosal fentanyl citrate. *J Clin Pharmacol.* 2007;47:343-350.

157. Panagiotou I, Mystakidou K. Intranasal fentanyl: from pharmacokinetics and bioavailability to current treatment applications. *Exp Rev Anticanc Ther.* 2010;10:1009-1021.

158. Varvel JR, Shafer SL, Hwang SS, et al. Absorption characteristics of transdermally administered fentanyl. *Anesthesiology.* 1989;70:928-934.

159. Bista SR, Haywood A, Hardy J, et al. Protein binding of fentanyl and its metabolite nor-fentanyl in human plasma, albumin and alpha-1 acid glycoprotein. *Xenobiotica.* 2015;45:207-212.

160. Takashina Y, Naito T, Mino Y, et al. Impact of CYP3A5 and ABCB1 gene polymorphisms on fentanyl pharmacokinetics and clinical responses in cancer patients undergoing conversion to a transdermal system. *Drug Metab Pharmacokinet.* 2012;27:414-421.

161. Park H-J, Shinn HK, Ryu SH, et al. Genetic polymorphisms in the *ABCB1* gene and the effects of fentanyl in Koreans. *Clin Pharmacol Therapeut.* 2007;81:539-546.

162. Volpe DA, McMahon Tobin GA, Mellon RD, et al. Uniform assessment and ranking of opioid Mu receptor binding constants for selected opioid drugs. *Regul Toxicol Pharmacol.* 2011;59:385-390.

163. Krzyzaniak N, Pawlowska I, Bajorek B. Review of drug utilization patterns in NICUs worldwide. *J Clin Pharm Therapeut.* 2016;41:612-620.

164. Cechvala MM, Christenson D, Eickhoff JC, et al. Sedative preference of families for lumbar punctures in children with acute leukemia: propofol alone or propofol and fentanyl. *J Pediatr Hematol Oncol.* 2008;30:142-147.

165. Moustafa MA. Nebulized lidocaine alone or combined with fentanyl as a premedication to general anesthesia in spontaneously breathing pediatric patients undergoing rigid bronchoscopy. *Pediatr Anesth.* 2013;23:429-434.

166. Tamura M, Nakamura K, Kitamura R, et al. Oral premedication with fentanyl may be a safe and effective alternative to oral midazolam. *Eur J Anesth.* 2003;20:482-486.

167. Epstein RH, Mendel HG, Witkowski TA, et al. The safety and efficacy of oral transmucosal fentanyl citrate for preoperative sedation in young children. *Anesth Analg.* 1996;83:1200-1205.

168. Dsida RM, Wheeler M, Birmingham PK, et al. Premedication of pediatric tonsillectomy patients with oral transmucosal fentanyl citrate. *Anesth Analg.* 1998;86:66-70.

169. Galinkin JL, Fazi LM, Cuy RM, et al. Use of intranasal fentanyl in children undergoing myringotomy and tube placement during halothane and sevoflurane anesthesia. *Anesthesiology.* 2000;93:1378-1383.

170. Borland M, Milsom S, Esson A. Equivalency of two concentrations of fentanyl administered by the intranasal route for acute analgesia in children in a paediatric emergency department: a randomized controlled trial. *Emerg Med Australas.* 2011;23:202-208.

171. Duncan HP, Cloote A, Weir PM, et al. Reducing stress responses in the pre-bypass phase of open heart surgery in infants and young children: a comparison of different fentanyl doses. *Br J Anaesth.* 2000;84:556-564.

172. Christensen ML, Wang WC, Harris S, et al. Transdermal fentanyl administration in children and adolescents with sickle cell pain crisis. *J Pediatr Hematol Oncol.* 1996;18:372-376.

173. Kim JG, Sohn SK, Kim DH, et al. Effectiveness of transdermal fentanyl patch for treatment of acute pain due to oral mucositis in patients receiving stem cell transplantation. *Transplant Proc.* 2005;37:4488-4491.

174. Hunt A, Goldman A, Devine T, et al. Transdermal fentanyl for pain relief in a paediatric palliative care population. *Palliat Med.* 2001;15:405-412.

175. Finkel JC, Finley A, Greco C, et al. Transdermal fentanyl in the management of children with chronic severe pain: results from an international study. *Cancer.* 2005;104:2847-2857.

176. Dewhirst E, Naguib A, Tobias JD. Chest wall rigidity in two infants after low-dose fentanyl administration. *Pediatr Emerg Care.* 2012;28:465-468.

177. Elakkumanan LB, Punj J, Talwar P, et al. An atypical presentation of fentanyl rigidity following administration of low dose fentanyl in a child during intraoperative period [Letter to the Editor]. *Pediatr Anesth.* 18:1102-1143.

178. Lindemann R. Respiratory muscle rigidity in a preterm infant after use of fentanyl during Caesarean section. *Eur J Pediatr.* 1998;157:1012-1013.

179. Eventov-Friedman S, Rozin I, Shinwell ES. Case of chest-wall rigidity in a preterm infant caused by prenatal fentanyl administration. *J Perinatol.* 2010;30:149-150.

180. Bagley JR, Thomas SA, Rudo FG, et al. New 1-(heterocyclylalkyl)-4-(proprionanilido)-4-piperidinyl methyl ester and methylene methyl ether analgesics. *J Med Chem.* 1991;34:827-841.

181. Kharasch ED, Walker A, Isoherranen N, et al. Influence of CYP3A5 genotype on the pharmacokinetics and pharmacodynamics of the cytochrome *P*450 3A probes alfentanil and midazolam. *Clin Pharmacol Therapeut.* 2007;82:410-426.

182. Kharasch ED, Hoffer C, Walker A, et al. Disposition and miotic effects of oral alfentanil: a potential noninvasive probe for first-pass cytochrome P450 3A activity. *Clin Pharmacol Therapeut.* 2003;73:199-208.

183. Schwagmeier R, Boerger N, Meissner W, et al. Pharmacokinetics of intranasal alfentanil. *J Clin Anesth.* 1995;7:109-113.

184. Willsie SK, Evashenk MA, Hamel LG, et al. Pharmacokinetic properties of single- and repeated-dose sufentanil sublingual tablets in healthy volunteers. *Clin Therapeut.* 2015;37:145-155.

185. Helmers JH, Noorduin H, Van Peer A, et al. Comparison of intravenous and intranasal sufentanil absorption and sedation. *Can J Anaesth.* 1989;36:494-497.

186. Bosilkovska M, Walder B, Besson M, et al. Analgesics in patients with hepatic impairment: pharmacology and clinical implications. *Drugs.* 2012;72:1645-1669.

187. Saari TI, Ihmsen H, Mell J, et al. Influence of intensive care treatment on the protein binding of sufentanil and hydromorphone during pain therapy in postoperative cardiac surgery patients. *Br J Anaesth.* 2014;113:677-687.

188. Meistelman C, Benhamou D, Barre J, et al. Effects of age on plasma protein binding of sufentanil. *Anesthesiology.* 1990;72:470-473.

189. Lundeberg S, Roelofse JA. Aspects of pharmacokinetics and pharmacodynamics of sufentanil in pediatric practice. *Pediatr Anesth.* 2011;21:274-279.

190. Klees TM, Sheffels P, Dale O, et al. Metabolism of alfentanil by cytochrome P4503A (CYP3A) enzymes. *Drug Metab Dispos.* 2005;33:303-311.

191. Guitton J, Buronfosse T, Desage M, et al. Possible involvement of multiple cytochrome P450S in fentanyl and sufentanil metabolism as opposed to alfentanil. *Biochem Pharmacol.* 1997;53:1613-1619.

192. Meuldermans W, Van Peer A, Hendrickx J, et al. Alfentanil pharmacokinetics and metabolism in humans. *Anesthesiology.* 1988;69:527-534.

193. Meuldermans W, Hendrickx J, Lauwers W, et al. Excretion and biotransformation of alfentanil and sufentanil in rats and dogs. *Drug Metab Dispos.* 1987;15:905-913.

194. Ahonen J, Olkkola KT, Hynynen M, et al. Comparison of alfentanil, fentanyl and sufentanil for total intravenous anaesthesia with propofol in patients undergoing coronary artery bypass surgery. *Br J Anaesth.* 2000;85:533-540.

195. Antmen B, Sasmaz I, Birbicer H, et al. Safe and effective sedation and analgesia for bone marrow aspiration procedures in children with alfentanil, remifentanil and combinations with midazolam. *Pediatr Anesth.* 2005;15:214-219.

196. Chiaretti A, Ruggiero A, Barone G, et al. Propofol/alfentanil and propofol/ketamine procedural sedation in children with acute lymphoblastic leukaemia: safety, efficacy and their correlation with pain neuromediator expression. *Eur J Canc Care.* 2010;19:212-220.

197. Kwak HJ, Min SK, Kim JS, et al. Prevention of propofol-induced pain in children: combination of alfentanil and lidocaine vs alfentanil or lidocaine alone. *Br J Anaesth.* 2009;103:410-412.

198. Oh AY, Seo KS, Goo EK, et al. Prevention of withdrawal movement associated with injection of rocuronium in children: comparison of remifentanil, alfentanil and fentanyl. *Acta Anaesthesiol Scand.* 2007;51:1190-1193.

199. Kim JY, Kwak HJ, Kim JY, et al. Prevention of rocuronium-induced withdrawal movement in children: a comparison of remifentanil with alfentanil. *Pediatr Anesth.* 2008;18:245-250.

200. Tan Y, Shi Y, Ding H, et al. Mu-opioid agonists for preventing emergence agitation under sevoflurane anesthesia in children: a meta-analysis of randomized controlled trials. *Pediatr Anesth.* 2016;26:139-150.

201. Pokela ML, Ryhanen PT, Koivisto ME, et al. Alfentanil-induced rigidity in newborn infants. *Anesth Analg.* 1992;75:252-257.

202. Saarenmaa E, Huttunen P, Leppaluoto J, et al. Alfentanil as procedural pain relief in newborn infants. *Arch Dis Childhood.* 1996;75:F103-F107.

203. Glenski JA, Friesen RH, Berglund NL, et al. Comparison of the hemodynamic and echocardiographic effects of sufentanil, fentanyl, isoflurane, and halothane for pediatric cardiovascular surgery. *J Cardiothorac Anesth.* 1988;2:147-155.

204. Moore RA, Yang SS, McNicholas KW, et al. Hemodynamic and anesthetic effects of sufentanil as the sole anesthetic for pediatric cardiovascular surgery. *Anesthesiology.* 1985;62:725-731.

205. Nielsen BN, Friis SM, Romsing J, et al. Intranasal sufentanil/ketamine analgesia in children. *Pediatr Anesth.* 2014;24:170-180.

206. Wang T, Xiang Q, Liu F, et al. Effects of caudal sufentanil supplemented with levobupivacaine on blocking spermatic cord traction response in pediatric orchidopexy. *J Anesth.* 2013;27:650-656.

207. Cho JE, Kim JY, Kim JE, et al. Epidural sufentanil provides better analgesia from 24h after surgery compared with

epidural fentanyl in children. *Acta Anaesthesiol Scand.* 2008;52:1360-1363.

208. Woloszczuk-Gebicka B, Grabowski T, Borucka B, et al. Pharmacokinetics of sufentanil administered with 0.2% ropivacaine as a continuous epidural infusion for postoperative pain relief in infants. *Pediatr Anesth.* 2014;24:962-967.

209. Verghese ST, Hannallah RS, Brennan M, et al. The effect of intranasal administration of remifentanil on intubating conditions and airway response after sevoflurane induction of anesthesia in children. *Anesth Analg.* 2008;107:1176-1181.

210. Benet LZ, Hoener B. Changes in plasma protein binding have little clinical relevance *Clin Pharmacol Therapeut.* 2002;71:115-121.

211. Dershwitz M, Hoke JF, Rosow CE, et al. Pharmacokinetics and pharmacodynamics of remifentanil in volunteer subjects with severe liver disease. *Anesthesiology.* 1996;84:812-820.

212. Ross AK, Davis PJ, De Lisle Dear G, et al. Pharmacokinetics of remifentanil in anesthetized pediatric patients undergoing elective surgery or diagnostic procedures. *Anesth Analg.* 2001;93:1393-1401.

213. Glass PSA, Hardman D, Kamiyama Y, et al. Preliminary pharmacokinetics and pharmacodynamics of an ultrashort-acting opioid: remifentanil (GI87084B). *Anesth Analg.* 1993;77:1031-1040.

214. Manullang J, Egan TD. Remifentanil's effect is not prolonged in a patient with pseudocholinesterase deficiency. *Anesth Analg.* 1999;89:529-530.

215. Pitsiu M, Wilmer A, Bodenham A, et al. Pharmacokinetics of remifentanil and its major metabolite, remifentanil acid, in ICU patients with renal impairment. *BrJ Anaesth.* 2004;92:493-503.

216. Hoke JF, Cunningham F, James MK, et al. Comparative pharmacokinetics and pharmacodynamics of remifentanil, its principle metabolite (GR90291) and alfentanil in dogs. *J Pharmacol Exp Therapeut.* 1997;281:226-232.

217. Pereira e Silva Y, Gomez RS, De Oliveira Marcatto J, et al. Early awakening and extubation with remifentanil in ventilated premature neonates. *Pediatr Anesth.* 2008;18:176-183.

218. Kamata M, Tobias JD. Remifentanil: applications in neonates. *J Anesth.* 2016;30:449-460.

219. Angst MS. Intraoperative use of remifentanil for TIVA: postoperative pain, acute tolerance, and opioid-induced hyperalgesia. *J Cardiothorac Vasc Anesth.* 2015;29:S16-S22.

220. Kim SH, Lee MH, Seo H, et al. Intraoperative infusion of 0.6-0.9 mcg/kg/min remifentanil induces acute tolerance in young children after laparoscopic ureteroneocystostomy. *Anesthesiology.* 2013;118:337-343.

221. Kars MS, Mori BV, Ahn S, et al. Fentanyl versus remifentanil-based TIVA for pediatric scoliosis repair: does it matter? *Reg Anesth Pain Med.* 2019;44(6):627-631.

222. Buck ML. Is meperidine the drug that just won't die? [Editorial]. *J Pediatr Pharmacol Therapeut.* 2011;16:167-169.

223. Latta KS, Ginsberg B, Barkin RL. Meperidine: a critical review. *Am J Therapeut.* 2002;9:53-68.

224. Glynn CJ, Mather LE. Clinical pharmacokinetics applied to patients with intractable pain: studies with pethidine. *Pain.* 1982;13:237-246.

225. Pond SM, Tong T, Benowitz NL, et al. Enhanced bioavailability of pethidine and pentazocine in patients with cirrhosis of the liver. *Aust N Z J Med.* 1980;10:515-519.

226. Clark RF, Wei EM, Anderson PO. Meperidine: therapeutic use and toxicity. *J Emerg Med.* 1995;13:797-802.

227. Beckwith MC, Fox ER, Chandramouli J. Removing meperidine from the health-system formulary: frequently asked questions. *J Pain Palliat Care Pharmacother.* 2002;16:45-59.

228. Benner KW, Durham SH. Meperidine restriction in a pediatric hospital. *J Pediatr Pharmacol Therapeut.* 2011;16:185-190.

229. American Academy of Pediatrics Committee on Psychosocial Aspects of Child and Family Health, American Pain Society Task Force on Pain in Infants, Children, and Adolescents. The assessment and management of acute pain in infants, children, and adolescents. *Pediatrics.* 2001;108:793-797.

230. Lugo RA, Satterfield KL, Kern SE. Pharmacokinetics of methadone. *J Pain Palliat Care Pharmacother.* 2005;19:13-24.

231. Dale O, Sheffels P, Kharasch ED. Bioavailabilities of rectal and oral methadone in healthy subjects. *Br J Clin Pharmacol.* 2004;58:156-162.

232. Dale O, Hoffer C, Sheffels P, et al. Disposition of nasal, intravenous, and oral methadone in healthy volunteers. *Clin Pharmacol Therapeut.* 2002;72:536-545.

233. Ward RM, Drover DR, Hammer GB, et al. The pharmacokinetics of methadone and its metabolites in neonates, infants, and children. *Pediatr Anesth.* 2014;24:591-601.

234. Kharasch ED, Hoffer C, Whittington D, et al. Methadone pharmacokinetics are independent of cytochrome P4503A (CYP3A) activity and gastrointestinal drug transport: insights from methadone interactions with ritonavir/indinavir. *Anesthesiology.* 2009;110:660-672.

235. Mitchell TB, Dyer KR, Newcombe D, et al. Fluctuations in (R, S)-methadone pharmacokinetics and response among long-term methadone maintenance patients. *Addict Biol.* 2006;11:170-174.

236. Li Y, Kantelip JP, Gerritsen-van Schieveen P, et al. Interindividual variability of methadone response: impact of genetic polymorphism. *Molec Diagn Ther.* 2008;12:109-124.

237. Ansermot N, Albayrak O, Schlapfer J, et al. Substitution of (R, S)-methadone by (R)-methadone: impact on QTc interval. *Arch Intern Med.* 2010;170:529-536.

238. Ebert B, Thorkildsen C, Andersen S, et al. Opioid analgesics as noncompetitive N-methyl-D-aspartate (NMDA) antagonists. *Biochem Pharmacol.* 1998;56:553-559.

239. Hewitt DJ. The use of NMDA-receptor antagonists in the treatment of chronic pain. *Clin J Pain.* 2000;16:S73-S79.

240. Salpeter SR, Buckley JS, Bruera E. The use of very-low-dose methadone for palliative pain control and the prevention of opioid hyperalgesia. *J Palliat Med.* 2013;16:616-622.

241. Moulin DE, Boulanger A, Clark AJ, et al. Pharmacological management of chronic neuropathic pain: revised consensus statement from the Canadian Pain Society. *Pain Res Manag.* 2014;19:328-335.

242. Bagley SM, Wachman EM, Holland E, et al. Review of the assessment and management of neonatal abstinence syndrome. *Addict Sci Clin Pract.* 2014;9:1-10.

243. Berde CB, Beyer JE, Bournaki MC, et al. Comparison of morphine and methadone for prevention of postoperative pain in 3- to 7-year-old children. *J Pediatr.* 1991;119:136-141.

244. Stemland CJ, Witte J, Colquhoun DA, et al. The pharmacokinetics of methadone in adolescents undergoing posterior spinal fusion. *Pediatr Anesth.* 2013;23:51-57.

245. Sharma A, Tallchief D, Blood J, et al. Perioperative pharmacokinetics of methadone in adolescents. *Anesthesiology.* 2011;115:1153-1161.

246. Singhal NR, Jones J, Semenova J, et al. Multimodal anesthesia with the addition of methadone is superior to epidural analgesia: a retrospective comparison of intraoperative

anesthetic techniques and pain management for 124 pediatric patients undergoing the Nuss procedure. *J Pediatr Surg.* 2016;51:612-616.

247. Rasmussen VF, Lundberg V, Jespersen TW, et al. Extreme doses of intravenous methadone for severe pain in two children with cancer. *Pediatr Blood Canc.* 2015;62:1087-1090.

248. Kirchheiner J, Keulen JT, Bauer S, et al. Effects of the CYP2D6 gene duplication on the pharmacokinetics and pharmacodynamics of tramadol. *J Clin Psychopharmacol.* 2008;28:78-83.

249. Ardakani YH, Rouini MR. Pharmacokinetics of tramadol and its three main metabolites in healthy male and female volunteers. *Biopharmaceut Drug Dispos.* 2007;28:527-534.

250. Lintz W, Barth H, Osterloh G, et al. Pharmacokinetics of tramadol and bioavailability of enteral tramadol formulations. 3rd communication: suppositories. *Arzneimittelforschung.* 1998;48:889-899.

251. Lassen D, Damkier P, Brosen K. The pharmacogenetics of tramadol. *Clin Pharmacokinet.* 2015;54:825-836.

252. Bressolle F, Rochette A, Khier S, et al. Population pharmacokinetics of the two enantiomers of tramadol and O-demethyl tramadol after surgery in children. *Br J Anaesth.* 2009;102:390-399.

253. Tzvetkov MV, Saadatmand AR, Lotsch J, et al. Genetically polymorphic OCT1: another piece in the puzzle of the variable pharmacokinetics and pharmacodynamics of the opioidergic drug tramadol. *Clin Pharmacol Therapeut.* 2011;90:143-150.

254. Schnabel A, Reichl SU, Meyer-Friebem C, et al. Tramadol for postoperative pain treatment in children. *Cochrane Database Syst Rev.* 2015;(3):CD009574.

255. Taheri R, Shayeghi S, Razavi SS, et al. Efficacy of bupivacaine-neostigmine and bupivacaine-tramadol in caudal block in pediatric inguinal herniorrhaphy. *Pediatr Anesth.* 2010;20:866-872.

256. Inanoglu K, Ozcengiz D, Gunes Y, et al. Epidural ropivacaine versus ropivacaine plus tramadol in postoperative analgesia in children undergoing major abdominal surgery: a comparison. *J Anesth.* 2010;24:700-704.

257. Akkaya T, Bedirli N, Ceylan T, et al. Comparison of intravenous and peritonsillar infiltration of tramadol for postoperative pain relief in children following adenotonsillectomy. *Eur J Anaesth.* 2009;26:333-337.

258. Borazan H, Sahin O, Kececioglu A, et al. Prevention of propofol injection pain in children: a comparison of pretreatment with tramadol and propofol-lidocaine mixture. *Int J Med Sci.* 2012;9:492-497.

259. Neri E, Maestro A, Minen F, et al. Sublingual ketorolac versus sublingual tramadol for moderate to severe post-traumatic bone pain in children: a double-blind, randomized, controlled trial. *Arch Dis Childhood.* 2013;98:721-724.

260. Erhan E, Inala MT, Aydin Y, et al. Tramadol infusion for the pain management in sickle cell disease: a case report. *Pediatr Anesth.* 2007;17:84-86.

261. Marzulli P, Caligari's L, Barba E. Tramadol can selectively manage moderate pain in children following European advice limiting codeine use. *Acta Paediatr.* 2014;103:1110-1116.

262. Palash TJ, Gill CJ. Butorphanol and nalbuphine: a pharmacologic comparison. *Oral Surg.* 1985;59:15-20.

263. Shah B, Ramchandani Y, Misran A. Development and evaluation of oral osmotic pump of butorphanol tartrate. *Pharmaceut Dev Technol.* 2014;19:868-880.

264. Shy WC, Morgenthau EA, Baraiya RH. Pharmacokinetics of butorphanol nasal spray in patients with renal impairment. *Br J Clin Pharmacol.* 1996;41:397-402.

265. Shy WC, Morgenthau EA, Pittman KA, et al. The effects of age and sex on the systemic availability and pharmacokinetics of transnasal butorphanol. *Eur J Clin Pharmacol.* 1994;47:57-60.

266. Vachharajani NN, Shyu WC, Greene DS, et al. The pharmacokinetics of butorphanol and its metabolites at steady state following nasal administration in humans. *Biopharmaceut Drug Dispos.* 1997;18:191-202.

267. Singh V, Pathak M, Singh GP. Oral midazolam and oral butorphanol premedication. *Indian J Pediatr.* 2005;72:741-744.

268. Pappas AL, Fluder EM, Creech S, et al. Postoperative analgesia in children undergoing myringotomy and placement equalization tubes in ambulatory surgery. *Anesth Analg.* 2003;96:1621-1624.

269. Bennie RE, Boehringer LA, Dierdorf SF, et al. Transnasal butorphanol is effective for postoperative pain relief in children undergoing myringotomy. *Anesthesiology.* 1998;89:385-390.

270. Lawhorn CD, Stoner JM, Schmitz ML, et al. Caudal epidural butorphanol plus bupivacaine versus bupivacaine in pediatric outpatient genitourinary procedures. *J Clin Anesth.* 1997;9:103-108.

271. Singh V, Kanaujia A, Singh GP. Efficacy of caudal butorphanol. *Indian J Pediatr.* 2006;73:147-150.

272. Gunter JB, McAuliffe J, Gregg T, et al. Continuous epidural butorphanol relieves pruritus associated with epidural morphine infusions in children. *Paediatr Anaesth.* 2000;10:167-172.

273. Radvansky BM, Puri S, Sofonios AN, et al. Ketamine: a narrative review of its uses in medicine. *Am J Therapeut.* 2016;23:e1414-e1426.

274. Mion G, Villevieille T. Ketamine pharmacology: an update (pharmacodynamics and molecular aspects, recent findings). *CNS Neurosci Therapeut.* 2013;19:370-380.

275. Dayton PG, Stiller RL, Cook DR, et al. The binding of ketamine to plasma proteins: emphasis on human plasma. *Eur J Clin Pharmacol.* 1983;24:825-831.

276. Rao LK, Flaker AM, Friedel CC, et al. Role of cytochrome P4502B6 polymorphisms in ketamine metabolism and clearance. *Anesthesiology.* 2016;125:1103-1112.

277. Alletag MJ, Auerbach MA, Baum CR. Ketamine, propofol, and ketofol use for pediatric sedation. *Pediatr Emerg Care.* 2012;28:1391-1398.

278. Roelofse JA. The evolution of ketamine applications in children. *Pediatr Anesth.* 2010;20:240-245.

279. Fredriksson A, Ponten E, Gordh T, et al. Neonatal exposure to a combination of N-methyl-D-aspartate and gamma-aminobutyric acid type A receptor anesthetic agents potentiates apoptotic neurodegeneration and persistent behavioral deficits. *Anesthesiology.* 2007;107:427-436.

280. Dong C, Anand KJS. Developmental neurotoxicity of ketamine in pediatric clinical use. *Toxicol Lett.* 2013;220:53-60.

281. Anand KJS, Garg S, Rovnaghi CR, et al. Ketamine reduces the cell death following inflammatory pain in newborn rat brain. *Pediatr Res.* 2007;62:283-290.

Hypnotics

Sapan Amin

FOCUS POINTS

1. Body composition is different in children than in adults, with children having a higher proportion of total body water than fat and muscle.
2. Egg allergy does not preclude propofol use (egg lecithin) because the usual allergy is due to egg albumin.
3. Prolonged propofol infusions (24 hours) can lead to propofol infusion syndrome (PRIS), which is a syndrome defined by metabolic acidosis, rhabdomyolysis, lipemia, and hepatomegaly.
4. Among the hypnotics, only ketamine has both amnestic and analgesic properties and is considered the most complete anesthetic.
5. Ketamine should be used with caution in patients that are sympathetically depleted (ICU patients) because it has direct myocardial depressant effects.
6. Etomidate provides hemodynamic stability upon administration but can cause adrenal insufficiency even after a single dose.
7. Midazolam is the most common premedication in adults intravenously, and in children orally.
8. Methohexital can be used for maintenance of anesthesia instead of propofol in patients with mitochondrial disorders. It should be used with caution in patients with seizure history.

INTRODUCTION

Hypnotics are drugs that have dose-dependent effects extending from reduction of anxiety to a sleep-like state. Due to differences in drug distribution between adults and children, dosing needed to exert similar clinical effects may vary. Parameters such as body composition, metabolism, regional blood flow, and clinical state affect distribution and thus effect.

Body composition is different in children than in adults, with children having a higher proportion of total body water than fat and muscle. Total body water is significantly larger in neonates and infants, especially preterm infants. Preterm infants and neonates have other differences in metabolism when compared to older children and adults. They have immature hepatic and renal function and decreased protein binding of drugs.

Regional blood flow plays a significant role in the effects of hypnotic drugs. The brain, heart, and liver are the main organs that first receive the drug. The next group to receive blood flow is the less perfused muscle group. The last group made up of the poorly perfused tissues is fat. Fat in turn acts as a reservoir and can release the drug into the bloodstream, maintaining higher drug concentration levels and prolonging drug effects.

As children get older, the renal and hepatic function increases as a larger fraction of cardiac output goes toward the liver and kidneys. Thus, the half-life of many medications in children over 2 years is shorter than in adults.

Sicker children especially in states of hemodynamic instability may need to have drug dosages reduced and/or given at a slower rate to prevent further cardiovascular deterioration.

As clinicians became more experienced with hypnotic drugs, more drug combinations have been considered to both decrease individual drug doses and improve side effect profile of individual drugs. An example of this is the use of ketamine along with propofol ("ketofol").

PROPOFOL

Propofol is the most commonly used intravenous induction agent because of its desirable properties of fast onset, clear headedness upon awakening, and less incidence of postoperative nausea and vomiting (infused at a low dose).[1] Propofol is a phenol derivative that is insoluble in water and is dissolved in 1.2% egg lecithin, 10% soybean oil, and 2.25% glycerol. The lipid solution can lead to microbial growth and contains ethylenediaminetetraacetic acid (EDTA) or metabisulfite. Propofol should be administered within 6 hours of opening the vial. An egg allergy does not contraindicate the use of propofol since most egg allergies are due to egg albumin (egg white), and egg lecithin is taken from egg yolk.[2]

Clinical Uses

1. Induction of anesthesia
2. Procedural sedation
3. Laryngospasm to deepen the patient
4. Total intravenous anesthesia (TIVA) or balanced anesthesia (in combination with opioids)
5. Prevention of postoperative nausea and vomiting[3]

Mechanism of Action

Propofol acts by facilitating GABA(A) receptor, which leads to increased influx of chloride ions causing hyperpolarization of neurons rendering them resistant to activation. It is only available for intravenous injection. It is fast-acting with short initial distribution half-life, leading to a quick wake-up. Even after long infusions, it has a relatively short context-sensitive half-time.[4,5] It can cause discomfort when given through a peripheral vein most likely due to the medication's intrinsic properties (pH and emulsion composition), a side effect that may be relieved with the administration through a larger vein or with the addition of lidocaine in advance or administration.

Induction Dose

2.5 to 3.5 mg/kg–higher doses than that of adults are needed[6,7]

Continuous intravenous sedation dose 200 to 300 mg/kg/min when used for TIVA

Elimination

Conjugation occurs in the liver, which leads to inactive metabolites that are renally excreted. Clearance is greater than hepatic blood flow and the high clearance can lead to rapid recovery after infusions.

Medication Profile

1. *Cardiovascular effects*: Propofol decreases blood pressure by lowering systemic vascular resistance, increasing venous capacitance, and decreasing cardiac contractility (decreasing sympathetic tone).[8] Factors associated with hypotension are prematurity, large doses, rapid bolusing, and patients that have poor LV contractility. Fall in systemic vascular resistance can lead to a decreased pulmonary blood flow (Qp<Qs) and arterial desaturation in patients with congenital heart disease that have a cardiac shunt.[9]

2. *Respiratory effects*: Propofol inhibits the response of the respiratory centers to hypercarbia and hypoxia.[10] It causes dose-dependent decrease in tidal volume, minute ventilation, and ventilatory drive and at induction doses extreme respiratory depression leading to apnea. Propofol can cause profound loss of muscle tone in the upper airway causing obstruction, while also depressing airway reflexes, useful in the treatment of laryngospasm. Although it can cause histamine release, it mostly causes bronchodilation and therefore has a lower incidence of wheezing than etomidate or thiopental.

3. *CNS effects*: Propofol decreases cerebral metabolic activity and oxygen demand, causing decreases in cerebral blood flow and intracranial pressure.[11] Due to its effect on blood pressure, leading to hypotension, propofol can lower cerebral perfusion pressure. Cerebral autoregulation and CO_2 vascular reactivity are maintained.[12] Propofol is an excellent hypnotic but a poor analgesic. Propofol has antiepileptic properties and can be used for patients that are acutely seizing and has been used in the treatment of status epilepticus. It has been known to cause dystonia.

Caution

Prolonged propofol infusions (24 hours) can lead to propofol infusion syndrome (PRIS), which is a syndrome defined by metabolic acidosis, rhabdomyolysis, lipemia, hepatomegaly, and possibly an increase in serum lactate and can often times be fatal. It is hypothesized that propofol can cause either direct inhibition of the mitochondrial respiratory chain or deficient mitochondrial fatty acid metabolism.[13] This syndrome has the propensity to occur in patients who are concurrently treated with catecholamines and steroids.[14]

Propofol inhibits multiple mitochondrial pathways and should be used judiciously (single induction dose) in patients with mitochondrial disease.

KETAMINE

Ketamine is a phencyclidine derivative and has multiple effects throughout the central nervous system (CNS).

Clinical Uses

1. *Procedural sedation*: It is used frequently in the emergency department for procedural sedation. When added in a low dose with propofol, it can decrease the respiratory depression associated with propofol.[15]

2. *Induction of general anesthesia*: It is used in patients with increased sympathetic activity whereby the sympathetic reserve is not depleted. It is also used in situations where hemodynamic instability is evident and heart

rate is desired to be elevated (ie, hypotension in cardiac tamponade), or when the patient needs to be spontaneously breathing (difficult airway).[16]

3. *Analgesia*: It has been used perioperatively for analgesia in lower doses either as a bolus or as infusion and to decrease opioid requirements and opioid-induced hyperalgesia.[17] It is also used in the treatment of complex regional pain.

Mechanism of Action

It is an NMDA receptor antagonist and primarily works by dissociating the thalamus from the limbic cortex, known as "dissociative anesthesia." The S(+) isomer has increased potency due to its greater affinity for the NMDA receptor but is unavailable in the United States.

Pharmacokinetics

Absorption

Ketamine is usually given intravenously but can also be administered intramuscularly especially in the case of special needs children or for IV placement when the child is agitated.

Distribution

Ketamine is very lipid soluble, which leads to rapid brain uptake and distribution. Awakening occurs due to redistribution peripherally.

Biotransformation

Ketamine has very high hepatic clearance with an extraction ratio of 0.9. It is biotransformed into different metabolites, one of which is norketamine that exhibits anesthetic activity. Tolerance can develop to ketamine.

Excretion

Ketamine is mostly metabolized in the liver and the products of ketamine biotransformation are excreted renally.

Medication Profile

1. *Cardiovascular effects*: Ketamine causes increased blood pressure, heart rate, and cardiac output. These effects are due to increased sympathetic stimulation and inhibition of norepinephrine reuptake. Ketamine should be given cautiously in patients with uncontrolled hypertension because of its sympathetic tone stimulation. In patients that are sympathetically depleted, ketamine has direct myocardial depressant effects. Although there have been concerns for increased pulmonary vascular resistance due to ketamine, studies suggest that if ventilation is maintained, there is not an increase in pulmonary vascular resistance.[16,18,19]

2. *Respiratory effects*: The respiratory system is minimally affected by doses of ketamine, but rapid IV bolus can still cause apnea. Racemic ketamine is an extremely potent bronchodilator, but the S(+) enantiomer produces minimal bronchodilation. Laryngeal reflexes are usually left intact though laryngospasm may occur due to increased salivation, which can be attenuated with an antisialagogue.

3. *CNS effects*: Ketamine is associated with increased cerebral oxygen demand, and cerebral blood flow. It has been associated with increased intracranial pressure in the past, but more recent data debunked that association. Ketamine increases somatosensory evoked potentials. Patients' eyes may remain open with spontaneous eye movements and nystagmus. Ketamine is the most complete anesthetic in that it provides amnesia as well as analgesia. It causes hallucinations and bad dreams. Hallucinations can be attenuated with a dose of midazolam or propofol.

Caution

Ketamine has a higher incidence of nausea than either propofol or thiopental (barbiturate).

ETOMIDATE

Etomidate works by mimicking the inhibitory effects of GABA. Etomidate binds to GABA(A) receptor and increases the receptor's affinity for GABA. Etomidate contains a carboxylated imidazole ring and is dissolved in propylene glycol for injection. This solution causes pain on injection, which can be pretreated with lidocaine, but is still painful for many.

Pharmacokinetics

Absorption

Available only for intravenous injection with immediate action.

Distribution

Very rapid onset of action due to its lipid solubility and large nonionized fraction at physiological pH. Redistribution is the primary cause of decreasing plasma levels after injection and reawakening.

Biotransformation

Hepatic microsomal enzyme system and plasma esterases rapidly hydrolyze etomidate to an inactive metabolite.

Excretion

Hydrolyzed end products are excreted in the urine.

Medication Profile

1. *Cardiovascular effects*: It is noted to be a very stable cardiovascular induction agent.[20,21] Cardiac output and myocardial contractility usually remain unhindered.

2. *Respiratory effects*: Ventilation is less affected with etomidate than other induction agents.

3. *CNS effects*: It decreases cerebral metabolic activity, cerebral blood flow, and intracranial pressure. Etomidate increases the evoked potentials of somatosensory evoked potentials (SSEPs).

4. *Endocrine*: Etomidate hinders production of cortisol and aldosterone by reversibly inhibiting enzymes involved in their synthesis (11 beta-hydroxylase). Critically ill patients may be disserviced by etomidate administration, the one induction agent that is considered to maintain hemodynamic stability. Even one dose in pediatric patients produces decreased adrenal function and 11 beta-hydroxylase activity for a minimum of 24 hours.[22–24] Therefore, it is prudent to consider an alternative to etomidate in the critically ill patient.

Caution

Myoclonus can be observed due to disinhibitory effects on the extrapyramidal system.

Postoperative nausea and vomiting are more common than with other induction agents. Etomidate lacks analgesic properties.

DEXMEDETOMIDINE

Dexmedetomidine is a more selective alpha-2 adrenergic agonist and eight times more selective than clonidine. It mimics natural sleep and reduces sympathetic activity. Dexmedetomidine causes analgesia at the level of the spinal cord and hypnosis by stimulation of the locus coeruleus. It is most commonly administered intravenously and intranasally. It undergoes rapid hepatic metabolism by hydroxylation and conjugation.

Clinical Uses

1. *Premedication*: –Intranasal administration 0.5 to 1 mcg/kg.[25]

2. *Procedural sedation for radiological procedures*: MRI/CT (1–2 mcg/kg).

3. Facilitating sedated intubation in children.

4. *As an anesthetic adjunct*: Decreases intraoperative narcotic requirements, helps to maintain spontaneous ventilation.

5. Prophylaxis for or treatment of emergence delirium.

Medication Profile

1. *Cardiovascular effects*: Dexmedetomidine causes decreased HR and increased blood pressure due to increased systemic vascular resistance when given as a bolus. The decreased HR is a response to increased systemic vascular resistance and increased blood pressure most likely due to increased postsynaptic alpha-2 receptor stimulation on vascular smooth muscle.[26] As the central alpha-2 effects take hold, the SVR will come down with a slow increase in the HR.

2. *Respiratory effects*: Dexmedetomidine causes very little respiratory depression and the ventilatory response to hypercarbia is minimal. Upper airway obstruction can occur during sedation.

3. *CNS effects*: Dexmedetomidine decreases cerebral blood flow without significant changes in intracranial hemodynamics.

Caution

Dexmedetomidine's context-sensitive half-time increases considerably with increasing duration of the infusion.

BENZODIAZEPINES

Benzodiazepines are sedative-hypnotics that contain a benzene ring fused with a diazepine ring. The three commonly used benzodiazepines are midazolam (short acting), lorazepam (intermediate acting), and diazepam (long acting).

Midazolam's imidazole ring allows it to be water soluble at low pH.

Diazepam and lorazepam are insoluble in water and therefore are dissolved in propylene glycol which can cause irritation upon injection.

Clinical Uses

1. *Premedication*: Midazolam is the most commonly administered premedication. It is usually given orally in pediatric patients without an intravenous catheter in place. It can also be administered intramuscularly or intranasally. Intranasal administration can be irritating.

2. *Procedural sedation*

3. *Treatment of seizures*: Benzodiazepines all decrease seizure activity and can be used in the treatment of seizures.

4. *Induction of anesthesia*: Infrequent use with the addition of opioids.

Pharmacokinetics

Metabolism

Metabolized by the liver through microsomal oxidation or glucuronide conjugation.

Absorption

Benzodiazepines are administered orally (midazolam 40%, lorazepam/diazepam 90%), intramuscularly, and intravenously.

Distribution

Midazolam is highly lipid soluble, which leads to quick redistribution going from the brain to peripheral inactive sites.

Pharmacodynamics

Benzodiazepines bind to GABA(A) receptor and change the conformation of the GABA receptor causing it to have more affinity for GABA molecules, increasing chloride ions. They have a favorable safety profile with less respiratory and cardiovascular depression when compared to barbiturates and propofol. Benzodiazepines also have a short-acting antagonist (flumazenil) used to reverse sedative effects when needed.

Medication Profile

1. *Cardiovascular effects*: Benzodiazepines can cause peripheral vasodilation with little change in cardiac output. In conjunction with fentanyl they can decrease blood pressure.
2. *Respiratory effects*: They cause a decrease in respiration due to a decrease in response to arterial carbon dioxide.
3. *CNS effects*: Benzodiazepines decrease $CMRO_2$ and cerebral blood flow, but less than barbiturates. They have a ceiling effect and are unable to cause an isoelectric EEG; therefore, they are not used in cerebral protection during focal injuries. They act as antiepileptics and can be used in the treatment of status epilepticus.

Midazolam Dosing

0.3 to 0.5 mg/kg orally (max 10–15 mg).

0.1 mg/kg intravenously.

0.2 mg/kg intranasally/intramuscularly.

Caution

Intravenous induction of general anesthesia takes a much higher dose and is slower than propofol, thiopental, or etomidate. The delayed awakening when compared to other agents makes the use of midazolam or diazepam for induction much less common.

BARBITURATES

Barbiturates used to be the most common intravenous anesthetic drugs prior to the advent of propofol. Barbiturates come from derivatives of barbituric acid. Substitutions at N1, C2, and C5 lead to different properties for each of the drugs in this class. The only intravenous anesthetic commonly used in the United States is methohexital (oxybarbiturate). Barbiturate solutions can precipitate with acidic drugs (non-depolarizing neuromuscular blockers-e.g.-vecuronium, rocuronium, cisatracurium) since they are alkaline with a pH of 10 which in turn can lead to crystallization of intravenous lines. Arterial injection or intravenous infiltration can lead to severe pain and tissue injury.

Clinical Uses

1. *Induction of anesthesia*: The short-acting methohexital can be used for induction of general anesthesia.
2. Total intravenous anesthesia (TIVA).

Pharmacokinetics

Thiopental is highly lipid soluble and its high nonionized fraction leads to rapid uptake in the brain. If there is hypoalbuminemia, hypovolemia, or acidosis, there can be higher concentrations delivered to the brain and heart.

Biotransformation

Hepatic oxidation is the primary route of elimination to inactive water-soluble metabolites which are excreted by the kidneys. The exception to this is phenobarbital which is primarily excreted by renal excretion.

Medication Profile

1. *Cardiovascular effects*: Thiopental tends to cause a reduction in MAP by centrally mediated inhibition of the sympathetic nervous system and direct myocardial inhibition.[27] The reduction in MAP is less than that of propofol.[28] There is vasodilation of the peripheral capacitance vessels due to depression of the medullary vasomotor center. Tachycardia occurs due to reflex response to blood pressure. There may be an exaggerated fall in blood pressure in patients with hypovolemia, congestive heart failure, and beta-blockade.
2. *Respiratory effects*: Depression of the medullary ventilatory center leads to decreased responses to hypercapnia and hypoxia. Barbiturates depress upper airway tone and lead to upper airway obstruction and apnea. Minute ventilation is decreased along with a decrease in tidal volumes and respiratory rate. Thiopental can rarely cause bronchoconstrictive effects (cholinergic nerve stimulation) especially in patients with asthma but methohexital does not share that characteristic.
3. *Cerebral*: Barbiturates decrease cerebral metabolic rate, cerebral blood flow, cerebral blood volume, and intracranial pressure but increase cerebral vasoconstriction. Cerebral perfusion pressure is usually maintained due to a greater reduction of intracranial pressure than mean arterial blood pressure. Barbiturates at higher doses can lead to burst suppression and electrical silence. Barbiturates do not have analgesic properties at induction doses.

Thiopental is mentioned above as one of the representatives of the barbiturate class, but it is NO longer available for use in the United States.

METHOHEXITAL

It is an ultrashort-acting barbiturate with a protein binding of about 70%. It is cleared rapidly by the liver after demethylation and oxidation and subsequent renal elimination.

Administration: Intravenous, intramuscular, rectal.

Redistribution of methohexital leads to awakening just like thiopental. An induction intravenous dose can lead to reawakening within 5 to 10 minutes. It can be given in place of propofol for induction in patients in whom there is possible concern with propofol, eg, mitochondrial disorders, propofol allergy.[29]

Caution

Methohexital potentiates cerebral evoked potentials, decreases seizure threshold, and can cause seizures unlike the other barbiturates.

On IV administration it can cause patients to hiccup, become apneic, and have dystonic movements.

REFERENCES

1. Unlugenc H, Guler T, Gunes Y, Isik G. Comparative study of the antiemetic efficacy of ondansetron, propofol, and midazolam in the early postoperative period. *Eur J Anaesthesiol.* 2004;21(1):60-65.
2. Murphy A, Campbell DE, Baines D, Mehr S. Allergic reactions to propofol in egg-allergic children. *Anesth Analg.* 2011;113(1):140-144.
3. Gan TJ, Diemunsch P, Habib AS, et al. Consensus guidelines for the management of postoperative nausea and vomiting. *Anesth Analg.* 2014;118: 85-113.
4. Glass PS. Half-time or half-time: what matters for recovery from intravenous anesthesia? *Anesthesiology.* 2010;112:1266-1269.
5. Hughes MA, Glass PS, Jacobs JR. Context-sensitive half-time in multi-compartment pharmacokinetic models for intravenous anesthetic drugs. *Anesthesiology.* 1992;76:334-341.
6. Rigouzzo A, Girault L, Louvet N, et al. The relationship between bispectral index and propofol during target-controlled infusion anesthesia. *Anesth Analg.* 2008;106(4):1109-1116.
7. McFarlan CS, Anderson BJ, Short TG. The use of propofol infusions in pediatric anesthesia: a practical guide. *Paediatr Anesth.* 1999;9(3):209-216.
8. Robinson BJ, Ebert TJ, OBrien TJ, Colinco MD, Muzi M. Mechanisms whereby propofol mediates peripheral vasodilation in humans: sympathoinhibition or direct vascular relaxation? *Anesthesiology.* 1997;86(1):64-72.
9. Williams GD, Jones TK, Hanson KA, Morray JP. The hemodynamic effects of propofol in children with congenital heart disease. *Anesth Analg.* 1999;89(6):1411-1416.
10. Jonsson MM, Lindahl SG, Eriksson LI. Effect of propofol on carotid body chemosensitivity and cholinergic chemotransduction. *Anesthesiology.* 2005;102(1):110-116.
11. Szabo EZ, Liginbuehl I, Bissonette B. Impact of anesthetic agents on cerebrovascular physiology in children. *Paediatr Anesth.* 2009;19(2):108-118.
12. Matta BF, Lam AM, Strebel S, Mayberg TS. Cerebral pressure autoregulation and carbon dioxide reactivity during propofol-induced EEG suppression. *Br J Anesth.* 1995;74(2):159-163.
13. Kam PC, Cardone D. Propofol infusion syndrome. *Anesthesia.* 2007;62(7):690-7015.
14. Vasile B, Rasulo F, Candiani A, Latronico N. The pathophysiology of propofol infusion syndrome: a simple name for a complex syndrome. *Intensive Care Med.* 2003;29(9):1417-1425.
15. Montero RF, Clark LD, Tolan MM, Metz RJ, Tsueda K, Sheppard RA. The effects of small-dose ketamine on propofol sedation: respiration, postoperative mood, perception, cognition, and pain. *Anesth Analg.* 2001;92(6):1465-1469.
16. Morray JP, Lynn AM, Stamm SJ, Herndon PS, Kawabori I, Stevenson J. Hemodynamic effects of ketamine in children with congenital heart disease. *Anesth Analg.* 1984;63(10):895-899.
17. Himmelseher S, Durieux M. Ketamine for perioperative pain management. *Anesthesiology.* 2005;102:211-220.
18. Hickey PR, Hansen DD, Cramolini GM, Vencent RN, Lang P. Pulmonary and systemic hemodynamic responses to ketamine in infants with normal and elevated pulmonary vascular resistance. *Anesthesiology.* 1985;62(3):287-293.
19. Williams GD, Philip BM, Chu LF, et al. Ketamine does not increase pulmonary vascular resistance in children with pulmonary hypertension undergoing sevoflurane anesthesia and spontaneous ventilation. *Anesth Analg.* 2007;105(6):1578-1584.
20. Sarkar M, Laussen PC, Zurakowski D, et al. Hemodynamic responses to etomidate on induction of anesthesia in pediatric patients. *Anesth Analg.* 2005;101(3):645-665.
21. Guldner G, Schultz J, Sexton P, et al. Etomidate for rapid sequence intubation in young children: hemodynamic effects and adverse events. *Acad Meg Med.* 2003;10(2):134-139.
22. de Jong FH, Mallios C, Jansen C, et al. Etomidate suppresses adrenocortical function by inhibition of 11 beta-hydroxylation. *J Clin Endocrinol Metab.* 1984;59:1143-1147.
23. den Brinker M, Joosten KFM, Liem O, et al. Adrenal insufficiency in meningococcal sepsis: bioavailability cortisol levels and impact of interleukin-6 levels and intubation with etomidate on adrenal function and mortality. *J Clin Endocrinol Metab.* 2005;90:5110-5117.
24. den Brinker M, Hokken-Koelega ACS, Hazelzet JA, et al. One single dose of etomidate negatively influences adrenocortical performance for at least 24 hours in children with meningococcal sepsis. *Intensive Care Med.* 2008;34:163-168.
25. Yuen VM, Hui TW, Irwin MG, Yuen MK. A comparison of intranasal dexmedetomidine and oral midazolam for premedication in pediatric anesthesia: a double-blinded randomized controlled trial. *Anesth Analg.* 2008;106:1715-1721.
26. Dyck JB, Maze M, Haack C, et al. The pharmacokinetics and hemodynamic effects of intravenous and intramuscular dexmedetomidine hydrochloride in adult human volunteers. *Anesthesiology.* 1993;78(5):813-820.
27. Komai H, Rusy BF. Effect of thiopental on Ca^{+2} release from sarcoplasmic reticulum in intact myocardium. *Anesthesiology.* 1994;81:946-952.
28. Aun CS, Sung RY, O'Meara ME, et al. Cardiovascular effects of i.v. induction in children: comparison between propofol and thiopentone. *Br J Anaesth.* 1993;70(6):647-653.
29. Jones NE, Kelleman MS, Simon HK, et al. Evaluation of methohexital as an alternative to propofol in a high-volume outpatient pediatric sedation service. *Am J Emerg Med.* 2017;35(8):1101-1105.

Muscle Relaxants

Albert C. Yeung

FOCUS POINTS

1. Neuromuscular blocking drugs (NMBDs) are quaternary ammonium compounds that have structural similarities to acetylcholine (Ach).
2. The *potency* of a NMBD is a measure of the dose required to produce the corresponding twitch suppression.
3. The *onset time* is the time from administration to maximum blockade.
4. The *duration of action* is the time to return to 25% of baseline single twitch height (T25).
5. Succinylcholine is the only clinically available depolarizing NMBD and is hydrolyzed by plasma cholinesterase (also referred to as butyrylcholinesterase or pseudocholinesterase).
6. The efficacy of a patient's plasma cholinesterase can be expressed by the dibucaine number.
7. Contraindications to succinylcholine administration include personal or family history of malignant hyperthermia, known or suspected myopathy, hyperkalemia, and medical conditions that result in increased extrajunctional acetylcholine receptors such as burns, trauma, and immobility.
8. The routine use of succinylcholine in infants and children should be avoided due to the risk of hyperkalemic cardiac arrest in patients with undiagnosed skeletal muscle myopathy.
9. There are two chemical classes of clinically available nondepolarizing NMBDs: the aminosteroid compounds (pancuronium, vecuronium, rocuronium) and the benzylisoquinolinium compounds (atracurium, cisatracurium, mivacurium).

10. There are two classes of agents for reversal of neuromuscular blockade: anticholinesterases and cyclodextrins.

PHYSIOLOGY OF THE NEUROMUSCULAR JUNCTION

The neuromuscular junction consists of the prejunctional motor neuron, synaptic cleft, and postsynaptic endplate of the skeletal muscle membrane (Figure 7-1).[1] Neuromuscular transmission begins when an action potential in the prejunctional motor neuron reaches the nerve terminal. The arrival of the action potential triggers the opening of voltage-gated calcium channels, leading to the influx of calcium ions. The increase in calcium results in fusion of vesicles containing acetylcholine (ACh) molecules with the membrane of the nerve terminal, thus releasing ACh into the synaptic cleft by exocytosis. ACh serves as the neurotransmitter at the neuromuscular junction and is synthesized and stored in vesicles at the motor nerve terminal.[2]

ACh released into the synaptic cleft diffuses to the motor endplate and binds to nicotinic ACh receptors. The ACh receptor consists of five subunits arranged in a rosette to form an ion channel. The simultaneous binding of two ACh molecules to the two α subunits of the ACh receptor causes the channel to open, allowing inward movement of sodium ions and outward movement of potassium ions. The increase in intracellular sodium depolarizes the membrane, generating an action potential that propagates along the length of the muscle fiber, leading to muscular contraction. Once in the synaptic cleft, ACh is rapidly hydrolyzed by acetylcholinesterase. The motor nerve ending also reuptakes ACh.[3]

ACh receptors are located at prejunctional, postjunctional, and extrajunctional locations and have different

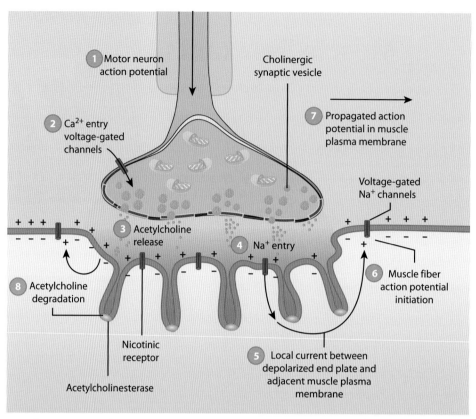

▲ Figure 7-1. The neuromuscular junction. (Adapted with permission, from Widmaier EP, Raff H, Strang KT: *Vander's Human Physiology: The Mechanisms of Body Function.* 11th ed. 2008. Copyright © McGraw Hill LLC. All rights reserved.)

composition of subunits. The prejunctional ACh receptors are composed of two α3 and three β2 subunits and are thought to modulate ACh release via a positive feedback system to mobilize ACh vesicles. The adult postjunctional ACh receptor is composed of two α1, one β1, one δ, and one ε subunit (α2βδε) (Figure 7-2).[4,5] In the fetal ACh receptor, the ε subunit is replaced by a γ subunit (α2βδγ) (Figure 7-3).[6] During early development, fetal ACh receptors are present throughout the length of the muscle fiber. Late in fetal development, the γ subunit is replaced by the ε subunit, such that at term a neonate has both adult and fetal ACh receptors, with a predominance of adult ACh receptors.[7] Extrajunctional ACh receptors are located outside of the neuromuscular junction and have the same structure as fetal ACh receptors. Synthesis of extrajunctional receptors is suppressed under normal conditions.

NEUROMUSCULAR TRANSMISSION IN THE NEONATE

Neuromuscular transmission in the neonate differs from older children and adults. At birth, infants have both fetal and adult ACh receptors. The adult subtype replaces the fetal subtype during the first 2 to 4 years of life. Compared to the adult subtype, the fetal ACh receptor is a low-conductance channel. The fetal subtype has a slower response to ACh and has a prolonged open channel time once it is depolarized.[8] The fetal receptor is more sensitive to succinylcholine and more resistant to nondepolarizing neuromuscular blockers compared to the adult subtype. Neonates younger than 2 months deplete acetylcholine reserves faster than older infants in response to tetanic nerve stimulation.[9,10]

NEUROMUSCULAR MONITORING

Neuromuscular junction function is assessed by visual, tactile, or recording of the response of a peripheral nerve to electrical stimulation. Neuromuscular monitoring assesses the depth and recovery of blockade after administration of a NMBD. Superficial electrodes are placed over a peripheral nerve and various patterns of supra-maximal electrical stimulation are applied. Commonly, the adductor pollicis muscle of the thumb is monitored by

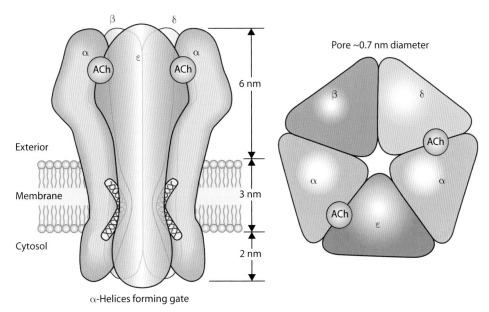

▲ **Figure 7-2.** The adult acetylcholine receptor composed of two α, one β, one δ, and one ε subunits (α2βδε) arranged in a rosette. (Reproduced with permission, from Mashour GA, Lydic R, eds. *The Neuroscientific Foundations of Anesthesiology.* 2011. Copyright © Oxford University Press. All rights reserved.)

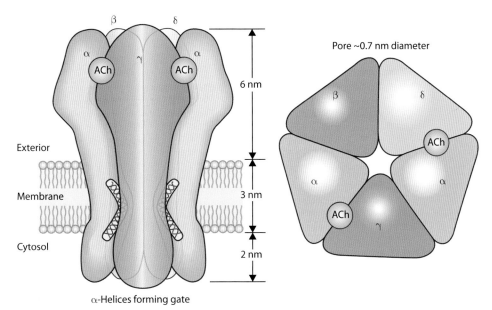

▲ **Figure 7-3.** The fetal acetylcholine receptor is similar in structure to the adult acetylcholine receptor, except the ε subunit is replaced by a γ subunit (α2βδγ). Extrajunctional acetylcholine receptors have the same composition. (Reproduced with permission, from Mashour GA, Lydic R, eds. *The Neuroscientific Foundations of Anesthesiology.* 2011. Copyright © Oxford University Press. All rights reserved.)

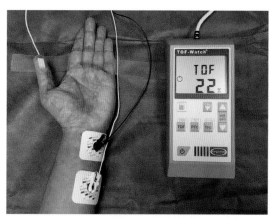

▲ **Figure 7-4.** Nerve monitoring based on acceleromyography provides a quantitative assessment of neuromuscular blockade. The display shows the train of four ratio as a percentage. (Photo courtesy of Dr. Albert C. Yeung.)

stimulation of the ulnar nerve. Other muscles such as the orbicularis oculi muscle of the face and the flexor hallucis muscle of the foot can also be monitored. NMBDs have different effects on various muscle groups with respect to time of onset, depth, and duration of action. For example, the dose of pancuronium in infants and children for blockade of the diaphragm is higher than for the adductor pollicis.[11] Recovery of the central muscles is also faster than for peripheral muscles. In this regard, recovery of peripheral neuromuscular function suggests that the vocal cords and diaphragm are at a more advanced state of recovery.

Assessment of the response to a stimulus can be qualitative or quantitative. The easiest and least expensive method is qualitative with visual or tactile evaluation. However, even experienced anesthesiologists may be unable to detect fade using subjective evaluation of train-of-four stimulation.[12] Various methods can be used for objective monitoring. Commercially available monitors for quantitative measurement are based on the acceleration of the muscle response (acceleromyography) (Figure 7-4), the electrical response of the muscle (electromyography), and the evoked electrical response from a piezoelectric sensor attached to the muscle (kinemyography).[13]

PATTERNS OF STIMULI

Modes of stimulation in clinical practice include single twitch, train-of-four ratio, tetanic stimulation, post-tetanic stimulation, and double burst suppression (Figure 7-5).[14] In single twitch, a single stimulus at intervals greater than 10 seconds is applied to a nerve. The amplitude response after administration of a NMBD is compared to the baseline twitch before neuromuscular blockade. The depth of blockade is expressed as the percentage block from baseline. Clinical use of single twitch monitoring is limited because a control value is required.

Train-of-four (TOF) stimulation is the most commonly used pattern of monitoring for nondepolarizing neuromuscular blockade. Unlike single twitch, no baseline measurement is required. TOF stimulation consists of four supramaximal stimuli given every 0.5 seconds. Each successive stimulus depletes ACh, resulting in a "fade" in the setting of partial neuromuscular blockade. The TOF ratio is the amplitude of the fourth twitch compared to the first twitch. Prior to administration of a NMBD, the TOF ratio should be 1.0. Full-term infants under 1 month of age and premature infants have a reduced ratio, likely reflective of the immature neuromuscular junction. By the age of 2 months, the TOF ratio is near 1.0.[15] In clinical practice, a TOF ratio of >0.9 indicates adequate recovery from neuromuscular blockade.[16]

With TOF monitoring, the depolarizing block from succinylcholine initially produces what is referred to as a phase 1 block. As twitches return after a single dose of succinylcholine, all four twitches are decreased by a similar amount such that there is no fade and the TOF ratio remains near 1.0 (Figure 7-6).[17] With increasing doses of succinylcholine, such as with a large single dose or repeated doses, a phase 2 block can develop. A phase 2 block shows fade with TOF stimulation like a nondepolarizing blockade.[18]

Tetanus is the rapid delivery of electrical stimulus, most commonly for 5 seconds at 50 hertz (Hz). At baseline, such a stimulus does not result in fade. In the presence of nondepolarizing neuromuscular blockade, tetanic fade is present. Tetanic stimulation can be used to detect residual neuromuscular blockade but is painful in an unanesthetized patient. Tetanic stimulation increases quantities of ACh in the neuromuscular junction, producing post-tetanic facilitation with a brief period of increased twitch tension after tetanic stimulation.[19]

Post-tetanic count (PTC) stimulation can be used to monitor the degree of neuromuscular blockade after a large dose of a nondepolarizing NMBD. With profound blockade, there is no contractile response to single twitch or TOF stimulus. PTC is based on the principle of post-tetanic facilitation. To assess PTC, a tetanic stimulus is followed by a 3-second pause and then a series of single-twitch stimuli at 1 Hz. As the profound block dissipates, post-tetanic twitches will be visible. In children who have received 1 mg/kg of rocuronium, the presence of one PTC twitch predicts the return of response to TOF stimulation in 7 minutes.[20]

Double-burst stimulation (DBS) is two short tetanic stimulations at 50-Hz separated by 750 milliseconds. The ratio of the second to the first stimulus is assessed for fade. DBS was developed as a method to manually detect fade that cannot be perceived in TOF monitoring. The ability of the anesthesiologist to manually detect fade in both children and adults is greater with DBS than with TOF

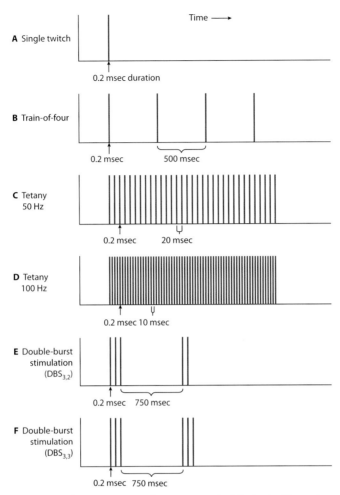

A Single twitch

0.2 msec duration

B Train-of-four

0.2 msec   500 msec

C Tetany
50 Hz

0.2 msec   20 msec

D Tetany
100 Hz

0.2 msec 10 msec

E Double-burst
stimulation
(DBS$_{3,2}$)

0.2 msec   750 msec

F Double-burst
stimulation
(DBS$_{3,3}$)

0.2 msec 750 msec

▲ **Figure 7-5.** Modes of stimulation for monitoring of neuromuscular blockade. (Reproduced with permission, from Butterworth IV JF, Mackey DC, Wasnick JD. eds. *Morgan & Mikhail's Clinical Anesthesiology,* 6th ed. 2013. http:// accessanesthesiology.mhmedical.com. Copyright © McGraw Hill LLC. All rights reserved.)

monitoring.[21] However, the absence of fade with DBS is not an indicator that the TOF ratio is >0.9.

MECHANISM OF ACTION OF NEUROMUSCULAR BLOCKING DRUGS

NMBDs are quaternary ammonium compounds that have structural similarities to ACh. The drugs can be classified as depolarizing or nondepolarizing NMBDs. Succinylcholine is the only depolarizing NMBD in clinical use. It is composed of two ACh molecules linked together by their methyl groups and mimics ACh by binding to the ACh receptor, resulting in opening of the ion channel. Depolarization of the postjunctional membrane generates muscle contraction (fasciculations), followed by a period of relaxation as the motor end plate remains depolarized. Unlike ACh, succinylcholine is not hydrolyzed by acetylcholinesterase at the neuromuscular junction and is instead eliminated in the plasma by plasma cholinesterase (also referred to as butyrylcholinesterase or pseudocholinesterase).[22]

Nondepolarizing NMBDs impair neuromuscular transmission primarily as competitive antagonists of ACh by blocking the binding of endogenous ACh to its postjunctional receptor.[23] They competitively bind the α subunit of postjunctional ACh receptors, preventing depolarization. No fasciculations occur with the onset of blockade.[24]

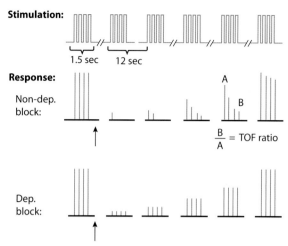

Stimulation:

1.5 sec   12 sec

Response:

Non-dep.
block:

$\dfrac{B}{A}$ = TOF ratio

Dep.
block:

▲ Figure 7-6. Train-of-four monitoring after administration of nondepolarizing and depolarizing NMBDs. (Reproduced with permission, from Freeman BS, Berger JS. eds. *Anesthesiology Core Review: Part One Basic Exam.* 2014. http://accessanesthesiology.mhmedical.com. Copyright © McGraw Hill LLC. All rights reserved.)

PHARMACOLOGIC PROPERTIES OF NEUROMUSCULAR BLOCKING DRUGS

The *potency* of a NMBD is a measure of the dose required to produce the corresponding twitch suppression. The effective dose 95 (ED95) of a NMBD is the dose that produces a 95% depression of the single twitch height. In general, a dose of two to three times the ED95 is suggested to achieve intubating conditions. Recommended maintenance doses are ¼ to ⅓ of the intubating dose. The *onset time* is the time from administration to maximum blockade. Potent drugs have a slower onset time compared to less potent ones. The *duration of action* is the time to return to 25% of baseline single twitch height (T25). Medications that have rapid plasma clearance have a shorter duration of action compared to agents that are slowly eliminated from the plasma. The *recovery index* is the duration between 25% and 75% recovery of twitch height.[25,26]

Infants and children exhibit some differences compared to adults in their pharmacologic responses to NMBDs. The factors contributing to the variations may be due to age-related differences in the maturity of the neuromuscular junction, the volume of distribution, and clearance. In particular, infants are more sensitive to NMBDs compared to children and adults.[27] The onset time tends to be faster in infants compared to older children and adults, but the duration of action and recovery index are longer in infants compared to children.[28] The ED95 value tends to be higher in children than in infants and adults.[29]

DEPOLARIZING NEUROMUSCULAR BLOCKING DRUG: SUCCINYLCHOLINE

Succinylcholine is the only clinically available depolarizing NMBD. It binds the ACh receptor at the neuromuscular junction, resulting in depolarization of the postjunctional membrane. Succinylcholine has a rapid onset time and a short duration of action in most individuals, which makes it an ideal drug for a rapid-sequence induction for intubation. Depolarization of the postjunctional membrane manifests as general skeletal muscle contractions known as fasciculations, followed by relaxation.

► Pharmacology of Succinylcholine

The dose requirement for succinylcholine is higher in infants and children compared to adults. The ED90 in neonates and infants are 517 and 608 mcg/kg, respectively, compared to 290 mcg/kg in adults. The higher ED90 may be reflective of the higher volume of distribution in infants and children. The suggested intubating dose is 3 mg/kg for infants and 1.5 to 2 mg/kg for children, compared to 1 mg/kg in adults.[30] Succinylcholine can also be administered intramuscularly. For children, 3 to 4 mg/kg of intramuscular succinylcholine will provide relaxation for intubation.[31] For treatment of laryngospasm, a much lower dose (such as 0.1 mg/kg) may be sufficient to allow positive pressure ventilation.[32] As succinylcholine both rapidly reaches the neuromuscular junction and becomes hydrolyzed by plasma cholinesterase, the maximum effect is achieved quickly. The elimination half-life is less than 1 minute.

The duration of action for succinylcholine is prolonged in patients with decreased or abnormal plasma cholinesterase. Plasma cholinesterase is synthesized by the liver. Plasma cholinesterase deficiency in the setting of severe disease may lead to moderate increases in the duration of action. Patients with atypical variants of plasma cholinesterase that result in decreased enzyme activity or quantity will experience prolonged blockade after administration of

Table 7-1. Dibucaine Number and Response to Succinylcholine

Type of Plasma Cholinesterase	Homozygous Typical	Heterozygous	Homozygous Atypical
Dibucaine number (% inhibition)	70–80	50–60	20–30
Duration of blockade	Normal	Lengthened 50–100%	Lengthened 4–8 h

succinylcholine.[33] In patients who are heterozygous with one atypical allele of plasma cholinesterase, the duration of the block from succinylcholine may be lengthened 50% to 100%. A patient who is homozygous for atypical plasma cholinesterase may have blockade for several hours.[34]

The efficacy of a patient's plasma cholinesterase can be expressed by the dibucaine number (Table 7-1). Dibucaine is a local anesthetic that inhibits the activity of normal plasma cholinesterase by about 70% to 80%.[35] The dibucaine number is expressed as the percent inhibition of this enzyme. Thus, a patient with normal enzymatic activity will have a dibucaine number of 70 to 80. Patients heterozygous for atypical plasma cholinesterase will have inhibition of 50% to 60% and those who are homozygous will have inhibition of about 20% to 30%.

Side Effects of Succinylcholine

While useful for rapid neuromuscular blockade, succinylcholine has multiple adverse side effects that limit its routine use in pediatric anesthesia (Table 7-2).

Cardiac

Due to its structural relationship to ACh, succinylcholine stimulates cholinergic autonomic receptors. Arrhythmias such as bradycardia, junctional rhythms, tachycardia, and ventricular dysrhythmias can occur from administration of succinylcholine.[36] The bradycardia and junctional rhythms may be due to activation of cardiac postganglionic muscarinic receptors, with succinylcholine mimicking the effects of ACh. Bradyarrhythmias can be more pronounced when a second dose of succinylcholine is given but do not seem to occur after intramuscular injection. Administration of an anticholinergic such as atropine can prevent the bradycardic response to succinylcholine.[37] Succinylcholine can also increase catecholamine levels, resulting in tachycardia and ventricular dysrhythmias.

Hyperkalemia

Binding of succinylcholine to the ACh receptor opens the voltage-gated sodium channel, resulting in the influx of sodium ions and the efflux of potassium ions. Administration of succinylcholine results in an increase of up to 1 mEq/L of plasma potassium in children.[38] Patients with denervation injuries, prolonged immobilization, or burn injuries may have upregulation of extrajunctional

Table 7-2. Adverse Side Effects of Succinylcholine

Cardiac
- Bradyarrhythmia
- Junctional rhythm
- Ventricular dysrhythmia
- Tachycardia

Hyperkalemia

Increased intracranial pressure

Increased intraocular pressure

Myalgia

Myoglobinemia

Trismus

Triggering agent for malignant hyperthermia

acetylcholine receptors, leading to an exaggerated hyperkalemic response to succinylcholine. Life-threatening hyperkalemia after succinylcholine can occur in patients with neuromuscular diseases such as muscular dystrophy, upper and lower motor neuron lesions, burns, trauma, and prolonged immobilization from critical illness.[39]

Hyperkalemic cardiac arrest after succinylcholine has been reported in apparently healthy children who were subsequently diagnosed with muscular dystrophy.[40] This led the United States Food and Drug Administration (FDA) to issue a warning that "the use of succinylcholine in pediatric patients should be reserved for emergency intubation or instances where immediate securing of the airway is necessary, eg, laryngospasm, difficult airway, full stomach, or for intramuscular use when a suitable vein is inaccessible."[41]

Increased Intracranial Pressure and Intraocular Pressure

Succinylcholine can increase intracranial pressure. The increase in intracranial pressure may be attenuated by pretreatment with a nondepolarizing NMBD.[42] Intraocular pressure increases about 1 minute after administration of succinylcholine and returns to baseline in 5 to 10 minutes. The increase in intraocular pressure has led to the recommendation that succinylcholine be avoided in patients with an open-eye injury. However, there is scant evidence that use of succinylcholine leads to extrusion of ocular contents in such patients.[43]

Fasciculations, Myalgia, and Myoglobinemia

Fasciculations can be observed in children and adolescents and less commonly in infants. Pretreatment with a low dose (10–30% of ED95) of a nondepolarizing NMBD can prevent fasciculation and may ameliorate resulting muscle pain.[44] Myoglobinemia can occur but is rarely of clinical significance.[45]

Trismus and Malignant Hyperthermia

Masseter jaw rigidity can occur after succinylcholine administration, particularly with halothane anesthesia. In extreme cases, trismus can be so severe that strong force may be required to open the mouth for intubation. Incomplete jaw relaxation can be seen in up to 4.4% of children receiving succinylcholine during halothane anesthesia.[46] Masseter muscle rigidity can be seen with malignant hyperthermia, but masseter spasm alone is not diagnostic. While some have advocated taking malignant hyperthermia precautions if masseter jaw rigidity develops, others propose that masseter spasm alone is not an indication to switch to a non-triggering anesthetic.[47] Succinylcholine is a trigger for malignant hyperthermia in susceptible patients.

INDICATIONS AND CONTRAINDICATIONS FOR SUCCINYLCHOLINE USE IN INFANTS AND CHILDREN

The rapid onset and short duration of action make succinylcholine an ideal agent for rapid-sequence tracheal intubation and for treatment of laryngospasm. With a dose of 2 mg/kg, twitch suppression of 95% occurs within 36 seconds in infants and children.[48] Due to the potential for bradyarrhythmias, administration of atropine 0.01 to 0.02 mg/kg prior to succinylcholine should be considered especially in children with Trisomy 21. An alternative to succinylcholine for a rapid sequence induction is rocuronium 1.2 mg/kg, which can produce intubating conditions similar to those after succinylcholine in children.[49]

The routine use of succinylcholine in infants and children is not advised due to the risk of cardiac arrest and hyperkalemia in children with undiagnosed Duchenne's muscular dystrophy, particularly in males 8 years of age or younger. The FDA has a "black box" warning stating that succinylcholine use in pediatric patients should be limited to emergency airway control. Contraindications to succinylcholine are personal or family history of malignant hyperthermia, known or suspected myopathy, hyperkalemia, and medical conditions that result in increased extrajunctional acetylcholine receptors such as burns, trauma, and immobility.

NONDEPOLARIZING NEUROMUSCULAR BLOCKADE DRUGS

Nondepolarizing NMBDs compete with endogenous ACh at the neuromuscular junction, preventing postjunctional depolarization required for muscle contraction. There are several nondepolarizing NMBDs available for clinical use. Selection of one drug over another should take into account the onset, duration of action, side effects, metabolism, and clearance of the individual medication.

Nondepolarizing NMBDs can be classified according to onset, duration of action, or chemical class. The onset is inversely related to the potency of the drug (Table 7-4). At equipotent doses the onset time is more rapid in drugs with lower potency.[50] The duration of action can be classified as short-acting (duration 10–20 minutes), intermediate-acting (duration 20–50 minutes), and long-acting (duration >50 minutes) (Table 7-3). There are two chemical classes of clinically available nondepolarizing NMBDs: the aminosteroid compounds (pancuronium, vecuronium, rocuronium) and the benzylisoquinolinium compounds (atracurium, cisatracurium, mivacurium).

There are various side effects associated with nondepolarizing NMBDs.[51] An increase in heart rate can be seen with administration of pancuronium and rocuronium. A vagolytic effect appears to occur with pancuronium. With rocuronium, it is unclear whether the increase in heart rate is due to pain on injection (pH adjusted with acetic acid and/or sodium hydroxide) or a direct chronotropic effect. Histamine release, with transient flushing and hypotension, is most frequently associated with benzylisoquinolinium drugs. NMBDs are the most common medication class in anesthetic-related hypersensitivity reactions[52] with anaphylaxis being an uncommon but serious complication. Despite sharing structural similarities to steroids, the aminosteroids do not possess hormonal activity.

Nondepolarizing NMBDs have various modes of metabolism (Table 7-5). The benzylisoquinolinium compounds undergo organ-independent degradation. Mivacurium is metabolized by plasma cholinesterase, atracurium is metabolized by plasma esterase, and both atracurium and cisatracurium undergo Hoffman elimination. The

Table 7-3. Classification of Nondepolarizing NMBDs

Short-acting (duration 10–20 min)
• Mivacurium
Intermediate-acting (duration 20–50 min)
• Atracurium
• Cisatracurium
• Rocuronium
• Vecuronium
Long-acting (duration >50 min)
• Pancuronium

Table 7-4. Comparison of NMBDs for Intubation

Drug	Intubating Dose (mg/kg)	Onset Time (minutes)
Succinylcholine	3 (infant)	0.5–1
	1.5–2 (children)	
Mivacurium	0.25	1.5–2
Atracurium	0.5	1–1.4
Cisatracurium	0.15	2–3
Rocuronium	0.45 (infant)	1.5
	0.6 (children)	
	1.2 (rapid sequence induction in children)	0.7
Vecuronium	0.1	1–2
Pancuronium	0.1	3

aminosteroids depend on organ function for metabolism and clearance, and some have active metabolites. Vecuronium and pancuronium undergo partial hepatic metabolism, and both have active metabolites. Rocuronium is not metabolized. Elimination of the aminosteroids is dependent on the kidney and liver to various degrees (Table 7-5).[53]

SHORT-ACTING NONDEPOLARIZING NMBD

Mivacurium

Mivacurium is a short-acting benzylisoquinolinium that is hydrolyzed by plasma cholinesterase. Mivacurium is

not available in the United States because production was discontinued in 2006, but the drug continues to be in use in Europe. It consists of three isomers, two of which are active. Compared to adults, infants and children have a higher ED95 for mivacurium. The ED95 in children is about 90 mcg/kg. An intubating dose of 0.25 mg/kg has an onset of 1.5 to 2 minutes, with complete recovery in 15 to 20 minutes.[54] Mivacurium undergoes degradation by plasma cholinesterase at a rate slower than that of succinylcholine. This may account for the longer duration of mivacurium compared to succinylcholine. Patients with decreased plasma cholinesterase activity will exhibit a prolonged duration of neuromuscular blockade with mivacurium.[55]

INTERMEDIATE-ACTING NONDEPOLARIZING NMBDS

Atracurium

Atracurium is an intermediate-acting benzylisoquinolinium consisting of 10 stereoisomers. Atracurium undergoes both spontaneous degradation and enzymatic hydrolysis. Under physiologic temperature and pH, atracurium is cleaved into inactive metabolites by the nonenzymatic Hofmann elimination reaction. Ester hydrolysis also occurs by nonspecific plasma esterases that are distinct from the plasma cholinesterase involved in degradation of succinylcholine. Thus, the duration of action of atracurium is not affected in patients with renal impairment, cirrhosis, or atypical plasma cholinesterase.[56] Laudanosine and acrylates are the major metabolites of atracurium from both degradation pathways. At high, nonclinical concentrations, laudanosine stimulates the central nervous system.

Table 7-5. Metabolism and Elimination of NMBDs

Drug	Metabolism	Metabolites	Elimination
Succinylcholine	Plasma cholinesterase (>98%)	Monoester, choline	Kidney (<2%)
Mivacurium	Plasma cholinesterase (>95%)	Monoester, quaternary alcohol	Kidney (<5%)
Atracurium	Plasma esterase, Hoffman elimination (60–90%)	Laudanosine, acrylates, alcohols, acids	Kidney (10–40%)
Cisatracurium	Hoffman elimination (77%)	Laudanosine, acrylates	Kidney (16%)
Rocuronium	None	None	Kidney(10–25%)
			Liver (>70%)
Vecuronium	Liver (30–40%)	3-OH vecuronium	Kidney (40–50%)
			Liver (50–60%)
Pancuronium	Liver (10–20%)	3-OH pancuronium	Kidney (85%)
			Liver (15%)

The adverse effects of laudanosine are unlikely at clinically relevant doses of atracurium.[57]

The ED95 of atracurium is higher in children (195 mcg/kg) than in neonates and infants (119 and 163 mcg/kg, respectively). With an intubating dose of 0.5 mg/kg, depression of twitch height by 95% occurs within 1 minute in neonates and infants and 1.4 minutes in children.[58] Recovery to 10% control twitch height occurs within 30 minutes in infants and children. Adverse effects with atracurium are related to histamine release, notably at higher doses. Hypotension, tachycardia, or bronchospasm can occur at doses greater than twice the ED95.

Cisatracurium

Cisatracurium is the *1R-Cis, 1'-R-Cis* stereoisomer of atracurium but unlike atracurium, cisatracurium does not undergo degradation by nonspecific esterases. Cisatracurium primarily undergoes Hofmann elimination. The organ-independent clearance of cisatracurium makes it an appropriate choice for patients with renal or hepatic dysfunction. Hofmann elimination of cisatracurium produces laudanosine and quaternary acrylates, which are inactive metabolites. As cisatracurium is more potent than atracurium, less laudanosine is produced at equipotent doses. Unlike atracurium, cisatracurium is not associated with significant histamine release.[59]

The ED95 of cisatracurium is similar in infants and children during nitrous oxide–narcotic anesthesia (43 and 47 mcg/kg, respectively).[60] After an intubating dose of 0.15 mg/kg, maximal blockade occurred at 2 minutes in infants and 3 minutes in children.[61] Time to recovery to 25% control twitch height was longer in infants compared to children (43.3 and 36.0 minutes, respectively). The rate of recovery is similar in infants and children. Due to its organ-independent clearance, cisatracurium is suitable for maintenance of neuromuscular blockade in the intensive care setting. In children receiving cisatracurium at a rate of 3.9 ± 1.3 mcg/kg/min, TOF ratio recovery of 70% occurred in 52 minutes on average.[62]

Rocuronium

Rocuronium is a monoquarternary aminosteroid NMBD of intermediate duration. The relative lower potency and consequent higher dose requirement of rocuronium compared to other NMBDs account for its more rapid onset of action at equipotent doses. The higher dose results in more drug molecules available to diffuse to the neuromuscular junction, thus hastening onset. A large dose (three to four times the ED95) of rocuronium can be used as an alternative to succinylcholine in situations where a rapid sequence induction is indicated. Rocuronium is not metabolized to any significant degree and is eliminated through hepatobiliary excretion in bile and feces. Approximately 10% is renally eliminated in urine. In cirrhosis or end-stage renal disease, the duration of action of rocuronium is prolonged.[63,64]

A transient increase in heart rate can be observed at the higher dose range. It is unclear if the heart rate increase is due to pain on injection or a chronotropic effect.

The ED95 of rocuronium under nitrous oxide–opioid anesthesia in infants, children, and adults are 251, 409, and 350 mcg/kg, respectively.[65] A dose of 0.6 mg/kg provides intubating conditions within 1 minute in children 18 to 72 months.[66] A lower dose of 0.3 mg/kg provides intubating conditions in 95% of children 2 to 7 years within 2 minutes.[67] At this lower dose, recovery of TOF ratio to 0.8 was on average 24 minutes. In situations where rapid intubation is indicated, 1.2 mg/kg of rocuronium provides intubating conditions similar to 2 mg/kg of succinylcholine in children ages 2 to 10 years.[68] At 1.2 mg/kg in this age group, the time for 25% recovery of twitches is 41 minutes. In situations where intravenous access is unavailable, intramuscular rocuronium is an alternative, but the onset is slow and insufficient for emergencies. An intramuscular dose of 1 mg/kg in infants and 1.8 mg/kg in children provides ≥98% blockade in 7.4 and 8 minutes, respectively.[69] At 3 minutes, intubating conditions were inadequate for the majority of patients after an intramuscular dose.

Neonates and infants are more sensitive to the effects of rocuronium and require longer time to recovery than children and adolescents. Neonates and infants receiving 0.6 mg/kg rocuronium at 0 to 1 month, 2 to 4 months, and 5 to 12 months required 61, 49, and 44 minutes, respectively, for recovery to 25% control twitch height.[70] In comparison, 1- to 5-year-old children receiving the same dose (0.6 mg/kg) required 27 minutes for recovery to 25% of control twitch height.[71]

Vecuronium

Vecuronium, a derivative of pancuronium, was the first nondepolarizing NMBD with intermediate duration introduced into clinical use. Vecuronium is primarily eliminated in bile and urine. A portion also undergoes hepatic degradation into several metabolites. The 3-OH vecuronium metabolite has about 60% the activity of vecuronium and undergoes renal clearance. In the pediatric intensive care setting, decreased clearance of vecuronium and its 3-OH metabolite may be responsible for prolonged neuromuscular blockade.[72] Patients with severe hepatic or renal dysfunction may have increased duration of action. Compared to the other aminosteroids, pancuronium and rocuronium, vecuronium does not have cardiovascular effects even at doses several times the ED95.[73]

The potency, onset, and duration of action of vecuronium vary between infants, children, and adolescents. Children have a higher dose requirement and shorter duration of action compared to neonates and adolescents. The ED95 is 47 mcg/kg in neonates and infants, 81 mcg/kg in children 3 to 10 years, and 55 mcg/kg in adolescents 13 years and older.[74] The onset of vecuronium is faster is infants compared to children and adolescents. In infants under 1, onset time after 0.1 mg/kg is 68 seconds, compared to 107 seconds in children 3 to 10 years old, and 93 seconds in children 10 to 15 years.[75] Overall, a dose of 0.1 mg/kg provides intubating conditions within 90 seconds in children 1 to 13 years.[76] Vecuronium can be considered a long-acting NMBD in patients under 1 year. A dose of 0.1 mg/kg produces >90% neuromuscular blockage from 57 to 60 minutes in children under 1 year, compared to 18 to 39 minutes in children ranging from 1 to 17 years.[77]

LONG-ACTING NONDEPOLARIZING NMBD

Pancuronium

Pancuronium is the only long-acting NMBD in clinical use. About 10% to 20% undergoes hepatic metabolism into three metabolites, the most important of which is 3-desacetylpancuronium which is about half as potent as pancuronium. Pancuronium is eliminated primarily by the kidney, with a small portion cleared by the liver. In the presence of severe hepatic or renal impairment, the duration of action is prolonged.[78,79] Pancuronium induces tachycardia due to a vagolytic effect at muscarinic receptors.[80] The vagolytic effect may be advantageous in infants, in whom bradycardia is not well tolerated. Pancuronium may also have a role in cardiac surgery, where the tachycardia may offset the bradycardia from high-dose opioids. Other effects include an increase in blood pressure and catecholamine release. Pancuronium does not produce histamine release.

The ED95 of pancuronium in infants is 45 to 52 mcg/kg in infants 3 to 12 months and 62 mcg/kg in children 13 to 83 months.[81] With a dose of 0.1 mg/kg, intubating conditions are good to excellent at 151 seconds in children 2 to 8 years.[82] The time to 25% twitch recovery at a dose of 0.12 mg/kg is 60 minutes in children 1 to 8 years.[83]

DRUG INTERACTIONS AND FACTORS AFFECTING NEUROMUSCULAR BLOCKADE

Various medications and factors can potentiate the effect of NMBDs.[84] Volatile inhaled anesthetics potentiate the effects of NMBDs and can reduce the dose requirement for maintenance of neuromuscular blockade. The exact mechanism is unknown but may be related to an effect at the acetylcholine receptor. In children 3 to 11 years old, the infusion rate of rocuronium to maintain greater than 90% twitch depression is reduced by 20% with halothane and isoflurane anesthesia, and by 50% with sevoflurane anesthesia.[85] Nitrous oxide appears to have minimal to no effect on neuromuscular blockade. Local anesthetics such as lidocaine enhance the effects of NMBDs. Antibiotics such as aminoglycosides, polymyxins, lincomycin, and clindamycin have minor effects in prolonging blockade. Magnesium decreases the onset of action and increases the duration of action of cisatracurium and rocuronium. Hypothermia prolongs the effect of NMBDs.

Resistance to the effects of nondepolarizing NMBDs can be observed in patients under long-term antiepileptic therapy. Rocuronium and vecuronium have a shorter duration of action in children on chronic carbamazepine and phenytoin therapy.[86,87] The effect of chronic anticonvulsant therapy on atracurium and cisatracurium is less apparent. Antiepileptics induce the cytochrome P450 system, which may account for more rapid clearance of the aminosteroid NMBDs. Calcium can decrease sensitivity to NMBDs.

ANTAGONISM OF NEUROMUSCULAR BLOCKING AGENTS

Adequate recovery from neuromuscular blockade must be present prior to extubation. Residual neuromuscular blockade increases the risk of perioperative complications such as hypoxemia and airway obstruction.[88] Recovery of respiratory muscle function may be especially important in infants and children due to their higher oxygen requirement. Clinical evaluation of muscle tone by the anesthesiologist may underestimate the degree of residual neuromuscular blockade. The degree of recovery should be assessed prior to extubation and traditionally, a TOF ratio of 0.7 was considered adequate neuromuscular recovery. However, a TOF ratio <0.9 is associated with pharyngeal dysfunction, laryngeal aspiration, and airway obstruction.[89] There is abundant data that a TOF ratio of >0.9 is required for complete recovery. Administration of anticholinesterase for antagonism of neuromuscular blockade should be delayed until a TOF count of two or greater is present.[90] A portion of patients who receive neostigmine with a TOF count of 1 will have inadequate return of neuromuscular function at 20 minutes after reversal.[91]

There are two classes of agents for reversal of neuromuscular blockade: anticholinesterases and cyclodextrins.

Anticholinesterases

Anticholinesterases are agents that inhibit acetylcholinesterase. Inhibition of acetylcholinesterase prevents breakdown of ACh in the neuromuscular junction. ACh competes with a nondepolarizing NMBD for binding with the receptor. The increased concentration of ACh at the motor end plate alters the balance in favor of neuromuscular transmission.

The effects of increased ACh are not limited to the neuromuscular junction. Activation of muscarinic ACh receptors of the parasympathetic system can result in bradycardia, salivation, bronchospasm, increased gastrointestinal motility, and nausea and vomiting.[92] To counter the muscarinic effects, an antimuscarinic such as glycopyrrolate (5–10 mcg/kg) or atropine (10–20 mcg/kg) should be administered with an anticholinesterase.

The three anticholinesterases traditionally available for reversal of nondepolarizing NMBDs are edrophonium, neostigmine, and pyridostigmine. Among their differences is the time to onset. Edrophonium is the most rapid with peak effect within 2 minutes, while pyridostigmine is the slowest.[93] Although the rapid onset of edrophonium may be clinically useful, it is not as effective as neostigmine in antagonizing profound blockade of greater than 90% twitch suppression.[94] Compared to neostigmine, edrophonium has greater variability in individual patient response. Furthermore, the duration of action of edrophonium is shorter than that of neostigmine, such that there is a concern of recurarization, or a return of neuromuscular blockade after a period of recovery. Pyridostigmine, with a slower onset time than neostigmine, has fallen out of favor as a reversal agent. Neostigmine is the most commonly used anticholinesterase for antagonism of neuromuscular blockade and has been advocated as the anticholinesterase for use in pediatrics.[95]

Neostigmine

Neostigmine is a quaternary ammonium compound that forms a covalent bond with acetylcholinesterase. It is cleared by the kidney, such that clearance is prolonged in patients with severe renal disease. The time to onset is 5 to 10 minutes in infants, children, and adults.[96] The duration of action of approximately 1 to 2 hours is comparable between age groups. The elimination half-life is faster in infants compared with children and adults. The dose for reversal varies from 0.03 to 0.07 mg/kg. In infants and children with 90% twitch depression from atracurium, a dose of 0.05 mg/kg produces a TOF ratio of 0.9 or greater at 13 minutes, with neonates and infants under 1 year showing the fastest recovery.[90] In children 2 to 12 years and adults with 90% twitch depression from rocuronium, a dose of 0.07 mg/kg of neostigmine results in a TOF ratio of 0.9 or greater within 8 minutes, with children showing a shorter time to reversal.[97] When reversing patients with a low degree of residual blockade (such as the presence of four twitches and TOF ratio of 0.4–0.6), a smaller dose of 0.02 to 0.03 mg/kg of neostigmine may be adequate.[98]

Edrophonium

Edrophonium inhibits acetylcholinesterase by forming a reversible ionic bond. It is less potent than neostigmine and has a faster onset of action. A reversal dose of 0.5 to 1 mg/kg has an onset of action within 2 minutes.[88] In infants and children with 90% twitch depression from pancuronium, initial recovery of neuromuscular function was faster with edrophonium compared to neostigmine. Recovery is comparable at 10 minutes.[99] The effects of edrophonium are more variable than those of neostigmine, and the final TOF ratio reached is less with edrophonium compared to neostigmine.[90] Edrophonium is less effective at reversing profound neuromuscular blockade than neostigmine.[89]

▶ Cyclodextrins

Sugammadex

Sugammadex is a γ-cyclodextrin that can reverse aminosteroid NMBDs. Sugammadex is an oligosaccharide arranged in a ring. Rocuronium, and to a lesser extent vecuronium and pancuronium, binds the center of the ring structure, forming a complex that is renally excreted.[100] Administration of 2 mg/kg sugammadex at the reappearance of the second twitch results in recovery to a TOF ratio of 0.9 within 0.6 minutes for infants and 1.2 minutes in children.[101] Recovery is faster in infants than in children and adults. Sugammadex has the ability to quickly reverse profound block from rocuronium. In adults, 16 mg/kg sugammadex given 3 minutes after 1.2 mg/kg rocuronium results in recovery to a TOF ratio of 0.9 within 3 minutes after administration of sugammadex.[102] In infants 2 to 12 months with a TOF ratio of 0 at the end of surgery, a dose of 3 mg/kg sugammadex results in a TOF ratio of >0.9 within 2 minutes.[103] The FDA initially deferred approval for sugammadex, requesting additional data on hypersensitivity, but granted approval in 2015.

REFERENCES

1. Barrett KE, Barman SM, Boitano S, Brooks HL. Synaptic & junctional transmission. In: Barrett KE, Barman SM, Boitano S, Brooks HL, eds. *Ganong's Review of Medical Physiology*. 25th ed. New York: McGrawHill; 2016.
2. Fagerlund MJ, Eriksson LI. Current concepts in neuromuscular transmission. *Br J Anaesth*. 2009;103(1):108-114.
3. Naguib M, Flood P, McArdle JJ, Brenner HR. Advances in neurobiology of the neuromuscular junction: implications for the anesthesiologist. *Anesthesiology*. 2002;96(1):202-231.
4. Hughes BW, Kusner LL, Kaminski HJ. Molecular architecture of the neuromuscular junction. *Muscle Nerve*. 2006;33(4):445-461.
5. Aniskevich S, Brull SJ, Naguib M. Neuromuscular blocking agents. In: Johnson KB, ed. *Clinical Pharmacology for Anesthesiology*. New York: McGraw-Hill; 2015.
6. Gu Y, Franco AJr, Gardner PD, Lansman JB, Forsayeth JR, Hall ZW. Properties of embryonic and adult muscle acetylcholine receptors transiently expressed in COS cells. *Neuron*. 1990;5(2):147-157.
7. Naguib M, Flood P, McArdle JJ, Brenner HR. Advances in neurobiology of the neuromuscular junction: implications for the anesthesiologist. *Anesthesiology*. 2002;96(1):202-231.
8. Meakin GH. Neuromuscular blocking drugs in infants and children. *Contin Educ Anaesth Crit Care Pain*. 2007;7(5):143-147.
9. Fisher DM. Neuromuscular blocking agents in paediatric anaesthesia. *Br J Anaesth*. 1999;83(1):58-64.
10. Goudsouzian NG, Standaert FG. The infant and the myoneural junction. *Anesth Analg*. 1986;65(11):1208-1217.
11. Laycock JR, Baxter MK, Bevan JC, Sangwan S, Donati F, Bevan DR. The potency of pancuronium at the adductor pollicis and diaphragm in infants and children. *Anesthesiology*. 1988;68(6):908-911.
12. Capron F, Fortier LP, Racine S, Donati F. Tactile fade detection with hand or wrist stimulation using train-of-four, double-burst stimulation, 50-hertz tetanus, 100-hertz tetanus, and acceleromyography. *Anesth Analg*. 2006;102(5):1578-1584.
13. Fuchs-Buder T, Schreiber JU, Meistelman C. Monitoring neuromuscular block: an update. *Anaesthesia*. 2009;64(suppl 1): 82-89.

14. Butterworth JF IV, Mackey DC, Wasnick JD. Noncardiovascular monitoring. In: Butterworth JF IV, Mackey DC, Wasnick JD, eds. *Morgan & Mikhail's Clinical Anesthesiology*. 6th ed. New York: McGraw-Hill; 2018.

15. Goudsouzian NG. Maturation of neuromuscular transmission in the infant. *Br J Anaesth*. 1980;52(2):205-214.

16. Lien CA, Kopman AF. Current recommendations for monitoring depth of neuromuscular blockade. *Curr Opin Anaesthesiol*. 2014;27(6):616-622.

17. Price SW, Ved S. Monitoring neuromuscular function. In: Freeman BS, Berger JS, eds. *Anesthesiology Core Review: Part One Basic Exam*. New York: McGraw-Hill; 2014.

18. Ramsey FM, Lebowitz PW, Savarese JJ, Ali HH. Clinical characteristics of long-term succinylcholine neuromuscular blockade during balanced anesthesia. *Anesth Analg*. 1980;59(2):110-116.

19. Gissen AJ, Katz RL. Twitch, tetanus and posttetanic potentiation as indices of nerve-muscle block in man. *Anesthesiology*. 1969;30(5):481-487.

20. Baykara N, Woelfel S, Fine GF, Solak M, Toker K, Brandom BW. Predicting recovery from deep neuromuscular block by rocuronium in children and adults. *J Clin Anesth*. 2002; 14(3):214-217.

21. Saddler JM, Bevan JC, Donati F, Bevan DR, Pinto SR. Comparison of double-burst and train-of-four stimulation to assess neuromuscular blockade in children. *Anesthesiology*. 1990;73(3):401-403.

22. Martyn J, Durieux ME. Succinylcholine: new insights into mechanisms of action of an old drug. *Anesthesiology*. 2006;104(4):633-634.

23. Bovet D. Some aspects of the relationship between chemical constitution and curare-like activity. *Ann N Y Acad Sci*. 1951;54(3):407-437.

24. Martyn JA, Fagerlund MJ, Eriksson LI. Basic principles of neuromuscular transmission. *Anaesthesia*. 2009;64(suppl 1):1-9.

25. Donati F. Neuromuscular blocking drugs for the new millennium: current practice, future trends—comparative pharmacology of neuromuscular blocking drugs. *Anesth Analg*. 2000;90(5 suppl):S2-S6.

26. Fuchs-Buder T, Claudius C, Skovgaard LT, Eriksson LI, Mirakhur RK, Viby-Mogensen J; 8th International Neuromuscular Meeting. Good clinical research practice in pharmacodynamic studies of neuromuscular blocking agents II: the Stockholm revision. *Acta Anaesthesiol Scand*. 2007;51(7):789-808.

27. Meretoja OA, Wirtavuori K, Neuvonen PJ. Age-dependence of the dose-response curve of vecuronium in pediatric patients during balanced anesthesia. *Anesth Analg*. 1988;67(1):21-26.

28. Driessen JJ, Robertson EN, Van Egmond J, Booij LH. The time-course of action and recovery of rocuronium 0.3 mg · kg⁻¹ in infants and children during halothane anaesthesia measured with acceleromyography. *Paediatr Anaesth*. 2000;10(5):493-497.

29. Meretoja OA. Neuromuscular blocking agents in paediatric patients: influence of age on the response. *Anaesth Intensive Care*. 1990;18(4):440-448.

30. Meakin G, McKiernan EP, Morris P, Baker RD. Dose-response curves for suxamethonium in neonates, infants and children. *Br J Anaesth*. 1989;62(6):655-658.

31. Liu LM, DeCook TH, Goudsouzian NG, Ryan JF, Liu PL. Dose response to intramuscular succinylcholine in children. *Anesthesiology*. 1981;55(5):599-602.

32. Alalami AA, Ayoub CM, Baraka AS. Laryngospasm: review of different prevention and treatment modalities. *Paediatr Anaesth*. 2008;18(4):281-288.

33. Levano S, Ginz H, Siegemund M, et al. Genotyping the butyrylcholinesterase in patients with prolonged neuromuscular block after succinylcholine. *Anesthesiology*. 2005;102(3):531-535.

34. Viby-Mogensen J, Hanel HK. Prolonged apnoea after suxamethonium: an analysis of the first 225 cases reported to the Danish Cholinesterase Research Unit. *Acta Anaesthesiol Scand*. 1978;22(4):371-380.

35. Kalow W, Genest K. A method for the detection of atypical forms of human serum cholinesterase; determination of dibucaine numbers. *Can J Biochem Physiol*. 1957;35(6):339-346.

36. Barreto RS. Effect of intravenously administered succinylcholine upon cardiac rate and rhythm. *Anesthesiology*. 1960;21:401-404.

37. Lerman J, Chinyanga HM. The heart rate response to succinylcholine in children: a comparison of atropine and glycopyrrolate. *Can Anaesth Soc J*. 1983;30(4):377-381.

38. Keneally JP, Bush GH. Changes in serum potassium after suxamethonium in children. *Anaesth Intensive Care*. 1974;2(2):147-150.

39. Martyn JA, Richtsfeld M. Succinylcholine-induced hyperkalemia in acquired pathologic states: etiologic factors and molecular mechanisms. *Anesthesiology*. 2006;104(1):158-169.

40. Larach MG, Rosenberg H, Gronert GA, Allen GC. Hyperkalemic cardiac arrest during anesthesia in infants and children with occult myopathies. *Clin Pediatr (Phila)*. 1997;36(1):9-16.

41. Succinylcholine chloride injection, USP: A short-acting depolarizing skeletal muscle relaxant. Available at https://www.accessdata.fda.gov/drugsatfda_docs/label/2010/008845s065lbl.pdf. Accessed August 20, 2019.

42. Minton MD, Grosslight K, Stirt JA, Bedford RF. Increases in intracranial pressure from succinylcholine: prevention by prior nondepolarizing blockade. *Anesthesiology*. 1986;65(2):165-169.

43. Vachon CA, Warner DO, Bacon DR. Succinylcholine and the open globe. *Teach Anesthesiol*. 2003;99(1):220-223.

44. Schreiber JU, Lysakowski C, Fuchs-Buder T, Tramèr MR. Prevention of succinylcholine-induced fasciculation and myalgia: a meta-analysis of randomized trials. *Anesthesiology*. 2005;103(4):877-884.

45. Ryan JF, Kagen LJ, Hyman AI. Myoglobinemia after a single dose of succinylcholine. *N Engl J Med*. 1971;285(15): 824-827.

46. Hannallah RS, Kaplan RF. Jaw relaxation after a halothane/succinylcholine sequence in children. *Anesthesiology*. 1994;81(1):99-103; discussion 28A.

47. Littleford JA, Patel LR, Bose D, Cameron CB, McKillop C. Masseter muscle spasm in children: implications of continuing the triggering anesthetic. *Anesth Analg*. 1991;72(2):151-160.

48. Meakin G, Walker RW, Dearlove OR. Myotonic and neuromuscular blocking effects of increased doses of suxamethonium in infants and children. *Br J Anaesth*. 1990;65(6):816-818.

49. Mazurek AJ, Rae B, Hann S, Kim JI, Castro B, Coté CJ. Rocuronium versus succinylcholine: are they equally effective during rapid-sequence induction of anesthesia? *Anesth Analg*. 1998;87(6):1259-1262.

50. Kopman AF, Klewicka MM, Kopman DJ, Neuman GG. Molar potency is predictive of the speed of onset of neuromuscular block for agents of intermediate, short, and ultrashort duration. *Anesthesiology*. 1999;90(2):425-431.

51. Naguib M, Magboul MM. Adverse effects of neuromuscular blockers and their antagonists. *Drug Saf.* 1998;18(2):99-116.
52. Hepner DL, Castells MC. Anaphylaxis during the perioperative period. *Anesth Analg.* 2003;97(5):1381-1395.
53. Naguib M, Lien CA, Meistelman C. Pharmacology of neuromuscular blocking drugs. In: Miller RD, ed. *Miller's Anesthesia.* 8th ed. Philadelphia, PA: Elsevier/Saunders; 2015.
54. Goudsouzian NG. Mivacurium in infants and children. *Paediatr Anaesth.* 1997;7(3):183-190.
55. Ostergaard D, Jensen FS, Jensen E, Skovgaard LT, Viby-Mogensen J. Mivacurium-induced neuromuscular blockade in patients with atypical plasma cholinesterase. *Acta Anaesthesiol Scand.* 1993;37(3):314-318.
56. Miller RD. Pharmacokinetics of atracurium and other non-depolarizing neuromuscular blocking agents in normal patients and those with renal or hepatic dysfunction. *Br J Anaesth.* 1986;58(suppl 1):11S-13S.
57. Fodale V, Santamaria LB. Laudanosine, an atracurium and cisatracurium metabolite. *Eur J Anaesthesiol.* 2002;19(7):466-473.
58. Meakin G, Shaw EA, Baker RD, Morris P. Comparison of atracurium-induced neuromuscular blockade in neonates, infants and children. *Br J Anaesth.* 1988;60(2):171-175.
59. Doenicke A, Soukup J, Hoernecke R, Moss J. The lack of histamine release with cisatracurium: a double-blind comparison with vecuronium. *Anesth Analg.* 1997;84(3):623-628.
60. de Ruiter J, Crawford MW. Dose-response relationship and infusion requirement of cisatracurium besylate in infants and children during nitrous oxide-narcotic anesthesia. *Anesthesiology.* 2001;94(5):790-792.
61. Taivainen T, Meakin GH, Meretoja OA, et al. The safety and efficacy of cisatracurium 0.15 mg·kg⁻¹ during nitrous oxide-opioid anaesthesia in infants and children. *Anaesthesia.* 2000;55(11):1047-1051.
62. Burmester M, Mok Q. Randomised controlled trial comparing cisatracurium and vecuronium infusions in a paediatric intensive care unit. *Intensive Care Med.* 2005;31(5):686-692.
63. Robertson EN, Driessen JJ, Booij LH. Pharmacokinetics and pharmacodynamics of rocuronium in patients with and without renal failure. *Eur J Anaesthesiol.* 2005;22(1):4-10.
64. van Miert MM, Eastwood NB, Boyd AH, Parker CJ, Hunter JM. The pharmacokinetics and pharmacodynamics of rocuronium in patients with hepatic cirrhosis. *Br J Clin Pharmacol.* 1997;44(2):139-144.
65. Taivainen T, Meretoja OA, Erkola O, Rautoma P, Juvakoski M. Rocuronium in infants, children and adults during balanced anaesthesia. *Paediatr Anaesth.* 1996;6(4):271-275.
66. Scheiber G, Ribeiro FC, Marichal A, Bredendiek M, Renzing K. Intubating conditions and onset of action after rocuronium, vecuronium, and atracurium in young children. *Anesth Analg.* 1996;83(2):320-324.
67. Eikermann M, Hunkemöller I, Peine L, et al. Optimal rocuronium dose for intubation during inhalation induction with sevoflurane in children. *Br J Anaesth.* 2002;89(2):277-281.
68. Woolf RL, Crawford MW, Choo SM. Dose-response of rocuronium bromide in children anesthetized with propofol: a comparison with succinylcholine. *Anesthesiology.* 1997;87(6):1368-1372.
69. Kaplan RF, Uejima T, Lobel G, et al. Intramuscular rocuronium in infants and children: a multicenter study to evaluate tracheal intubating conditions, onset, and duration of action. *Anesthesiology.* 1999;91(3):633-638.
70. Rapp HJ, Altenmueller CA, Waschke C. Neuromuscular recovery following rocuronium bromide single dose in infants. *Paediatr Anaesth.* 2004;14(4):329-335.
71. Woelfel SK, Brandom BW, Cook DR, Sarner JB. Effects of bolus administration of ORG-9426 in children during nitrous oxide-halothane anesthesia. *Anesthesiology.* 1992;76(6):939-942.
72. Reich DL, Hollinger I, Harrington DJ, Seiden HS, Chakravorti S, Cook DR. Comparison of cisatracurium and vecuronium by infusion in neonates and small infants after congenital heart surgery. *Anesthesiology.* 2004;101(5):1122-1127.
73. Tullock WC, Diana P, Cook DR, et al. Neuromuscular and cardiovascular effects of high-dose vecuronium. *Anesth Analg.* 1990;70(1):86-90.
74. Meretoja OA, Wirtavuori K, Neuvonen PJ. Age-dependence of the dose-response curve of vecuronium in pediatric patients during balanced anesthesia. *Anesth Analg.* 1988;67(1):21-26.
75. Kalli I, Meretoja OA. Duration of action of vecuronium in infants and children anaesthetized without potent inhalation agents. *Acta Anaesthesiol Scand.* 1989;33(1):29-33.
76. Ferres CJ, Crean PM, Mirakhur RK. An evaluation of Org NC 45 (vecuronium) in paediatric anaesthesia. *Anaesthesia.* 1983;38(10):943-947.
77. Meretoja OA. Is vecuronium a long-acting neuromuscular blocking agent in neonates and infants? *Br J Anaesth.* 1989;62(2):184-187.
78. Duvaldestin P, Agoston S, Henzel D, Kersten UW, Desmonts JM. Pancuronium pharmacokinetics in patients with liver cirrhosis. *Br J Anaesth.* 1978;50(11):1131-1136.
79. Gramstad L. Atracurium, vecuronium and pancuronium in end-stage renal failure. Dose-response properties and interactions with azathioprine. *Br J Anaesth.* 1987;59(8):995-1003.
80. Saxena PR, Bonta IL. Mechanism of selective cardiac vagolytic action of pancuronium bromide. Specific blockade of cardiac muscarinic receptors. *Eur J Pharmacol.* 1970;11(3):332-341.
81. Blinn A, Woelfel SK, Cook DR, Brandom BW, Cohen IT. Pancuronium dose-response revisited. *Paediatric Anaesthesia.* 1992;2:153-155.
82. Cunliffe M, Lucero VM, McLeod ME, Burrows FA, Lerman J. Neuromuscular blockade for rapid tracheal intubation in children: comparison of succinylcholine and pancuronium. *Can Anaesth Soc J.* 1986;33(6):760-764.
83. Montgomery CJ, Steward DJ. A comparative evaluation of intubating doses of atracurium, d-tubocurarine, pancuronium and vecuronium in children. *Can J Anaesth.* 1988;35(1):36-40.
84. Feldman S, Karalliedde L. Drug interactions with neuromuscular blockers. *Drug Saf.* 1996;15(4):261-273.
85. Woloszczuk-Gebicka B, Lapczynski T, Wierzejski W. The influence of halothane, isoflurane and sevoflurane on rocuronium infusion in children. *Acta Anaesthesiol Scand.* 2001;45(1):73-77.
86. Soriano SG, Sullivan LJ, Venkatakrishnan K, Greenblatt DJ, Martyn JA. Pharmacokinetics and pharmacodynamics of vecuronium in children receiving phenytoin or carbamazepine for chronic anticonvulsant therapy. *Br J Anaesth.* 2001;86(2):223-229.
87. Soriano SG, Kaus SJ, Sullivan LJ, Martyn JA. Onset and duration of action of rocuronium in children receiving chronic anticonvulsant therapy. *Paediatr Anaesth.* 2000;10(2):133-136.

88. Murphy GS, Szokol JW, Marymont JH, Greenberg SB, Avram MJ, Vender JS. Residual neuromuscular blockade and critical respiratory events in the postanesthesia care unit. *Anesth Analg.* 2008;107(1):130-137.

89. Murphy GS, Brull SJ. Residual neuromuscular block: lessons unlearned. Part I: definitions, incidence, and adverse physiologic effects of residual neuromuscular block. *Anesth Analg.* 2010;111(1):120-128.

90. Kopman AF, Eikermann M. Antagonism of non-depolarising neuromuscular block: current practice. *Anaesthesia.* 2009;64(suppl 1):22-30.

91. Kopman AF, Kopman DJ, Ng J, Zank LM. Antagonism of profound cisatracurium and rocuronium block: the role of objective assessment of neuromuscular function. *J Clin Anesth.* 2005;17(1):30-35.

92. Bevan DR, Donati F, Kopman AF. Reversal of neuromuscular blockade. *Anesthesiology.* 1992;77(4):785-805.

93. Ferguson A, Egerszegi P, Bevan DR. Neostigmine, pyridostigmine, and edrophonium as antagonists of pancuronium. *Anesthesiology.* 1980;53(5):390-394.

94. Rupp SM, McChristian JW, Miller RD, Taboada JA, Cronnelly R. Neostigmine and edrophonium antagonism of varying intensity neuromuscular blockade induced by atracurium, pancuronium, or vecuronium. *Anesthesiology.* 1986;64(6):711-717.

95. Kirkegaard-Nielsen H, Meretoja OA, Wirtavuori K. Reversal of atracurium-induced neuromuscular block in paediatric patients. *Acta Anaesthesiol Scand.* 1995;39(7):906-911.

96. Fisher DM, Cronnelly R, Miller RD, Sharma M. The neuromuscular pharmacology of neostigmine in infants and children. *Anesthesiology.* 1983;59(3):220-225.

97. Bevan JC, Collins L, Fowler C, et al. Early and late reversal of rocuronium and vecuronium with neostigmine in adults and children. *Anesth Analg.* 1999;89(2):333-339.

98. Fuchs-Buder T, Meistelman C, Alla F, Grandjean A, Wuthrich Y, Donati F. Antagonism of low degrees of atracurium-induced neuromuscular blockade: dose-effect relationship for neostigmine. *Anesthesiology.* 2010;112(1):34-40.

99. Meakin G, Sweet PT, Bevan JC, Bevan DR. Neostigmine and edrophonium as antagonists of pancuronium in infants and children. *Anesthesiology.* 1983;59(4):316-321.

100. Hunter JM, Flockton EA. The doughnut and the hole: a new pharmacological concept for anaesthetists. *Br J Anaesth.* 2006;97(2):123-126.

101. Plaud B, Meretoja O, Hofmockel R, et al. Reversal of rocuronium-induced neuromuscular blockade with sugammadex in pediatric and adult surgical patients. *Anesthesiology.* 2009;110(2):284-294.

102. Lee C, Jahr JS, Candiotti KA, Warriner B, Zornow MH, Naguib M. Reversal of profound neuromuscular block by sugammadex administered three minutes after rocuronium: a comparison with spontaneous recovery from succinylcholine. *Anesthesiology.* 2009;110(5):1020-1025.

103. Ozmete O, Bali C, Cok OY, et al. Sugammadex given for rocuronium-induced neuromuscular blockade in infants: a retrospective study. *J Clin Anesth.* 2016;35:497-501.

Local Anesthetics

Cassandra Wasson and Stacy Peterson

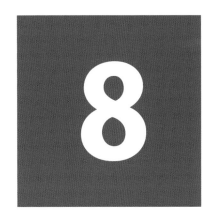

FOCUS POINTS

1. In infants, amide local anesthetics are not metabolized at a regular rate. This is especially important to remember when running infusions either intravenously or via regional or neuraxial anesthesia.
2. Ester local anesthetics are metabolized by pseudocholinesterases in the plasma. Amide local anesthetics are metabolized in P450 dependent pathways.
3. Maximum dose of local anesthetic varies based on the local anesthetics and sometimes the addition of epinephrine.
4. Treatment of local anesthetic systemic toxicity has two arms—one is supportive care and another is treatment with intralipid 20% at 1.5 mL/Kg.
5. Systemic absorption depends on location of injection, with intercostal injection leading to the highest blood levels.

HISTORY OF LOCAL ANESTHETICS

Cocaine is the first local anesthetic to be discovered. It remains the only naturally occurring local anesthetic. In regions where the coca leaf grows, such as Peru, the leaf has a long history of being dried and chewed. Reports of cocaine "making the tongue numb" existed. Carl Koller, an ophthalmologist, had sampled this and believed that cocaine could potentially be applied to the eye for surgery. He studied this on animals in the laboratory, then upon his own eye and eventually on patients. In 1884, he used cocaine to provide local anesthesia for glaucoma surgery,

the first report of use of a local anesthetic for surgical anesthesia.[1] Until 1905, cocaine was the only available local anesthetic. In 1905, Alfred Einhorn synthesized procaine, another ester local anesthetic.

William Halstead is another pioneer in the area of local anesthetics. He is credited with performing the first regional block, a dental nerve block. He performed many blocks and held weekly teaching sessions of regional anesthesia with the use of cocaine. This led to him becoming a habitual user of cocaine and much of his work was not reported.

Following this, the use of local anesthetic developed in the hands of pioneers such as Leonard Corning, Heinrich Quincke, and Karl Bier.

MECHANISM OF ACTION

Nerve Anatomy

To understand how local anesthetics exert their action it is important to understand nerve cell conduction and to have a basic understanding of the nerve itself. Nerve fibers consist of axons that are encased in endoneurium. Nerve fibers are then collected into fascicles, which are surrounded by specialized connective tissues known as perineurium. Finally, the fascicles are grouped and bound by another layer of connective tissue known as the epineurium (Figure 8-1).[2] An important difference between the epineurium and the perineurium is that the perineurium is capable of protecting neurons from chemical injury.[3]

Nerves are then classified based on presence or absence of the myelin sheath. Nerves are also classified based on their function, conduction velocity, or size (Table 8-1).

The myelin sheath is not continuous, rather it is interrupted at regular intervals by regions knows as the nodes of Ranvier.[4] These areas are required for transmission of electrical impulses. Myelinated nerves are capable of faster

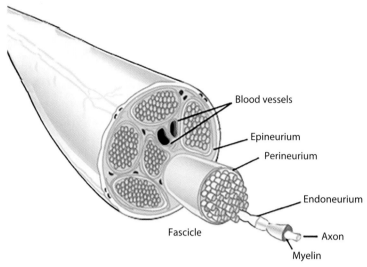

▲ **Figure 8-1.** Nerve anatomy. (Adapted with permission, from Siemionow M, Brzezicki G. Chapter 8 current techniques and concepts in peripheral nerve repair. *Int Rev Neurobiol*. 2009;87:141-72. https://www.sciencedirect.com/journal/international-review-of-neurobiology.)

Table 8-1. Neve Characteristics Including Local Anesthetic Sensitivity

Class	Aα	Aβ	Aγ	Aδ	B	C
Function	Motor	Touch/pressure	Proprioception/motor tone	Pain/temperature	Preganglionic autonomic	Pain/temperature
Myelin	+++	+++	++	++	+	–
Diameter (μm)	12–20	5–12	1–4	1–4	1–3	0.5–1
Conduction speed (m/sec)	70–120	30–70	10–30	12–30	10–15	0.5–1.2
Local anesthetic sensitivity	‡‡	‡‡	‡‡‡	‡‡‡	‡‡	‡

+++, Heavy myelinated; ++, moderately myelinated; +, lightly myelinated; ‡‡‡, most susceptible to impulse blockade; ‡‡, moderately susceptible; and ‡, least susceptible.
Source: Adapted from Strichartz G, Pastijn E, and Sugimoto K. Neural physiology and local anesthetic action. In: Cousins MJ, Carr DB, Adapted with permission, from Cousins MJ, Carr DB, Horlocker TT, et al. eds. *Cousins & Bridenbaugh's Neural Blockade in Clinical Anesthesia and Pain Medicine*, 4th ed. 2008. Copyright © Lippincott Williams & Wilkins. All rights reserved.

conduction of nerve impulses secondary to salutatory conduction where impulses skip from one node of Ranvier to the next. Unmyelinated nerves are, in general, smaller in diameter and transmit electrical impulses slower than their myelinated counterparts.

The various types of nerves are not equally blocked by local anesthetics. In general, local anesthetics first work on temperature sensation then proprioception, motor function, sharp pain, and light touch. This was thought to be due to the nerve's diameter, but the correlation between nerve diameter and onset of blockade does not entirely hold true. Large A delta fibers are blocked before small C fibers which are unmyelinated.[2]

▶ Voltage-Gated Sodium Channel

Neurons maintain a resting membrane potential via use of a Na^+-K^+-ATPase pump that exchanges three sodium ions for every two potassium ions that are imported. This leads to a resting membrane potential of –70 mV. In order for an action potential to be generated, depolarization must occur. This is accomplished by activation of voltage-gated sodium channels following an influx of sodium ions leading to creation of an action potential. Specifically, they reversibly bind the intracellular portion of the sodium channel. Following depolarization and the action potential, there is a drop in sodium permeability and an increase in potassium influx via voltage-gated potassium channels, which works to return the membrane to its resting potential.

Local anesthetics provide anesthesia by blocking nerve impulses and thus altering sensation. Nerve impulses are blocked via blocking voltage-gated sodium channels, which alternate between several conformational states, including activated and inactivated states, leading to interruption of impulses in nerve axons. Specifically, local anesthetics bind the alpha subunit of the sodium channels intracellularly and thus block the influx of sodium that is necessary to cause depolarization and subsequent impulse conduction.[5]

Classes of Local Anesthetics

There are two major classes of local anesthetics, the amino esters and the amino amides (Table 8-2). Local anesthetics consist of a lipophilic aromatic ring attached to a tertiary hydrophilic amine. The bond that connects these defines whether the local anesthetic is an amide or an ester. Those anesthetics that are connected by an ester (–C–O) are esters and those connected by an amide link (–NHC–) are amides.

The classes differ in their metabolism, excretion, as well as the risk of allergy. The ester class local anesthetics are metabolized by pseudocholinesterase. The metabolites are then excreted in the urine. Two esters, procaine and benzocaine, are metabolized to *p*-aminobenzoic acid or PABA. This metabolite has been associated with allergic reactions. In addition to this, those individuals with pseudocholinesterase deficiencies will metabolize the ester local anesthetics more slowly, which will increase the chance of untoward effects. Cocaine, an ester, differs as it is partially metabolized in the liver by *N*-methylation and excreted unchanged in the urine.

Amide local anesthetics are metabolized via *N*-dealkylation and hydroxylation by P450 enzymes in the liver. The rate varies with local anesthetic and occurs more slowly than ester hydrolysis.

Para-aminobenzoic acid is not a metabolite of amides and reports of allergic reactions to amide type local anesthetics are quite rare.

Clinical Pharmacology

When choosing a local anesthetic for use in clinical practice, it is important to be aware of the properties of the drug that are relevant. Key factors that should be considered include speed of onset, potency, duration of action, and motor vs. sensory blockad. In addition to factors inherent to the local anesthetics themselves, it is also important to be mindful of additional factors that affect their activity in vivo. Such factors include dosage of local anesthetics, addition of substances such as vasoconstrictors or other agents, and using mixtures of local anesthetics.

Onset and Duration of Action

The anesthetic agent itself is a huge determinate of the onset and duration of blockade. With regards to onset,

agents that are moderately hydrophobic, such as lidocaine, have a faster onset of action than highly hydrophobic or hydrophilic agents.

Onset of action also depends on each anesthetic agent's pK_a, also known as the dissociation constant. The pK_a is the pH at which the ratio of the ionized water-soluble form is equal to the nonionized lipid soluble form. Local anesthetics that have a pK_a close to the pH where they are injected will have a faster onset because more local anesthetic is unionized, allowing the local anesthetic to cross and become intracellular. It is important to note that pK_a is not the only determining factor for clinical onset, thus agents with similar pK_a may have varying onset times and local anesthetics may act faster or slower than expected based on their pK_a. For example, chloroprocaine has a pK_a of 9.0 yet has a very rapid onset.

Duration of action is in part determined by the hydrophilic or hydrophobic nature of the local anesthetic. Agents that are more hydrophobic, such as bupivacaine, are more potent and in general produce longer lasting blocks.

Potency

The main determinant of anesthetic agent potency is hydrophobicity. Agents that are more hydrophobic, such as bupivacaine, are more highly potent and thus require a lower concentration to achieve a block. This correlation does not hold 100% true in clinical practice as other factors such as intrinsic vasoconstrictor/vasodilator properties and local anesthetic charge also affect potency.[6]

Sensory and Motor Blockade

Use of local anesthetics may lead to both sensory and motor blockade, but the amount of blockade of each varies with the specific agent used as well as the concentration of the agent utilized.

Bupivacaine has long been favored for use in epidurals as it provides reliable sensory blockade at low concentrations with minimal motor blockade. This is especially true when used in low concentrations such as 0.125%. In contrast, when given epidurally, etidocaine produces equal motor and sensory blockade.[6] More recently, use of ropivacaine has come in to favor given its ability to produce even less of a motor blockade compared to bupivacaine while maintaining adequate sensory blockade.

PHARMACOKINETICS

Systemic Absorption

Rate of absorption depends on the local anesthetic, the location of the injection, as well as the presence of additives such as vasoconstrictors (Figure 8-2). Local anesthetics that are highly protein bound dissociate from the nerve at a slower rate, which results in slower absorption and increased duration of action.[5]

Epinephrine may be added to local anesthetics. The addition of epinephrine leads to local vasoconstriction and

Table 8-2. Common Local Anesthetics

Drug and Chemical Structure	Classification	pK_a	Onset (min)	Duration (min)	Maximum Dose for Plain Solution (mg/kg)	Maximum Dose with Epinephrine (mg/kg)
Bupivacaine	Amide	8.1	5–11	240–360	2	2.5
Chloroprocaine	Ester	8.7	6–12	30–60	10	15
Cocaine	Ester	8.6	5–10	30–60	3	NA
Lidocaine	Amide	7.8	2–4	60–120	5	7
Mepivacaine	Amide	7.6	2–4	90–180	5	7
Prilocaine	Amide	7.8	2–4	30 60	7	8
Procaine	Ester	8.9	7–8	30–60	8	10
Ropivacaine	Amide	8.1	10–15	180–300	3	3
Tetracaine	Ester	8.5	5–9	90–360	1.5	2

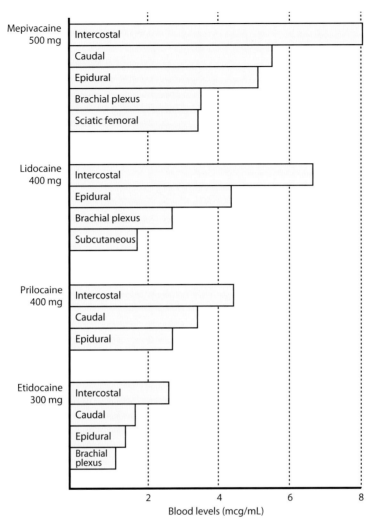

▲ **Figure 8-2.** Local anesthetic blood levels based on injection site. (Adapted with permission, from Covino BD, Vassals HG. *Local Anesthetics: Mechanism of Action in Clinical Use.* 1976. Grune & Stratton. Copyright © Elsevier. All rights reserved.)

subsequently decreased absorption of the local anesthetic. This increases neuronal uptake and prolongs the duration of action via activation of α_2-adrenergic receptors. This effect is more pronounced with shorter-acting local anesthetics such as lidocaine, especially when used in areas that are highly vascular.[5]

Onset also reflects the vascularity of the tissue into which it is injected. Tissues that are highly vascularized such as the trachea or intercostal area have a higher rate of systemic absorption.

Biotransformation and Excretion

Metabolism varies based on local anesthetic class as discussed in section "Special Pharmacokinetic Considerations." Aminoamide drugs are primarily transformed in the liver and excretion occurs via the kidney. Given metabolism by the liver, it is important to remember that severe liver disease can alter the transformation of amide local anesthetics. As discussed below age is a factor in the elimination process.

Ester class local anesthetics are hydrolyzed by pseudocholinesterase in the plasma.

Special Pharmacokinetic Considerations: Dosing in Neonates and Infants

At birth the P450 hepatic enzyme system is not mature. As a result, amide type local anesthetics are metabolized at a slower rate.[7] This is seen with single doses of these anesthetics, but is particularly notable when neonates and infants are receiving continuous infusions of local anesthetics.[8] As they have decreased metabolism, they are at increased risk for elevated plasma levels and thus at an increased risk of experiencing local anesthetic toxicity if this is not taken into account. Bupivacaine has a half-life of 3.5 hours in adults, but in infants and neonates the half-life may be as long as 12 hours.[6]

In addition to immature hepatic P450 systems, neonates also have low levels of α_1-acid glycoprotein. This leads to decreased local anesthetic plasma binding capacity, which subsequently leads to increased levels of the free drug.

Bupivacaine

Bupivacaine use in infants has been studied. In the early 1990s local anesthetic toxicity in infants with the use of continuous epidural bupivacaine infusions was reported. Following these reports and an investigation by the Anesthesia Patient Safety Foundation, new recommendations came about to limit infusion rates of bupivacaine in infants to ≤ 0.2 mg/kg/h.[9] Following this recommendation, further study has shown that even at this recommended dosing plasma levels of bupivacaine can continue to rise beyond 48 hours of continuous infusion. Given this, thought should be given to its clinical use in neonates.

Bupivacaine exists in a racemic form with l and d enantiomers, with the dextrorotary form having a higher risk of cardiotoxicity.[5] Currently, levobupivacaine is not commercially available in the United States despite its wide use in Europe and better safety profile.

Recently, a liposomal form of bupivacaine has also been released with approval for use in adults for incisional pain with studies showing pain relief for up to 72 hours. Although not approved for use in children, one should be aware of this preparation, as it could be beneficial to the practice of anesthetic in pediatrics in the future.

Liposomal bupivacaine (Exparel®) was originally approved by the US Food and Drug Administration (FDA) in October 2011 for use as a local anesthetic by wound infiltration for hemorrhoidectomies and bunionectomies. Liposomal bupivacaine is based on DepoFoam technology, which encapsulates drugs in a liposomal platform and releases them over an extended period of time. By doing so, the toxic dose of bupivacaine decreases and potentially provides a greater safety profile. For example, a study by Boogaerts et al[10] compared plain bupivacaine to liposomal bupivacaine in rabbits and illustrated that more than twice the dose of liposomal bupivacaine was needed compared to plain bupivacaine to produce seizures and ventricular arrhythmias.

Since its original approval, the use of liposomal bupivacaine has expanded greatly to include transversus abdominis plane (TAP) blocks, infiltration in mammoplasties, total knee arthroplasties, and many other procedures. The use in neuraxial blocks and peripheral nerve blocks is also under investigation. The results of the studies are promising and show clinically meaningful lower cumulative pain scores, reduced opioid requirements, faster hospital discharges, and reduced hospital costs.[11]

Ropivacaine

Ropivacaine is an l-enantiomer that has less cardiac and neurologic toxicities compared to bupivacaine.[5] Ropivacaine, as with bupivacaine, has clearance that is age-dependent and decreased in neonates. However, unlike bupivacaine, ropivacaine was not found to have increased accumulation in neonates on prolonged infusions.[7] Although it has not been found to have the same accumulation as bupivacaine, one should still be mindful of the possibility of local anesthetic toxicity especially in neonates and infants given that clearance is age-dependent and the potential for higher than expected plasma concentrations exists.

In comparison to bupivacaine, ropivacaine also exhibits less motor blockade.

Topical Anesthetics

The primary topical anesthetic used currently is EMLA (eutectic mixture of local anesthetics). EMLA is a mixture of 2.5% lidocaine and 2.5% prilocaine that is unique in its ability to penetrate intact skin. This is particularly useful in the pediatric practice. It is used for procedures such as intravenous access, lumbar puncture, circumcision, or removal of small lesions. To achieve effective cutaneous anesthesia it must be placed under an occlusive bandage for 45 to 60 minutes prior to the painful stimuli. EMLA has been used in infants and children and has been shown to be safe. Other topical formulations such as tetracaine gel and liposomal lidocaine are also available.[12,13]

Other forms of topical anesthesia such as TAC (tetracaine, epinephrine, and cocaine) are also available, but are ineffective through intact skin. This is particularly useful in pediatrics when anesthetizing lacerations for suture repair. Given concerns for diversion and toxicity with TAC, other forms of anesthetics such as LET (lidocaine-epinephrine-tetracaine) have largely replaced TAC.[6]

Adjuvants

The use of local anesthetics is limited by its duration of action and the dose-dependent adverse effects.[14] Prolongation of local anesthetic peripheral nerve blocks can be achieved by utilizing catheter-based techniques. However, these can post challenges, such as catheter displacement and potential for increased infection risk.[15] An alternative is to use adjuvants to prolong the effect of local anesthetics and limit the cumulative dose requirements of the local anesthetic, thus improving the efficacy of perineural blocks and decreasing local anesthetic toxicity (Table 8-3).[14] Many adjuvants have been used in adult medicine, but all are off-label use and no adjuvant has been approved by the FDA for prolongation of peripheral nerve blocks.[15]

Table 8-3. Local Anesthetic Adjuncts

Class	Drug	Route	Adverse Effects
Opioid	Morphine	Intrathecal and epidural	Respiratory depression (early and late), nausea, vomiting, pruritus, urinary retention
Opioid	Fentanyl	Intrathecal and epidural	Same as for morphine, but decreased severity
Opioid	Sufentanil	Intrathecal and epidural	Sedation, bradycardia, and hypotension
Opioid	Hydromorphone	Intrathecal and epidural	Preferred in patients with renal insufficiency rather than morphine
Partial opioid agonist	Buprenorphine	Intrathecal and epidural	
Weak opioid with sodium and potassium channel blocking actions and serotonin and norepinephrine reuptake inhibition	Tramadol	Intrathecal and epidural	
Sympathomimetic	Epinephrine	Intrathecal and epidural	Tachycardia, hypertension
Alpha-2 adrenoreceptor antagonists	Clonidine	Intrathecal, epidural, and peripheral nerve blocks	Sedation, bradycardia, and hypotension
Alpha-2 adrenoreceptor antagonists	Dexmedetomidine	Intrathecal, epidural, and peripheral nerve blocks	Hypotension and bradycardia
Steroid	Dexamethasone	Intrathecal, epidural, and peripheral nerve blocks	
Benzodiazepine	Midazolam	Intrathecal and epidural	
Anticholinesterase inhibitor	Neostigmine	Intrathecal and epidural	Nausea, vomiting, bradycardia, agitation, restlessness
N-methyl-D-aspartate (NMDA) receptor antagonist	Ketamine	Intrathecal and epidural	Psychotomimetic sequelae (hallucinations, drowsiness, nausea)
NMDA receptor antagonist and inhibitor of voltage-gated calcium channel	Magnesium sulfate	Intrathecal and epidural	Bradycardia, hypotension, sedation, headache, disorientation

Various drugs have been used as adjuncts, including opioids, epinephrine, α_2-adrenergic antagonists, steroids, anti-inflammatory drugs, midazolam, ketamine, magnesium sulfate, and neostigmine.[14]

Opioids are the most frequently used local anesthetic adjuvant.[14] They potentiate antinociception of local anesthetics by G protein–coupled receptor mechanisms by causing hyperpolarization of the afferent sensory neurons.[14]

Preservative free morphine has been used extensively in neuraxial blocks across all age groups.[14] Morphine is hydrophilic, which results in a cephalad spread leading to an increased area of analgesia.

Epinephrine is one of the oldest additives to local anesthetic solutions.[14] It is believed to prolong the duration by its vasoconstrictive properties that prevent systemic reabsorption of local anesthetics.[15] It is useful for detecting intravascular injections of presumed epidural catheters.[14,15] However, epinephrine has not been shown to prolong peripheral nerve blocks, so it is not recommended for this use.[15]

Toxicity

Systemic toxicity to local anesthetics can occur with overdose of local anesthetics or with accidental intravascular injection. The primary effects seen are central nervous system (CNS) and cardiovascular changes.

In addition to the specific effects on the central nervous and cardiovascular systems discussed next, hypercapnia,

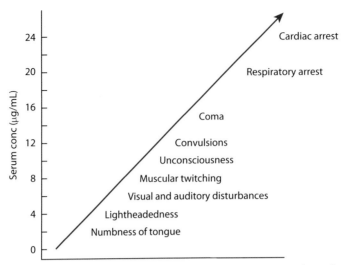

▲ **Figure 8-3.** Local anesthetic toxicity symptoms based on serum concentration. (Adapted with permission, from Hoffman RS, Howland M, Lewin NA, Nelson LS, Goldfrank LR. eds. *Goldfrank's Toxicologic Emergencies*, 10th ed. 2015. https://accesspharmacy.mhmedical.com. Copyright © McGraw Hill LLC. All rights reserved.)

acidosis, and hypoxia have further untoward effects on these systems. The hypercapnia and acidosis that may occur with local anesthetic toxicity lead to potentiation of the negative chronotropic and inotropic actions in cardiac tissue while it leads to increased free drug and thus the amount available to the CNS with resulting exacerbation of CNS toxicity.

Central Nervous System Toxicity

Often the first symptoms of local anesthetic toxicity are in the CNS system and may be vague such as a sense of feeling light-headed or dizzy. Tinnitus may also be present as an early sign. It is important to note that these early findings can be difficult to assess in infants and small children, as they may be unable to verbalize what they are experiencing. This makes it important to watch for objective signs of CNS toxicity that might occur. These signs include muscle twitches and tremors and may progress to generalized seizure activity. Following this period of excitement, CNS depression may occur and lead to respiratory failure.

Cardiovascular Toxicity

In addition to CNS effects, local anesthetic toxicity also directly and indirectly affects the cardiovascular system. Local anesthetics work to decrease the rate of depolarization in the ventricular muscle by decreasing the rate of depolarization in the fast conducting Purkinje fibers.[16]

Local anesthetics also produce negative inotropic action of the cardiac muscle. They can also lead to vasodilation of

peripheral vasculature in high concentrations. Cocaine is the one exception to this in that it exerts a vasoconstrictor effect at all doses via inhibition of norepinephrine uptake and thus causing neurogenic vasoconstriction.[6]

As briefly discussed above, special attention should be given to bupivacaine's cardiovascular toxicity. Discussion of this is important, as reversal of cardiovascular collapse from bupivacaine is particularly difficult to reverse. The dose of bupivacaine required to produce irreversible cardiovascular collapse is closer to the dose necessary to produce CNS toxicity compared to lidocaine where the difference between the doses required to produce irreversible cardiovascular collapse is significantly more than that required to produce CNS toxicity.[17]

Treatment of Local Anesthetic Toxicity

It is imperative if local anesthetics are being utilized that one knows how to treat local anesthetic toxicity. Treatment is based on two things—supportive care (including resuscitation) and intralipid. Intralipid 20% at 1.5 mL/kg should be initiated immediately if a patient develops cardiovascular compromise secondary to local anesthetic toxicity. Beyond this, one should be prepared to administer an infusion of 0.25 mL/kg/min for 10 minutes following the initial bolus. Additional supportive care with basic life support (BLS), advanced cardiac life support (ACLS), and resuscitation drugs should be used as necessary. Use of lidocaine to treat arrhythmias related to local anesthetic toxicity is of course not recommended (Figure 8-3).

Methemoglobinemia

Methemoglobinemia is a unique side effect that can occur with the use of the local anesthetic prilocaine. This occurs when hepatic metabolism of prilocaine leads to production of O-toluidine, which in turn oxidizes hemoglobin to methemoglobin. As noted earlier, although EMLA contains prilocaine it has been shown to generally be safe in term newborns. Although it is generally considered safe, there are reports of methemoglobinemia following use of EMLA in infants.[18]

Direct Nerve Toxicity

Neurologic injury after peripheral nerve blocks is multifactorial. At the site of injection, nerve damage can be due to needle injury, hematoma, or local anesthetic toxicity.[3] Utilization of nerve stimulation techniques does not prevent intraneural injections, and intraneural injections do not necessarily result in injury. Injection inside the epineurium with low initial pressures (<5 psi) maintains normal neurologic function. Initial injection pressures less than 12 psi results in return of neurologic function to baseline within 24 hours after injection. However, high injection pressures (>20 psi) intrafascicularly leads to fascicular injury, neurologic deficits, and persistent neurologic dysfunction.[19]

Needle type may also play a role. Short bevel needles less frequently produce fascicular damage than long bevel needles.[19] However, the injuries that do occur from short bevel needles are usually more severe than those from long bevel needles.[3] Additionally, orientation of the needle affects severity of injury; injuries caused by needle bevels perpendicular to the nerve fibers are more severe than those by bevels aligned parallel.[19]

Toxicity of local anesthetics themselves is time and dose dependent. Local anesthetics can induce direct nerve injury at clinical concentrations. Toxicity levels differ among local anesthetics and can be caused by the local anesthetic itself or its additives.[3]

Patient factors also contribute to nerve injury. Those with underlying nerve pathology, such as chemotherapy-related neurotoxicity or diabetic neuropathies, are more susceptible to peripheral nerve complications.[19]

REFERENCES

1. Fink BR. Leaves and needles: the introduction of surgical local anesthesia. *Anesthesiology*. 1985;63(1):77-83.
2. Lin, Y.a.L., S.S. Local Anesthetics. Barash PG, Cullen BF, Stoelting RK, et al., eds. *Clinical Anesthesia*, 8th ed. Philadelphia, PA: Wolters Kluwer, 2017..
3. Verlinde M, Hollmann MW, Stevens MF, Hermanns H, Werdehausen R, Lirk P. Local anesthetic-induced neurotoxicity. *Int J Mol Sci.* 2016;17(3):339.
4. Waxman SG, Ritchie JM. Organization of ion channels in the myelinated nerve fiber. *Science*. 1985;228(4707):1502-1507.
5. Thomas JM, Schug SA. Recent advances in the pharmcokinetics of local anesthetics. *Clin Pharmacokinet.* 1999;36(1):67-83.
6. Berde CB, Strichartz GR. Local anesthetics. In Miller RD, et al. eds. *Miller's Anesthesia.* 7th ed. Philadelphia, PA: Churchill Livingstone Elsevier; 2010:913-940.
7. Veneziano G, Tobias JD. Chloroprocaine for epidural anesthesia in infants and children. *Paediatr Anaesth.* 2017;27(6):581-590.
8. Peutrell JM, Holder K, Gregory M. Plasma bupivacaine concentrations associated with continuous extradural infusions in babies. *Br J Anaesth.* 1997;78(2):160-162.
9. Berde CB. Convulsions associated with pediatric regional anesthesia. *Anesth Analg.* 1992;75(2):164-166.
10. Boogaerts JG, Lafont ND, Luo H, Legros FJ. Plasma concentrations of bupivacaine after brachial plexus administration of liposome-associated and plain solutions to rabbits. *Can J Anaesth.* 1993;40(12):1201-1204.
11. Malik O, Kaye AD, Kaye A, Belani K, Urman RD. Emerging roles of liposomal bupivacaine in anesthesia practice. *J Anaesthesiol Clin Pharmacol.* 2017;33(2):151-156.
12. Eichenfield LF, Funk A, Fallon-Friedlander S, Cunningham BB. A clinical study to evalute the efficacy of ELA-max (4% liposomal lidocaine) as compared with eutectic mixture of local anesthetics cream for pain reduction of veinpuncture in children. *Pediatrics.* 2002;109(6):1093-1099.
13. Browne J, Awad I, Plant R, McAdoo J, Shorten G. Topical amethocaine (Ametop) is superior to EMLA for intravenous cannulation. Eutectic mixture of local anesthetics. *Can J Anaesth.* 1999;46(11):1014-1018.
14. Swain A, Nag DS, Sahu S, Samaddar DP. Adjuvants to local anesthetics: current understanding and future trends. *World J Clin Cases.* 2017;5(8):307-323.
15. Kirksey MA, Haskins SC, Cheng J, Liu SS. Local anesthetic peripheral nerve block adjuvants for prolongation of analgesia: a systematic qualitative review. *PLoS One.* 2015;10(9):e0137312.
16. Clarkson CW, Hondeghem LM. Mechanism for bupivacaine depression of cardiac conduction: fast block of sodium channels during the action potential with slow recovery from block during diastole. *Anesthesiology.* 1985;62(4):396-405.
17. de Jong RH, Ronfeld RA, DeRosa RA. Cardiovascular effects of convulsant and supraconvulsant doses of local amide local anesthetics. *Anesth Analg.* 1982;61(1):3-9.
18. Larson A, Stidham T, Banerji S, Kaufman J. Seizures and methemoglobinemia in an infant after excessive EMLA application. *Pediatr Emerg Care.* 2013;29(3):377-379.
19. Jeng CL, Rosenblatt MA. Intraneural injections and regional anesthesia: the knowna dn the unknown. *Minerva Anaesthesiol.* 2011;77(1):54-58.

Vasoactive Medications

Stylianos Voulgarelis

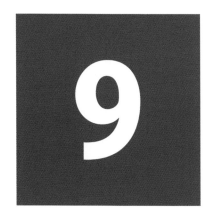

FOCUS POINTS

1. The increased metabolic rate of children comparing to adults requires a different selection of vasoactive drugs to restore and maintain the oxygen delivery to the tissues and support the circulation during periods of stress or sepsis.
2. Phenylephrine has a very narrow therapeutic spectrum in the pediatric population, mostly limited for patients with tetralogy of Fallot (TOF) and hypertrophic obstructive cardiomyopathy (HOCM)
3. Milrinone is used in pediatric patients with congenital heart disease, cardiomyopathy, and heart failure and in patients with increased pulmonary vascular resistance (PVR).
4. Dopamine is still used to improve tissue perfusion and urine output in neonates and premature infants.
5. Newborn myocardium contractility depends significantly on serum calcium levels. Hypocalcemia needs to be promptly identified and corrected.

SYMPATHOMIMETIC DRUGS, INOTROPES, AND VASOACTIVE DRUGS

Epinephrine

Epinephrine is an endogenous catecholamine that is being produced and secreted in the blood stream by the adrenal medulla after direct stimulation from sympathetic efferent fibers. It combines with pre- and postsynaptic adrenergic receptors in the periphery to generate a stress response. Epinephrine has more pronounced β1 and β2 receptor effect and less α1 and α2 effect. It produces a positive inotropic and chronotropic effect on the heart and causes splanchnic vasoconstriction and vasodilation of the skeletal muscle vascular bed in order to facilitate the flight or fight response. Additionally, it increases gluconeogenesis and glycogenolysis, supplying the body with the nutrients to meet the high metabolic demands associated with the stress state. As a β1-agonist, it is a very effective bronchodilator.

In clinical practice, epinephrine is used as an infusion for patients with left ventricular systolic dysfunction or right heart failure in order to increase the oxygen delivery to the body. It increases the oxygen consumption of the myocardium, which can be a limitation on its use for older adult patients with coronary artery disease. The absence of coronary artery disease in the pediatric population makes epinephrine the choice of preference.

The infants and children have high metabolic demands with an oxygen consumption of 10 to 14 mL/kg for infants dropping to 5 to 7 mL/kg after the first year. The oxygen demand increases even more in critically ill or septic patients, and a pharmacologic support that increases the cardiac output helps the cardiovascular system meet this demand.[1,2]

Most common uses of epinephrine in pediatric patients are as follows:

Sepsis and hypotension in the ICU: Epinephrine is the first drug of choice for critically ill patients with a wide range of doses. The effects of the treatment on the oxygen delivery can be indirectly assessed by measuring the blood pressure or directly measured by the mixed venous saturation (SvO_2) or using NIRS (near-infrared spectroscopy). When the pharmacological treatment fails, patients may require extracorporeal membrane oxygenation (ECMO) support. Most of these patients have been on high doses of epinephrine for at least 48 hours resulting in downregulation of their adrenergic receptors. The abrupt discontinuation of the adrenergic drugs may result in severe hypoglycemia. It may be beneficial to continue a low-dose 0.01 to 0.03 mcg/kg/min epinephrine infusion and slowly wean to prevent such hypoglycemic events. Steroid administration may also be required for pediatric patients to augment the response to the catecholamines and maintain better hemodynamic stability.[3]

Anaphylaxis: Epinephrine is used as an intramuscular (IM) or intravenous (IV) (10 mcg/kg for pediatric patients) bolus injection for severe anaphylactic reactions or shock. The initial bolus has to be followed by an infusion with rates of up to and even higher than 1 mcg/kg/min. Epinephrine not only counteracts the effects of histamine but also stabilizes the mast cells in order to prevent further histamine release.[4] The infusion should be titrated to the effects (blood pressure, bronchospasm) and be accompanied with the administration of H1/H2 blockers, steroids, and cessation of the allergenic triggering factor.

Pediatric Advanced Life Support (PALS): Epinephrine is part of the PALS protocol for patients with a nonperfusing rhythm. The dose is 10 mcg/kg IV or intraosseous (IO) repeated every 3 to 5 minutes. For administration of the epinephrine through the endotracheal tube the dose is not known with recommendations varying from 3 to 10 times higher than the IV dose followed by a flush of 2 to 5 mL of saline (depending on the size of the patient) followed by a couple of breaths so that the medication can reach the alveoli.

Anesthesia: All the anesthetic agents have direct or indirect negative inotropic and/or vasoplegic effects. A low dose of 0.02 to 0.05 mcg/kg/min of epinephrine can counteract these effects especially for congenital cardiac patients undergoing noncardiac procedures. This can also minimize the necessary fluid administration. This infusion can be weaned at emergence from anesthesia with no hemodynamic instability especially if the patient did not need it preoperatively.

Norepinephrine

Norepinephrine is an endogenous catecholamine being secreted by all the postganglionic sympathetic neurons. In clinical practice it is being used as an infusion for patients with profound hypotension. It directly binds mainly to the $\alpha 1$ and less to the $\beta 1$ receptors (Table 9-1).

It has strong vasopressor effects (increases the systolic, diastolic, and mean arterial pressure) and intermediate inotropic effects. It may cause a reflex decrease of the heart rate or maintain it at the same levels.

It is being used in the pediatric population in combination with epinephrine when the mean arterial blood pressure is not sufficient for the perfusion of critical organs such as the brain and kidneys, or the diastolic pressure is not sufficient for myocardial perfusion.

The dose of administration varies from low doses of 0.02 to 0.05 mcg/kg/min up to 0.3 mcg/kg/min. At these high doses, clinicians choose to add another agent such as vasopressin in the treatment plan to maintain hemodynamic stability.

Table 9-1 Vasoactive Drugs

Medication	Receptors Affected	Bolus	Infusion
Calcium chloride		30 mg/kg	
Calcium gluconate		10 mg/kg	
Epinephrine	Mainly β_1 and β_2	1–10 mcg/kg	0.01–0.5 mcg/kg/min
Dopamine	Dopamine		0.5–5 mcg/kg/min
	β_1		5–15 mcg/kg/min
	α		>15 mcg/kg/min
Labetalol	Nonselective β, α_1	0.25–1 mg/kg	0.2–1 mg/kg/h
Milrinone	cAMP phosphodiesterase inhibition	25–50 mcg/kg	0.125–0.5 mcg/kg/min
Norepinephrine	α_1 and β_1		0.02–0.3 mcg/kg/min
Nicardipine	Calcium		0.5–10 mcg/kg/min
Phenylephrine	α_1	10 mcg/kg	0.1–1 mcg/kg/min
Vasopressin	V_1 and V_2		0.2–0.5 mU/kg/min

Vasopressin

Vasopressin is a hormone secreted by the posterior pituitary grand. The osmoreceptors of the hypothalamus sense an increase of serum osmolality causing secretion of vasopressin in the bloodstream. Vasopressin subsequently acts on the collecting ducts of the kidneys, mostly via the V2 receptors, increasing free water retention, resulting in increased intravascular volume and decreased serum osmolality. Other mechanisms that stimulate the secretion of vasopressin are the decreased vascular volume/pressure, pain, and stress.

Vasopressin action on the V1 receptors offers a different mechanism than the adrenergic one, augmenting vascular tone but lacking any inotropic effects. Its action is based on the IP3/DAG pathway (inositol triphosphate/diacylglycerol), which causes an increase in the ionized calcium.

Vasopressin and its analogue DDAVP also stimulate the endothelium to secret von Willebrand factor through the cAMP pathway.

The pulmonary vasculature lacks vasopressin receptors. Patients with increased pulmonary vascular resistance (PVR) and reduced systemic vascular resistance benefit the most by the administration of vasopressin. The infusion rate is 0.2 to 0.5 mU/kg/min up to 0.04 U/min.

Vasopressin is part of the Advanced Cardiac Life Support (ACLS) protocol for a nonperfusing rhythm and a 40-U bolus can replace the epinephrine in one of the first two boluses. In the Pediatric Advanced Life Support (PALS) cardiac arrest, it is not routinely recommended because there is no clear evidence of improving the ROSC (Return of Spontaneous Circulation).[5–12]

Phenylephrine

Phenylephrine is a pure $\alpha 1$ agonist. It increases systemic vascular resistance and may cause a profound reflex bradycardia. Although it has no inotropic effects and for that reason is a poor choice for the pediatric population who respond to stress with a high cardiac output state, phenylephrine has still a very important role in the management of some pediatric diseases such as tetralogy of Fallot (ToF). This congenital heart disease is characterized by an overriding aorta, perimembranous ventricular septal defect, right ventricular hypertrophy, and pulmonary stenosis. ToF patients may require much higher doses per kilogram (up to 10 mcg/kg bolus) of phenylephrine than adults especially during their intraoperative management. Increase of the heart rate in the preoperative area from anxiety and decrease of the systemic vascular resistance (SVR) on induction can cause right to left shunt and cyanosis refractory to oxygen administration. The drug of choice is phenylephrine because it lacks any inotropic effect, increases SVR, and causes reflex bradycardia.

Another pediatric population that may require phenylephrine administration is children with dynamic or fixed left ventricular outflow tract (LVOT) obstruction. In the presence of subaortic membrane, hypertrophic obstructive cardiomyopathy, congenital aortic valve stenosis, or supravalvular aortic stenosis (William's syndrome), the preservation of the afterload maintains the perfusion of the coronary arteries making phenylephrine an ideal medication for emergencies and intraoperative management. Additionally, in the presence of dynamic obstruction the preservation of the afterload prevents the almost complete emptying of the left ventricle (LV) which worsens that LVOT obstruction and the gradient across it.

Milrinone

Milrinone is a drug with intracellular action. It inhibits the cAMP phosphodiesterase (PDE) isoenzyme peak III in the myocyte and increases the ionized calcium levels as a result of increased cAMP. Milrinone has a positive inotropic and lusitropic effect on the myocardium. In the peripheral vascular system, the intracellular increase of the cAMP causes a decrease in the vascular tone. In the pulmonary vasculature, milrinone directly reduces pulmonary vascular resistance. Although not as effective as inhaled nitric oxide (iNO) or the cGMP PDE inhibitors, the combined pulmonary vasodilatory and inotropic effect on the right ventricle can improve the cardiac output and systemic perfusion for patients with pulmonary hypertension and/or right heart failure.

It has no direct diuretic effects but the increase in the cardiac output may cause an increase in the urine output.

Milrinone has a half-life of 2.3 hours and it is 70% bound on plasma proteins. The dose used in clinical practice is 25 to 50 mcg/kg bolus over 10 minutes followed by infusion of 0.125 to 0.5 mcg/kg/min up to 0.75 mcg/kg/min in rare clinical conditions.

High doses of 0.5 to 0.75 mcg/kg/min may cause profound vasoplegia (reduced SVR in the setting of normal or elevated cardiac output) in adults. Other side effects with such high-dose administration include flushing and headaches.

In the pediatric population milrinone is a commonly used drug in high doses without any side effects seen in adults. Pediatric patients with cardiomyopathy and heart failure (eg, enterovirus cardiomyopathy), patients with increased PVR [hypoplastic lung due to congenital diaphragmatic hernia, persistent pulmonary hypertension of the newborn (PPHN)], and congenital heart patients are the main populations that benefit from the use of milrinone.

Dopamine

Dopamine is an adrenoreceptor with a dose-dependent action and affinity to receptors. At low dose (0.5–5 mcg/kg/min) dopamine activates the dopamine-specific receptors located in the renal vascular bed causing vasodilation and diuresis. At intermediate dose (5–15 mcg/kg/min) dopamine has a β_1 agonist action increasing contractility and heart rate, whereas in high doses (>15 mcg/kg/min) it activates α-adrenoceptors increasing systemic vascular resistance.

The use of dopamine has been limited to the last decade as it has not been proven to reduce the incidence of renal failure. Some studies support its use in the NICU because of increase in urine production for low birth weight and premature neonates.[13]

Digoxin

Digoxin is a glucoside with positive inotropic and negative chronotropic effects on the heart. It is frequently used for patients with congenital heart disease with circulation in parallel (eg, Norwood physiology) or series (eg, Fontan physiology) and patients with dilated cardiomyopathy.

Digoxin inhibits the Na^+/K^+ adenosine triphosphatase (Na^+/K^+ pump) competing with potassium for the same binding area. This is the reason that the levels of serum potassium affect the action of the digoxin. Potassium levels and digoxin levels should be measured frequently especially at the beginning of the treatment and periodically after initiation of treatment.

Digoxin has a very low therapeutic index meaning that the safety window between therapeutic and toxic doses is very narrow. The signs of toxicity can be gastrointestinal in nature, cardiac dysrhythmias, or mental status changes. Digoxin can be given IV but most frequently is given PO postoperatively or through a nasogastric tube. The most common clinical dose is 3 to 6 mcg/kg/day divided in 2 doses/day.

Ionized Calcium

Newborns are prone to hypocalcemia during their first days of life. Risk factors include prematurity, small for gestational age (SGA), maternal diabetes, and perinatal asphyxia/hypoxia. The latter causes reduction in circulating calcium by an increase in calcitonin levels which inhibit calcium release from the bones.

Immature sarcoplasmic reticulum unable to regulate calcium levels makes the also immature myocardium dependent on influx of calcium through the sarcolemma and serum ionized calcium.

Hypocalcemia can be a bigger concern during surgical procedures that require administration of albumin or citrated blood products. Citrate is primarily metabolized in the liver to bicarbonate. In infancy the hepatic enzymes are immature, and the liver is unable to remove the citrate from the blood stream resulting frequently in citrate intoxication during transfusion. Citrate intoxication can also occur during massive transfusion in pediatric trauma patients with rapid administration of blood products. The first clinical signs that will alert the anesthesiologist are QT prolongation, hypotension, increased central venous pressure (CVP), and coagulopathy.[14]

Calcium comes in two preparations: calcium chloride and gluconate. To date there has been no difference in outcome between administration of calcium chloride versus calcium gluconate. Studies in the 1980s and 1990s during anhepatic phase of liver transplant patients have shown that calcium gluconate does not depend on hepatic metabolism to release calcium. The main difference providers should be aware of is that calcium chloride carries three times more calcium ions per milligram. They can both be given as a bolus or infusion. Bolus should not exceed 10 mg/kg for calcium chloride or 30 mg/kg for calcium gluconate due to the risk of cardiac dysrhythmias. In awake patients, an intravenous calcium bolus may cause dysphoria and flushing, both transient effects. Calcium gluconate can also be given as a PO supplement.

Levosimendan

Levosimendan is a newer drug that has been used in Europe and Asia for more than a decade but has not yet been Food and Drug Administration (FDA) approved in the United States (as of August 2019). It is a calcium sensitizer that acts at a molecular level on the cardiac myofilament and exhibits positive inotropic effects. It also causes vasodilation in the periphery, the coronary arteries, and the pulmonary arteries. PO administration has been studied but there is only IV formulation available.

Initially, levosimendan was developed for use in adults with acute or decompensated chronic heart failure. In the last decade this has been used in younger patients, even infants, exhibiting a safe profile. Currently, it is frequently used in pediatric patients with either congenital heart disease or cardiomyopathy. There have also been case reports for its use in sepsis-related heart failure in infants, but the vasodilatory effects have to be carefully considered.[15]

The dose is 6 to 12 mcg/kg bolus followed by an infusion of 0.1 mcg/kg/min. The elimination half-life of the drug is 1 hour but the active metabolite has a half-life of 80 hours.

PARASYMPATHOMIMETIC DRUGS AND VASODILATORS

Phenoxybenzamine

Phenoxybenzamine is an oral α-adrenergic antagonist that has been traditionally used in the preoperative preparation of patients with pheochromocytoma.

After the initiation of the α blockade process a β-blocker may need to be added in the regimen to ameliorate tachycardia. β-Blockers should not be added unless α blockade has been established because their initiation may potentiate hypertension ($β_2$ blockade of skeletal muscle vasodilation).

Patients are expected to respond with a decrease in arterial pressure and increased weight due to the replenishment of the intravascular volume. Common side effects include orthostatic hypotension, nasal congestion, and flushing.

Phenoxybenzamine has a half-life of 24 hours. The dose for pediatric patients is 0.25 to 1 mg/kg/day divided into 2 to 3 doses.

Phentolamine

Phentolamine is a pure α-adrenergic blocking agent. It has a half-life of 19 minutes. The dose range is 0.2 to 2 mcg/kg/min. In pediatrics it is used for the following cases:

Pheochromocytoma: preoperative preparation or intraoperative management of hypertension.

Extravasation of norepinephrine (or other vasoactive drugs) followed by skin necrosis: The dose is 0.1 to 0.2 mg/kg up to 10 mg, diluted in normal saline and infiltrated locally.

Single ventricle patients: It has been shown that α blockade in the intraoperative and postoperative period of the first stage of Norwood palliation helps in balancing the Qp:Qs and improves systemic perfusion.

Cardiopulmonary bypass (CPB): Phentolamine can be used to facilitate homogeneous and fast cooling during CPB.

Captopril

Angiotensin-converting enzyme (ACE) inhibitors block the transformation of angiotensin I to angiotensin II and prevent the production of aldosterone. The primary effect is afterload reduction, but it is also proven that ACE inhibitors improve outcome by inhibiting the remodeling process and prevent the left ventricular enlargement for patients with cardiomyopathy, heart failure, and congenital heart disease.

It is often being administered with a selective aldosterone antagonist (spironolactone) to prevent hypokalemia and its dysrhythmia side effects.

Captopril is being used orally with a starting dose of 0.3 mcg/kg/day up to 4 to 6 mcg/kg/day divided in 3 to 4 doses.[16,17]

Labetalol

Labetalol is a nonselective β-blocker with combined α$_1$ blocking activity. It can be administered PO or IV as a bolus or drip. The half-life is approximately 6 hours. The pediatric dose is 0.25 to 1 mg/kg IV or 0.2 to 1 mg/kg/h. The peak effect of a single dose is 15 minutes, so redosing to effect should take that into consideration.

Because of its dual adrenoreceptor effects, special attention should be paid in children with history of reactive airway disease and pediatric patients with increase in QT interval and AV blocks.

Nitroglycerin

Nitroglycerin acts by releasing nitric oxide (NO) and by increasing the cGMP in the smooth muscles of vessels, causing primarily venous and coronary dilation.

The dose is 0.2 to 1 mcg/kg/min. The use of nitroglycerin in the pediatric population is very limited.

Sodium Nitroprusside

Sodium nitroprusside is an intravenous agent with very potent vasodilatory effects. It mainly acts on arterioles and less on the venous system with no direct cardiac effect.

It acts through the NO pathway with a half-life of only 2 minutes. The duration of the treatment is limited especially in patients with decreased renal function because cyanide ions can be accumulated to toxic levels. The regular dose is 0.2 to 4 mcg/kg/min (maximum 10 mcg/kg/min). The use of nitroprusside is not very common for pediatric patients.

Some providers use it immediately postoperatively after the second-stage palliation for single ventricle patients (Glenn procedure) or during aortic coarctation repair for afterload reduction.

It can also be used in low doses for patients undergoing deep hypothermic cardiac arrest to achieve more even and quicker cooling or rewarming.[18,19]

Nicardipine

Nicardipine is a calcium channel blocker with a selective action mainly in the systemic arterial bed and coronary arteries and minimal effect on the myocardium.

It can be administered PO or IV, is 95% bound on proteins, is metabolized by the liver, and has a half-life of 8.6 hours. The initial dose for an infusion is 0.5 mcg/kg/min increased up to 5 to 10 mcg/kg/min. For teenagers or young adults, the dose can be given starting at 1 mg/h and going up to 15 mg/h.

It can be used for patients that undergo procedures with vascular anastomosis or manipulation and need tight blood pressure control. It is also the drug of choice for blood pressure control of neurosurgical patients or patients with traumatic brain injury.

Frequently, patients on immunosuppression after a transplant or chemotherapy may exhibit increased systemic vascular resistance and require blood pressure control, which can be achieved effectively by nicardipine while they are nothing per Os (NPO) or still need titration of their medications.

Nimodipine

Nimodipine is an orally administered lipophilic calcium channel blocker with high selectivity for the cerebral arteries. It is used to prevent cerebral vasospasm following subarachnoid hemorrhage that has potentially devastating outcomes. Its mechanism of action is not quite clear in humans. Although the neurologic outcomes are significantly better, the angiographic evidence is not always in agreement. It is highly possible that the neuroprotective effects of nimodipine are related to the prevention of calcium influx in the damaged cells that promotes apoptosis.[20]

In children, the dose is not clear and careful titration is required to avoid hypotension. Nimodipine is also being studied for migraine prevention in the pediatric population.

Clevidipine

Clevidipine is a newer ultrashort acting calcium channel blocker that is being used perioperatively for blood pressure control or controlled hypotension. The half-life is 1 minute. It is rapidly hydrolyzed by esterases in the blood and extravascular tissue. Its use in the pediatric population has been studied with infusion rates reported to be in the 0.5 to 5 mcg/kg/min range.[21,22]

REFERENCES

1. U.S. Food and Drug Administration, 10903 New Hampshire Avenue, Silver Spring, MD 20993, USA. Available at: https://www.fda.gov/media/105790/download.
2. Health Canada, Address Locator 0900C2, Ottawa, Ontario, K1A 0K9, Canada. Available at: https://www.fda.gov/media/105790/download.
3. van der Laan ME, Schat TE, Olthuis AJ, Boezen HM, Bos AF, Kooi EM. The association between multisite near-infrared spectroscopy and routine hemodynamic measurements in relation to short-term outcome in preterms with clinical sepsis. *Neonatology*. 2015;108(4):297-304.
4. Kay LJ, Peachell PT. Mast cell β12-adrenoceptors. *Chem Immunol Allergy*. 2005;87:145-153.
5. Wallace AW, Tunin CM, Shoukas AA. Effects of vasopressin on pulmonary and systemic vascular mechanics. *Am J Physiol*. 1989;257(4 pt 2):H1228-H1234.
6. Swieringa F, Lancé MD, Fuchs B, et al. Desmopressin treatment improves platelet function under flow in patients with postoperative bleeding. *J Thromb Haemost*. 2015;13(8):1503-1513.
7. Kamath SA, Laskar SR, Yancy CW. Novel therapies for heart failure: vasopressin and selective aldosterone antagonists. *Congest Heart Fail*. 2005;11(1):21-29.
8. Kleinman ME, Chameides L, Schexnayder SM, et al. Part 14: Pediatric Advanced Life Support. 2010 American Heart Association Guidelines for Cardiopulmonary Resuscitation and Emergency Cardiovascular Care. *Circulation*. 2010;122(18 suppl 3):S876-S908.
9. Holmes CL, Landry DW, Granton JT. Science review: vasopressin and the cardiovascular system part 2—clinical physiology. *Critical Care*. 2004;8:15-23.
10. Callaway CW, Hostler D, Doshi AA, et al. Usefulness of vasopressin administered with epinephrine during out-of-hospital cardiac arrest. *Am J Cardiol*. 2006;98:1316-1321.
11. Gueugniaud PY, David JS, Chanzy E, et al. Vasopressin and epinephrine vs. epinephrine alone in cardiopulmonary resuscitation. *N Engl J Med*. 2008;359:21-30.
12. Lindner KH, Prengel AW, Brinkmann A, Strohmenger HU, Lindner IM, Lurie KG. Vasopressin administration in refractory cardiac arrest. *Ann Intern Med*. 1996;124:1061-1064.
13. Crouchley JL, Smith PB, Cotten CM, et al. Effects of low-dose dopamine on urine output in normotensive very low birth weight neonates. *J Perinatol*. 2013;33(8):619-621.
14. Cho WI, Yu HW, Chung HR, et al. Clinical and laboratory characteristics of neonatal hypocalcemia. *Ann Pediatr Endocrinol Metab*. 2015;20(2):86-91.
15. Joshi RK, Aggarwal N, Aggarwal M, Pandey R, Dinand V, Joshi R. Successful use of levosimendan as a primary inotrope in pediatric cardiac surgery: an observational study in 110 patients. *Ann Pediatr Cardiol*. 2016;9(1):9-15.
16. Bonaduce D, Petretta M, Arrichiello P, et al. Effects of captopril treatment on left ventricular remodeling and function after anterior myocardial infarction: comparison with digitalis. *J Am Coll Cardiol*. 1992;19(4):858-863.
17. Momma K. ACE inhibitors in pediatric patients with heart failure. *Paediatr Drugs*. 2006;8(1):55-69.
18. Scheffer T, Sanders DB. The neurologic sequelae of cardiopulmonary bypass-induced cerebral hyperthermia and cerebroprotective strategies. *J Extra Corpor Technol*. 2003;35(4):317-321.
19. Ambesh SP, Chattopadhyaya M, Saxena PV, Mahant TS, Ganjoo AK. Combined use of isoflurane and sodium nitroprusside during active rewarming on cardiopulmonary bypass: a prospective, comparative study. *J Postgrad Med*. 2000;46(4):253-257.
20. Heffren J, McIntosh AM, Reiter PD. Nimodipine for the prevention of cerebral vasospasm after subarachnoid hemorrhage in 12 children. *Pediatr Neurol*. 2015;52(3):356-360.
21. Deeks ED, Keating GM, Keam SJ. Clevidipine: a review of its use in the management of acute hypertension. *Am J Cardiovasc Drugs*. 2009;9(2):117-134.
22. Tobias JD, Hoernschemeyer DG. Clevidipine for controlled hypotension during spinal surgery in adolescents. *J Neurosurg Anesthesiol*. 2011;23(4):347-351.

Anesthetic Practice

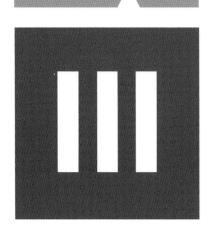

Preoperative Evaluation

Lynne R. Ferrari

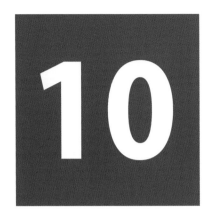

INTRODUCTION

There is an increasing desire among patients and families to be involved in the perioperative decision-making process.[1] Informed consent in pediatric surgical and interventional procedures requiring general anesthesia involves a shared decision-making process between the multidisciplinary physicians, patient, and family. Shared decision making has the potential to increase satisfaction with care, reduce decisional conflict and regret, improve understanding of and participation in care, and thereby improve health-related quality of life. It is important that the anesthesiologist should be able to accurately estimate and describe the risks of the proposed anesthetic management to the family. Pediatric risk assessment tools may be used to communicate these patient-specific risks.[2]

Anesthetic risk can be decreased by maximizing the information known about the patient's health prior to induction of anesthesia. The overall incidence of cardiac arrest in children under 18 years of age has been reported to be 2.9–4.95/10,000 and of these 18.28/10,000 or 0.18% were below 1 year of age.[3] Since there is no substitute for the long-term relationship that pediatrician, family, and patient have, it is the responsibility of the perioperative anesthesia care team to assess the patient's current health status as it compares with the usual state of health. Both acute and chronic diseases should be evaluated and optimized prior to anesthesia. The choice of anesthetic agent and mode of delivery is a multifactorial decision; however, state of health, both current and prior, is the major determinant. Appropriate laboratory examination should be performed prior to the time of surgery to provide adequate opportunity to adjust or optimize a patient's current health status. If consultation by another specialist is warranted, this can be planned and accomplished prior to anesthesia and surgery. Not only will this planning optimize anesthetic risk factors, but will also prevent cancellation as a consequence of inadequate documentation of health status or data that cannot be retrieved.

PSYCHOLOGICAL PREPARATION

The understanding of and response to illness is affected by a child's maturity. The medical practitioner should anticipate the child's needs and concerns and be able to interpret the child's nonverbal expressions and actions when the child's communication skills are not highly developed. Diseases carry with them different psychosocial aspects for children as compared to adults. For many healthy children who undergo elective surgery, the emotional disruption may surpass the medical issues. Children respond to the prospect of surgery in a varied and age-dependent manner, and the anesthesiologist must consider this during the preoperative interview.

The toddler's greatest fear is the loss of control for actions and choices. The preschooler fears injury, loss of control, the unknown, and abandonment. The preschooler interprets words literally and is unable to differentiate between what is heard and what is implied. The words adults use with children are as important as the messages they try to convey. Because preschoolers are unable to distinguish between reality and fantasy and exist in a world of magical thinking, they cannot recognize the difference between safe sleep during anesthesia and the kind of "sleep" from which their animal did not awaken. The school-aged child fears loss of control, injury, inability to meet the expectations of adults, and death. Between the ages of 6 and 12, children begin to think more logically; yet they may nod with understanding and listen intently, when in fact they do not fully grasp the explanation. These children may fail to ask questions or admit a lack of knowledge because they feel that they should know the information. Adolescents fear loss of control, an altered body image, and segregation from peers. They are usually convinced that the anesthesiologist will not be able to put them to sleep and that, if the anesthesiologist does succeed, they will never wake up.[4]

PAST MEDICAL HISTORY

The child's prior anesthetic experience should be explored during the preoperative visit, since reactions to previous anesthetics may guide the choice of techniques to utilize or avoid. Was general anesthesia previously induced with a mask? Was the parent present for induction? Was premedication used? Was the induction stormy? Were there any sequelae after the hospital experience, such as nightmares, regression to earlier behavior, or new fears of odors? Family history should be explored for anesthesia-related events. Malignant hyperthermia (MH) is always a concern in the pediatric age group and high fevers or unusual perioperative events in the operating room or in family members should be investigated.[5] Although most pediatric anesthesiologists refrain from routinely using succinylcholine, questions about prolonged paralysis or mechanical ventilation after general anesthesia in family members should be asked. If there is a possible history of pseudocholinesterase deficiency, laboratory examination should be performed to determine if that child is at risk. Family members should be queried for a history of unexpected death, sudden infant death syndrome (SIDS), genetic defects, or familial conditions such as muscular dystrophy, cardiomyopathy, cystic fibrosis, sickle cell disease, bleeding tendencies, or human immunodeficiency virus (HIV) infection.

A complete review of systems should be included with emphasis placed on medical comorbidity, which might influence either the choice or outcome of the anesthetic. The presence of cough, asthma, or a recent upper respiratory infection might predispose the child to laryngospasm, bronchospasm, atelectasis, or pneumonia. The new onset of a heart murmur, cyanosis, hypertension, exercise intolerance, or a history of rheumatic fever might suggest an evolving problem which could become exacerbated during the administration of an anesthetic or with a surgical procedure. Parents should be questioned for the presence of vomiting, diarrhea, malabsorption, black stools, gastroesophageal reflux, or jaundice to reveal electrolyte imbalance, dehydration, hypoglycemia, anemia, or the need for a rapid sequence induction. The presence of seizures, head trauma, or swallowing problems may indicate a metabolic derangement, increased intracranial pressure, or sensitivity to muscle relaxants and the anesthetic plan should be altered accordingly. The presence of a urinary tract abnormality should be sought in an attempt to evaluate the state of hydration and integrity of renal function. Abnormal development, alterations in serum glucose levels, or a history of chronic steroid use may indicate an endocrinopathy, diabetes mellitus, hypothyroidism, or adrenal insufficiency. Finally, a history of anemia, bruising, or excess bleeding may suggest a transfusion requirement or coagulopathy, which should be investigated prior to the time of surgery.

PREGNANCY TESTING

The decision to require pregnancy testing prior to administration of anesthesia is institution dependent. Most hospitals do, however, have guidelines for mandatory pregnancy testing for all post-menarchal females prior to anesthesia.[6]

The rate of undiagnosed pregnancy in adolescent females is approximately 1%. Fetal exposure to some anesthetic agents may increase the risk of spontaneous miscarriage, teratogenic effects, and apoptosis in the rapidly developing brain. For these reasons it has been suggested that elective surgery should be postponed in pregnant female patients.[7,8]

FASTING GUIDELINES

Liberalization of oral intake results in a less anxious child, calmer parents, better maintenance of hemodynamic parameters, and less risk of intraoperative hypoglycemia. Fasting guidelines for children before general anesthesia have been modified to recommend that restricting children to fasting after midnight is no longer common practice and children should be encouraged to drink clear fluids up to 2 hours prior to the time of general anesthesia.[9]

In general, most institutions allow the ingestion of clear fluids until 2 to 3 hours before the time of surgery. These include water, electrolyte solutions (Pedialyte), glucose water, apple juice, white grape juice, and frozen pops without fruit pulp. Clear fluids are defined as any fluid through which a newspaper can be read. No evidence exists that volume has an impact on gastric emptying time or residual volume; therefore, the quantity of clear fluids is not limited.

Formula and breast milk are not clear fluids. Breast milk is considered to be intermediate between clear fluids and formula usually restricted for 4 hours prior to general anesthesia. Clear policies regarding formula, breast milk, and solids should be established for each institution.

MEDICATIONS, ALLERGIES, ADJUNCT THERAPY, AND BEYOND

The parent should be questioned for current use of antibiotics, antihistamines, or other medicines. Many children have never been on medications, some only have been exposed to antibiotics for a simple illness yet others may have received many medications for complex disease processes. It is essential to obtain a full medication history including nonprescription medications administered for minor illness since many over-the-counter (OTC) cold remedies contain aspirin, nonsteroidal anti-inflammatory drugs (NSAIDs), or other compounds which may interfere with coagulation and platelet function. The use of alternative therapies as well as herbal remedies should be documented since these may complicate the anesthetic management. The American Society of Anesthesiologists does not have a formal position on phytopharmaceuticals or other forms of alternative therapy; however, taking "all natural" agents during the perioperative period may put a patient at risk for untoward events. Weight loss aids may augment sympathetic function, and agents designed to enhance muscle growth (eg, creatine) may alter hepatic and renal functions. It should be common practice during the preoperative interview to document intake of any herbal therapies and determine if an alteration in anesthetic technique is warranted. Similarly, the practice of body piercing is becoming increasingly more common. Metal objects in the skin during surgery and anesthesia increase the risk of burn injury if there is an intraoperative electrocautery malfunction. Additionally, metal objects may become caught on equipment in the OR resulting in tearing of skin and subcutaneous tissue. Large metal objects pierced through the midline of the tongue may interfere with effective laryngoscopy and make securing the airway unnecessarily challenging. These objects may also tear nondisposable laryngeal mask airways. Patients, especially adolescents, should be counseled to remove all metal objects and disclose any body piercing that can't be seen during the preoperative interview.

Queries regarding known drug allergies should be made in children just like in adults. Inquiry regarding primary and secondhand smoke exposure should be made since there is evidence to suggest that these result in an increase in perioperative airway complications.[10,11] Inquiry regarding illicit drug use should also be included in the adolescent population.

Several groups of pediatric patients are at increased risk for latex allergy including children with spina bifida. Adverse reactions to bananas, latex balloons, other latex-containing toys, or the rubber dam used by a dentist should alert the practitioner to the possibility of latex allergy.[12] Allergy consultation and preoperative RAST testing and skin prick testing should be considered in children with a high index of suspicion. Latex sensitization in general pediatric surgical patients is becoming more common; therefore, there is a need for increased screening of patients.[13]

Most regular medications (exceptions maybe drugs such as diuretics and antihypertensives) should be taken on the morning of surgery with a sip of water including oral suspensions. For children who cannot ingest oral medication without food, a spoonful of grape or apple jelly may be substituted as an acceptable alternative.

SPECIAL CONSIDERATIONS

Anesthesia-Induced Neurotoxicity

There have been recent allegations that commonly used anesthetic drugs are deleterious to the developing brain. Most of the epidemiological studies are retrospective and include significant confounders of underlying pathology and surgery.[14,15]

Animal studies have demonstrated that commonly used anesthetic, sedative, and analgesic agents are associated with neuroapoptosis and neurobehavioral deficits; however, the mechanisms underlying the neurotoxic effects have not been elucidated. It is likely that the group of patients potentially susceptible to the effects of prolonged exposure to anesthetics and sedatives are premature infants requiring neonatal intensive care and complex pediatric patients undergoing long, complicated procedures.[16]

Obstructive Sleep Apnea and Sleep-Disordered Breathing

Obstruction of the oropharyngeal airway by hypertrophied tonsils leading to apnea during sleep is an important clinical entity. Despite only mild-to-moderate tonsillar enlargement on physical examination, these patients have upper airway obstruction while awake and apnea during sleep.[17] In children with long-standing hypoxemia and hypercarbia, increased airway resistance can lead to cor pulmonale. Patients may have electrocardiographic evidence of right ventricular hypertrophy, and radiographic evidence consistent with cardiomegaly.[18] These patients often have dysfunction in the medulla or hypothalamic areas of the central nervous system causing persistently elevated CO_2, despite relief of airway obstruction as well as a hyperreactive pulmonary vascular bed. The increased pulmonary vascular resistance and myocardial depression in response to hypoxia, hypercarbia, and acidosis are far greater than what is expected for that degree of physiologic alteration in the normal population. A thorough investigation of this is essential in children who are at risk.

Sleep-disordered breathing (SDB) is a spectrum of disorders ranging from primary snoring to obstructive sleep apnea syndrome (OSAS). SDB affects 10% of the population but only 1% to 4% will progress to OSAS.[19] Proper screening for and diagnosis of obstructive sleep apnea prior to surgery is important in reducing the associated risks. The STOP-BANG questionnaire which has been developed as a tool to screen adult patients for obstructive sleep apnea (Snoring, Tiredness, Observation of apnea during sleep, high blood Pressure, BMI >35 kg/m², Age >50, Neck size, Gender) is not applicable to children.[20] The STBUR questionnaire has been proposed as an alternative for pediatric patients. It screens for Snoring, Trouble Breathing and whether a child is Un-Refreshed after sleep and has potential to be a reliable predictor of children at risk for perioperative respiratory events.[21,22] Repetitive arousal from sleep to restore airway patency is a common feature as are episodic sleep-associated oxygen desaturations, hypercarbia, and cardiac dysfunction as a result of airway obstruction. Individuals who experience obstruction during sleep may have snoring loud enough to be heard through closed doors or observed pauses in breathing during sleep and the presence of these findings should be documented. Obesity changes craniofacial anthropometric characteristics; therefore, a body mass index of a greater than or equal of 95% for age or greater is a predisposing physical characteristic that increases the risk of developing OSAS.[23] Children with craniofacial abnormalities including a small maxilla and mandible, a large tongue for a given mandibular size, and a thick neck have a similar increased risk.

A history of sleep-disordered breathing should be sought. The physical examination should begin with observation of the patient. The presence of audible respirations, mouth breathing, nasal quality of the speech, and chest retractions should be noted. Mouth breathing may be the result of chronic nasopharyngeal obstruction. An elongated face, a retrognathic mandible, and a high-arched palate may be present. The oropharynx should be inspected for evaluation of tonsillar size to determine the ease of mask ventilation and tracheal intubation. The presence of wheezing or rales on auscultation of the chest may be a lower respiratory component of upper airway infection. The presence of inspiratory stridor or prolonged expiration may indicate partial airway obstruction from hypertrophied tonsils or adenoids.

Chest radiographs and electrocardiograms (ECGs) are not required unless specific abnormalities are elicited during the history, such as recent pneumonia, bronchitis, upper respiratory infection (URI), or history consistent with cor pulmonale, which is seen in children with obstructive sleep apnea syndrome. In those children with a history of cardiac abnormalities, an echocardiogram may be indicated.

The Child with a Cold

Children usually experience three to nine episodes of respiratory infection each year. It is, therefore, likely that especially during the winter months a child has an acute upper respiratory infection, is just recovering from one, or is about to have another. The risks vary from minor complications to death under anesthesia as a result of pathophysiology associated with a respiratory infection.[24,25] Children with a respiratory tract infection have a 2- to 7-fold increase in perioperative respiratory complications and an 11-fold increase if endotracheal intubation is performed.[26] Complications include atelectasis, oxygen desaturation, bronchospasm, croup, laryngospasm, and postoperative pneumonia.[27] Although definitive criteria for cancelling surgery have not been established, the decision is often subjective. Decisions to cancel or postpone surgery should be made in conjunction with the surgeon and be based on the type of procedure, the urgency of the procedure, and the child's overall medical condition.[28]

Criteria which are suggestive of cancellation include the necessity of endotracheal intubation, parental observation that the child is acutely ill on the day of surgery, the presence of nasal congestion, cough and active sputum production, and whether the child is exposed to passive smoke. If the airway can be adequately maintained with a face mask or laryngeal mask airway, the possible morbidity associated with the respiratory infection may be minimized.

Cough is a sign of lower respiratory involvement and should be evaluated for origin (upper airway or bronchial) and quality (wet or dry). Most children will have clear breath sounds when auscultated during quiet respirations. It is during coughing and crying that rales and rhonchi will best be detected. Bronchial hyperreactivity may exist for up to 7 weeks after the resolution of URI symptoms; although it is often impossible to delay surgery for this length of time, most anesthesiologists would agree that surgery may be scheduled after the acute symptoms have resolved and no sooner than 3 weeks after the initial evaluation.

Asthma

Asthma is a leading cause of chronic illness in the pediatric population and consists of bronchoconstriction, hypersecretion of mucus, mucosal edema, and desquamation of inflammatory cells. The hyperreactive airways are very sensitive to stimuli and endotracheal intubation is one of the most potent stimuli for this.

A thorough history should be taken and must include the age of onset of symptoms, the severity of symptoms, the frequency of wheezing, prior steroid therapy, the frequency of emergency room visits, and the number of hospital admissions for pulmonary problems including necessity of mechanical ventilation. The current medical therapy should be noted as well as any additional therapy which is required during acute exacerbations of the disease. It is important to note if a child is on maximal medical therapy and if wheezing persists despite this. It may not be possible for some children to be free of wheezing prior to the administration of general anesthesia.

All medications, both inhaled and oral, should be administered up to and including the morning of surgery. If children are not on maintenance therapy and only require treatment during acute exacerbations, this therapy should be considered for the 24 hours prior to anesthesia even if the child has no respiratory symptoms. This provides an added protection against intraoperative pulmonary complications.

Cystic Fibrosis

Cystic fibrosis is an inherited multisystem disorder and the major cause of severe chronic lung disease in children. It is characterized by chronic obstruction and inflammation of the airway as well as exocrine gland dysfunction. Children with cystic fibrosis may also have nasal polyps, pansinusitis, rectal prolapse, pancreatitis, cholelithiasis, and insulin-dependent diabetes mellitus. An attempt should be made to optimize pulmonary function prior to general anesthesia. This may be accomplished through the use of bronchodilator therapy, antibiotics, and vigorous pulmonary toilet. Recent pulmonary function tests (PFTs) should be reviewed so that the baseline pulmonary status may be documented. Children as young as 5 years of age can cooperate and complete PFT and these should be checked within 6 months of the planned procedure.

Cardiac Disease

Most children with significant cardiac disease are followed regularly by a cardiologist and should have an interval evaluation by the cardiologist in the preoperative period to detect and document any change. Children who have corrected congenital heart disease should have a description of the repair and current anatomy documented and made available to the anesthesia team. If a defect still exists, management recommendations should be requested from the cardiologist. All current cardiac catheterization data should be reviewed. Children with cardiac disease can be divided into two categories: those who have structural congenital heart disease (corrected and uncorrected) and those who have a heart murmur without structural abnormalities (previously diagnosed or new)

and this should be clarified. Heart murmurs in children should be identified as innocent or pathologic and this is easily accomplished by a screening echocardiogram. If a murmur is pathologic, the degree of physiologic and hemodynamic compromise should be determined and the need for antibiotic prophylaxis should be assessed during the preoperative visit.

The Former Premature Infant

Premature infants frequently have complex medical histories and require surgery for a variety of reasons. Many former premature infants have developed bronchopulmonary dysplasia (BPD), which is the result of prematurity itself, mechanical ventilation, and respiratory distress syndrome early in the neonatal period. These infants may have interstitial fibrosis, increased airway resistance, decreased pulmonary compliance, fluid retention, and hyperinflation of the lungs. They may require supplemental oxygen, steroids, and diuretics and should have preoperative radiologic documentation of their pulmonary status. Spinal anesthesia is recommended for appropriate surgical procedures.

Apnea associated with bradycardia is another entity frequently observed in former premature infants. Apnea is usually central in origin and is the result of brainstem immaturity which predisposes these infants to more significant apnea during the postoperative period. This risk is less than 1% in a child born at 35 weeks' gestation if surgery is delayed until after 54 weeks postconceptual age.[29] If surgery cannot wait, then postanesthetic apnea monitoring is required for 24 hours. Postanesthetic apnea has been reported in full-term infants less than 4 weeks of age, so similar monitoring is required. A hematocrit less than 30 is associated with an increased risk of postanesthetic apnea in the former preterm infant; therefore, a preoperative hematocrit is warranted in all patients.[30] The presence of retinopathy of prematurity should be sought and documented as well as a history of intraventricular hemorrhage requiring ventriculoperitoneal shunt placement.

CENTRAL NERVOUS SYSTEM DISORDERS

Myelomeningocele

The incidence of myelomeningocele is 1 per 1000 live births and although 75% of lesions occur in the lumbosacral region, affected children may present with a defect anywhere along the neuraxis.[31]

Dysfunction of the skeletal system, skin, genitourinary tract, and peripheral and central nervous systems may also be present so these organ systems should be fully evaluated during the preoperative visit. There is high incidence of sensitivity to latex-containing products, so an attempt to limit exposure to latex should be made. This caution should be noted during the preoperative visit and "Latex Sensitivity" should be posted clearly in the child's chart.

Seizure Disorders

Seizures are a frequently encountered component of many childhood illnesses and afflictions and occur in 4 to 6 children per 1000. They are a symptom of an underlying central nervous system disorder that must be fully investigated and understood. The history should provide a detailed description of the seizure, including the type, frequency, and severity of symptoms as well as the characteristics of the postictal state so that it may easily be recognized by the OR team should it occur during the perioperative period. All anticonvulsant therapy should be recorded and serum drug levels should be checked. All anticonvulsants should be taken up to and including the morning of surgery. If the child has seizures despite adequate therapy, this should be noted.

Cervical Spine Instability

Children who have had significant trauma as well as children who have a variety of congenital abnormalities are at risk for cervical spine instability. Altered mucopolysaccharide metabolism may predispose children to deformities of the odontoid process resulting in cervical spine instability. Atlantoaxial instability and superior migration of the odontoid process may occur in children with rheumatoid arthritis and skeletal dysplasia. Children with Trisomy 21 have laxity of the transverse ligament and abnormal development of the odontoid process which results in cervical spine instability in 15% of cases. Symptoms include clinical manifestations of cord compression which usually are not manifested until after 5 years of age. Although there are no uniform guidelines regarding preoperative testing in these children, it has been suggested that children who are symptomatic have flexion-extension radiographs of the cervical spine and a neurological consultation. If cervical abnormalities are noted, intubation of the trachea should be undertaken in a neutral head position or with somatosensory evoked potential (SSEP) monitoring of the upper extremities.[32]

HEMATOLOGIC DISORDERS

Sickle Cell Disease

Sickle cell disease is a genetically transmitted autosomal recessive disorder that occurs in 8% of the African American population in the heterozygous form and 0.16% in the homozygous form.[33] Heterozygous sickle cell trait does not affect anesthetic management or perioperative outcome, whereas homozygous sickle cell disease increases the risk of perioperative acute chest syndrome, stroke, myocardial infarction, and sickle cell crises. Preoperative preparation should include a measurement of hemoglobin or hematocrit to ascertain deviation from baseline (usually in the 7–8 g/dL range) with the need for presurgical procedure blood transfusion. Partial exchange transfusion should be performed in order to decrease the level of Hgb S to less than 30% to 40% or transfusing to 10 grams of hemoglobin in severe cases where anemia is severe or there is a history of prior stroke or acute chest syndrome. Patients should be admitted to the hospital 12 to 24 hours in advance of their scheduled procedure and receive vigorous intravenous hydration to optimize intravascular flow.

Hemophilia

Hemophilia is the most common and serious of the inherited coagulation disorders. It occurs in approximately 1 in 10,000 males since the defective gene is carried on the X chromosome. Since factor VIII does not cross the placenta, bleeding during the neonatal period suggests the diagnosis. Ninety percent of children have had a significant bleeding episode by the end of the first year of life. The hallmark of the disease is hemarthrosis so children frequently present to the operating room for surgical treatment of this as well as other emergent and routine surgical procedures.

Factor VIII levels should be measured during the preoperative period and orders for replacement therapy should be written when indicated. A consultation with a pediatric hematologist is advisable to determine if therapy with desmopressin (DDAVP) is indicated in addition to guiding factor replacement. The partial thromboplastin time (PTT) will be prolonged but platelet count and prothrombin time will be normal so routine measurement is not necessary. An order for topical analgesic cream or use of pressurized injectable lidocaine (j-tip) should be provided so that preoperative intravenous cannulation will be less painful if preoperative Factor VIII or DDAVP administration is required. These children exhibit an increased frequency of hematoma formation; therefore, intramuscular premedication should be avoided. Due to the high probability of prior blood component therapy, the HIV and hepatitis status of all patients with hemophilia should be documented so that proper precautions may be taken by caregivers.

von Willebrand Disease (vWD)

This bleeding disorder occurs equally in both sexes and is inherited as an autosomal dominant trait. Clinical manifestations include nosebleeds, bleeding from gums, prolonged bleeding from bruises and lacerations, and increased bleeding during surgery. In contrast to hemophilia, hemarthrosis is rare in vWD. The defect is in the platelet binding protein but the platelet count is normal. The prothrombin time (PT) is normal and the partial thromboplastin time (PTT) may be slightly prolonged. Consultation with a pediatric hematologist is suggested to obtain specialized tests to identify the type of vWD to guide therapy during the perioperative period. Therapy consists of DDAVP or replacement therapy with von Willebrand factor from either fresh frozen plasma or cryoprecipitate.

ENDOCRINE DISORDERS

Diabetes Mellitus

The prevalence of diabetes mellitus in school aged children is 1.9 per 1000. The goal of perioperative glucose management is to maintain serum glucose as close to the patient's usual level despite the effects of stress on serum hormonal levels and fasting. It is essential that the physician (pediatrician or endocrinologist) who manages the child's glucose control on a regular basis should be consulted for input on the acceptable range of serum glucose values in each specific patient and how those are best achieved. There should also be clear guidelines for glucose and insulin management if serum glucose measurement either increases or decreases from the acceptable range. Diabetic children should be scheduled as the first morning case to minimize the period of fasting. The serum glycosylated hemoglobin (HbA1C) should be measured during the preoperative period to determine the efficacy of long-term glucose control. Age-appropriate fasting guidelines should be observed and serum glucose should be measured on the morning of surgery.

Diabetes Insipidus

Children with diabetes insipidus may be effectively managed in a variety of ways during the perioperative period and consultation with an endocrinologist at the specific institution is suggested. One effective method of maintaining electrolyte balance without the compounded difficulty of over- or underhydration involves a two-tiered process. Surgery in children with diabetes insipidus should be scheduled as the first case of the day. All patients should have serum electrolytes and osmolality documented preoperatively to establish a baseline. For children who are scheduled for ambulatory or minor surgery, DDAVP should be administered at the usual time and in the usual dose on the day prior to and morning of surgery.

For children who are scheduled for major surgery in which a significant blood loss or fluid shift is anticipated, the DDAVP administration should be modified. A complete history of the dose and timing of DDAVP should be documented as well as the time that urinary breakthrough occurs. If a child receives DDAVP twice a day, the evening dose should be administered prior to surgery but the morning dose should be omitted. If a patient receives a single daily dose it should be omitted on the day of surgery if it is usually taken in the morning but administered as half the usual dose in the evening prior to surgery if it is usually administered at night. In children who have had their DDAVP omitted preoperatively, intraoperative fluid management may be aided by the administration of intravenous vasopressin. Postoperative observation in the ICU should be arranged during the preoperative visit.

Neuromuscular Disorders

Diseases of the motor unit are not uncommon in children and since the combination of certain muscular diseases and specific anesthetic agents may be lethal, identification of these children during the preoperative period is essential. The specific association of malignant hyperthermia and hyperkalemia and certain muscular dystrophies remains unclear; however, the opportunity for the OR team to use a "clean" non-triggering technique should be explored as well. Children with Duchenne muscular dystrophy, central core disease, and other myopathies are in this category.

All children who have either a presumed or confirmed diagnosis of myopathy should have a preoperative electrocardiogram and chest radiograph to identify a rhythm disturbance or dilated cardiac chambers which might be suggestive of an associated cardiomyopathy. In children with a heart murmur or those less than a year of age, a consultation with a pediatric cardiologist should be sought. Poor neuromuscular function may result in compromised respiratory function. Pulmonary function testing may be helpful in predicting which children will have difficulty with extubation at the conclusion of surgery. If postoperative ventilation is considered, appropriate discussion with the family as well as an arrangement for appropriate postoperative disposition should be made. Children who have a diagnosis of mitochondrial myopathy may have metabolic derangements if NPO status is maintained for a prolonged period of time. These children should be specifically instructed to drink glucose containing clear fluids up to 2 hours prior to the time of surgery.

Oncologic Disease

Children with current or prior malignancy should have their chemotherapy documented. The anthracycline class of drugs may cause myocardial dysfunction and others such as mitomycin and bleomycin may cause pulmonary dysfunction. Children who have received chemotherapy regimens which include anthracycline agents require echocardiographic evaluation if the cumulative dose is greater than 150 mg/m^2. Any child with a history of congestive heart failure, who has not had a post-chemotherapy echocardiogram or who has not had an echocardiogram within 2 years prior to the time of anesthesia irrespective of length of time since completion of therapy, requires a preoperative echocardiogram.

Specific chemotherapeutic agents may cause toxicity and abnormal function in other organ systems including renal, hepatic, and the central nervous system. Specific laboratory testing and imaging should be completed preoperatively when compromised function is suspected.

The Child of a Jehovah's Witness Parent

The belief of Jehovah's Witnesses that requires them to refuse transfused blood is based on scriptural passages that define the "life force" as residing in the blood. Many

Jehovah's Witness patients would rather die than receive blood or blood products. Although adult Jehovah's Witness patients may choose to refuse lifesaving blood transfusions, pediatric patients as minor children do not have that same right. It is, therefore, the responsibility of the anesthesiologist to define a plan with the parents in the event that blood is required.[34]

The anesthesiologist should explore the particular family beliefs of each patient since some Jehovah's Witness patients will allow the use of blood conservation in an attempt to minimize intraoperative blood loss and transfusion requirement. Perioperative volume expanders (ie, albumin), hemodilution, and blood salvage are acceptable to some individuals depending on their interpretation of biblical passages, while others will not allow their administration.[35]

Most medical personnel are in agreement that in an emergency situation it is unacceptable for a parent to make a conscious decision that could result in the loss of the minor child's life and in such cases appropriate medical therapy, including transfusion or blood and/or blood products are administered against the wishes of the family. In most circumstances, the courts have intervened to allow blood transfusions over the religious objections of the parents. No child of Jehovah's Witness parents should die for lack of transfused blood, as courts have uniformly intervened to allow hospitals to give blood transfusions to minors irrespective of the religious objections of Jehovah's Witness parents. Thus, if a minor requires blood and the parents object, the anesthesiologist may contact the Office of General Counsel to obtain a court order authorizing the blood transfusion. In the event of an emergency, the blood can be administered while the Office of General Counsel is simultaneously being contacted. This process should be disclosed during the preoperative discussion. Additional preoperative preparation includes optimization of hemoglobin with oral iron therapy 2 to 3 weeks prior to surgery.

Autism

Autism is a heterogenous neurodevelopmental disorder that impairs social communication capabilities as well as the way an individual perceives his or her surroundings. Children present early in life with deficits in their information processing skills and their ability to cope with stress. The initial interview provides valuable information regarding patient's behavior, likes and dislikes, favorite activities, triggers for negative behaviors, modeling, and coping techniques. It is widely accepted that collecting information from parents regarding their child's behavioral patterns and needs, and previous anesthetic experiences lead to a more successful anesthetic experience. A connection can be established with some autistic children; however, low-functioning patients present a significant challenge to the anesthesiologist. Establishing

good rapport with the family is helpful since gaining parental trust, acknowledging their anxiety and previous experiences, willingness to listen to their concerns, and formulating management plan together can all contribute to a smooth anesthetic course. Collecting pertinent information about the behavioral profile of the patient including baseline behaviors, triggers of emotional outbursts, and signs of escalating anxiety during the preoperative interview is beneficial to the anesthesia team in planning the perioperative anesthetic management. The family should be encouraged to bring favorite toys, electronic devices, and comforting items on the day of the procedure. In addition careful detailed discussion with the surgical team regarding the plan and workflow is important to the design of the perioperative plan.[36]

Immunization

Frequently, children present for general anesthesia shortly after an immunization has been administered. Post-immunization effects include fever, pain at the injection site, malaise, and irritability. These clinical symptoms must not be confused with perioperative complications. The effect of anesthesia on the immune response during elective surgery is minor and usually persists for 48 hours and there is no contraindication to the immunization of healthy children scheduled for elective surgery. However, a delay prior to anesthesia of 2 days for inactivated vaccines such as diphtheria-pertussis-tetanus (DPT) or 14 to 21 days for live attenuated vaccines such as measles-mumps-rubella (MMR) immunization may be prudent.[37] The time interval between immunizations and procedures may be important in preventing misinterpretation of vaccine-driven adverse events as postoperative/postprocedure complications. This includes, but is not limited to, routine scheduled vaccines as well as seasonal and flu vaccine. When a vaccine is administered within 7 days of a scheduled procedure or in the case of unplanned procedures, both the anesthesiologist and surgeon should be informed. Cases should not be automatically cancelled but left to the discretion of the anesthesiologist and/or surgeon based on individual patient considerations.

Concussion

Sport- or recreation-related concussion may occur in the setting of trauma requiring surgical intervention under general anesthesia especially in adolescents. The effect of surgery and general anesthesia on brain recovery, either favorable or unfavorable, in this population is unknown. There is no evidenced-based, clinical pathway describing the optimal timing of surgery and anesthesia for semi-elective surgical procedures following a concussion. The decision to proceed with surgery in patients with known concussion is based on individual clinician's judgment. Elective surgery is often delayed in patients with known concussion until the patient is cleared to "return to play" or "free of symptoms." Rest and avoidance of second or recurrent collisions are essential to the patient's recovery; however, there is no clear clinical definition of "rest" or how much time is needed for full recovery.[38]

Physical Examination

The physical examination of the pediatric patient must begin with simple observation from a distance since the infant or child may become frightened when approached directly. A great deal may be learned about physical findings that relate to the anesthetic without touching the child. The color of the skin including the presence of pallor, cyanosis, rash, jaundice, unusual markings, or prior surgical scars may reveal the presence of organ system dysfunction. Since one congenital abnormality is often associated with others, abnormal facies should be explored as an indication of a syndrome.

The respiratory system should be evaluated by noting the rate and quality of respirations, the presence of noisy breathing, coughing, purulent nasal discharge, stridor, and wheezing. Signs of an acute upper respiratory infection should be evaluated. The ease of mouth opening should be determined as well as the presence of loose teeth.

If a heart murmur is detected on the cardiovascular examination there are specific concerns that must be addressed. An innocent murmur may be due to turbulent blood flow during a growth spurt, whereas a pathologic murmur is usually due to a structural abnormality; this distinction must be made. Lesions in which bacterial endocarditis prophylaxis or protection from paradoxical air embolus are required must be documented.

The patient's neurologic evaluation should include the level of consciousness, presence of an intact gag reflex, and adequate cervical spine movement. General muscle tone and the presence of signs of an increase in intracranial pressure should also be noted.

Diagnostic Testing

It is important to remember that phlebotomy is often traumatic for children and an event that they do not easily forget. For this reason, it is best to limit the number of invasive tests performed. The diagnostic studies should be selected based on the general medical health of the patient and the procedure being performed. In general, measurement of hematocrit in a healthy child undergoing elective surgery is unnecessary. If significant blood loss is anticipated or if the child is less than 6 months of age or was born prematurely a hematocrit should be measured. Neither the routine measurement of the coagulation profile nor a history of "easy bruising" is reliable in predicting surgical bleeding. The presence of prior hematoma, bleeding from circumcision, or large bruises should prompt an investigation; however, a negative history for bruising in an otherwise healthy child would require no further testing. Routine preoperative urinalysis is not indicated in children and serum chemistry analysis should only be performed when an abnormality is suspected. Children who are treated with anticonvulsants should have these medication levels checked and an electrocardiogram or chest radiograph should only be ordered if the general medical condition warrants. Routine pregnancy testing is controversial and the policy of the specific medical facility should be followed.

REFERENCES

1. Kraemer K, Cohen ME, Liu Y, et al. Development and evaluation of the American College of Surgeons NSQIP pediatric surgical risk calculator. *J Am Coll Surg.* 2016;223(5):685-693.
2. Nasr VG, DiNardo JA, Faraoni D. Development of a pediatric risk assessment score to predict perioperative mortality in children undergoing noncardiac surgery. *Anesth Analg.* 2017;124(5):1514-1519.
3. Ahmed A, Ali M, Khan M, Khan F. Perioperative cardiac arrests in children at a university teaching hospital of a developing country over 15 years. *Paediatr Anaesth.* 2009;19(6):581-586.
4. Moynihan R, Kurker C. The perioperative environment and the pediatric patient. In: Ferrari LR, ed. *Anesthesia and Pain Management for the Pediatrician.* Baltimore, MD: Johns Hopkins Press; 1999.
5. Wappler F. Anesthesia for patients with a history of malignant hyperthermia. *Curr Opin Anaesthesiol.* 2010;23(3):417-422.
6. Wetzel RC. Routine pregnancy testing in adolescents: to test or not to test—what is the answer? *Seminars in Anesthesia, Perioperative Medicine and Pain.* 2007;26(3):120-125.
7. Azzam FJ, Padda GS, DeBoard JW, Krock JL, Kolterman SM. Preoperative pregnancy testing in adolescents. *Anesth Analg.* 1996;82(1):4-7.
8. Committee on Standards and Practice Parameters, Apfelbaum JL, Connis RT, et al. Practice advisory for preanesthesia evaluation: an updated report by the American Society of Anesthesiologists Task Force on Preanesthesia Evaluation. *Anesthesiology.* 2012;116(3):522-538.
9. American Society of Anesthesiologists Committee. Practice guidelines for preoperative fasting and the use of pharmacologic agents to reduce the risk of pulmonary aspiration: application to healthy patients undergoing elective procedures: an updated report by the American Society of Anesthesiologists Committee on Standards and Practice Parameters. *Anesthesiology.* 2017;126(3):376-393.
10. Caffarelli C, Stringari G, Pajno GB, et al. Perioperative allergy: risk factors. *Int J Immunopathol Pharmacol.* 2011;24(3 suppl):S27-S34.
11. Skolnick ET, Vomvolakis MA, Buck KA, Mannino SF, Sun LS. Exposure to environmental tobacco smoke and the risk of adverse respiratory events in children receiving general anesthesia. *Anesthesiology.* 1998;88(5):1144-1153.
12. De Queiroz M, Combet S, Bérard J, et al. Latex allergy in children: modalities and prevention. *Paediatr Anaesth.* 2009;19(4):313-319.
13. Meric F, Teitelbaum DH, Geiger JD, Harmon CM, Groner JI. Latex sensitization in general pediatric surgical patients: a call for increased screening of patients. *J Pediatr Surg.* 1998;33(7):1108-1111; discussion 1111-2.
14. McCann ME, Soriano SG. Perioperative central nervous system injury in neonates. *Br J Anaesth.* 2012;109(suppl 1):i60-i67.

15. Davidson AJ, Disma N, de Graaff JC, et al. Neurodevelopmental outcome at 2 years of age after general anaesthesia and awake-regional anaesthesia in infancy (GAS): an international multicentre, randomised controlled trial. *Lancet.* 2016;387(10015):239-250. Erratum in: *Lancet.* 2016;387(10015):228.

16. Ko WR, Liaw YP, Huang JY, et al. Exposure to general anesthesia in early life and the risk of attention deficit/hyperactivity disorder development: a nationwide, retrospective matched-cohort study. *Paediatr Anaesth.* 2014;24(7):741-748.

17. Section on Pediatric Pulmonology, Subcommittee on Obstructive Sleep Apnea Syndrome. American Academy of Pediatrics. Clinical practice guideline: diagnosis and management of childhood obstructive sleep apnea syndrome. *Pediatrics.* 2002;109(4):704-712.

18. Blum RH, McGowan FX Jr. Chronic upper airway obstruction and cardiac dysfunction: anatomy, pathophysiology and anesthetic implications. *Paediatr Anaesth.* 2004;14(1):75-83.

19. Lerman J. Unraveling the mysteries of sleep-disordered breathing in children. *Anesthesiology.* 2006;105(4):645-647.

20. Chung SA, Yuan H, Chung F. A systemic review of obstructive sleep apnea and its implications for anesthesiologists. *Anesth Analg.* 2008;107(5):1543-1563.

21. Tait AR, Voepel-Lewis T, Christensen R, O'Brien LM. The STBUR questionnaire for predicting perioperative respiratory adverse events in children at risk for sleep-disordered breathing. *Paediatr Anaesth.* 2013;23(6):510-516.

22. Tait AR, Bickham R, O'Brien LM, Quinlan M, Voepel-Lewis T. The STBUR questionnaire for identifying children at risk for sleep-disordered breathing and postoperative opioid-related adverse events. *Paediatr Anaesth.* 2016;26(7):759-766.

23. Coté CJ, Posner KL, Domino KB. Death or neurologic injury after tonsillectomy in children with a focus on obstructive sleep apnea: Houston, we have a problem! *Anesth Analg.* 2014;118(6):1276-1283.

24. Von Ungern-Sternberg BS, Habre W. Pediatric anesthesia—potential risks and their assessment: part I. *Paediatr Anaesth.* 2007;17(3):206-215.

25. Von Ungern-Sternberg BS, Habre W. Pediatric anesthesia - potential risks and their assessment: part II. *Paediatr Anaesth.* 2007;17(4):311-320.

26. Becke K. Anesthesia in children with a cold. *Curr Opin Anaesthesiol.* 2012;25(3):333-339.

27. Mamie C, Habre W, Delhumeau C, Argiroffo CB, Morabia A. Incidence and risk factors of perioperative respiratory adverse events in children undergoing elective surgery. *Paediatr Anaesth.* 2004;14(3):218-224.

28. Tait AR, Malviya S. Anesthesia for the child with an upper respiratory tract infection: still a dilemma? *Anesth Analg.* 2005;100(1):59-65.

29. Coté CJ, Zaslavsky A, Downes JJ, et al. Postoperative apnea in former preterm infants after inguinal herniorrhaphy. A combined analysis. *Anesthesiology.* 1995;82(4):809-822.

30. Welborn LG, Hannallah RS, Luban NL, Fink R, Ruttimann UE. Anemia and postoperative apnea in former preterm infants. *Anesthesiology.* 1991;74(6):1003-1006.

31. Adzick NS. Fetal surgery for spina bifida: past, present, future. *Semin Pediatr Surg.* 2013;22(1):10-17.

32. Cunningham MJ, Ferrari LR, Kerse LA, McPeck K. Intraoperative somatosensory evoked potential monitoring in achondroplasia. *Pediatr Anesth.* 1994 4(2):129-132.

33. Quinn CT. Sickle cell disease in childhood: from newborn screening through transition to adult medical care. *Pediatr Clin North Am.* 2013;60(6):1363-1381.

34. Campbell YN, Machan MD, Fisher MD. The Jehovah's Witness population: considerations for preoperative optimization of hemoglobin. *AANA J.* 2016;84(3):173-178.

35. Mason CL, Tran CK. Caring for the Jehovah's Witness parturient. *Anesth Analg.* 2015;121(6):1564-1569.

36. Vlassakova BG, Emmanouil DE. Perioperative considerations in children with autism spectrum disorder. *Curr Opin Anaesthesiol.* 2016;29(3):359-366.

37. Siebert JN, Posfay-Barbe KM, Habre W, Siegrist CA. Influence of anesthesia on immune responses and its effect on vaccination in children: review of evidence. *Paediatr Anaesth.* 2007;17(5):410-420.

38. Thomas DG, Apps JN, Hoffmann RG, McCrea M, Hammeke T. Benefits of strict rest after acute concussion: a randomized controlled trial. *Pediatrics.* 2015;135(2):213-223.

Pre-procedure Medications

Sarah Reece-Stremtan and Claude Abdallah

INTRODUCTION

In the preoperative period, children have significant anxiety and behavioral and pharmacological interventions are used to mitigate these symptoms prior to surgery. Although this is true for adults as well, in the young pediatric patient it is related to a limited understanding of the nature of the illness, the need for surgery, and the unfamiliarity of the environment. Anxiolysis is the primary aim of premedication use, although other clinical goals include amnesia, optimization of preoperative conditions, and prevention of physiological stress.

Nearly 50% of children demonstrate signs of significant preoperative fear and anxiety.[1] Heart rate and blood pressure measurements correlate with behavioral ratings of anxiety.[2] Anesthesiologists may use either parental presence or sedative premedication to alleviate physiological and psychological effects of preoperative anxiety, since separation from parents and induction of anesthesia are considered the most stress-inducing phases of the perioperative experience. Anesthesiologists who favor parental presence during induction of anesthesia tend to use sedative premedications least frequently, and vice versa.[3,4] Both approaches are considered appropriate depending on the clinical scenario.

The most popular premedicant available in the past were long acting (eg, morphine and pentobarbital) but their administration delayed postoperative recovery and increased the incidence of postoperative nausea and vomiting. In addition, these medications were not available via oral route. This resulted in underuse of sedative premedication in many children with anxiety compromising their psychological welfare for the goal of efficiency and rapid discharge. The introduction of oral midazolam as premedication is the main reason pharmacological sedation has regained popularity in modern pediatric anesthesia practice, especially in the ambulatory setting. Oral midazolam remains the most commonly used premedication for pediatric practice, with several other medications (eg, alpha agonists) available depending on the specific clinical needs.

Premedication versus Parental Presence for Induction

Early studies suggested reduced anxiety and improved patient cooperation if parents were present during induction.[5,6] The majority of parents prefer to be present during induction of anesthesia regardless of the child's age or previous surgical experience,[7] and regardless of their experience with prior parental presence or premedication of their child in the case of repeated surgery.[8] Concerns regarding parental presence for induction (PPI) do include a negative behavioral response to stress when a parent is present, and an upsetting experience for the parents, especially when watching their child become unconscious or needing to leave their child after induction.[9,10] This experience correlates with an increase in heart rate and skin conductance levels in mothers.[11] Oral midazolam has been shown to be more effective in reducing a child's anxiety than PPI, and parental presence combined with oral midazolam was not superior in reducing a child's anxiety than sedation alone.[12] PPI is most helpful in children older than 4 years of age who share a calm baseline personality with the accompanying parent.[13,14] However, limitations to controlled studies such as these may be that randomization in subject recruitment may not reflect the everyday practice of anesthesiologists who largely individualize their approach to each child and parents.

If PPI is deemed to be in the child's best interest, a clear explanation that describes what the parent can expect to witness during the peri-induction period can significantly decrease parental anxiety and increase their level of satisfaction, which may be reflected in the child's behavior.[15-17] Predictive characteristics for children who would probably benefit from sedative premedication include children between the ages of 2 and 6 years, who have a history of prior stressful medical encounters, who are shy and inhibited, and who were accompanied by an anxious parent.[7,18] In the extremely anxious child, premedication is indicated to avoid a traumatic anesthetic induction and consequently a possible postoperative psychological disturbance.[19]

PREMEDICATIONS

The major objectives of preanesthetic medications are to decrease the stress response with preservation of hemodynamic parameters, facilitate anesthesia induction, and produce amnesia. The child's age, body weight, medication history, allergic status, and underlying medical or surgical conditions are factors that need to be taken into consideration prior to administration of any premedication. In most cases, oral or nasal medications are preferred over rectal, intramuscular, or IV routes if no IV access is already in place. Oral premedication administration does not increase the risk of aspiration pneumonia.[20] A variety of different medications and classes may be used as premedication.

BENZODIAZEPINES

Midazolam is the most commonly used sedative premedicant in the preoperative holding area.[3] After appropriate administration of midazolam, the following is expected: sedation, induction of sleep, reduction in anxiety,

anterograde amnesia, muscle relaxation, and anticonvulsant effects.[21]

Midazolam can be administered orally, intranasally, intravenously, rectally, and intramuscularly.

When administered orally its favorable characteristics are the short onset and offset of action. Bioavailability is highly sensitive to changes in pH. As a standard syrup preparation, midazolam exists in both an open and a closed ring structure. The closed ring formulation is lipophilic and physiologically active, and its proportion in the preparation is dependent on pH values.[22] The drawback is its bitter taste. The most common oral dose used is 0.5 mg/kg, but ranges from 0.25 to 1 mg/kg have been described. Higher doses of midazolam appear not to offer any additional benefits and may cause more side effects. Commercially prepared oral midazolam formulation is rapidly absorbed with most patients demonstrating a satisfactory degree of sedation and anxiolysis within 10 minutes of consumption, with an even higher percentage appropriately sedated at 20 minutes after administration. The dose of oral midazolam should be adjusted in children taking depressants or inducers of the cytochrome oxidase system, such as anticonvulsants or barbiturates. All doses should be administered under direct supervision with the patient placed in a closely monitored bed space in the preoperative holding area.

The bioavailability of different routes of administration and suggested doses are as given in Table 11-1.

A sublingual route of administration (0.2mg/kg) has also been described.[23-29]

After IV administration, the time to peak central nervous system (CNS) electroencephalographic effect is 4.8 minutes. It is preferable to wait this interval of time prior to administering any additional dose of midazolam to avoid oversedation. To avoid the added trauma of venipuncture, IV midazolam is best reserved for children who already have a functioning IV line.

When administered intranasally, peak plasma concentrations of midazolam occurs in only 10 minutes; however, discomfort due to irritation has been associated with this route. Intranasal midazolam with preservative has been shown to induce neurotoxic effects in an animal model.[30] A preservative-free midazolam preparation is recommended when using this route of administration.

Table 11-1. Bioavailability and Suggested Doses of Midazolam

	Oral	Nasal	Intramuscular	Rectal
Bioavailability (%)	30	57	90	40–50
Suggested dose (mg/kg)	0.25–0.75	0.2	0.1-0.2	1

There is synergism between propofol and midazolam on gamma-aminobutyric acid (GABA) receptors.[31] Oral midazolam decreases the infusion requirements of propofol by one-third during a propofol-based anesthetic.[32] After premedication with oral midazolam (0.5 mg/kg), in children 1 to 3 years of age post-adenoidectomy after induction of anesthesia with propofol, and maintenance with sevoflurane, emergence and early recovery were shown to be delayed with no change in discharge times.[33] Spontaneous eye opening and discharge time were delayed as compared with placebo after 25 minutes of sevoflurane anesthesia.[34] Extubation, awakening, and discharge times were not affected after sevoflurane anesthesia in children 1 to 10 years of age receiving a similar dose of oral midazolam.[35]

Midazolam has the advantage of producing anterograde amnesia. Memory usually becomes impaired within 10 minutes after oral administration.[36] This effect is beneficial in children who require repetitive interventions. Midazolam, like other benzodiazepines, increases the seizure threshold for CNS toxicity but does not affect the threshold for cardiovascular toxicity. Therefore, cardiovascular collapse after regional anesthesia toxicity may occur unrelatedly to CNS symptoms of toxicity after a patient has received premedication with midazolam or another benzodiazepine. Other secondary effects of midazolam may include a paradoxical effect with behavioral changes: anxiety, agitation, involuntary movements, aggressive or violent behavior, uncontrollable crying or verbalization, and hiccups. These adverse effects may occur independently of the mode of administration, ie, rectal, nasal, or oral. They seem to be related to the altered state of consciousness or disinhibition produced by the drug. To directly reverse such midazolam, flumazenil, a competitive benzodiazepine antagonist[37], can be administered. TP mitigate side effects, ketamine at 0.5 mg/kg IV[38] or antipsychotic medications such as haloperidol can be administered.

Lorazepam can be administered orally, intravenously, or intramuscularly. It has a slow onset and offset of action and may be better used for inpatients. It is metabolized by the liver to inactive metabolites. The usual dose is 0.05 mg/kg administered orally or intravenously to older children; however, a dose of 0.025 mg/kg has been shown to be adequate for decreasing preoperative anxiety.[39] Lorazepam has good amnestic properties and produces less tissue irritation than diazepam.

Diazepam has a greater fat solubility than midazolam and a faster CNS effect after IV administration (1.6 minutes). Diazepam undergoes oxidative metabolism to pharmacologically active metabolites by demethylation, hydroxylation, and glucuronidation in the liver. The main active metabolite is desmethyldiazepam (nordiazepam) with pharmacologic activity equal to the parent compound.[40] Other active metabolites include temazepam and oxazepam. Diazepam has a biphasic half-life of about 1 to 3 days, and 2 to 7 days for the active metabolite desmethyldiazepam.[41] Diazepam is a less popular choice as a preoperative premedicant in young children because of their immature liver function that may lead to a prolonged half-life. The average oral dose for premedicating healthy children with diazepam ranges from 0.1 to 0.3 mg/kg. When administered rectally, diazepam appears to be less effective than rectal midazolam.[42] The intramuscular route is not recommended because it is painful and absorption is erratic.[43] Use of diazepam should be avoided in individuals with ataxia, severe hypoventilation, acute narrow-angle glaucoma, severe hepatic and renal deficiencies, severe sleep apnea, severe depression, particularly when accompanied by suicidal tendencies, psychosis, myasthenia gravis, and hypersensitivity or allergy to any drug in the benzodiazepine class. Paradoxical side effects have been reported, including nervousness, irritability, excitement, insomnia, worsening of seizures, and muscle cramps. These adverse reactions are more likely to occur in children, the elderly, and individuals with a history of drug or alcohol abuse and/or aggression.[44] In some patients, diazepam may increase the tendency toward self-harming behaviors.[45]

BARBITURATES

Barbiturates have become less commonly used for premedication in children since the advent of shorter-acting benzodiazepines. IV **methohexital**, still in use, has a relatively short elimination half-life (3.9 ± 2.1 hours) than thiopental (9 ± 1.6 hours) because of a faster hepatic metabolism.[46] A major disadvantage of barbiturates is hyperalgesia, which can induce agitation in children who experience postoperative pain. Methohexital, in a rectal dose of 20 to 30 mg/kg, may result in sleep/sedation in 15 to 20 minutes but has unpredictable systemic absorption and side effects including hiccups, apnea, airway obstruction, laryngospasm, seizures, and possible allergic reaction.[47,48] An increase in absorption through rectal mucosa abnormality may lead to cardiorespiratory arrest. Contraindications to methohexital include porphyria, hypersensitivity, and temporal lobe epilepsy.[49]

NONBARBITURATE SEDATIVES

Chloral hydrate is an orally administered nonbarbiturate (20 to 75 mg/kg with a total maximum dose of 2 g). It is devoid of analgesic properties and has a bitter taste. Its principal advantage is that it can be administered orally or rectally with relatively good sedation within 30 to 45 minutes. Its use is less frequent than midazolam as a premedicant because of its slow onset and long elimination half-life.[50] It is not recommended in neonates and patients with liver disease because of impaired metabolism, and the potential accumulation of toxic metabolites leading to metabolic acidosis, renal failure, and hypotonia.[51] The active metabolite of chloral hydrate, trichloroethanol, has a long half-life in toddlers and in preterm infants (39.8 ± 14.3 hours) with a risk for residual drug effect and prolonged sedation or resedation.[52] Airway obstruction may occur in children with tonsillar hypertrophy.[53] Deaths after administration of chloral hydrate for sedation have been reported.[54] Concerns for potential carcinogenicity with chronic administration exist. Other adverse effects include irritation of the skin, mucous membranes, and gastrointestinal tract, possibly in relation to the metabolism of chloral hydrate to trichloroacetic acid.

Phenothiazines

Promethazine (0.25 mg to 0.5 mg/kg intravenously, intramuscularly, or orally) possesses several beneficial properties. It is sedating, and it is an antihistamine (H1 blocker), an antiemetic/anti-motion sickness medication, and an anticholinergic. However, it is not a popular premedicant in pediatric ambulatory anesthesia because of ineffective sedative effects as sole premedication and because of long elimination half-life (8 to 12 hours). It may also cause dystonic reactions.

Ketamine

Ketamine is a phencyclidine derivative that antagonizes the *N*-methyl-D-aspartate (NMDA) receptor (NMDAR). The principal effect of ketamine is due to the central dissociation of the cortex from the limbic system. Ketamine provides good sedation and analgesia while preserving upper airway muscular tone and respiratory drive. Ketamine also relaxes the smooth musculature of the airway stimulated by the release of histamine, an effect with the potential risk for bronchoconstriction. The most common adverse reaction to ketamine is postoperative vomiting, which occurs in 33% of children.[55] The dextro-isomer of ketamine has more potent analgesia and a reduced incidence of side effects.[56] Other side effects associated with the administration of ketamine include sialorrhea and hallucinations. It is recommended to administer an antisialagogue (atropine or glycopyrrolate) with ketamine in order to decrease the amount of oral secretions that may occur and therefore to decrease the risk of laryngospasm. Hallucinations during recovery from ketamine may occur mostly in older children, although oral ketamine has been reported to reduce emergence delirium. Coadministration of benzodiazepines or subsequent administration of general anesthetic agents reduces the incidence of hallucinations to approximately 4%.[57] It is preferable to recover patients who have received ketamine in a quiet environment with the least stimulation in order to help decrease the incidence of undesirable effects such as hallucinations, nightmares, and delirium.

NMDAR antagonism is responsible for the anesthetic, amnestic, dissociation, and hallucinogenic effects of ketamine. Activation of k-opioid receptors and possibly sigma and mAch receptors may also contribute to its hallucinogenic properties.[58] The mechanism of action for the possible antidepressant effects of ketamine at lower doses is being investigated.[59] Ketamine blocks voltage-dependent calcium and sodium channels, attenuating hyperalgesia; it alters cholinergic neurotransmission and inhibits the reuptake of serotonin and norepinephrine.[60]

Ketamine can be administered via the oral, intramuscular, and nasal routes. Bioavailability and peak concentrations for each route are as mentioned in Table 11-2. After oral administration, ketamine undergoes first-pass metabolism, where it is biotransformed in the liver by CYP3A4, CYP2B6, and CYP2C9 isoenzymes into norketamine, hydroxynorketamine, and finally dihydronorketamine.[61] Norketamine is the major metabolite of ketamine and is one-third to one-fifth as potent, and plasma levels of this metabolite are three times higher than ketamine following oral administration.[62]

Peak plasma concentrations of ketamine are reached within a minute intravenously, but in 5 to 15 minutes when administered intramuscularly.[60]

IV ketamine has a fast onset of effect (<1 minute). Duration of action of a single IV dose is 5 to 8 minutes (α-elimination half-life of 11 minutes and a β-elimination half-life of 2.5 to 3 hours).[63] Ketamine is administered in very low doses intravenously (0.25 to 0.5 mg/kg) or intramuscularly (1 to 2 mg/kg) preferably in combination with low-dose midazolam (0.05 mg/kg) along with atropine (0.02 mg/kg) for sedation. The dose of ketamine needed to prevent gross movement in infants younger than 6 months of age is four times greater than in children 6 years of age.[64]

The intramuscular route of administration is very useful for children who are uncooperative, refuse oral medications, and become combative. These children become adequately calm in around 3 minutes and will then accept a mask inhalation induction of anesthesia. There is no documentation of prolongation of the hospital discharge times after IM ketamine administration (2 mg/kg) even after brief surgical procedures and there is only a minimal likelihood of delirium or bad dreams during recovery.[65] However, the combination of intramuscular ketamine (2 mg/kg) and midazolam (0.1 to 0.2 mg/kg) may prolong recovery and discharge times after brief ambulatory procedures.[66] A larger dose (4 to 5 mg/kg) sedates children with 2 to 4 minutes, and a dose of 10 mg/kg usually produces deep sedation. Larger and repeated doses are associated with hallucinations, nightmares, vomiting, and a prolonged recovery from anesthesia.

Table 11-2. Bioavailability and Peak Concentrations of Ketamine

	Oral	Intramuscular	Intranasal
Bioavailability (%)	17	93	25–50
Peak plasma concentration (minutes)	30	5–15	10–15

Oral ketamine alone and in combination with midazolam have been used for premedication in healthy children and those with congenital heart defects. Sedation is usually achieved after a dose of 5 to 6 mg/kg of oral ketamine in most children within 12 minutes; the depth of sedation is sufficient to obtain IV access in more than half of children. Larger doses may prolong recovery from anesthesia. The combination of oral midazolam (0.5 mg/kg) and ketamine (3 mg/kg) is synergistic in its efficiency for preoperative sedation and does not seem to prolong recovery time for procedures longer than 30 minutes.[67]

Only preservative-free ketamine should be given intranasally to avoid neurotoxicity, and the 100 mg/mL concentration is preferable to minimize volume administered.[68] Nasal transmucosal ketamine at a dose of 6 mg/kg is also effective in sedating children within 20 to 40 minutes before induction of anesthesia.

Rectal ketamine administration has a bioavailability of only 25% and can result in an unpredictable effect.[69]

Ketamine should be used with caution in any child with a history of psychiatric or seizure disorder because of its psychotropic and epileptogenic effects. Although ketamine was considered to increase intracranial pressure (ICP) as a result of cerebral vasodilation, with adequate ventilation this effect may be minimal. Ketamine was also thought to produce an increase in intraocular pressure (IOP), although this effect is clinically not significant.

Opioids

Opioids are a useful preanesthetic medication for children with preoperative pain, as preemptive analgesia. However, common opioid-related side effects such as respiratory depression, dysphoria, pruritus, and nausea/vomiting should be considered when these medications are administered. If opioids are used in combination with other sedatives such as benzodiazepines, the dose of each drug should be appropriately adjusted to avoid the risk of respiratory depression. Neonates are very sensitive to the respiratory depressant effects of opioids, and they are rarely used to premedicate in this age group.

Fentanyl may be administered by parenteral, transdermal, nasal, and oral routes. The optimal oral dose as a preanesthetic medication with minimal desaturation and preoperative nausea appears to be 10 to 15 mcg/kg. Children begin to show signs of sedation within 10 minutes after receiving this dose. Recovery is similar to that after 2 mcg/kg given intravenously. Doses greater than 15 mcg/kg are not recommended because of opioid side effects, particularly respiratory depression. Fentanyl may also be administered nasally (1 to 2 mcg/kg) as a premedication, but it is most frequently utilized after induction of anesthesia as a means of providing analgesia in children without IV access.

Sufentanil is 10 times more potent than fentanyl. Several instances of reduced chest wall compliance have been reported in children after nasal sufentanil, as well as a higher incidence of nausea and vomiting and a prolonged discharge time when compared to nasally administered midazolam.[70] These potential side effects and prolonged hospital stay after nasal sufentanil makes it an unpopular choice for premedication.

Morphine sulfate may be administered intramuscularly (0.1 to 0.2 mg/kg) or intravenously (0.05 to 0.1 mg/kg) or orally.

Codeine has been a commonly prescribed oral opioid, which must undergo O-demethylation in the liver to produce morphine to provide effective analgesia. Five percent to 10% of children lack the cytochrome isoenzyme (CYP2D6) required for this conversion and therefore do not derive analgesic benefit. The combination of codeine with acetaminophen is effective in relieving mild to moderate pain but its use in the United States has fallen out of favor because of several deaths in pediatric patients; the Food and Drug Administration (FDA) in 2017 recommended against the use of this medication in pediatric patients.[71]

Alpha-2 Agonists

Clonidine causes dose-related sedation by its effect in the locus coeruleus through inhibition of adenylate cyclase and reduction in norepinephrine release. Clonidine acts both centrally and peripherally to reduce blood pressure and therefore it attenuates the hemodynamic response to intubation. The plasma concentration peaks at 60 to 90 minutes after oral administration.[72,73] The need to administer clonidine 60 minutes before induction of anesthesia makes its use impractical in most clinical settings. An oral dose of 3 mcg/kg given 45 to 120 minutes before surgery produces comparable sedation to that of diazepam or midazolam.[74] Clonidine if given at 4 mcg/kg is effective in the reduction of postoperative pain. In most studies reviewed, the side effects were minimal, but some investigators added atropine to prevent bradycardia and hypotension.

Dexmedetomidine is a newer, more highly selective alpha-2 agonist than clonidine, with more favorable pharmacokinetics. Commonly used in the intraoperative period to smooth emergence and reduce opioid use, dexmedetomidine also demonstrates utility when used as an anesthetic premedication. Meta-analyses recommend its use as superior to midazolam in that it produces better preoperative sedation and parental separation, and reduction of postoperative pain.[75,76] It can be given intravenously or intranasally with onset of action of 5 to 30 minutes, respectively. It is most commonly administered via nasal route at 1 to 2 mcg/kg with ease of separation from parents for the majority of patients at 30 minutes after administration.[77] Statistically but not clinically significant reductions in heart rate and blood pressure may be seen, but discharge time from the recovery room is not prolonged in comparison with midazolam.[75,76]

Antihistamines

Antihistamines are not commonly used because their sedative effects are somewhat variable. **Diphenhydramine** is an H1 blocker with mild sedative and antimuscarinic effects. The dosage for children is 0.5 mg/kg intravenously or intramuscularly.[78] Although the duration of action is 4 to 6 hours, it does not appear to interfere with recovery from anesthesia. **Hydroxyzine** has antiemetic, antihistaminic, and antispasmodic effects with minimal respiratory and circulatory changes. It is usually administered intramuscularly at a dose of 0.5 to 1 mg/kg.

ANTICHOLINERGIC DRUGS

Anticholinergic agents were commonly used in the past to prevent the undesirable bradycardia associated with some anesthetic agents (halothane and succinylcholine), and to minimize autonomic vagal reflexes and reduce secretions. Current inhalational anesthetics are not associated with bradycardia and do not stimulate salivary or tracheobronchial secretions; therefore, the routine use of an anticholinergic drug is not generally needed prior to induction. In the majority of cases, anticholinergics are given after IV access is established.

Atropine (0.02 mg/kg) and **scopolamine** (0.01 mg/kg) both have CNS effects, although the sedating effects of scopolamine is 5 to 15 times greater than atropine. The central sedative effects of both atropine and scopolamine may be antagonized with physostigmine. Atropine is more commonly used and is a better vagolytic agent than scopolamine, whereas scopolamine is a better sedative, antisialagogue, and amnestic. **Glycopyrrolate** is a quaternary amine and as such it does not cross the blood-brain barrier and does not produce CNS side effects including sedation. When compared to atropine, it is less effective in attenuating bradycardia during induction.

Anticholinergic agents are very useful as an adjuvant to ketamine anesthesia because of their antisialagogue and central sedative effects. The recommended doses of anticholinergics are scopolamine 0.005 to 0.01 mg/kg, atropine 0.01 to 0.02 mg/kg, and glycopyrrolate 0.01 mg/kg intravenously or intramuscularly.

TOPICAL ANESTHETICS

Topical anesthetic applications are commonly used as an attractive alternative to intradermal local anesthetic infiltration for obtaining IV access when this is indicated prior to induction of anesthesia.

EMLA cream (eutectic mixture of local anesthetic, Astra Zeneca, Wilmington DE) is a mixture of two local anesthetics (2.5% lidocaine and 2.5% prilocaine). One-hour application of EMLA cream to intact skin with an occlusive dressing provides adequate topical anesthesia for an IV catheter insertion. However, EMLA causes venoconstriction and skin blanching, making IV cannulation more difficult. Methemoglobinemia may occur secondary to prilocaine.[79] A 1-hour application of EMLA cream and a maximum dose of 1 g did not induce methemoglobinemia when applied to intact skin of full-term neonates younger than 3 months of age.[80]

Ametop, a 4% tetracaine topical preparation, has the advantage of no venoconstriction or skin blanching and no risk of methemoglobinemia. Its onset time is 30 to 40 minutes.

ELA-Max (4% lidocaine) decreases pain associated with IV catheter insertion after only a 30-minute application with lesser skin blanching and better vein dilation compared to EMLA cream. There is no risk of methemoglobinemia with this formulation.

Synera is a eutectic mixture of lidocaine and tetracaine (70 mg of each per patch) that uses a controlled heating system to accelerate delivery and analgesic effect of the local anesthetic. An application time of 20 minutes lessens pain associated with venipuncture in children and is associated with only mild and transient local erythema and edema and no skin blanching.[81] Methemoglobinemia has not been reported with this formulation.

The **J-tip Needle-Free Injection System** (National Medical Products, Irvine CA) uses a carbon dioxide–driven dispersion method to distribute lidocaine 1% into the intradermal space. It demonstrates equivalent to superior analgesia as compared with EMLA when used for peripheral venous access, with analgesia achieved in 1 to 2 minutes.[82,83]

The primary goal of premedication in children is to reduce anxiety by facilitating a smooth separation from parents and ease the induction of anesthesia. Other pharmacological effects (amnesia, prevention of physiologic stress, reduction of total anesthetic requirements, decrease in risk of aspiration of acidic stomach content, and analgesia) may also be achieved. Special considerations for patients with deteriorating mental status, with airway obstruction, or patients with hemodynamic instability/intolerance to hypercapnia (such as those with significant increases in pulmonary artery pressure/pulmonary arteriolar resistance) or with systemic organ failure should be taken into account prior to administration of premedication. In these cases, parental presence may be the preferable choice. Pediatric premedication should be administered with caution, and under supervision and close monitoring. Skilled staff should be immediately available to rescue the airway and initiate resuscitation should it be needed.

REFERENCES

1. Kain ZN, Caldwell-Andrews AA. Preoperative psychological preparation of the child for surgery: an update. *Anesthesiol Clin N Am.* 2005;23(4):597-614.
2. Williams JGL. Psychophysiological responses to anesthesia and operation. *JAMA.* 1968;203(6):127-129.

3. Kain ZN, Mayes LC, Bell C, Weisman S, Hofstadter MB, Rimar S. Premedication in the united states: a status report. *Anesth Analg.* 1997;84(2):427-432.

4. Kain ZN, Ferris CA, Mayes LC, Rimar S. Parental presence during induction of anaesthesia: practice differences between the United States and Great Britain. *Paediatr Anaesth.* 1996;6(3):187-193.

5. Schulman JL, Foley JM, Vernon DT, Allan D. A study of the effect of the mother's presence during anesthesia induction. *Pediatrics.* 1967;39(1):111-114.

6. Hannallah RS, Rosales JK. Experience with parents' presence during anaesthesia induction in children. *Can Anaesth Soc J.* 1983;30(3 pt 1):286-289.

7. Ryder IG, Spargo PM. Parents in the anaesthetic room. A questionnaire survey of parents' reactions. *Anaesthesia.* 1991;46(11):977-979.

8. Kain ZN, Caldwell-Andrews AA, Wang SM, Krivutza DM, Weinberg ME, Mayes LC. Parental intervention choices for children undergoing repeated surgeries. *Anesth Analg.* 2003;96(4):970-975, table of contents.

9. Kain ZN, Caldwell-Andrews AA, Krivutza DM, Weinberg ME, Wang SM, Gaal D. Trends in the practice of parental presence during induction of anesthesia and the use of preoperative sedative premedication in the United States, 1995–2002: results of a follow-up national survey. *Anesth Analg.* 2004;98(5):1252-1259, table of contents.

10. Shaw EG, Routh DK. Effect of mother presence on children's reaction to aversive procedures. *J Pediatr Psychol.* 1982;7(1):33-42.

11. Bowie JR. Parents in the operating room? *Anesthesiology.* 1993;78(6):1192-1193.

12. Kain ZN, Mayes LC, Wang SM, Caramico LA, Hofstadter MB. Parental presence during induction of anesthesia versus sedative premedication: which intervention is more effective? *Anesthesiology.* 1998;89(5):1147-1156; discussion 9A-10A.

13. Kain ZN, Mayes LC, Wang SM, Caramico LA, Krivutza DM, Hofstadter MB. Parental presence and a sedative premedicant for children undergoing surgery: a hierarchical study. *Anesthesiology.* 2000;92(4):939-946.

14. Kain ZN, Mayes LC, Caramico LA, et al. Parental presence during induction of anaesthesia. A randomized controlled trial. *Anesthesiology.* 1996;84(5):1060-1067.

15. American Academy of Pediatrics Committee on hospital care: child life programs. *Pediatrics.* 1993;91(3):671-673.

16. Kain ZN, Caldwell-Andrews AA, Mayes LC, et al. Family-centered preparation for surgery improves perioperative outcomes in children: a randomized controlled trial. *Anesthesiology.* 2007;106(1):65-74.

17. Melamed BG, Dearborn M, Hermecz DA. Necessary considerations for surgery preparation: age and previous experience. *Psychosom Med.* 1983;45(6):517-525.

18. Kain ZN, Mayes LC, Caramico LA. Preoperative preparation in children: a cross-sectional study. *J Clin Anesth.* 1996;8(6):508-514.

19. O'Byrne KK, Peterson L, Saldana L. Survey of pediatric hospitals' preparation programs: evidence of the impact of health psychology research. *Health Psychol.* 1997;16(2):147-154.

20. Riva J, Lejbusiewicz G, Papa M, et al. Oral premedication with midazolam in paediatric anaesthesia: effects on sedation and gastric contents. *Paediatr Anaesth.* 1997;7(3):191-196.

21. Olkkola KT, Ahonen J. Midazolam and other benzodiazepines. *Handb Exp Pharmacol.* 2008;(182):335-360. doi(182):335-360.

22. Cote CJ, Cohen IT, Suresh S, et al. A comparison of three doses of a commercially prepared oral midazolam syrup in children. *Anesth Analg.* 2002;94(1):37-43, table of contents.

23. Feld LH, Negus JB, White PF. Oral midazolam preanesthetic medication in pediatric outpatients. *Anesthesiology.* 1990;73(5):831-834.

24. Rita L, Seleny FL, Mazurek A, Rabins SY. Intramuscular midazolam for pediatric preanesthetic sedation: a double-blind controlled study with morphine. *Anesthesiology.* 1985;63(5):528-531.

25. Saint-Maurice C, Landais A, Delleur MM, Esteve C, MacGee K, Murat I. The use of midazolam in diagnostic and short surgical procedures in children. *Acta Anaesthesiol Scand Suppl.* 1990;92:39-41; discussion 47.

26. Saarnivaara L, Lindgren L, Klemola UM. Comparison of chloral hydrate and midazolam by mouth as premedicants in children undergoing otolaryngological surgery. *Br J Anaesth.* 1988;61(4):390-396.

27. Wilton NC, Leigh J, Rosen DR, Pandit UA. Preanesthetic sedation of preschool children using intranasal midazolam. *Anesthesiology.* 1988;69(6):972-975.

28. Walbergh EJ, Wills RJ, Eckhert J. Plasma concentrations of midazolam in children following intranasal administration. *Anesthesiology.* 1991;74(2):233-235.

29. Griffith N, Howell S, Mason DG. Intranasal midazolam for premedication of children undergoing day-case anaesthesia: comparison of two delivery systems with assessment of intraobserver variability. *Br J Anaesth.* 1998;81(6):865-869.

30. Malinovsky JM, Cozian A, Lepage JY, Mussini JM, Pinaud M, Souron R. Ketamine and midazolam neurotoxicity in the rabbit. *Anesthesiology.* 1991;75(1):91-97.

31. Alternative routes of drug administration—advantages and disadvantages (subject review). american academy of pediatrics. committee on drugs. *Pediatrics.* 1997;100(1):143-152.

32. Martlew RA, Meakin G, Wadsworth R, Sharples A, Baker RD. Dose of propofol for laryngeal mask airway insertion in children: effect of premedication with midazolam. *Br J Anaesth.* 1996;76(2):308-309.

33. Viitanen H, Annila P, Viitanen M, Yli-Hankala A. Midazolam premedication delays recovery from propofol-induced sevoflurane anesthesia in children 1-3 yr. *Can J Anaesth.* 1999;46(8):766-771.

34. Viitanen H, Annila P, Viitanen M, Tarkkila P. Premedication with midazolam delays recovery after ambulatory sevoflurane anesthesia in children. *Anesth Analg.* 1999;89(1):75-79.

35. Brosius KK, Bannister CF. Effect of oral midazolam premedication on the awakening concentration of sevoflurane, recovery times and bispectral index in children. *Paediatr Anaesth.* 2001;11(5):585-590.

36. Kain ZN, Hofstadter MB, Mayes LC, et al. Midazolam: effects on amnesia and anxiety in children. *Anesthesiology.* 2000;93(3):676-684.

37. Mancuso CE, Tanzi MG, Gabay M. Paradoxical reactions to benzodiazepines: literature review and treatment options. *Pharmacotherapy.* 2004;24(9):1177-1185.

38. Golparvar M, Saghaei M, Sajedi P, Razavi SS. Paradoxical reaction following intravenous midazolam premedication in pediatric patients—a randomized placebo controlled trial of ketamine for rapid tranquilization. *Paediatr Anaesth.* 2004;14(11):924-930.

39. McCall JE, Fischer CG, Warden G, et al. Lorazepam given the night before surgery reduces preoperative anxiety in children undergoing reconstructive burn surgery. *J Burn Care Rehabil.* 1999;20(2):151-154.

40. Mandelli M, Tognoni G, Garattini S. Clinical pharmacokinetics of diazepam. *Clin Pharmacokinet.* 1978;3(1):72-91.

41. Riss J, Cloyd J, Gates J, Collins S. Benzodiazepines in epilepsy: pharmacology and pharmacokinetics. *Acta Neurol Scand.* 2008;118(2):69-86.

42. Roelofse JA, van der Bijl P. Comparison of rectal midazolam and diazepam for premedication in pediatric dental patients. *J Oral Maxillofac Surg.* 1993;51(5):525-529.

43. Mattila MA, Ruoppi MK, Ahlstrom-Bengs E, Larni HM, Pekkola PO. Diazepam in rectal solution as premedication in children, with special reference to serum concentrations. *Br J Anaesth.* 1981;53(12):1269-1272.

44. Marrosu F, Marrosu G, Rachel MG, Biggio G. Paradoxical reactions elicited by diazepam in children with classic autism. *Funct Neurol.* 1987;2(3):355-361.

45. Berman ME, Jones GD, McCloskey MS. The effects of diazepam on human self-aggressive behavior. *Psychopharmacology (Berl).* 2005;178(1):100-106.

46. Hudson RJ, Stanski DR, Burch PG. Pharmacokinetics of methohexital and thiopental in surgical patients. *Anesthesiology.* 1983;59(3):215-219.

47. Yemen TA, Pullerits J, Stillman R, Hershey M. Rectal methohexital causing apnea in two patients with meningomyeloceles. *Anesthesiology.* 1991;74(6):1139-1141.

48. Liu LM, Liu PL, Moss J. Severe histamine-mediated reaction to rectally administered methohexital. *Anesthesiology.* 1984;61(1):95-97.

49. Rockoff MA, Goudsouzian NG. Seizures induced by methohexital. *Anesthesiology.* 1981;54(4):333-335.

50. Beekman RP, Hoorntje TM, Beek FJ, Kuijten RH. Sedation for children undergoing magnetic resonance imaging: efficacy and safety of rectal thiopental. *Eur J Pediatr.* 1996;155(9):820-822.

51. Reimche LD, Sankaran K, Hindmarsh KW, Kasian GF, Gorecki DK, Tan L. Chloral hydrate sedation in neonates and infants—clinical and pharmacologic considerations. *Dev Pharmacol Ther.* 1989;12(2):57-64.

52. Malviya S, Voepel-Lewis T, Prochaska G, Tait AR. Prolonged recovery and delayed side effects of sedation for diagnostic imaging studies in children. *Pediatrics.* 2000;105(3):E42.

53. Biban P, Baraldi E, Pettenazzo A, Filippone M, Zacchello F. Adverse effect of chloral hydrate in two young children with obstructive sleep apnea. *Pediatrics.* 1993;92(3):461-463.

54. Cote CJ, Karl HW, Notterman DA, Weinberg JA, McCloskey C. Adverse sedation events in pediatrics: analysis of medications used for sedation. *Pediatrics.* 2000;106(4):633-644.

55. Hollister GR, Burn JM. Side effects of ketamine in pediatric anesthesia. *Anesth Analg.* 1974;53(2):264-267.

56. White PF, Ham J, Way WL, Trevor AJ. Pharmacology of ketamine isomers in surgical patients. *Anesthesiology.* 1980;52(3):231-239.

57. Tamminga RY, Noordhoek M, Kroon J, Faber-Nijholt R. Ketamine anesthesia with or without diazepam premedication for bone marrow punctures in children with acute lymphoblastic leukemia. *Pediatr Hematol Oncol.* 2000;17(5):383-388.

58. Kohrs R, Durieux ME. Ketamine: teaching an old drug new tricks. *Anesth Analg.* 1998;87(5):1186-1193.

59. Abdallah CG, Sanacora G, Duman RS, Krystal JH. Ketamine and rapid-acting antidepressants: a window into a new neurobiology for mood disorder therapeutics. *Annu Rev Med.* 2015;66:509-523.

60. Quibell R, Prommer EE, Mihalyo M, Twycross R, Wilcock A. Ketamine*. *J Pain Symptom Manage.* 2011;41(3):640-649.

61. Sinner B, Graf BM. Ketamine. *Handb Exp Pharmacol.* 2008;(182):313-333.

62. Aroni F, Iacovidou N, Dontas I, Pourzitaki C, Xanthos T. Pharmacological aspects and potential new clinical applications of ketamine: reevaluation of an old drug. *J Clin Pharmacol.* 2009;49(8):957-964.

63. Wieber J, Gugler R, Hengstmann JH, Dengler HJ. Pharmacokinetics of ketamine in man. *Anaesthesist.* 1975;24(6):260-263.

64. Lockhart CH, Nelson WL. The relationship of ketamine requirement to age in pediatric patients. *Anesthesiology.* 1974;40(5):507-508.

65. Hannallah RS, Patel RI. Low-dose intramuscular ketamine for anesthesia pre-induction in young children undergoing brief outpatient procedures. *Anesthesiology.* 1989;70(4):598-600.

66. Verghese ST, Hannallah RS, Patel RI, Patel KM. Ketamine and midazolam is an inappropriate preinduction combination in uncooperative children undergoing brief ambulatory procedures. *Paediatr Anaesth.* 2003;13(3):228-232.

67. Funk W, Jakob W, Riedl T, Taeger K. Oral preanaesthetic medication for children: double-blind randomized study of a combination of midazolam and ketamine vs midazolam or ketamine alone. *Br J Anaesth.* 2000;84(3):335-340.

68. Weksler N, Ovadia L, Muati G, Stav A. Nasal ketamine for paediatric premedication. *Can J Anaesth.* 1993;40(2):119-121.

69. van der Bijl P, Roelofse JA, Stander IA. Rectal ketamine and midazolam for premedication in pediatric dentistry. *J Oral Maxillofac Surg.* 1991;49(10):1050-1054.

70. Binstock W, Rubin R, Bachman C, Kahana M, McDade W, Lynch JP. The effect of premedication with OTFC, with or without ondansetron, on postoperative agitation, and nausea and vomiting in pediatric ambulatory patients. *Paediatr Anaesth.* 2004;14(9):759-767.

71. U.S. Food and Drug Administration. FDA drug safety communication: FDA restricts use of prescription codeine pain and cough medicines and tramadol pain medicines in children; recommends against use in breastfeeding women. Available at https://www.fda.gov/Drugs/DrugSafety/ucm549679.htm. Updated 2017. Accessed May 17, 2017.

72. Lambert P, Cyna AM, Knight N, Middleton P. Clonidine premedication for postoperative analgesia in children. *Cochrane Database Syst Rev.* 2014 Jan 28;(1):CD009633.

73. Nishina K, Mikawa K, Shiga M, Obara H. Clonidine in paediatric anaesthesia. *Paediatr Anaesth.* 1999;9(3):187-202.

74. Ramesh VJ, Bhardwaj N, Batra YK. Comparative study of oral clonidine and diazepam as premedicants in children. *Int J Clin Pharmacol Ther.* 1997;35(5):218-221.

75. Peng K, Wu SR, Ji FH, Li J. Premedication with dexmedetomidine in pediatric patients: a systematic review and meta-analysis. *Clinics (Sao Paulo).* 2014;69(11):777-786.

76. Feng JF, Wang XX, Lu YY, Pang DG, Peng W, Mo JL. Effects of dexmedetomidine versus midazolam for premedication in paediatric anaesthesia with sevoflurane: a meta-analysis. *J Int Med Res.* 2017;45(3):912-923.

77. Kumar L, Kumar A, Panikkaveetil R, Vasu BK, Rajan S, Nair SG. Efficacy of intranasal dexmedetomidine versus oral midazolam for paediatric premedication. *Indian J Anaesth.* 2017;61(2):125-130.

78. Simons KJ, Watson WT, Martin TJ, Chen XY, Simons FE. Diphenhydramine: pharmacokinetics and pharmacodynamics in elderly adults, young adults, and children. *J Clin Pharmacol.* 1990;30(7):665-671.

79. Nilsson A, Engberg G, Henneberg S, Danielson K, De Verdier CH. Inverse relationship between age-dependent erythrocyte activity of methaemoglobin reductase and prilocaine-induced methemoglobinemia during infancy. *Br J Anaesth.* 1990;64(1):72-76.

80. Brisman M, Ljung BM, Otterbom I, Larsson LE, Andreasson SE. Methaemoglobin formation after the use of EMLA cream in term neonates. *Acta Paediatr.* 1998;87(11): 1191-1194.

81. Sethna NF, Verghese ST, Hannallah RS, Solodiuk JC, Zurakowski D, Berde CB. A randomized controlled trial to evaluate S-caine patch for reducing pain associated with vascular access in children. *Anesthesiology.* 2005;102(2): 403-408.

82. Jimenez N, Bradford H, Seidel KD, Sousa M, Lynn AM. A comparison of a needle-free injection system for local anesthesia versus EMLA for intravenous catheter insertion in the pediatric patient. *Anesth Analg.* 2006;102(2):411-414.

83. Spanos S, Booth R, Koenig H, Sikes K, Gracely E, Kim IK. Jet injection of 1% buffered lidocaine versus topical ELA-max for anesthesia before peripheral intravenous catheterization in children: a randomized controlled trial. *Pediatr Emerg Care.* 2008;24(8):511-515.

Fluids and Acid-Base Management

Rita Saynhalath

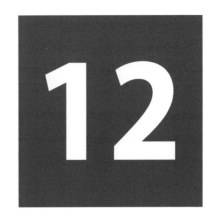

Fluid management in the operating room is as important as the medications administered to achieve anesthesia and analgesia. Fasting times can significantly affect infants and toddlers, and subsequently lead to hemodynamic instability under general anesthesia. Furthermore, in the pediatric population, physiological buffer systems are still immature making the patient more prone to acid-base disturbances. This chapter will review the main principles of fluid management, the different strategies for fluid repletion, including the transfusion of blood products, the physiology behind acid-base homeostasis, and the diagnostic approach to acid-base disturbances.

FLUID MANAGEMENT

One of the first considerations when evaluating a pediatric patient who presents to the preoperative area is to inquire about fasting times. This allows the anesthesiologist to calculate the fluid deficit already present prior to induction. The Holliday-Segar formula, developed in the 1950s,[1] is used to calculate the rate of maintenance fluids; it is more commonly known as the "4-2-1" rule. For the first 10 kg of a patient's weight, the patient requires 4 mL/kg/h. For the next 10 kg, the patient should receive an additional 2 mL/kg/h. Lastly, for each kilogram thereafter, 1 mL/kg/h should be administered in addition to the 60 mL/h calculated for the first 20 kg. This holds true for an otherwise healthy patient, or even a patient with comorbid conditions that are medically optimized, presenting for an elective procedure. In a patient who is acutely sick and likely dehydrated, other clinical signs can guide fluid resuscitation perioperatively. There are several criteria obtained from a physical examination that can help classify a patient's status into mild, moderate, or severe dehydration (Table 12-1). Fluid resuscitation can then be carried out accordingly prior to induction, then continued intraoperatively to achieve hemodynamic stability.

There is a wide variety of intravenous fluids that are used as maintenance fluids perioperatively depending on the patient's comorbid conditions and the indicated surgical procedure. The difference between these fluids lies in the osmolarity of the fluid and content of electrolytes.

CRYSTALLOIDS VERSUS COLLOIDS

▸ Lactated Ringer's

The most common type of intravenous fluid used in the operating room for the pediatric population is lactated Ringer's. The osmolarity of lactated Ringer's, at 273 milliOsmoles per liter (mOsm/L), is similar to plasma

Table 12-1. Clinical Criteria to Classify Dehydration[2]

	Mild (3% - 5%)	Moderate (6% - 9%)	Severe (> 10%)
Mental status	Well-appearing	Ill-appearing, nontoxic	Lethargic, toxic
Heart rate	Normal to increased	Tachycardia	Marked tachycardia
Breathing	Normal	Increased	Increased, deep
Pulse	Normal quality	Normal to decreased quality	Poor quality
Capillary refill	Normal (<2 sec)	Normal to slightly prolonged (2–4 sec)	Markedly prolonged
Perfusion	Warm	Cool	Cool, mottled
Blood pressure	Normal	Normal	Hypotensive
Eyes	Normal	Slightly sunken	Very sunken
Tears	Normal	Decreased	Absent
Mucous membranes	Moist	Sticky	Very dry
Skin turgor (recoil)	Instant recoil	Delayed (2 sec)	Very prolonged
Urine output	Normal to slightly decreased	Decreased	Minimal

Source: Used with permission of EB Medicine. Mark A. Hostetler. Gastroenteritis: an evidence-based approach to typical vomiting, diarrhea, and dehydation. *Pediatric Emergency Medicine Practice.* 2004;1(5):1-20 © 2004 EB Medicine. www.ebmedicine.net.

Table 12-2. Composition of Commonly Used Crystalloid Solutions

Fluid	pH	Na$^+$ (mEq/L)	K$^+$ (mEq/L)	Cl$^-$ (mEq/L)	Ca^{2+} (mEq/L)	Other	Osmolality (mOsm/L)
Lactated Ringer's	6.5	130	4	109	3	Lactate 28 mEq/L	273
Normal saline	5.6	154	–	154	–	–	308
Plasma-Lyte®	5.5	140	5	98	–	Magnesium 3 mEq/L Acetate 27 mEq/L Gluconate 23 mEq/L	294
5% Dextrose and 0.9% sodium chloride	4.3	154	–	154	–	Dextrose 50 g/L	560
5% Dextrose and 0.45% sodium chloride	4.4	77	–	77	–	Dextrose 50 g/L	405

osmolarity, which ranges from 275 to 290 mOsm/L (Table 12-2). The concentration of electrolytes is also comparable to physiologic plasma concentrations, making it an ideal fluid to achieve euvolemia perioperatively. However, one must keep in mind that lactated Ringer's contains lactate and must be avoided in conditions where lactate metabolism may be compromised or the administration of lactate itself may be detrimental. Such conditions include severe liver disease, anoxic states, and severe metabolic acidosis

or alkalosis. A common misconception is that the patient in renal failure may develop life-threatening hyperkalemia due to the concentration of potassium present in lactated Ringer's. O'Malley has conducted a prospective, randomized, double-blind trial comparing lactated Ringer's to normal saline in the setting of renal transplantation. The group who received Lactated Ringer's had a lower incidence of hyperkalemia requiring treatment (defined as a potassium level greater than 6 mEq/L) and metabolic acidosis.[3] Lactated Ringer's also contains calcium and should not be used during the transfusion of blood products due to the presence of citrate. It is incompatible with ceftriaxone because precipitates can form with calcium leading to significant morbidity and mortality.

0.9% Sodium Chloride

The second most common intravenous fluid used in the pediatric population is 0.9% sodium chloride solution, or normal saline. This fluid is favored during neurosurgical cases because infusion of a large amount of lactated Ringer's can result in cerebral edema due to its hypo-osmolarity compared to plasma osmolarity. Normal saline has an osmolarity of 309 mOsm/L and contains equal but supraphysiologic concentrations of sodium and chloride, at 154 mEq/L. Therefore, when infused in large quantities, it can lead to a hyperchloremic metabolic acidosis. Another important consideration to keep in mind when usi ng normal saline is the lack of electrolytes such as potassium, magnesium, calcium, or glucose, because a prolonged infusion can result in electrolyte imbalances or hypoglycemia.

Plasma-Lyte®

Plasma-Lyte has emerged as an alternative for fluid maintenance, especially in the critical care population, and during the transfusion of blood products. Each liter of Plasma-Lyte has an osmolarity of 294 mOsm and contains 140 mEq of sodium, 5 mEq of potassium, 98 mEq of chloride, 3 mEq of magnesium, 27 mEq of acetate, and 23 mEq of gluconate. The acetate and gluconate ions inside the solution are metabolized to carbon dioxide and water through the consumption of hydrogen ions, thus leading to an overall metabolic alkalosis. Therefore, it may not be ideal in patients already in respiratory or metabolic alkalosis. Similarly, to lactated Ringer's, it must be used with caution in patients with hyperkalemia or renal failure due to its potassium content.[4]

Albumin 5%

When to transition from crystalloids to colloids? There is a concern when crystalloids are used exclusively for fluid resuscitation or in the setting of excessive blood loss. Over time, only a transient response will be appreciated because only 30% of the crystalloid solution stays in the intravascular space. Alternatively, an infusion of colloids will remain mostly in the intravascular space, instead of expanding the interstitial fluid space. The rule-of-thumb during fluid resuscitation is to replace the estimated volume of blood lost in a 3 to 1 ratio when using crystalloids, but a 1 to 1 ratio when using colloids. The most common colloid solution used intraoperatively is albumin 5%. It is dispensed in a sterile glass bottle as a slightly yellow and viscous liquid. Large pools of human plasma are used to manufacture this colloid solution. Other components of albumin 5% include

sodium, potassium, N-acetyl-DL-tryptophan, and caprylic acid. Sodium levels should be monitored if large volumes of albumin 5% are administered. The United States Food and Drug Administration (US FDA) issued a warning regarding the use of this solution because it is derived from human plasma and thus may contain infectious agents that can be transmitted to the recipient and cause disease. However, it is pasteurized at 60°C and there are no reported cases of viral hepatitis from an infusion of albumin 5%. It is classified as Category C for use in pregnant women. Lastly, using a large volume of albumin 5% after significant blood loss can lead to hemodilution, dilution of coagulation factors, and electrolyte disturbances.[5]

TRANSFUSION OF BLOOD PRODUCTS

During invasive surgeries where significant blood loss is anticipated, it is important to calculate a patient's estimated blood volume and the allowable blood loss (Table 12-3). Assuming that the patient has a hematocrit within normal limits preoperatively, the calculated allowable blood loss can serve as a guide to determine the necessity for transfusion of blood products. It is very important to monitor the ongoing blood loss during a surgical procedure. This can be done by keeping track of the amount of fluids collected in the suction canister, the number of sponges used on the field, and the amount of blood absorbed into the drapes. The three most common sponges used in the operating room are as follows: a 4 × 4 piece of gauze that holds 10 mL of blood, a Ray-Tec® sponge that holds up to 20 mL of blood, a pediatric lap sponge that holds 50 mL of blood, and an adult lap sponge that holds 100 mL of blood. Irrigation fluids are also often used to irrigate wounds or body cavities to assist during procedures such as a cystoscopy or arthroscopy, and when certain instruments are used such as coblation wands. The total amount of irrigation fluids used during the operation must be subtracted to ensure a correct estimation of blood loss.

If a transfusion is highly likely during the surgical procedure, a type and crossmatch must be obtained preoperatively to ensure that the appropriate blood products

Table 12-3. Estimated Blood Volume and Allowable Blood Loss Formulas

Patient's Age	Estimated Blood Volume (mL/kg)
Preterm neonate	100
Full-term neonate	90
Infant	80
Child	75
Teenager/Adult	70

Allowable blood loss = Estimated blood volume × ($Hct_{initial}$ − $Hct_{allowable}$)/ $Hct_{initial}$

will be readily available. Blood type is classified into four major groups: A, B, AB, and O. For instance, a person with blood group A carries the A antigen and will mount an immune response with anti-B antibodies when exposed to blood group B or blood group AB, which both carry the B antigen. Furthermore, blood types are further subclassified into Rh D antigen positive or negative. To avoid detrimental effects from a blood transfusion, compatibility between the donor's blood and the recipient's blood must be verified. The first step involves determining the patient's blood type, meaning his or her ABO type and Rh D status. A crossmatch is then performed to rule out possible adverse reactions to other antigens. This involves mixing a small volume of the recipient's serum with a small volume of red blood cells from the donor's blood. Examination under a microscope will reveal if antibodies from the recipient cause agglutination of the donor red blood cells. If agglutination occurs, the transfusion is deemed incompatible and the recipient will not receive that specific unit of blood. On the other hand, a type and screen can also be performed. This is only recommended if the possibility of transfusion is low. The test determines the patient's blood type and screens for the most commonly found unexpected antibodies. However, because there is no actual compatibility test between the recipient's and the donor's blood samples, a transfusion reaction can still occur. A type and crossmatch can take between 45 and 60 minutes. Therefore, results must be obtained prior to transferring a patient to the operating room. This is especially crucial in a patient who has received multiple blood transfusions in the past, such as an oncology patient, or one with known rare antigens. In those cases, it might take longer before a compatible unit of blood can be identified. For the transfusion of other blood products such as platelets, fresh frozen plasma, or cryoprecipitate, a type and crossmatch are not necessary because they contain minimal amounts of red blood cells.[6]

ADVERSE REACTIONS TO BLOOD TRANSFUSION

There are several considerations to keep in mind when initiating the transfusion of blood products in the pediatric population. Adverse reactions can range from mild to severe; can be acute or delayed reactions; and can be categorized as immune- or non-immune-mediated events.

▶ Non-Immune-Mediated Reactions

Hypothermia

Blood products, except for platelets, are kept in coolers once they are released from the blood bank. Therefore, it is important to use a fluid warmer to administer them to prevent contributing to hypothermia in the pediatric patient. Hypothermia may lead to cardiac arrhythmias, platelet and clotting factors dysfunction, and increase in bleeding time.[7] Platelets, on the other hand, are stored at room

temperature.[8] A common misconception is that platelets cannot be transfused through a fluid warmer because it will affect their function. Konig et al have conducted a small-scale study that has refuted that belief. Their results "do not support the prohibition against mechanical platelet warming." However, they also state that further studies should be performed to investigate platelet activation.[9] Fluid warmers will warm fluids up to 42°C. Rao et al have demonstrated that warming platelets above 43 to 45°C has an adverse effect on platelet aggregation. Heat also affects the cytoskeletal proteins of platelets and surface membrane receptors, leading to altered function. The biochemical systems involved in activation events are however not impacted.[10] Blood products should be administered through a standard filter, usually a 170 to 260 μm filter.[8] The most common solution used as a priming fluid when administering blood products is normal saline. Plasma-Lyte is also a great alternative: it is compatible with blood products[4] and will not lead to a hyperchloremic metabolic acidosis compared to normal saline.

Volume Overload

The quantity of blood transfused should be determined meticulously to avoid volume overload and possible respiratory complications. A useful rule of thumb is that the transfusion of 4 to 5 mL/kg of packed red blood cells will increase the hemoglobin level by 1 g/dL. The transfusion of 5 mL/kg of platelets will increase the platelet count by 15,000 per microliter. Fresh frozen plasma is usually transfused 10 to 20 mL/kg at a time until bleeding improves clinically. One unit of cryoprecipitate per 7 kg of body weight will increase the fibrinogen level by 100 mg/dL. Once the decision has been made to start transfusing red blood cells, it is important to remember that coagulopathy can be associated with transfusions. To prevent this, it might be necessary to also transfuse fresh frozen plasma and platelets. More research is needed to determine the optimal ratio for a balanced transfusion strategy. In the meanwhile, most guidelines recommend transfusing in a PRBC:FFP:platelet ratio of 2:1:1.[11]

Electrolyte Disturbances

The two most common types of electrolyte disturbances from a blood transfusion involve potassium and calcium. Potassium is released from older, damaged red blood cells into the circulation during the transfusion process. The most serious complication from acute hyperkalemia is the development of cardiac arrhythmias.[6] This occurs rarely due to rapid dilution, redistribution into the cells, and excretion of excess potassium by the kidneys. Interestingly, hypokalemia is more common than hyperkalemia after a transfusion. The proposed mechanism is inward movement of potassium intracellularly into donor red blood cells. Citrate metabolism enhances this migration of potassium. During a massive transfusion, the release of catecholamines and loss of aldosterone in the urine also contribute to the development of hypokalemia.[7] Furthermore, citrate is the major anticoagulant used during the collection and storage process of packed red blood cells. Unfortunately, transfusion of large volumes of red blood cells can lead to hypocalcemia due to chelation by citrate. This would manifest clinically with muscle spasms, seizures, and cardiac arrhythmias.[6]

Transfusion-Associated Circulatory Overload

Another significant acute adverse reaction is transfusion-associated circulatory overload, or TACO. It is rare but is associated with considerable morbidity and mortality. The clinical symptoms are related to fluid overload, such as dyspnea, tachycardia, jugular venous distention, and edema. A hallmark sign is hypertension with a widened pulse pressure. Management consists mainly of treating the underlying etiology, mechanical ventilation, fluid restriction, and diuretic therapy.[7]

Infectious Diseases

Concern in the general population when faced with a possible transfusion is the risk of transmission of infectious diseases. Since the 1960s, blood banks have started universally screening donor's blood before it reaches the patient. Eligibility criteria are strict and anyone with a history of hepatitis or transfusions in the six preceding months is excluded from donating blood. The thorough evaluation of the donor, laboratory screening tests (including serologic testing and viral nucleic acid testing), and procedures to inactivate pathogens are the three main processes that serve to significantly decrease, but unfortunately cannot eradicate, the risk of transfusion-transmitted infections. The relative risk of transmission of the most frequent viruses has significantly decreased with time (Table 12-4). This has led to the risk of bacterial contamination being greater than the risk of a viral infection, at 1 in less than 40,000 when transfusing packed red blood cells and as high as 1 in 5000 when platelets are transfused. This can be explained by the

Table 12-4. Relative Risk of Transfusion-Transmitted Viral Disease in the United States[12]

Virus	Relative Risk of Transmission
Human immunodeficiency virus	1 in <2.2 million
Hepatitis C virus	1 in <2 million
Hepatitis B virus	1 in <300,000
West Nile virus	1 in 350,000
Human T cell lymphotrophic virus	1 in <3 million

Source: Data from Bihl F, Castelli D, Marincola F, Dodd RY, Brander C. Transfusion-transmitted infections. *J Transl Med.* 2007;5:25. https://translational-medicine.biomedcentral.com/.

storage conditions of platelets at room temperature where bacteria thrive better compared to the cold temperatures of 1 to 6°C that red blood cells require for storage.[12]

Immune-Mediated Reactions

Hemolytic Reactions

Immune-mediated blood transfusion reactions are defined by the substance that generates the immune response. Hemolytic transfusion reactions can be acute or delayed in onset. The acute reactions are further separated into intravascular or extravascular processes. Antigens present on the donor red blood cells are recognized by the recipient's immune system as foreign. This triggers antibody-medicated detection and destruction of the donor red blood cells. This can happen inside the blood vessels, or in the spleen and liver if the destruction is carried out by macrophages. Clinical signs include fever, chills, and back and flank pain. Unfortunately, the most common cause of this transfusion reaction is ABO incompatibility, most likely caused by human error. A hemolytic transfusion reaction can occur the day following the transfusion or 14 days later resulting in a delayed reaction. The reason for this "delay" is the low quantities of antibodies present in the circulation. The immune system will then produce more antibodies once the antigens are encountered, leading to extravascular hemolysis.[6,7]

Febrile Nonhemolytic Reactions

Febrile nonhemolytic reactions are acute in onset and are caused by the recipient's antibodies attacking HLA antigens on donor white blood cells. This is usually a mild reaction that presents as a rise in temperature of at least 1°C, chills, and rigors. Leukodepletion is a process that removes white blood cells from donated blood prior to storage and can prevent this reaction. Antipyretics can also be administered prophylactically before the transfusion occurs.[6,7]

Post-Transfusion Purpura

Post-transfusion purpura occurs when the recipient's platelet-specific antibody reacts with donor platelets leading to thrombocytopenia. It is a delayed reaction with an onset of 5 to 10 days and leads to the formation of purpura as well as an increased risk of bleeding. Unfortunately, during this process, the antibodies also attack the recipient's own platelets and the patient becomes thrombocytopenic. Treatment includes the infusion of intravenous immunoglobulins or plasmapheresis.[6,7]

Allergic Reactions

Allergic reactions can occur due to IgE or IgA antibodies. Urticaria, or hives, is caused by recipient or donor IgE antibodies that bind to a certain antigen leading to the activation of mast cells and basophils resulting in histamine release. This is more likely to happen in atopic patients such as those with seasonal allergies. Treatment is simple and consists of discontinuing the transfusion and administering antihistamines. In the case of a more severe reaction such as angioedema, steroids such as methylprednisolone or prednisone can be used. The transfusion can usually be resumed once the symptoms have resolved. If IgA antiplasma protein antibodies are involved, a life-threatening allergic reaction will develop, known as anaphylaxis. This reaction is more common in patients with IgA deficiency. Clinical symptoms include dyspnea, wheezing, coughing, nausea, or vomiting. This can rapidly progress to hypotension, loss of consciousness, respiratory arrest, and circulatory shock. Depending on the hemodynamic status of the patient, treatment includes discontinuing the transfusion, administering epinephrine, and even performing cardiopulmonary resuscitation.[6,7]

Transfusion-Associated Lung Injury

TRALI, or transfusion-associated lung injury, is among one of the most serious adverse reactions from the transfusion of blood products. It is rare but can become fatal. Donor antileukocyte antibodies attack the recipient's white blood cells leading to aggregation in the pulmonary vasculature. Inflammatory mediators are released and increase the permeability of the lung capillaries, resulting in pulmonary edema. It is a clinical diagnosis that manifests with the acute onset of shortness of breath within 6 hours of transfusion in the absence of preexisting lung pathology. A chest radiograph shows findings consistent with bilateral pulmonary edema and an echocardiogram should be obtained to rule out the presence of left atrial hypertension. An arterial blood gas reveals hypoxemia with a Pao_2 to Fio_2 ratio less than or equal to 300 or an oxygen saturation less than 90% on room air by pulse oximeter. In 80% of the cases, oxygenation improves within 48 to 96 hours and the lung injury resolves. Treatment is supportive and given the normal findings on echocardiogram, diuretics are not indicated.[6,7]

Transfusion-Associated Graft-Versus-Host Disease

The last important immune-mediated adverse reaction is TA-GVHD, or transfusion-associated graft-versus-host disease. This delayed adverse reaction occurs approximately 1 week after the transfusion due to donor T lymphocytes attacking the recipient's own cells that have the HLA antigen. Clinically, the patient will present with a fever, characteristic maculopapular rash that progresses to hemorrhagic bullae, and enterocolitis with diarrhea. Further evaluation reveals elevated liver function tests and pancytopenia indicating bone marrow failure. Unfortunately, the prognosis is grim with TA-GVHD and death occurs within a few weeks in 90% of the cases. High-risk patients include immunocompromised patients where the immune system is unable to eliminate the T cells in question. In that population, it is essential to limit blood transfusions when possible and use irradiated blood products if necessary.[6,7]

ACID-BASE MANAGEMENT

Homeostasis is defined as "a self-regulating process by which biological systems tend to maintain stability while adjusting to conditions that are optimal for survival."[13] In the human body, acid-base balance is achieved through buffer systems, excretion of carbon dioxide through ventilation, and elimination of acid by the kidneys.

Definitions

The Brønsted-Lowry definition of acids and bases states that an acid is a proton (or hydrogen ion) donor, and a base is a proton acceptor. A substance can be a strong or a weak acid or base, depending on how readily it donates or accepts a hydrogen ion, respectively. The Henderson-Hasselbalch equation can then be used to determine the acidity of a solution. The pK_a is the intrinsic value of a substance defined as the pH where it can be found in both its protonated and deprotonated forms in a 1:1 ratio.

$pH = pK_a + \log([A^-]/[HA])$, where pK_a represents the dissociation ionization constant, A^- the base, and HA the conjugate acid.

Regulation of Acid-Base Balance

The two main organs that allow regulation of acid-base balance are the lungs and the kidneys. The lungs allow elimination of carbon dioxide through alveolar ventilation to maintain arterial Pco_2 around 40 mm Hg. Two types of chemoreceptors help regulate the rate of alveolar ventilation. Central chemoreceptors are located on the anterolateral surface of the medulla oblongata. When carbon dioxide diffuses across the blood-brain barrier, the concentration of hydrogen ions in the cerebrospinal fluid increases leading to a decrease in pH. The chemoreceptors are sensitive to the change in pH and respond by increasing alveolar ventilation.[14] This relationship is linear except at the extremes of arterial $Paco_2$. Carbon dioxide narcosis occurs at very high arterial $Paco_2$ where alveolar ventilation no longer increases. On the other end of the spectrum, at very low arterial $Paco_2$, the apneic threshold is reached, and alveolar ventilation can no longer decrease. There are two groups of peripheral chemoreceptors: the carotid bodies at the bifurcation of the common carotid arteries in the carotid sinus, and the aortic bodies around the aortic arch. They are most sensitive to variation in Pao_2 but will also respond to changes in $Paco_2$, pH, and arterial perfusion pressure. A decrease in Pao_2, increase in $Paco_2$, or decrease in pH stimulates the carotid body chemoreceptors to send a signal via the glossopharyngeal nerves to the respiratory centers in the brainstem. A signal that originates from the aortic bodies travels via the vagus nerves to the cardiovascular centers in the brainstem. However, alveolar ventilation can only decrease to a certain extent because without supplemental oxygenation, hypoxia will inevitably ensue in response to significant hypoventilation. The decrease in Pao_2 stimulates chemoreceptors and limits the respiratory compensation to metabolic alkalosis.[15]

The kidneys also serve to preserve homeostasis, but these effects may take hours to days before they are observed clinically. There is an important chemical reaction necessary to understand the purpose of bicarbonate in the body:

$$CO_2 + H_2O \leftrightarrow H_2CO_3 \leftrightarrow HCO_3^- + H^+$$

This reaction is catalyzed by the enzyme carbonic anhydrase, which is located on the luminal side and inside the tubular cell. In the proximal tubule, bicarbonate is reabsorbed mainly through secretion of protons via the Na^+,H^+ antiporter. This exchange requires energy that is provided by the Na^+,K^+-ATPase. The reaction between carbon dioxide and water leads to the formation of bicarbonate and a hydrogen ion. Bicarbonate enters the bloodstream to be reabsorbed. The hydrogen ion is eliminated into the urine in exchange for sodium entering the tubular cell. It reacts with filtered bicarbonate present in the tubular lumen to form carbon dioxide and water. Carbon dioxide then reenters the tubular cell to start the cycle again. A third of bicarbonate reabsorption occurs via the H^+-ATPase. In the distal tubule, secretion of acid via the H^+-ATPase and H^+,K^+-ATPase serves to regenerate bicarbonate. Phosphate is the most abundant buffer present in the urine. It combines with a hydrogen ion to form phosphorous acid, which is excreted into the urine. Phosphate is thus considered a titratable acid because it is a weak acid anion present in the urine and used to maintain acid-base balance. Finally, ammonium excretion represents another mechanism that occurs in the kidneys. Inside the renal cell, glutamine is used to form NH_3, or ammonia, which is allowed to diffuse into the tubular lumen because it does not possess a charge. NH_3 in turn combines with a hydrogen ion to form NH^{4+}, or ammonium. Ammonium is then eliminated into the urine. There are a few factors that affect the amount of acid excreted in the distal tubule. Distal acidification is decreased in the setting of hyponatremia because the active transport of sodium creates a negative potential difference in the tubule, thus increasing the rate of proton excretion into the tubular lumen. Aldosterone modulates multiple processes occurring in the kidneys: it augments the rate of sodium reabsorption, stimulates Na^+,K^+-ATPase and H^+-ATPase, and enhances the production of ammonia. Therefore, an excess of aldosterone will significantly increase the quantity of acid excreted.[16]

Buffer Systems

A buffer system is defined as the presence of a weak base and its conjugate acid that serves to resist any extreme changes in the pH of the solution. This is important because a significant amount of acid is produced in the body, but it is essential to maintain the pH of body fluids within a narrow range for optimal conditions. There are four important buffer systems.

The bicarbonate–carbonic acid buffer system operates in the extracellular fluid. It starts with carbon dioxide reacting with water to form carbonic acid, with the help of the enzyme carbonic anhydrase as a catalyst. Since carbonic acid is a weak acid, it readily dissociates into bicarbonate and a hydrogen ion.

The hemoglobin buffer system is located in the red blood cells, a site that is abundant in carbonic anhydrase. This is important because the mechanism by which carbon dioxide travels to the lungs depends on the cooperation between the bicarbonate–carbonic acid and hemoglobin buffer systems. Carbon dioxide from tissues diffuses into the bloodstream to enter the red blood cells. Inside the cell, carbonic anhydrase catalyzes the chemical reaction to form bicarbonate and a hydrogen ion. The hydrogen ion combines with amino acid side chains in hemoglobin, while bicarbonate leaves the red blood cell in exchange for a chloride anion to maintain electroneutrality. The reverse occurs as the red blood cells travel toward the lungs, thus allowing for release of carbon dioxide into the alveoli to be eliminated through ventilation.

The last two buffer systems in the body, phosphate anions and proteins, exert their effect mainly in the intracellular fluid. Proteins are able to accept protons in a similar fashion to hemoglobin.[17]

Arterial Blood Gas Analysis

To apply the principles described above, it is essential to be able to interpret results of an arterial blood gas. However, if an arterial line is not warranted to monitor the patient during the surgical procedure, a venous blood gas can be acceptable in some circumstances. It is important to remember that a venous Pco_2 will be about 4 mm Hg higher than an arterial Pco_2 while the pH will be approximately 0.03 lower. This does not apply to a critical or hemodynamically unstable patient, and an arterial blood gas should be obtained for greater accuracy. A meta-analysis by Byrne et al found that venous Pco_2 does not consistently correlate with arterial Pco_2 and is not always greater as expected.[18] Furthermore, only the pH, Po_2, and Pco_2 are directly measured from the blood sample, while the concentration of bicarbonate and base excess are mathematically derived. The method used to obtain the arterial blood sample is critical. Depending on the size of the patient, it can be challenging to ensure that the blood sample is arterial, and not venous. Ideally, the sample should be analyzed within 30 minutes, or it should be collected in a glass syringe and placed in ice. Any delay could lead to erroneous results, especially in the setting of a shunt, elevated white blood cell, or platelet counts. Air bubbles present in the sample can also interfere with the accuracy of the results. Depending on the patient's oxygenation status when the sample was obtained, if the partial pressures of oxygen and carbon dioxide in the air bubble equilibrate with those in the blood sample, the values obtained could be falsely high or low.[19] Lastly, the patient's temperature affects the partial pressure of oxygen and carbon dioxide in blood, and therefore the pH of the blood sample. Hypothermia leads to increased solubility and therefore decreased partial pressures of oxygen and carbon dioxide.[20]

Once the results of an arterial or venous blood gas have been obtained, the next step is to diagnose the acid-base disturbance present. The disorder (acidosis or alkalosis) can be metabolic, respiratory, or mixed in etiology; acute or chronic in nature; and compensated or uncompensated. The first step is to look at the pH of the arterial or venous blood gas. Physiologic pH is maintained between 7.35 and 7.45. Acidosis is defined as a blood pH less than 7.35 and alkalosis is a blood pH above 7.45.

Metabolic Acidosis and Strong Ion Difference

Metabolic acidosis is differentiated from respiratory acidosis by the value of P_{CO_2}. When the pH is below 7.35, the concentration of bicarbonate is below 24 mEq/L, and P_{CO_2} is normal or below normal, the diagnosis is a metabolic acidosis resulting from the accumulation of acid in the body. The body attempts to maintain homeostasis by increasing ventilation to eliminate carbon dioxide and attempts to bring the pH closer to a normal value. There are two main categories of metabolic acidosis differentiated by the presence of an anion gap. The anion gap measures the difference between the concentration of cations (sodium) and anions (chloride and bicarbonate) in the serum. A normal anion gap is 12 ± 4 mEq/L. It is important to note that alterations in the concentration of unmeasured anions affect the anion gap. The concentration of plasma albumin has been shown to correlate linearly with plasma pH. Therefore, in the setting of hypoalbuminemia, the anion gap would be falsely lowered. The following formula can be used to possibly unmask a metabolic acidosis in a patient with hypoalbuminemia:

$$AG_{corrected} = AG + 0.25([albumin]_{reference} - [albumin]_{measured})$$

The mnemonic MUDPILES is commonly used to identify the underlying pathology causing an anion gap metabolic acidosis (Table 12-5). On the other hand, metabolic acidosis in the setting of a normal anion gap can be explained by the loss of bicarbonate and replacement

Table 12-5. Causes of Metabolic Acidosis

Anion Gap Metabolic Acidosis	Non-Anion Gap Metabolic Acidosis
Methanol	Infusion of normal saline, TPN
Uremia, chronic renal failure	
Diabetic, alcoholic, or starvation ketoacidosis	Gastrointestinal losses: diarrhea, vomiting, ileostomy, biliary or pancreatic fistula, ureteral diversion
Paraldehyde, propylene glycol	
Infection/sepsis, isoniazide, inborn errors of metabolism	Renal losses: renal tubular acidosis, Addison's disease
Lactic acidosis: congestive heart failure, cyanide toxicity	Drugs: potassium sparing diuretics, carbonic anhydrase inhibitors
Ethanol, ethylene glycol	
Salicylates	

by chloride. Gastrointestinal pathologies are a common etiology because gastrointestinal fluids are alkaline with a high concentration of bicarbonate. Renal disorders such as renal tubular acidosis result in the inability to acidify the urine and decreased excretion of acid. Another etiology is the use of normal saline for aggressive fluid resuscitation because a significant chloride burden will lead to impaired renal bicarbonate reabsorption. Table 12-5 describes the possible causes of metabolic acidosis.[21]

An alternative way of evaluating a metabolic acidosis is to calculate the strong ion difference, or SID. In the early 1980s, Peter Stewart developed a new method to evaluate acid-base disorders. He emphasized the importance of the water dissociation equation as the main determinant of the pH of any fluid, with the influence of several modifiers such as P_{CO_2}, weak acids, and electrolytes. He defined a new term, A_{TOT}, which represents the total concentration of nonvolatile weak acids. A_{TOT} is the sum of the concentration of a weak acid and its conjugate base, or $A_{TOT} = [HA] + [A^-]$. Therefore, it is a constant and is not affected by pH. A decrease or increase in pH reflects a shift toward an increase or a decrease in the concentration of the weak acid, respectively. He also characterized the strong ion difference as the difference between strong cations and strong anions present in body fluids. The normal value for SID is 42 mEq/L, reflecting excess of strong cations in the body. Stewart's method highlights the concept of electroneutrality in any body fluids. Strong cations in the body include sodium, potassium, magnesium, and calcium. Strong anions include chloride, lactate, and unidentified strong anions such as ketoacids and lactate. Urate is usually present at a concentration less than 0.2 mEq/L and is usually omitted from the equation. This leads to the following:

$$SID = [Na^+] + [K^+] + [Ca^{2+}] + [Mg^{2+}] - [Cl^-] - [lactate]$$

The simplified SID equation is as follows:

$$SID = [Na^+] + [K^+] - [Cl^-] - [lactate]$$

The significant deviation from traditional teaching that arises with Stewart's method is that there are only three independent variables: SID, A_{TOT}, and Pco_2. These can in turn affect the dependent variables: pH and concentration of bicarbonate, carbonate anion, and hydroxide. A metabolic alkalosis is represented by an increase in SID or a decrease in A_{TOT}, while a decrease in SID or an increase in A_{TOT} reflects a metabolic acidosis.[22]

Metabolic Alkalosis

Metabolic alkalosis is characterized by a pH greater than 7.45. It can be separated into two groups based on its response to chloride repletion. The underlying pathophysiology that causes a metabolic alkalosis is a gain of bicarbonate or a loss of nonvolatile acid. Acid can be lost from the gastrointestinal tract, such as in vomiting or nasogastric tube suctioning; from the kidneys, for example, primary aldosteronism and use of diuretics; or via intracellular shifts to compensate for hypokalemia. The body can experience excessive bicarbonate loads from alkali administration. Examples include milk alkali syndrome, lactate in intravenous fluids, acetate in total parenteral nutrition, and citrate during the transfusion of blood products.[16]

Respiratory Disorders

Respiratory disorders can be diagnosed when the change in pH can be explained by the deviation of $Paco_2$ from normal and the concentration of bicarbonate remains within normal limits. There is a mismatch between alveolar minute ventilation and carbon dioxide production leading to the acid-base disturbance. In the operating room, the patient is often mechanically ventilated and respiratory disorders can be corrected with simple changes of the ventilator settings. It is important to remember that the normal gradient between $Paco_2$ and end tidal CO_2 is around 5 mm Hg. Unless an arterial catheter is present, it is difficult to obtain $Paco_2$ values and readings from capnometry are used to estimate $Paco_2$. Furthermore, when a respiratory acid-base disorder has been diagnosed, it is important to determine whether it is an acute or a chronic process. If the disturbance occurred acutely, there will be a change in pH of 0.08 for every 10 mm Hg deviation from the normal value of 40 mm Hg. On the other hand, with a chronic process, the change in pH is decreased to 0.03.

Respiratory Acidosis

Respiratory acidosis occurs when the lungs are not able to eliminate enough carbon dioxide to match the amount produced by the body. This can be due to a decrease in elimination or an increase in production or both. This results in an increase in $Paco_2$ leading to a decrease in pH.

Circumstances where excess carbon dioxide is produced include exercise, fever, sepsis, burns, thyrotoxicosis, multi-organ failure, and overfeeding. Decreased elimination of carbon dioxide can be caused by a decrease in alveolar ventilation or ventilatory drive, or abnormal chest wall or respiratory muscles. General anesthesia with the administration of sedatives and opioids can lead to both alveolar and central hypoventilation. Mismatch between pulmonary perfusion and ventilation, such as in the presence of a pulmonary embolus, will also lead to alveolar hypoventilation. Other etiologies of central hypoventilation are as follows: central sleep apnea, obesity hypoventilation syndrome, central nervous system infection or trauma, and brainstem lesions. Disorders of the chest wall such as obesity and kyphoscoliosis, or respiratory muscle weakness can also cause respiratory acidosis. The three main categories of the latter include spinal cord injuries, neuromuscular junction disorders, and myopathies. Intraoperatively, respiratory muscle weakness can be caused by inadequate reversal of neuromuscular blockers.[23] Lastly, respiratory acidosis can also occur iatrogenically. During laparoscopic surgery, carbon dioxide is often used for insufflation and absorption will increase end-tidal and arterial CO_2 concentrations. Rebreathing can also cause an increase in carbon dioxide in the body and can be observed if the soda lime absorber is exhausted or the breathing machine has an incompetent one-way valve.

Respiratory Alkalosis

The reverse stands true for respiratory alkalosis: it is caused by increased minute ventilation or decreased production of carbon dioxide. There is a wide variety of pathologic states leading to hyperventilation. A few examples include hypoxia, intrinsic lung disease (parenchymal or bronchial), drugs, mechanical ventilation, pain, fever, hepatic disease, and diseases of the central nervous system. Hypoxia leads to stimulation of the chemoreceptors located on the carotid bodies resulting in hyperventilation.[24] It is also important to remember that end-tidal carbon dioxide levels can reflect cardiac output. An unanticipated decrease in end-tidal carbon dioxide with no recent change in ventilation should alert the anesthesiologist to possible cardiovascular compromise.

Compensatory Mechanisms

Compensation can occur in a chronic setting, where the lungs compensate for a metabolic disturbance or the kidneys compensate for a metabolic or respiratory disturbance. Winter's formula can be used to determine whether compensation or a mixed acid-base disorder is present. In the setting of a metabolic acidosis, the measured Pco_2 should be close to:

$$P_{CO_2} = (1.5 \times [HCO_3^-]) + 9$$

If it is greater, then there is both a respiratory and a metabolic acidosis. If it is less, the metabolic acidosis is compensated by a respiratory alkalosis. If the underlying disorder has been identified as a metabolic alkalosis, the following equation is used to estimate P_{CO_2}:

$$P_{CO_2} = (0.7 \times [HCO_3^-]) + 21$$

If it is greater than the measured P_{CO_2}, there is a compensatory respiratory acidosis. If it is less, there is both a respiratory and a metabolic alkalosis.

It is ideal but not realistic to expect the pH to remain within normal limits when a patient with multiple comorbidities undergoes a prolonged and invasive surgical procedure. While it is important to correctly identify the acid-base disturbance and treat the underlying etiology, electrolyte disturbances may occur before treatment can be completed. One of the most important electrolyte abnormalities is hyperkalemia. The body attempts to compensate for the metabolic acidosis by buffering the excess of hydrogen ions in the cells. However, to maintain electroneutrality, an exchange has to occur. Potassium ions are released into the extracellular fluid in exchange for hydrogen ions being reabsorbed into the cells. The main concern then becomes myocardial stability in the setting of hyperkalemia. Calcium supplementation is administered to stabilize myocardial cells and avoid any cardiac rhythm disturbances. This is not a long-term solution but simply serves to maintain the patient hemodynamically stable while the underlying acid-base disturbance and resulting electrolyte abnormalities are resolved.

REFERENCES

1. Holliday MA, Segar WE. The maintenance need for water in parenteral fluid therapy. *Pediatrics.* 1957;19:823-832.
2. Hostetler MA. Gastroenteritis: an evidence-based approach to typical vomiting, diarrhea, and dehydration. *Pediatr Emerg Med Prac.* 2004;1(5):1-19.
3. O'Malley CM, Frumento RJ, et al. Double-blind comparison of lactated Ringer's solution and 0.9% NaCl during renal transplantation. *Anesth Analg.* 2005;100:1518-1524.
4. Plasma-Lyte 148 Injection [package insert]. Baxter Healthcare Corporation, Deerfield, IL; December 2007. Available at https://www.accessdata.fda.gov/drugsatfda_docs/label/2009/017451s060,017378s065lbl.pdf. Accessed August 15, 2017.
5. Albumin (Human) 5% [package insert]. Octapharma USA, Inc., Centreville, VA; October 2006. Available at https://www.fda.gov/media/70406/download.
6. Dean L. Blood transfusions and the immune system. In: *Blood Groups and Red Cell Antigens* [Internet]. Bethesda, MD: National Center for Biotechnology Information; 2005:chap. 3.. Available at https://www.ncbi.nlm.nih.gov/books/NBK2265/. Accessed January 27, 2020.
7. Sahu S, Hemlata, Verma A. Adverse events related to blood transfusion. *Indian J Anaesth.* 2014;58(5):543-551.
8. American Society of Anesthesiologists Committee on Patient Blood Management. Platelets: An Update From COBM. Available at https://www.asahq.org/standards-and-guidelines/resources-from-asa-committees?&ct=c5d82a194c-b4e6a05b98a17d0cb95c87088881786d4d07ec050ab24d94d78e17ca99b1f9c06f959ae07f88f316f2f98faad9f1248e8aeb1-5870510381c34a4f6#bm. Accessed August 15, 2017.
9. Konig G, Yazer MH, Waters JH. Stored platelet functionality is not decreased after warming with a fluid warmer. *Anesth Analg.* 2013;117(3):575-578.
10. Rao GH, Smith CMII, Escolar G, White JG. Influence of heat on platelet biochemistry, structure, and function. *J Lab Clin Med.* 1993;122:455-464.
11. Blain S, Paterson N. Pediatric massive transfusion. *BJA Education.* 2016;16(8):269-275.
12. Bihl F, Castelli D, Marincola F, Dodd RY, Brander C. Transfusion-transmitted infections. *J Translat Med.* 2007;5:25.
13. The Editors of Encyclopaedia Britannica. "Homeostasis." *Encyclopaedia Britannica.* Encyclopaedia Britannica, Inc. Jun 29, 2017. Web: August 15, 2017.
14. Hamm LL, Nakhoul N, Hering-Smith KS. Acid-base homeostasis. *Clin J Am Soc Nephrol.* 2015;10:2232-2242.
15. Pittman RN. Chemical regulation of respiration. *Regulation of Tissue Oxygenation.* San Rafael, CA: Morgan & Claypool Life Sciences; 2011:chap. 5. Available at https://www.ncbi.nlm.nih.gov/books/NBK54106/.
16. Khanna A, Kurtzman NA. Metabolic alkalosis. *Respir Care.* 2001;46(4):354-365.
17. Lieberman M, Marks AD, Smith CM, Marks DB. *Marks' Essential Medical Biochemistry.* Philadelphia, PA: Lippincott Williams & Wilkins; 2007:30-33.
18. Byrne AL, Bennett M, Chatterji R, Symons R, Pace NL, Thomas PS. Peripheral venous and arterial blood gas analysis in adults: are they comparable? A systematic review and meta-analysis. *Respirology.* 2014;19(2):168-175.
19. Sood P, Paul G, Puri S. Interpretation of arterial blood gas. *Indian J Crit Care Med.* 2010;14(2):57-64.
20. Bacher A. Effects of body temperature on blood gases. *Intensive Care Med.* 2005;31:24-27.
21. Fidkowski C, Helstrom J. Diagnosing metabolic acidosis in the critically ill: bridging the anion gap, Stewart and base excess methods. *Can J Anesth.* 2009;56:247-256.
22. Morgan TJ. The stewart approach—one clinician's perspective. *Clin Biochem Rev.* 2009;30(2):41-54.
23. Epstein SK, Singh N. Respiratory acidosis. *Respir Care.* 2001;46(4):366-383.
24. Foster GT, Vaziri ND, Sassoon CSH. Respiratory alkalosis. *Respir Care.* 2001;46(4):384-491.

Pediatric Airway

Iolanda Russo-Menna

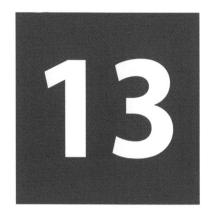

EMBRYOLOGY AND ANATOMY OF THE PEDIATRIC AIRWAY

The respiratory apparatus begins to form at the third gestational week when the laryngotracheal diverticulum (LTD) originates from the ventral wall of anterior primitive intestine. These structures are in communication until esophagotracheal septum separates the airways from the esophagus. The glottis region of larynx develops from the cranial portion of the LTD, while the caudal part forms the tracheal tube and the major bronchi. The supraglottis region will form the larynx and pharynx.

The LTD grows and extends caudally toward the future thoracic cavities, then splits into the two buds of the future main bronchi. The right will create the three bronchial lobes and the left the two lobes. The lobar bronchi form by dichotomous division during the sixth month of gestation and then expand to 23 bronchi by birth.

The respiratory tissue and vascular scaffolding derive from the mesoderm layer. The alveoli expand and form by breathing action, reaching full maturation by 5 to 8 years of age. During this very delicate developing embryologic phase, any pathogenic events may result in severe consequences with airway malformations as well as defects of the esophagus, duodenum, and gastric sac. Anomalies of the esophagotracheal septum may cause esophageal atresia, with or without tracheoesophageal fistula (TEF). Tracheal vascularity abnormalities may result in agenesis or complex tracheal stenosis.

AIRWAY MANAGEMENT IN CHILDREN

Children are not small adults, and it is important to remind to all anesthesia providers that only a few adult airway considerations are transferable to the pediatrics. For instance, the definition of difficult airways, ventilation, and some

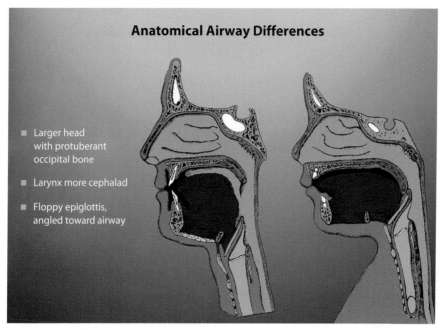

Anatomical Airway Differences

- Larger head with protuberant occipital bone
- Larynx more cephalad
- Floppy epiglottis, angled toward airway

▲ **Figure 13-1.** Anatomical airway differences in adult and child. (Reproduced with permission, from Sasaki CT, Isaacson GC. Functional anatomy of the larynx. *Otolaryngol Clin North Am.* 1988;21: 595-611. https://www.oto.theclinics.com.)

criteria of intubation may be like the adult difficult airway principles. The differences are related to functional anatomic structures in the pediatric patient, different availability of equipment adaptable to pediatric airways, and the extremely dynamic nature of pediatric airway problems because of patient size, weight, dimension, anatomy, as well as maturity and functions of organs and cardiorespiratory systems (Figure 13-1).

Understanding the important anatomical, physiological, and pathological features related to the pediatric airway as well as knowledge of the various tools and methods available are essential in airway management. The head of a pediatric patient is larger relative to body size, with a prominent occiput, large tongue, and short neck. These anatomic features predispose to airway obstruction in anesthetized children, because the neck is flexed when they lie on a flat surface. A folded towel or a gel pad is often required as a shoulder roll to achieve a neutral position of the neck and opening of the airway, as demonstrated in Figure 13-2.

The larger occiput combined with a shorter neck makes laryngoscopy relatively more difficult by providing obstacles to the alignment of the oral, laryngeal, and tracheal axes. The hypopharynx of the pediatric patient is relatively shorter in height and narrower in width. On cross section, the airway of an adult is more elliptical than that of the child, which has implications for supraglottic airway placement.[1]

The larynx is relatively higher in the neck in children. In some positions, the mandible may lie in line with the upper glottis structures. The cricoid ring is located approximately at the level of the C4 vertebrae at birth, C5 at age 6, and C6 as adult.[2]

The vocal cords are not typically found at a right angle (90°) to the tracheal rings. Instead, they are angled in an anterior-inferior to posterior-superior fashion, making insertion of an endotracheal tube challenging and sometime traumatic. If a suboptimal view is present the endotracheal tube will have a higher tendency to collide with or become obstructed on the anterior commissure of the vocal cords.[3]

Given the large tongue and "U" shape rigid epiglottis in children, many anesthesiologists prefer semi-straight laryngoscope blades such as a Miller, Wis-Hipple, and Phillips sizes 1 or 2, which are designed to directly lift the epiglottis and move the tongue at the left, out of view compared to a curved Macintosh blade which are designed to go into the vallecula (Figure 13-3).

▶ **Physiological Differences**

The physiological challenges predisposing children to hypoxemia are high oxygen consumption, the rate of 6 mL/kg/min in children vs 3 mL/kg/min in adults, combined with a lower functional residual capacity (FRC) and high closing capacity (CC). Oxygen desaturation

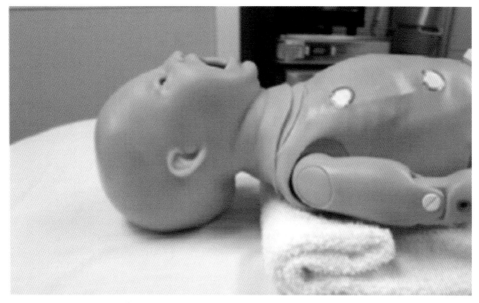

▲ **Figure 13-2.** Correct position of a toddler head, chin, and shoulder roll during inhalation induction. (Reproduced with permission, from Tintinalli JE, Ma O, Yealy DM, et al., eds. *Tintinalli's Emergency Medicine: A Comprehensive Study Guide*, 9th ed. 2020. https://accessmedicine.mhmedical.com. Copyright © McGraw Hill LLC. All rights reserved.)

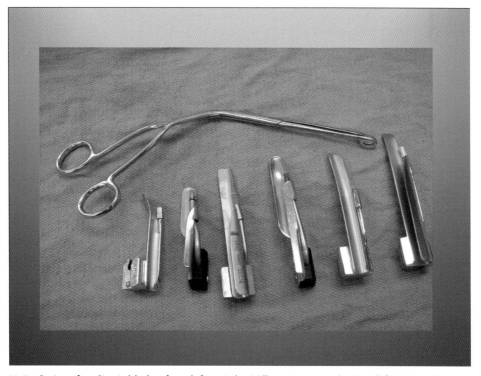

▲ **Figure 13-3.** Series of pediatric blades, from left to right: Miller 0, 1, 1.5, and a Magill forceps. (Photo courtesy of Dr. Iolanda Russo Menna.)

occurs quickly during apnea, long laryngoscopy, or a rapid sequence induction, despite best efforts at preoxygenation time.[4] CO_2 production is increased as well, on the order of 100 to 150 mL/kg/min compared to the 60 mL/kg/min in an adult. Since the tidal volume (per kg body weight) is relatively consistent with that of an adult, the respiratory rate increases in order to meet the higher oxygen consumption and need for rapid CO_2 elimination.[5]

The resistance to air flow in the airway is governed by Poiseulle's law: $R = 8\eta L/\pi r^4$. It is important to note that the inverse relationship to the radius of the airway raised to the fourth power, so a small amount of narrowing (due to edema, inflammation, etc.) in the already small pediatric airway may have severe consequences on respiratory function (Figure 13-4).

There are numerous causes of airway narrowing. Some pathological etiologies include hemangiomas, papillomas, thoracic masses, tracheomalacia, laryngomalacia, laryngeal clefts. Iatrogenic causes include vocal cord paralysis, subglottic stenosis from prolonged intubation[6] or the placement of an inappropriate endotracheal tube size.

Preparation to Induction and Intubation

The induction of general anesthesia in children is a critical time when difficulties and cardiorespiratory problems may occur. The experience of being separated from the parents is a crucial moment. In the past, a child was often forcefully detached from the caretaker and moved to the operating room, which could become a stressful experience not easily forgotten, especially when returning for repeated anesthesia and surgery.[7] The pediatric anesthesiologist must empathize and understand the young patient's and caregivers' psychological status and support their emotional needs. Parental presence in operating room may be desirable, as parents might be the best "premedication."[8,9]

Anxiety reduction may be approached not only by pharmacological strategies such as midazolam PO, ketamine IM, or dexmedetomidine intranasal, but also by the increasingly popular use of videos and television programs.[10] Familiarization with the mask and bringing along a favorite blanket or toy are also useful. These psychological approaches are effective to establish trust and reassurance between the patient and anesthesiology provider. This is especially important given the short duration of interaction prior to surgery.

Prior to the initiation of induction, the operating room must be ready to receive the patient, the machine should be checked, vaporizers filled, suction available, and all equipment available. This includes blades, endotracheal tubes, stylets, oral and nasal airways, nasal gastric tube, and IV catheters. Additionally, emergency medications such as succinylcholine, atropine, and epinephrine and also appropriate IV fluids should be available, and tubing should be cleared of air bubbles. The room should be warm, and anesthetic machine should be checked and prepared as should all the necessary monitors. Placement of monitors prior to induction may be challenging. Some providers choose to place monitors immediately after inhalational induction, while others induce with only pulse

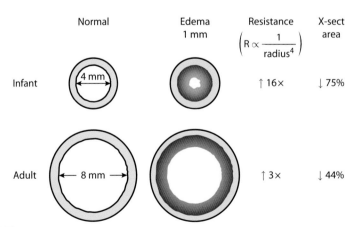

▲ **Figure 13-4.** Airway diameter relationship between infant and adult in normal status vs edema governed by Poiseulle's law: $R = 8\eta L/\pi r^4$. (Reproduced with permission, from Cote CJ, Lerman J, Todres ID. *A Practice of Anesthesia for Infants and Children.* 2009. Copyright © Saunders Elsevier. All rights reserved.)

oximeter on. On the other hand, in a small and sick infant it is imperative to place all the monitors before induction and review their baseline values, which are sometimes unexpectedly abnormal.

Induction techniques vary and can be performed via inhalational, intravenous, or intramuscular route. The most commonly used is inhalational, commonly called "mask induction," or "gas induction." This technique is often less objectionable in babies and toddlers, if they do not have already an IV catheter in place. The anesthesia provider must be flexible and consider the preexisting comorbidities and needs of each child, when choosing the method of induction.

Once in operating room, ambient noise should be minimized while the appropriate monitors placed. The child can be induced in the supine or sitting position. Adding a pleasant smell to the mask usually facilitates mask induction. It is often helpful to prime the machine with 70% nitrous oxide and 30% oxygen, and creating a closed circuit by blocking the outflow of the corrugate expiratory tube allows the breathing system to be saturated in 1 or 2 minutes. It is best to avoid an abrupt mask placement on the patient's face without warning. Engaging the child's imagination by singing a song or telling a story will decrease anxiety and allows a smoother induction. The appropriately sized mask is placed gently over the patient's face, and a few minutes of breathing will be enough to calm the child. It is imperative that the anesthesia provider carefully observes breathing and chest movements as the child passed through the hypnosis stage into deeper anesthesia. At the first sign of anesthetic induction (nystagmus maybe noted) sevoflurane is added gradually or quickly up to 7% to 8%. The transition through the excitation phase can result in laryngospasm that may be avoided by assisting the patient ventilation and deepening the anesthetic.[7,8] As soon as the patient is in adequate plane of anesthetic, monitors are immediately placed.

With a low blood-gas partition coefficient of 0.5, and nonirritable smell, sevoflurane is well tolerated by infants and children for inhalation induction. Rapid induction and emergence as well as relative safety make sevoflurane the most popular volatile agent for mask induction. Potential problems are degradation in soda lime, and biodegradation to the inorganic fluoride ion.[11] A problem that may be encountered during inhalation induction is an airway obstruction due to relaxation of the genioglossus and upper airway muscles. Oral and nasal airways may help to relieve the obstruction. Appropriate size, length, and lubricant usage may facilitate placement as well as prevent mucosal injury and epistaxis. The oral airway must be of correct size to prevent obstruction secondary to impacting the airway opening or pushing the tongue posteriorly into the pharynx.

If the insertion of an oropharyngeal or nasopharyngeal airway does not relieve the obstruction, the anesthesia provider should consider laryngospasm as a potential source of obstruction. Often, continuous positive pressure is enough to release vocal cords tightening. If this does not resolve vocal cords spasm, a muscle relaxant such as succinylcholine may be required. Succinylcholine may be given by intravenous (IV) injection of 2 mg/kg, or 4 mg/kg intramuscularly. This often quickly resolves the obstruction. Sublingual injection is not encouraged, as it may create swelling and complicate tracheal intubation. If recognized and managed appropriately, the effects of laryngospasm are transient and reversible. Prolonged obstruction could create negative pressure pulmonary edema, a severe respiratory complication.

Intravenous induction can be carried out with various agents including propofol, usually at a dose of 2 to 3 mg/kg followed by a small amount of fentanyl and muscle relaxant if indicated. Many providers also utilize a combination of IV induction in addition to 4% to 5% of sevoflurane, if the hemodynamics allow.

Emergency drugs including atropine (10 mcg/mL), succinylcholine, and epinephrine (10 mcg/mL) should be readily available. Older children may prefer intravenous to mask induction, others will fear the placement of an intravenous catheter and will require the "mask induction" approach. Pre-oxygenation should be started just before IV induction commences. Choosing an IV induction vs inhalation induction is highly dependent on the age of the patient and coexisting pathologies they present, such as dehydration, hypotension, type of surgical procedure, presence of full stomach, and how the patient will tolerate the needle stick.

PROCEDURES IN PEDIATRIC ANESTHESIA: ADVANCED AIRWAY TECHNIQUES

Initial airway assessment begins with a good history. Questions are directed toward indications of a potentially difficult airway, including complications of birth or delivery, history of prior trauma or surgery to the airway or adjacent structures, or prior difficult intubation. Additionally, one should inquire about current or recent symptoms suggesting upper respiratory infection (URI): speech, breathing, or feeding difficulty, hoarseness, snoring, and noisy breathing.

A history of snoring, day time drowsiness, or cessation of respiration during sleep may help identify children with obstructive sleep apnea which is very common and not well diagnosed. Many syndromes are associated with potentially difficult airway management (Table 13-1).

Numerous physical exam findings typically discussed in the adult difficult airway literature also apply to children.

Table 13-1. Comorbidities Associated to Difficult Airway

Medical Conditions Associated with Difficult Airways	
Microstomia	C-spine instability
Choanal Atresia	Mass Effect
Defective Malocclusion	Subglottic Stenosis
Macroglossia	Airway Trauma
Mandibular Retrognathia	Obesity

For example, limited head extension, reduced mandibular space, and increased tongue thickness have been shown to be reliable predictors of difficult intubation.[12] Case series have demonstrated a relationship between mandible length and lip to chin distance as associated with Cormack-Lehane view classification.[13] Micrognathia has been highly associated with a 42% incidence of difficult laryngoscopy.[14] However, even if no specific diagnosis is known, severity of disease or certain types of surgery as palate and craniofacial malformations are associated with increased risk for airway management complications.[6]

The fundamental maneuver in airway management is properly performed mask ventilation. As in adults, there are one- and two-hand techniques.

Upper airway obstruction, which may be encountered during simple mask ventilation, is often relieved by head tilt, chin lift, more than jaw thrust in children, and the application of continuous positive airway pressure.[15,16]

Additionally, the lateral position may also improve airway patency. This has been demonstrated in children undergoing surgery for adenotonsillary hypertrophy, a group that is more prone to upper airway obstruction.[17,18]

It is important to note that face mask ventilation increases dead space compared to ventilation via an endotracheal tube. In smaller children, this increase in volume becomes more significant due to the low absolute volumes of ventilation.[5] The use of an oral airway during spontaneous or positive pressure ventilation with a face mask helps relieve the obstruction that may be caused by posterior displacement of the tongue in the anesthetized child.[19,20]

The appropriate size of airway is important for an effective obstruction release. Nasopharyngeal airways may also be used to relieve upper airway obstruction during mask ventilation and are very useful in providing anesthetic gas, oxygen, and end tidal CO_2 monitoring while performing fiber-optic tracheal intubation in the child with a difficult airway.[21]

There are many tools to facilitate tracheal intubation. The standard is still direct laryngoscopy with various laryngoscope blade styles and sizes to choose from. Many anesthesiologists prefer the Macintosh blade, adapted from adult sizes, for older children. This blade is designed to be utilized with an indirect elevation of the epiglottis by placing the tip of the blade in the vallecula.

As mentioned earlier, in younger children the orientation of the epiglottis is in a more anterior-posterior plane, making this indirect method of elevating the epiglottis potentially less effective. Therefore, many pediatric anesthesiologists prefer the use of a straight or semi-curved blade designed to directly elevate the epiglottis in patients under the age of 4 years.[1,2]

In the past, uncuffed endotracheal tubes were used in this population to minimize resistance of the endotracheal tube while also minimizing pressure trauma to the subglottis, but it is now believed that cuffed tubes can provide better sealing and ventilating conditions while minimizing operating room gas pollution, and trauma to the delicate airway of pediatric patients. Therefore, it is increasingly common to use cuffed endotracheal tubes in children of all ages.

Checking for an air leak at an airway pressure of less than 20 cm H_2O is important. However, the utility of using an audible air leak has been called into question as being inadequate to prevent overinflation of endotracheal tube cuffs.

There are multiple options for induction of anesthesia in the anticipated difficult intubation. The use of inhalational induction tends not only to maintain spontaneous respirations but also depresses upper airway musculature and may worsen upper airway obstruction.[17,22]

Remifentanil has the advantage of being a short-acting opioid which can produce reasonable intubating conditions. Dexmedetomidine may help as an adjuvant while gas induction is obtained, reducing the gag reflex and allowing easier airway manipulation by fiber optics. Muscle relaxant use is discouraged unless the child's age allows the use of sugammadex; however, it has the limitation of not reversing anesthetic agents, and may not be sufficient for a patient to regain upper airway muscular tone in a failed airway attempt.[22]

In adults, awake fiberoptic intubation is often considered the gold standard method for the known or predicted difficult airway. It allows for the maintenance of spontaneous respirations until the trachea is intubated.[23]

However in the pediatric population, this option is more complex due to the need for significant cooperation on the part of the patient, which is usually impossible. Other approaches include fiber-optic intubation after induction. This can be done through a laryngeal mask airway (LMA), supraglottic device, or face mask.[24]

Another method involves placement of a supraglottic airway, followed by introduction of the fiberoptic bronchoscope into the trachea through the supraglottic airway. Once the fiberscope is in the trachea, a J-wire can be placed through the operating port of the scope.[25] The scope can then be removed and an airway exchange catheter advanced over the wire. Following the removal of the wire and supraglottic device, an endotracheal tube can be advanced over the exchange catheter.[26,27]

Newer devices designed to aid laryngoscopy include video laryngoscopes with pediatric blade sizes (Glidescope, Karl-Storz). Newer devices and ones with an endotracheal tube track to guide it into the trachea.[28,29] There is evidence that the video laryngoscopes provide better glottic views when compared to traditional direct laryngoscopy, especially when direct laryngoscopy is predicted to be challenging.[30]

The variety of airway devices are extremely useful in improving laryngeal views, higher likelihood of successful intubation, and a faster learning curve (Figures 13-3 and 13-4). They are important when difficult airways need to be secured, and have become an integral part of operating room equipment. The difficulty of airway management in children is usually related to either inadequate mask ventilation or difficulty in achieving tracheal intubation.

Anticipated difficult airways should be planned carefully with the appropriate equipment and staff. It may be prudent to have an ENT or pediatric surgeon in the operating room during airway management in the event the provider encounters a "cannot ventilate, cannot intubate" situation. The surgical colleagues can assist in cricothyroidotomy or tracheostomy. Even then it has been suggested that risk of complications from needle cricothyroidotomy is too high in children under the age of 5 or 6 years. In these situations, it is recommended to consider a tracheostomy.[31–33]

REFERENCES

1. Adewale L. Anatomy and assessment of the pediatric airway. *Paediatr Anaesth*. 2009;19(suppl 1):1-8.
2. Hudgins PA, Siegel J, Jacobs I, Abramowsky CR. The normal pediatric larynx on CT and MR. *Am J Neuroradiol*. 1997;18:239-245.
3. Carr RJ, Beebe DS, Belani KG. The difficult pediatric airway. *Sem Anesth Perioper Med Pain*. 2001;20:219-227.
4. Dalal PG, Murray D, Feng A, Molter D, McAllister J. Upper airway dimensions in children using rigid video-bronchoscopy and a computer software: description of a measurement technique. *Paediatr Anaesth*. 2008;18:645-653.
5. Bruce IA, Rothera MP. Upper airway obstruction in children. *Paediatr Anaesth*. 2009;19(suppl 1):88-99.
6. Nargozian C. The airway in patients with craniofacial abnormalities. *Paediatr Anaesth*. 2004;14:53-59.
7. Kain ZN, Wang SM, Mayes LC, Caramico LA, Hofstadter MB. Distress during the induction of anesthesia and postoperative behavioral outcomes. *Anesth Analg*. 1999;88(5):1042-1047.
8. Bevan JC, Johnston C, Haig MJ, et al. Preoperative parental anxiety predicts behavioural and emotional responses to induction of anesthesia in children. *Can J Anaesth*. 1990;37(2):177-182.
9. Hannallah RS, Rosales JK. Experience with parents' presence during anesthesia induction in children. *Can Anaesth Soc J*. 1983;30(3):286-289.
10. Sunder RA, Haile DT, Farrell PT, Sharma A. Pediatric airway management: current practices and future directions. *Paediatr Anaesth*. 2012;22:1008-1015.
11. Morio M, Fujii K, Satoh N. Reaction of sevoflurane and its degradation products with soda lime. *Anesthesiology*. 1992;77:1155.
12. Mirghassemi A, Soltani AE, Abtahi M. Evaluation of laryngoscopic views and related influencing factors in a pediatric population. *Paediatr Anaesth*. 2011;21:663-667.
13. Uezono S, Holzman RS, Goto T, Nakata Y, Nagata S, Morita S. Prediction of difficult airway in school-aged patients with microtia. *Paediatr Anaesth*. 2001;11:409-413.
14. Meier S, Geiduschek J, Paganoni R, Fuehrmeyer F, Reber A. The effect of chin lift, jaw thrust, and continuous positive airway pressure on the size of the glottic opening and on stridor score in anesthetized, spontaneously breathing children. *Anesth Analg*. 2002;94:494-499.
15. Litman RS, McDonough JM, Marcus CL, Schwartz AR, Ward DS. Upper airway collapsibility in anesthetized children. *Anesth Analg*. 2006;102:750-754.
16. Arai YC, Fukunaga K, Hirota S, Fujimoto S. The effects of chin lift and jaw thrust while in the lateral position on stridor score in anesthetized children with adenotonsillar hypertrophy. *Anesth Analg*. 2004;99:1638-1641.
17. Abramson Z, Susarla S, Troulis M, Kaban L. Age-related changes of the upper airway assessed by 3-dimensional computed tomography. *J Craniofac Surg*. 2009;20(suppl 1):657-663.
18. Holm-Knudsen R, Eriksen K, Rasmussen LS. Using a nasopharyngeal airway during fiberoptic intubation in small children with a difficult airway. *Paediatr Anaesth*. 2005;15:839-845.
19. Litman RS, Weissend EE, Shibata D, Westesson PL. Developmental changes of laryngeal dimensions in unparalyzed, sedated children. *Anesthesiology*. 2003;98:41-45.
20. Sims C, von Ungern-Sternberg BS. The normal and the challenging pediatric airway. *Paediatr Anaesth*. 2012;22:521-526.
21. White MC, Cook TM, Stoddart PA. A critique of elective pediatric supraglottic airway devices. *Paediatr Anaesth*. 2009;19(suppl 1):55-65.
22. Brooks P, Ree R, Rosen D, Ansermino M. Canadian pediatric anesthesiologists prefer inhalational anesthesia to manage difficult airways. *Can J Anaesth*. 2005;52:285-290.
23. Brambrink AM, Braun U. Airway management in infants and children. *Best Pract Res Clin Anaesthesiol*. 2005;19:675-697.
24. Walker RW. The laryngeal mask airway in the difficult paediatric airway: an assessment of positioning and use in fibreoptic intubation. *Paediatr Anaesth*. 2000;10:53-58.
25. Thomas PB, Parry MG. The difficult paediatric airway: a new method of intubation using the laryngeal mask airway, Cook airway exchange catheter and tracheal intubation fibrescope. *Paediatr Anaesth*. 2001;11:618-621.
26. Barch B, Rastatter J, Jagannathan N. Difficult pediatric airway management using the intubating laryngeal airway. *Int J Pediatr Otorhinolaryngol*. 2012;76:1579-1582.
27. Nagler J, Bachur RG. Advanced airway management. *Curr Opin Pediatr*. 2009;21:299-305.
28. Nandi PR, Charlesworth CH, Taylor SJ, Nunn JF, Doré CJ. Effect of general anaesthesia on the pharynx. *Br J Anaesth*. 1991;66:157-162.

29. Curtis R, Lomax S, Patel B. Use of sugammadex in a "can't intubate, can't ventilate" situation. *Br J Anaesth.* 2012;108:612-614.
30. Weiss M, Engelhardt T. Proposal for the management of the unexpected difficult pediatric airway. *Paediatr Anaesth.* 2010;20:454-464.
31. Coté CJ, Hartnick CJ. Pediatric transtracheal and cricothyrotomy airway devices for emergency use: which are appropriate for infants and children? *Paediatr Anaesth.* 2009;19(suppl 1):66-76.
32. Von Ungern-Sternberg BS, Boda K, Chambers NA, et al. Risk assessment for respiratory complications in paediatric anaesthesia: a prospective cohort study. *Lancet.* 2010; 376:773-783.
33. Heinrich S, Birkholz T, Ihmsen H, Irouschek A, Ackermann A, Schmidt J. Incidence and predictors of difficult laryngoscopy in 11,219 pediatric anesthesia procedures. *Paediatr Anaesth.* 2012;22:729-736.

Anesthesia for Neurosurgical Procedures

Jaya Varadarajan

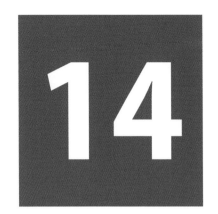

FOCUS POINTS

1. The cranial vault changes structurally from birth through the first 2 years of life. Eighty percent of the intracranial volume consists of brain and interstitial fluid, with blood and cerebrospinal fluid (CSF) making up the remainder. Intracranial compliance is the change in intracranial pressure (ICP) relative to the volume.

2. The open fontanelles and sutures in infancy results in increased intracranial compliance and allows for slow expansion of contents.

3. The Munro-Kellie hypothesis states that the sum of all intracranial volumes is always a constant. Infants are an exception to this rule because of the increased compliance and pliability of the skull. Mass effect of a slow growing tumor or hemorrhage can thus be masked by this compensation.

4. Acute changes in volume due to hemorrhage or obstruction of the CSF flow are not attenuated and can lead to life-threatening consequences.

5. Cerebral perfusion pressure (CPP), the pressure gradient across the brain, is the difference between mean arterial pressure (MAP) at the entrance to the brain and the mean exit pressure (i.e. central venous pressure), or intracranial pressure (ICP) if elevated. It is a more reliable estimate of cerebral perfusion.

6. In adults, cerebral autoregulation maintains a constant brain perfusion despite moderate changes in MAP or ICP. The lower absolute limits of cerebral autoregulation in infants and children is unclear and the range is believed to be narrower in neonates.

7. Acceptable MAP for a neonate is the gestational age in mmHg. Tight blood pressure control is essential in the management of neonates to minimize both cerebral ischemia with hypotension, and intraventricular hemorrhage with hypertension.

Certain pediatric disease states have specific anesthetic considerations and require tailoring of the intraoperative anesthetic management to the unique disease condition.

The practice of anesthesia for pediatric neurosurgical conditions requires understanding of the distinct differences in children compared to adults, and is made more challenging by the unique management considerations. There are age-related differences in the incidence, anatomy, and pathology of surgical lesions in this population, which translate into the need for an individualized approach to the pediatric neurosurgical patient. Differences in the physiological responses to surgery and anesthesia from adults are what set children apart, and make management decisions different from what is considered the norm of adult neuroanesthetic practice. Over the last couple of decades, the numerous technological advances in neurosurgery coupled with subspecialization, and a better understanding of the postoperative needs of pediatric patients have dramatically improved outcomes in infants and children with neurosurgical lesions.[1]

COMMON PEDIATRIC NEUROSURGICAL CONDITIONS

Congenital anomalies and malformations

Tumors

Hydrocephalus

Epilepsy

Craniosynostosis

Vascular anomalies—arteriovenous malformations, vein of
　Galen, moyamoya syndrome

Neuroimaging and interventional neuroradiological procedures

Neurotrauma

NEUROANATOMY, DEVELOPMENTAL CONSIDERATIONS, AND NEUROPHYSIOLOGY

The infant cranial vault undergoes several structural
and physiological changes in the first 2 years of life. The
intracranial space is compliant owing to open fontanelles
and sutures, allowing for a slow expansion of intracranial volume. The posterior fontanelle is the first to close
around 2 to 3 months of age, followed by the sphenoid
and mastoid fontanelles, with the anterior fontanelle
being the last to close about 2 to 3 years of age. The
infant brain triples its weight in the first year after birth.
Eighty percent of the intracranial volume consists of
brain and interstitial fluid, with blood and cerebrospinal
fluid (CSF) making up the remainder. CSF volume is
proportionately larger in infants and neonates (4 mL/kg)
compared to adults (2 mL/kg), but the rate of production
of CSF is similar.

The Munro-Kellie hypothesis states that the sum of all
intracranial volumes is always a constant. Infants demonstrate an exception to this hypothesis as the infant skull is
pliable up until 2 years of age.[2] The mass effect of a slow-
growing tumor or hemorrhage is thus often masked by
compensatory distension of the fontanelle and widening
of the cranial sutures. However, acute increases in volume
due to massive hemorrhage or an obstructed ventricular
system cannot be attenuated by this expansion, and can
result in life-threatening increases in intracranial pressure
(ICP) or herniation (Figure 14-1).[3]

Intracranial compliance is the change in ICP relative to
the intracranial volume. Once the fontanelles and sutures
have closed, children have a smaller cranial volume and
lower intracranial compliance than adults, putting them
at a higher risk for herniation (Figure 14-2).[4] A higher
ratio of brain water content, less CSF volume, and a higher
ratio of brain content to intracranial capacity are further
contributory factors.

There are unique differences in cerebrovascular physiology that distinguish children from adults. Cerebral
blood flow (CBF) is regulated to meet the brain's metabolic demands. Cerebral metabolic rate for oxygen
($CMRO_2$) is higher in children at about 5.8 mL/100 g/
min compared to adult levels of 3.5 mL/100 g/min. CBF
in healthy children is believed to be about 100 mL/100
g/min compared to adults at 50 mL/100 g/min. CBF is
tightly coupled to cerebral metabolism and $CMRO_2$ at
global and regional levels. Hypoxemia, hypercarbia, and

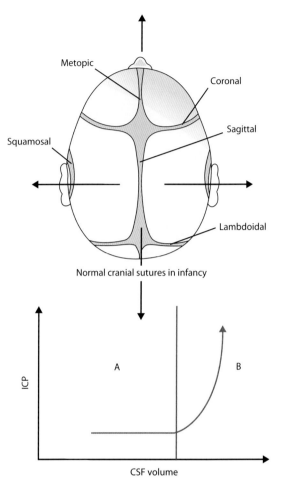

▲ **Figure 14-1.** Cranial sutures and fontanelle in
neonates and infants. Initially the compliant skull of the
neonate minimizes insidious increases in intracranial
volume. However, acute increases in intracranial
volume will lead to rapid rises in intracranial pressure.
(Reproduced with permission, from Davis P, Cladis FP,
eds. *Smith's Anesthesia for Infants and Children.* 8th ed.
2011. Copyright © Elsevier. All rights reserved.)

ischemia cause cerebral vasodilation, which increases
CBF. A decrease in brain metabolism similarly reduces
CBF. Both CBF and metabolic demand increase immediately after birth and thereafter, the changes mirroring
neuroanatomical and psychomotor growth, which in
turn reflect cognitive growth. CBF is 10% to 20% of the
cardiac output in the first 6 months of life, peaking at 55%
between ages 2 and 4 years, settling into adult levels of
15% by 7 to 8 years.[5]

Cerebral perfusion pressure (CPP) is a more practical estimate of the adequacy of cerebral circulation. It
is the pressure gradient across the brain, the difference
between MAP at the entrance to the brain and the mean

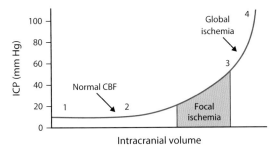

▲ **Figure 14-2.** Intracranial compliance curve. At normal intracranial volumes (1), ICP is low but compliance is high and remains so despite small increases in volume. As intracranial volume acutely rises (2), the ability to compensate is rapidly overwhelmed, even when the ICP is still within normal limits, but the compliance is low. At higher ICP (3), a threshold is quickly reached where further volume expansion leads to rapid and higher increase in ICP. Maximal intracranial volume and high ICP are shown by the number 4. (Reproduced with permission, from Davis P, Cladis FP, eds. *Smith's Anesthesia for Infants and Children*. 8th ed. 2011. Copyright © Elsevier. All rights reserved.)

exit pressure (ie, central venous pressure), or ICP if elevated. Autoregulation maintains a constant brain perfusion despite moderate changes in mean arterial pressure (MAP) or ICP. In adults, cerebral autoregulation ensures that CBF remains relatively constant within a MAP range of 50 to 150 mm Hg, outside of which CBF becomes pressure dependent. This autoregulation occurs at undefined lower absolute values in infants and children (Figure 14-3). There is data that children as young as 6 months of age autoregulate CBF as well as older children, but the lower limit of autoregulation (LLA) in healthy neonates is unclear. Neonates are believed to be especially vulnerable to cerebral ischemia and intraventricular hemorrhage due to a narrow autoregulatory range. However, previously held beliefs that the LLA is lower in infants than older children have been challenged.[6] Infants are also likely at increased risk for cerebral ischemia due to lower blood pressure reserve. Analysis of cerebral perfusion in infants and children undergoing cardiopulmonary bypass reveals a wide range in the lower limits of autoregulation suggesting individual variability, and highlights the limitations of currently available monitors to measure and optimize cerebral perfusion.[7] Diastolic blood pressure might be a better indicator of cerebral perfusion pressure (CPP) in this population.[8] Cerebral ischemia, heralded by EEG slowing, occurs at CBF values of about 25 to 40 mL/100 g/min and is followed by initially reversible neuronal damage. Rapid cell death occurs at a CBF less than 6 mL/100 g/min. The lower the CBF at ischemic levels, the shorter the duration allowable before irreversible neuronal damage. Tight blood pressure control is, therefore, essential in the management of neonates to minimize both cerebral ischemia with hypotension, and intraventricular hemorrhage with hypertension. A clinically accepted "rule of thumb" is that MAP for a neonate approximates the gestational age.

Despite these observations, the mechanism of normal cerebral autoregulation in healthy children and adaptations in acute disease are not completely understood. To complicate things further, both anatomical and physiological maturation might play a role in the development of a fully developed autoregulatory response as the child grows.

Vasoreactivity to CO_2 is believed to be higher in children than adults, and is well developed even in healthy preterm infants. Rapid diffusion of arterial CO_2 across the blood-brain barrier (BBB) leads to changes in extracellular pH, which in turn leads to cerebral vasodilation and increased CBF.[9] The relationship between $PaCO_2$ and CBF is linear. The mechanism of CO_2R, however, is complex and influenced by a variety of other mediators including nitric oxide, prostaglandin E2, and indomethacin. In comparison, the influence of PaO_2 is of much less clinical significance. There are minimal changes in CBF with changes in PaO_2 above 50 mm Hg. Below a PaO_2 of 50 mm Hg, cerebral vasodilation occurs and increases CBF to maintain adequate cerebral oxygen delivery.[10] This lower threshold of PaO_2 is lower in neonates. Hyperoxia is believed to decrease CBF; however, its influence is controversial.

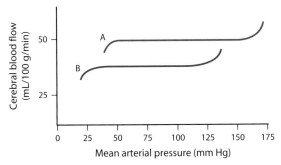

▲ **Figure 14-3.** Autoregulation of cerebral circulation in neonates (curve B) and adults (curve A). (Reproduced with permission, from Davis P, Cladis FP, eds. *Smith's Anesthesia for Infants and Children*. 8th ed. 2011. Copyright © Elsevier. All rights reserved.)

DRUGS AND THEIR EFFECTS ON NEUROPHYSIOLOGY

The ideal anesthetic agent would be one that decreases ICP and $CMRO_2$, and maintains CPP. There is insufficient data on the effects of commonly used anesthetic agents in infants and children. The changes seen in CBF, CPP, ICP, and $CMRO_2$ as summarized in Tables 14-1 and 14-2 are extrapolated from adult literature and should be used as a guideline.

Table 14-1. IV Anesthetics and their Effects on Cerebral Hemodynamics

	MAP	CBF	CPP	ICP	CMRO$_2$
Propofol	↓↓↓	↓↓↓	↑↑	↓↓	↓↓↓
Etomidate	0-↓	↓↓↓	↑↑	↓↓↓	↓↓↓
Ketamine	↑↑	↑↑↑	↓	↑↑↑	↑
Benzodiazepines	0-↓	↓↓	↑	0	↓↓
Opioids	0-↓	↓	↓↑	0-↓	↓

Table 14-2. Inhaled Anesthetics and their Effects on Cerebral Hemodynamics

	MAP	CBF	CPP	ICP	CMRO$_2$
Isoflurane	↓↓	↑	↓	↑	↓↓↓
Sevoflurane	↓↓	↑	0-↓	0-↑	↓↓↓
Desflurane	↓↓	↑	↓	↑	↓
Nitrous oxide	0-↓	↑-↑↑	↓	↑-↑↑	↓

Intravenous Agents

Propofol

Propofol maintains autoregulation and cerebral responsiveness to changes in $PaCO_2$, suppresses seizure activity, and may be neuroprotective. In the setting of elevated ICP, propofol may be a superior maintenance anesthetic compared to inhaled halogenated agents.

Opioids

Opioids have very minimal effects on CBF or ICP except in the setting of hypoventilation and elevated $Paco_2$. All opioids preserve cerebral autoregulation and CO_2 reactivity, and cause EEG slowing in a dose-dependent manner. Fentanyl has minimal effects, if any, on even the neonatal cerebral circulation and is used extensively. Sufentanil and alfentanil in dose ranges from 10 to 20 mcg/kg reduce both CBF and $CMRO_2$ by 25% to 30%.[11] Remifentanil is an ultra-short-acting opioid that is rapidly metabolized by plasma cholinesterases. It has a very short duration of action, because its context-sensitive half-life is independent of the duration of infusion.[12] This makes it especially suitable for lengthy procedures at the end of which an accurate neurological assessment is mandatory, the one caveat being that because analgesia is very brief after its discontinuation, it is imperative to administer a long-acting opioid analgesic in a timely manner to prevent severe pain and rebound hypertension.

Etomidate

Etomidate is often used in hemodynamically unstable patients as it causes less hypotension than propofol, but it is important to bear in mind that it can cause myoclonus.

Ketamine

Ketamine is unlike other induction agents. It is a potent cerebrovasodilator and increases CBF, with marked increase in ICP that is not prevented by hyperventilation. It is often not an appropriate choice for most neurosurgical patients, unless there is significant hemodynamic compromise.

Dexmedetomidine

Dexmedetomidine is a selective α_2 adrenergic agonist that is being increasingly used in anesthetic practice, either as a supplement to other agents during general anesthesia or as the sole agent for moderate to deep sedation. It was initially found especially useful in awake craniotomies in teenagers, but in recent years its use has encompassed other neurosurgical procedures also.[13,14] Small-scale studies report that it has a good safety profile.

Volatile Anesthetics

All inhalational agents uncouple CBF and $CMRO_2$, but to different degrees. They increase CBF and ICP by their vasodilatory effect, while decreasing $CMRO_2$. They also blunt the autoregulatory response in a dose-dependent manner. It is possible to minimally affect CBF and ICP by employing a balanced anesthetic technique with low concentrations of a volatile agent combined with intravenous agents, and a ventilatory strategy that maintains normocarbia or hypocarbia. Isoflurane and sevoflurane seem to maintain coupling to some degree, significantly decrease $CMRO_2$, and are often the agents of choice in neuroanesthetic practice.[15] It is worthwhile to note that isoflurane causes an isoelectric EEG at about 2.0 MAC compared to sevoflurane which causes dose-dependent epileptiform activity on EEG.

The use of nitrous oxide is controversial. The increased CBF and resultant increase in ICP can lead to complications especially in the presence of reduced intracranial compliance. Its effects are modified by other agents it is used with, and it is not an adequate anesthetic by itself. Some practitioners prefer to use it for the initial mask induction alone, reinstate it after the dura is opened, and then discontinue it prior to dural closure, as intracranial air can persist for up to 3 weeks after a craniotomy and the rapid expansion of air cavities can cause a tension pneumocephalus. However, it has also been used for entire procedures without detrimental effects and does have a long track record of safety. Most practitioners agree that it should be avoided in the situation where a child has had a recent craniotomy.[16] Its use is not contraindicated in sitting craniotomies; the fact that it might expand a venous air embolism (VAE) might even increase the sensitivity of monitoring for VAE by capnography in these cases.

PREOPERATIVE EVALUATION

A number of pediatric neurosurgical conditions are of an emergent nature. Despite this, a thorough preoperative evaluation and organ system review is essential to identify coexisting morbidities that might increase the likelihood of perioperative complications, and help anticipate physiological derangements. In the setting of emergent surgery, children with a preexisting upper or lower respiratory infection, a full stomach, gastrointestinal reflux, or ongoing emesis are at higher risk and appropriate precautions should be taken to prevent complications. Children presenting with repeated emesis, those who have had prolonged fasting periods, and those with polyuria secondary to diabetes insipidus are at risk for hypovolemia or hypoglycemia, both of which can cause hemodynamic and metabolic perturbations under anesthesia. Many neurosurgical patients have comorbidities that are part of a syndrome, and routinely return to the operating room for repeat procedures. It is useful to inquire about prior anesthetic experiences and issues in the postoperative period. The risk of latex allergy should be considered.

Premature infants are prone to postoperative apneic spells at baseline; this could be amplified by the neurological condition. Intraoperative management and postoperative disposition should take this into account. Craniofacial anomalies can make airway management a challenge; this should be anticipated, and special equipment and techniques utilized as necessary. Congenital heart disease might complicate the perioperative course, especially in the newborn. A thorough evaluation with input from a pediatric cardiologist, and an echocardiogram might be warranted to aid in optimizing cardiac function when the acuity of the condition allows. Children with suprasellar masses might need an endocrinological evaluation. There are certain neurological conditions that warrant special considerations in the preoperative period, as outlined in Table 14-3. Children might present with a vagal nerve stimulator, which might need to be deactivated for the anesthetic as it can cause repetitive vocal cord stimulation.

Preoperative physical examination should document the level of consciousness, motor and sensory function, cranial nerves, pupillary reflexes, and signs and symptoms of elevated ICP, which will serve as a baseline for postoperative assessment. The signs of raised ICP vary based on the age of the child, as outlined in Table 14-4. Irritability and altered consciousness are common signs, but papilledema may not be seen even in late stages of intracranial hypertension. Brainstem lesions can present with cranial nerve dysfunction such as impaired gag reflex and swallow, respiratory distress, diplopia, and aspiration. Visual

Table 14-3. Anesthetic Concerns for Pediatric Neurosurgery

Denervation injuries	Hyperkalemia after succinylcholine—use NDPMR Resistance to nondepolarizing muscle relaxants
Chronic exposure to antiseizure medications	Hepatic dysfunction Hematological abnormalities Increased metabolism of anesthetic agents Require increased doses and frequent redosing
Arteriovenous malformations Moyamoya disease	Potential for congestive heart failure Risk of perioperative ischemia
Neuromuscular disease	Malignant hyperthermia Respiratory failure Sudden cardiac death
Arnold-Chiari malformation	Postoperative apnea Aspiration pneumonia Postoperative stridor
Hypothalamic and pituitary lesions	Adrenal insufficiency/excess Thyroid abnormalities Diabetes insipidus/SIADH
Craniofacial abnormalities	Difficult airway Significant blood loss
Neural tube defects (myelomeningocele)	Latex sensitivity, allergy and risk of anaphylaxis

Table 14-4. Signs of Intracranial Hypertension in Infants and Children

Infants	Children	Infants and Children
Irritability	Headache	Decreased consciousness
Full fontanelle	Diplopia	Cranial nerve (III & IV) palsies
Widely separated sutures	Papilledema	Loss of upward gaze (setting sun sign)
Cranial enlargement	Vomiting	Signs of herniation, Cushing's triad, pupillary changes

field changes can occur with suprasellar masses. A clinical assessment of volume status is imperative. Preoperative laboratory tests should be tailored to the neurological condition, surgery being performed, anticipated blood loss, and general health of the child. Liver function tests and hematological profile may be necessary in children who are on chronic anticonvulsants. Type and cross-matched blood should be available for surgeries with large volumes of predicted blood loss, such as resection of large tumors, and craniofacial reconstructions. Unanticipated blood loss is a risk with interventional procedures for vascular malformations in the radiology suite. As blood-draws can be challenging in infants, it is reasonable to draw a hematocrit, PT, and PTT soon after induction in the operating room to minimize trauma to the child.

Premedication should be utilized judiciously in the pediatric patient requiring neurosurgery. In infants and younger children, it is best to administer this in the preoperative area, to ease separation from parents.[17,18] Premedication is especially necessary in certain conditions such as moyamoya disease to avoid agitation and crying, or in the case of an arteriovenous malformation that has recently bled. Oral midazolam is usually the drug of choice; it may be administered parenterally if an intravenous catheter is present, and titrated to effect under the direct supervision of a medical provider. The decision to premedicate should be weighed against the risk of oversedation in a neurologically impaired patient in whom hypoventilation might increase the risk of intracranial hypertension.

INTRAOPERATIVE AND POSTOPERATIVE CONSIDERATIONS

Induction technique and choice of induction agent are based on the preoperative status of the patient, a rapid sequence induction being mandatory in the somnolent child with signs of raised intracranial pressure owing to the risk of aspiration. The goal during induction is to minimize further increases in ICP. In general, as discussed earlier, most intravenous drugs decrease CBF, cerebral metabolism, and ICP. It may be necessary to use etomidate or ketamine in the setting of hemodynamic compromise; however, the use of ketamine in traumatic brain injury (TBI) is controversial. In neurologically stable patients, a mask induction with sevoflurane and nitrous oxide can be performed, followed by a muscle relaxant. Manual hyperventilation can be utilized if necessary to decrease ICP. Succinylcholine can result in life-threatening hyperkalemia in patients with denervating processes such as stroke, spinal cord injury, crush injuries, stroke, or muscular dystrophies, and should be avoided.

Positioning requirements vary among neurosurgical cases. Special attention should be paid during positioning to optimize access for both surgeon and anesthesiologist, while ensuring the safety of the patient. Many neurosurgical procedures require prone positioning, with the head of the bed turned 90 to 180 degrees away from the anesthesiologist. All the considerations for prone cases hold true. The head is secured in cranial fixation pins, or a Mayfield frame with the neck flexed or extended to facilitate surgical exposure. Extreme rotation of the head can impede

venous return or compromise cerebral perfusion; extreme flexion can cause migration of the endotracheal tube into a mainstem bronchus, or cause brainstem compression in posterior fossa lesions, while extreme extension can lead to unplanned extubation. Sometimes it is required that the head be higher than the torso to facilitate venous and CSF drainage from the surgical site, increasing the risk of venous air embolism (VAE).[19] In infants, VAE can occur even in the lateral, prone, or supine position, as the larger head rests above the heart.[20,21] The risk is increased in children with intracardiac shunts. Precordial Doppler is the earliest and most sensitive monitor to detect VAE but prone positioning may preclude its use on the anterior chest. In infants weighing less than 6 kg the Doppler could be placed on the posterior thorax between the scapulae. In addition to the characteristic changes in Doppler sounds, a sudden decrease in end-tidal CO_2, dysrhythmias, and ischemic changes on the EKG should alert one to the occurrence of VAE.

Two large peripheral venous catheters are usually sufficient for most cases. Central venous catheters are not routinely used unless needed for difficult access, as the narrow-gauge catheters used in children are often unsuccessful in aspirating air even in the event of a VAE. An arterial line is warranted for major craniotomies owing to the risk of hemodynamic instability from sudden hemorrhage, VAE, herniation, or cranial nerve manipulation. Currently, EEG is considered the most reliable intraoperative monitor for focal cerebral ischemia and is employed for cerebral aneurysm clipping and surgery for moyamoya disease. Near-infrared spectroscopy (NIRS) is increasingly proving useful for early detection of global cerebral ischemia. It provides a noninvasive assessment of venous oxy-Hb saturation and has been reported to correlate with jugular bulb saturation. EMG is useful in identification and dissection of functional nerve roots in tethered spinal cord syndrome. In surgeries involving the spine, SSEP monitoring is utilized to assess the dorsal sensory pathways of the spinal cord and MEP to monitor the integrity of the corticospinal tracts that transmit motor impulses. Electrocorticography (ECoG) is used for cortical stimulation in seizure surgery. Preoperative planning should include a discussion of the type and extent of neurophysiological monitoring to be used, as many anesthetic agents have a depressant effect on some monitors.

Maintenance of anesthesia is optimally achieved with an opioid-based balanced technique that includes low-dose volatile agent and a muscle relaxant. Muscle relaxation should be avoided in cases where intraoperative EMG, MEP, or muscle stimulation is utilized. As discussed, some prefer to avoid nitrous oxide completely while others reserve its use for certain portions of the surgery. Meticulous fluid management is essential and although there is no absolute formula, maintenance of normovolemia is key in most situations. Normal saline or Plasma-Lyte are commonly used as maintenance fluids. The use of colloids in the setting of a disrupted blood-brain barrier is controversial. The decision to transfuse blood is based on the type and duration of surgery, underlying condition of the child, and potential for ongoing blood loss. Brain swelling and raised ICP are managed with a combination of judicious hyperventilation, steroids, and hyperosmolar therapy that may include mannitol or hypertonic saline, along with furosemide.[22,23] Hypertonic saline may be associated with natriuresis, central pontine myelinolysis, and rebound increase in ICP, but it is being used increasingly in patients with elevated ICP from TBI.[24]

The decision to extubate after surgery is based on numerous factors. Airway edema is a concern in prolonged prone cases with significant blood loss requiring large volume replacement. The risk of postoperative apnea and vocal cord paralysis should be considered in surgeries involving the brainstem. If extubation in the operating room is planned, the anesthetic should be tailored to facilitate neurological assessment at or soon after emergence. Emergence and extubation should be smooth to prevent swings in blood pressure and ICP. Postoperative care for the large majority of neurosurgical cases is optimally provided in the intensive care unit for 1 to 3 days after surgery, where close monitoring of neurological status can be achieved. One should be alert to the occurrence of postoperative seizures; although the incidence is low, the effects can be devastating.[25] The routine use of prophylactic anticonvulsants for craniotomies is debatable. Levetiracetam is replacing phenytoin in some centers as the anticonvulsant of choice, as monitoring for therapeutic serum levels is not necessary, and risk of toxicity is lower.

CONSIDERATIONS FOR SPECIFIC DISEASE STATES AND SURGERIES

Certain neurological disease states are unique to infants and children. Understanding the natural course goes a long way in providing the optimal anesthetic, while minimizing complications. The general principles of intraoperative management may need to be modified for specific disease states.

Congenital Anomalies

Spinal dysraphism is a midline defect that can be minor involving only the superficial bone and membranous structures, or it may be more extensive involving malformed neural tissue; it can involve the head (encephalocele) or spine. Spina bifida refers to a spectrum of spine defects; a defect containing CSF alone is a meningocele; a defect that also includes neural tissue is a meningomyelocele. These are often associated with hydrocephalus and type II Arnold-Chiari malformations. Primary closure usually is undertaken on the first 1 to 2 days of life. Special attention is to be paid during induction to positioning; if intubation is attempted in the supine position a "donut"

ring is used to avoid pressure on the defect. In the case of large defects, intubation in the lateral position may be necessary. This is a field where in utero repair is increasingly being performed as the defect is frequently identified on prenatal ultrasound. These patients are at high risk of developing latex sensitivity and anaphylaxis, as they are repeatedly exposed to latex products, both in surgery for coexisting orthopedic and urological problems, and during routine care as in repeated bladder catheterizations. They may grow to develop a tethered spinal cord that can cause nerve root distortion, progressive neurological deficits, and chronic pain. Intraoperative EMG monitoring can help identify functional nerve roots and avoid inadvertent injury that can lead to fecal or urinary incontinence. Selective dorsal rhizotomy is a procedure performed for severe spasticity associated with cerebral palsy. This involves surgical division of dorsal rootlets to decrease afferent input to motor neurons in the spinal cord. The rootlets are identified by direct stimulation and noting of the corresponding muscle action potential with EMG. These patients have severe somatic pain postoperatively, along with dysesthesia, hyperesthesia, and muscle spasms. A multimodal postoperative pain management strategy is imperative.[26]

Arnold-Chiari Malformations

These consist of a bony abnormality of the posterior fossa and upper cervical spine, leading to varying degrees of caudad displacement of the cerebellar vermis and brainstem through the foramen magnum, often accompanied by myelodysplasia. Of the four types, children with type I have milder symptoms, type II often have coexisting hydrocephalus, type III have the most severe symptoms with long-term disability, and type IV is characterized by cerebellar hypoplasia or aplasia. Decompressive suboccipital craniectomy with cervical laminectomies is the surgical treatment. Care should be taken in these patients to avoid extreme head flexion during intubation as it can cause brainstem compression. Abnormal responses to hypoxia and hypercarbia should be anticipated as they have cranial nerve and brainstem dysfunction.

Tumors

Brain tumors are the second most common childhood malignancy, next to leukemias. The majority are infratentorial, occurring in the posterior fossa, and include medulloblastomas, cerebellar astrocytomas, brainstem gliomas, and ependymomas of the fourth ventricle. Infratentorial tumors can obstruct CSF flow early in the course, thereby leading to intracranial hypertension and hydrocephalus, in addition to causing cranial nerve palsies and ataxia. Supratentorial tumors account for 25% to 40% of brain tumors in children and include astrocytomas, oligodendrogliomas, ependymomas, and glioblastomas. Presenting symptom is often a seizure or focal neurological deficit.

Surgery for tumor resection is fraught with anesthetic challenges at every stage. Positioning is often prone or lateral decubitus with the head fixed in pins, and turned 90 to 180 degrees away from the anesthesiologist based on surgeon preference. Skull fractures, intracranial hematomas, and dural tears are risks during pinning. Sinus tears, VAE, and massive blood loss are risks during raising of the bone flap, and require constant vigilance. Elevated ICP is managed by altering ventilation techniques, administering mannitol, or both, or by the insertion of a ventricular or lumbar catheter by the surgeon. Arrhythmias and hemodynamic perturbations are not uncommon during brainstem manipulation. VAE can occur in any position as the head is often elevated to improve venous drainage. Postoperative concerns include apnea and airway obstruction from damage to the respiratory centers and cranial nerves, or airway edema from prolonged prone positioning.

Midbrain tumors seen in children include craniopharyngiomas, pituitary adenomas, optic nerve gliomas, hypothalamic tumors, and papillomas of the choroid plexus. Precocious puberty is often the presentation in hypothalamic tumors. Of the perisellar tumors, craniopharyngiomas are the most common and can be accompanied by endocrine derangements; steroids are often necessary as the hypothalamic-pituitary-adrenal axis is affected. Diabetes insipidus can occur anytime during the perioperative period. Urine output should be closely monitored along with serum electrolytes, and osmolality. The transsphenoidal approach is sometimes used in older children for pituitary adenoma resection; massive bleeding can occur and one should be prepared for urgent conversion to an open craniotomy. Optic nerve gliomas are common in children with neurofibromatosis. They are highly vascular and significant blood loss can occur. Choroid plexus papillomas are less common and usually arise from the lateral ventricle. The increased production of CSF and obstruction to flow can result in early hydrocephalus.

Stereotactic approaches to surgery involve application of a headframe that limits access to the airway, usually applied after induction in the operating room (OR), after which the anesthetized child is transported to the CT scanner, and then back to the OR. Newer thermolaser ablation for inoperable tumors involves transport to the MRI suite where the treatment is delivered with imaging guidance. It is necessary in these cases to have a secure airway, while maintaining TIVA during transport. Hybrid OR-MRI suites have made these procedures more manageable.

Hydrocephalus

Hydrocephalus is a condition of increased CSF volume as a result of mismatched CSF production and absorption, leading to increased intracranial pressure. It is the most common neurosurgical condition in pediatrics, most cases

resulting from the obstruction of CSF flow, or an inability to absorb CSF. In neonates, especially premies, intraventricular or subarachnoid hemorrhage is a common cause, as is congenital aqueductal stenosis. Other causes include trauma, infection, and posterior fossa tumors. Hydrocephalus may be nonobstructive (communicating) or obstructive (noncommunicating) based on whether there is unimpeded flow of CSF around the spinal cord. The acuity of presentation depends on the rapidity of development of hydrocephalus and the intracranial compliance. In the infant, the cerebral vault gradually expands to accommodate the increased CSF volume if hydrocephalus develops over time. In older children whose sutures are fused, the risk of herniation is higher as the skull cannot expand. These children present with increasing lethargy and vomiting, can rapidly develop cranial nerve dysfunction and bradycardia, and progress to brain herniation and death. They are definite aspiration risks. Following a rapid sequence induction, hyperventilation is instituted to control the ICP. Definitive treatment is correction of the cause, but immediate treatment involves placement of a ventricular drain or ventriculoperitoneal (VP) shunt with the goal of rapidly relieving the obstruction. VP shunts divert CSF from the ventricles to the peritoneal cavity. When absorption through the peritoneum is compromised, as in peritonitis, the distal end of the shunt is placed in the right atrium or pleural cavity. Shunts may need to be replaced as the child grows or the pathophysiology changes, requiring repeat trips to the operating room. Shunts with programmable valves help minimize this to some extent. Acute obstruction of a shunt needs to be treated urgently as it can have lethal consequences. Shunt infection is another possible risk; in this situation, the entire shunt system is removed and an external ventricular drain (EVD) established temporarily. A new shunt is placed after treatment of the infection. Transportation and moving of patients with EVDs require special attention to avoid sudden drainage of CSF or dislodgement of the tubing. Excess drainage of CSF can lead to slit ventricle syndrome.[27] Fluid overload should be avoided to minimize brain swelling. Endoscopic ventriculostomy is a procedure that creates an alternative route from one area of CSF to another, bypassing an area of obstruction. Common locations for a ventriculostomy are through the septum pellucidum allowing the lateral ventricles to communicate, or through the floor of the third ventricle into the CSF cisterns. Cauterization of the choroid plexus helps to reduce excessive CSF production. Damage to the basilar artery and its branches, or neural injuries are a concern with these procedures and can have dire consequences.

Epilepsy Surgery

Seizures are a common neurological disorder in children, and can be a component of various epilepsy syndromes. Vagal nerve stimulators inhibit seizures at the brainstem/

cortical levels. Surgical resection of the seizure focus is undertaken when a child has medically refractory epilepsy that has failed other treatment options, and involves serial craniotomies. The first is for insertion of intracranial grid-and-strip electrodes on the exposed cortex of the brain. During this first anesthetic, it is important to avoid agents that may suppress seizures during and after the procedure, that is, long-acting benzodiazepines. The patient is monitored for seizures in the electrophysiology unit to map the location of the seizure foci; the mapping then serves to guide the neurosurgeon for resection. This may take several days but typically the patient returns to the operating room in 2 to 3 days. Surgical risk and anesthetic concerns are dependent on the location of the seizure focus, its proximity to vital structures, and the age of the patient. Intraoperative neurophysiological monitoring is used to guide the resection; this might include cortical stimulation to identify the motor strip, EEG, and EMG. Advances in neurophysiological monitoring have made these procedures safer and more accurate. The anesthetic technique is tailored to the patient's specific requirements with the goal of not compromising the monitoring, especially when the seizure foci involve functional areas of the brain. A narcotic-based general anesthetic with low levels of volatile agent is optimal. Muscle relaxation is avoided if cortical stimulation of motor cortex or EMG is being used. Upregulation of the hepatic P450 enzymes from chronic use of anticonvulsants can result in rapid metabolism and clearance of neuromuscular blockers and opioids in these patients leading to the need for larger and repeated dosing, but also facilitates monitoring when needed.[28,29] A major risk during these procedures is harm to the "eloquent cortex," the area of the brain that controls speech, memory, and other vital functions. Awake craniotomies allow the patient to assist in the determination of the limits of safe cortical resection; they are rarely undertaken in children but may be considered in older cooperative teenagers. Anesthesia for an awake craniotomy can range from no sedation with local anesthesia alone to alternating "asleep-awake-asleep" techniques in which general anesthesia is limited to the period before and after functional testing.[30] Following induction of general anesthesia, the airway is secured with either an endotracheal tube or a laryngeal mask airway, and the patient is kept asleep for line placement, head pinning, and opening of skull and dura. The anesthetic is then discontinued, and the patient extubated and awakened for the period of functional neurological testing and resection, during which time a psychologist is also often present in the operating room. Once resection is completed, general anesthesia is reinstituted for the closure. This technique allows for the patient to be completely anesthetized for the painful parts of the surgery. A disadvantage is the unpredictability of the patient's emergence with pins in place, and reactions under surgical drapes. Deep sedation with a natural airway, using propofol and dexmedetomidine, combined with an opioid is an alternative. Not all older children are good candidates for an awake craniotomy; patient selection should take into consideration their maturity, psychological preparedness, and ability to cooperate with strangers in an unfamiliar environment. Developmentally delayed children and those with anxiety or other psychiatric disorders are clearly not candidates.

Lobectomy, corpus callostomy, and hemispherectomy are alternative procedures performed when focal resection is not an option. One should be prepared to manage large volumes of blood loss in these cases.

Craniosynostosis

Premature closure of one or more cranial sutures occurs in about 1 in 2000 births; it may be associated with a variety of syndromes, some of which are harbingers of a difficult airway. Uncorrected craniosynostosis can result in increased ICP and brain compression, with neurological sequelae. Correction is usually undertaken in the first 3 to 6 months of life, as brain growth is rapid during this period and the skull bones more malleable. The procedure may be a single strip craniectomy or a complete craniofacial reconstruction. These procedures fall into the purview of plastic surgery, but more extensive cranial exposures involve neurosurgeons. Although extradural, blood loss from the scalp and cranium can be significant, and VAE is a significant risk. Adequate venous access and invasive monitoring are imperative. The use of antifibrinolytics is controversial, but may have some utility. Less invasive neuroendoscopic techniques aim for smaller incisions, minimal dissection and blood loss, and fewer complications, allowing for less aggressive fluid replacement, less invasive hemodynamic monitoring, and possibly less mortality.[31,32]

Vascular Malformations

Vascular anomalies in children are rare, most being congenital lesions. Large arteriovenous malformations (AVMs), such as those of the vein of Galen in neonates, are associated with high-output congestive heart failure, with a poor prognosis. Initial treatment often consists of serial embolizations in the interventional radiology suite, followed by craniotomy for surgical excision, or Gamma Knife surgery.[33,34] Although advances in endovascular treatment have improved outcomes, embolization is still a very high-risk procedure. There are risks associated with the embolic agent, including cerebral hemorrhage or ischemia from total occlusion or extravasation, fluid overload in an infant that is already in high-output cardiac failure, and VAE. Vessel perforation requiring emergent conversion to a craniotomy, and leg ischemia from the femoral puncture site can be devastating. There very often is a need for inotropic support, or antihypertensive treatment with vasodilators during the procedure. Intracranial AVMs may be associated with vascular or lymphatic malformations in the spinal cord, or the face.

Moyamoya disease is a rare condition characterized by chronic progressive steno-occlusion of the arteries of the Circle of Willis, usually the intracranial portion of the internal carotid arteries, with collateral vessel formation at the base of the brain.[35] The syndrome can be associated with neurofibromatosis, tuberous sclerosis, Marfan syndrome, Noonan syndrome, homocystinuria, thalassemia, sickle cell disease, congenital heart disease, optic nerve gliomas, basal brain tumors, and chromosomal disorders such as Down, Williams, and Turner syndromes. These children present with frequent transient ischemic attacks or recurrent strokes. These patients require anesthesia for confirmatory angiography, followed by surgery. Surgical treatment aims to increase collateral flow by direct or indirect revascularization procedures, using the external carotid circulation as the donor supply. Indirect procedures are more common in children. In pial synangiosis, an intact superficial temporal artery is fixed to the pial surface with the creation of a wide opening of dura and arachnoid; over time, there is ingrowth of new vessels through the opening to the poorly perfused area of the brain. Perioperative ischemia is a significant risk both during angiography and surgery and thereafter as neovascularization can take several weeks to months; it is imperative to maintain normocapnia, normotension, normovolemia, and normothermia, concepts that are contrary to what is practiced for other neurosurgical cases, and continue them into the perioperative period.[36,37] Generous preoperative hydration and appropriate sedation to avoid agitation are key. Both hypercapnia and hypocapnia intraoperatively can be detrimental, a cerebral steal phenomenon diverting blood flow away from the compromised ischemic area of the brain. Anesthetic technique should not interfere with EEG monitoring. Measures to optimize cerebral perfusion should be continued into the postoperative period.

Neurotrauma

Traumatic brain injury is the leading cause of death and disability in children over 1 year of age in the United States. Spinal cord injury is often concurrent. Following blunt head trauma, diffuse cerebral edema is more common than intracranial hemorrhage, unlike adults. Most linear skull fractures do not require treatment but depressed skull fractures have a greater potential to harm underlying tissues, and may require urgent intervention. In children, cervical spine fractures can occur without neurological deficit, or present with delayed onset of symptoms; or deficits can occur without a radiological fracture.

Decreased perfusion to the brain and cerebral ischemia occur in the first 6 to 12 hours after a TBI, followed by hyperemia and raised ICP. Outcomes are better in children compared to adults but certain factors such as hypoxia, aggressive hyperventilation, hyperglycemia, hypotension, and intracranial hypertension predict poor outcome. Cerebral autoregulation may be impaired; the CPP threshold required to prevent cerebral hypoperfusion is not well understood. Current recommendation is to avoid CPP <40 mm Hg, although the threshold to prevent ischemia is likely age-dependent with older children requiring a higher CPP.[38] A systolic BP higher than normal may be needed to maintain adequate CPP, requiring the use of pressors. Ventricular catheters and fiber-optic transducers help in monitoring of ICP. Children with a GCS score less than 8 to 9 should be intubated for airway protection and management of raised ICP. Nasotracheal intubation should be avoided unless absolutely necessary in those with skull fractures. In the setting of cerebral edema, or when medical measures to decrease elevated ICP fail, decompressive craniectomy is the next option. The goal of surgery is to optimize viable brain recovery by removal of massive hemorrhages or lesions. Anesthetic goals include mild hyperventilation ($Paco_2$ about 35 mm Hg) to prevent brainstem herniation and intracranial hypertension. Adequate vascular access and invasive monitoring is necessary. Normothermia or mild hypothermia (Temperature 36–37°C) may be protective; hyperthermia should be avoided. There is a high risk of VAE and massive blood loss in craniotomies for evacuation of epidural or subdural hematomas.

Subdural hematomas can result from birth trauma or the occasional "shaken baby syndrome." When a child presents with a conglomeration of chronic and acute subdural hematomas, subarachnoid hemorrhage, skull fractures in various stages of healing, with or without other injuries out of proportion to the history, nonaccidental or inflicted trauma should be suspected. Outcomes are usually poor.

Neuroimaging and Interventions in Radiology Suites

Neurosurgical patients go through several imaging studies as part of their workup, including CT, MRI, PET, and nuclear medicine scans, for which younger children require sedation or general anesthesia. Dexmedetomidine has become established as a safe sedative drug for these studies and can be used alone or in conjunction with propofol.[39] Stereotactic procedures can start out in the radiology suite where the patient is often anesthetized prior to application of the frame and the anesthetized patient then transported to the operating room. The need for intraoperative MRI for procedures such as laser thermoablation has led to the construction of hybrid suites where imaging and surgery can be performed in a sterile environment. Access to the patient is a challenge in this situation, as is the need for MRI compatible or MRI conditional equipment. Some equipment, specifically Doppler ultrasounds, and fluid warmers are not MRI safe. This is a field that is rapidly evolving and will require the anesthesiologist to be flexible, while remaining vigilant to the need for sudden interventions.

SUMMARY

Pediatric neurosurgical anesthesia covers a wide spectrum of conditions across various age groups. The management of neurosurgical cases presents unique challenges to both surgeon and anesthesiologist, but also offers opportunities for close teamwork and collaboration. Understanding the age-related differences in this population is vital and goes a long way in avoiding complications. Formulating a thoughtful plan, understanding and being prepared for the complexities of the surgery, and maintaining open dialogue with the surgeon at all stages are essential to minimizing perioperative morbidity and mortality.

REFERENCES

1. Chumas P, Kenny T, Stiller C. Subspecialisation in neurosurgery—does size matter? *Acta Neurochir (Wien)*. 2011;153(6):1231-1236.
2. Mokri B. The Monro-Kellie hypothesis: applications in CSF volume depletion. *Neurology*. 2001;56(12):1746-1748.
3. Shapiro K, Marmarou A, Shulman K. Characterization of clinical CSF dynamics and neural axis compliance using the pressure-volume index: I. The normal pressure-volume index. *Ann Neurol*. 1980;7(6):508-514.
4. Vavilala M, Soriano S, Krane E. Anethesia for neurosurgery. In: Davis P, Cladis FP, eds. *Smith's Anesthesia for Infants and Children*. 8th ed. Philadelphia, PA: Elsevier; 2017:744-745.
5. Wintermark M, Lepori D, Cotting J, et al. Brain perfusion in children: evolution with age assessed by quantitative perfusion computed tomography. *Pediatrics*. 2004;113(6):1642-1652.
6. Vavilala MS, Lee LA, Lam AM. The lower limit of cerebral autoregulation in children during sevoflurane anesthesia. *J Neurosurg Anesthesiol*. 2003;15(4):307-312.
7. Brady KM, Mytar JO, Lee JK, et al. Monitoring cerebral blood flow pressure autoregulation in pediatric patients during cardiac surgery. *Stroke*. 2010;41(9):1957-1962.
8. Rhee CJ, Fraser CD, Kibler K, et al. The ontogeny of cerebrovascular pressure autoregulation in premature infants. *J Perinatol*. 2014;34(12):926-931.
9. Kontos HA, Raper AJ, Patterson JL. Analysis of vasoactivity of local pH, P_{CO_2} and bicarbonate on pial vessels. *Stroke*. 1977;8(3):358-360.
10. Ellingsen I, Hauge A, Nicolaysen G, Thoresen M, Walloe L. Changes in human cerebral blood flow due to step changes in $P_{A}O_2$ and $P_{A}CO_2$. *Acta Physiol Scand*. 1987;129(2):157-163.
11. Stephan H, Groger P, Weyland A, Hoeft A, Sonntag H. The effect of sufentanil on cerebral blood flow, cerebral metabolism and the CO_2 reactivity of the cerebral vessels in man. *Anaesthesist*. 1991;40(3):153-160.
12. Mertens MJ, Engbers FH, Burm AG, Vuyk J. Predictive performance of computer-controlled infusion of remifentanil during propofol/remifentanil anaesthesia. *Br J Anaesth*. 2003;90(2):132-141.
13. Ard J, Doyle W, Bekker A. Awake craniotomy with dexmedetomidine in pediatric patients. *J Neurosurg Anesthesiol*. 2003;15(3):263-266.
14. Bekker A, Sturaitis MK. Dexmedetomidine for neurological surgery. *Neurosurgery*. 2005;57(1 suppl):1-10; discussion 1-10.
15. Wong GT, Luginbuehl I, Karsli C, Bissonnette B. The effect of sevoflurane on cerebral autoregulation in young children as assessed by the transient hyperemic response. *Anesth Analg*. 2006;102(4):1051-1055.
16. Reasoner DK, Todd MM, Scamman FL, Warner DS. The incidence of pneumocephalus after supratentorial craniotomy. Observations on the disappearance of intracranial air. *Anesthesiology*. 1994;80(5):1008-1012.
17. McCann ME, Kain ZN. The management of preoperative anxiety in children: an update. *Anesth Analg*. 2001;93(1):98-105.
18. Kain ZN, Caldwell-Andrews AA, Krivutza DM, Weinberg ME, Wang SM, Gaal D. Trends in the practice of parental presence during induction of anesthesia and the use of preoperative sedative premedication in the United States, 1995-2002: results of a follow-up national survey. *Anesth Analg*. 2004;98(5):1252-1259, table of contents.
19. Grady MS, Bedford RF, Park TS. Changes in superior sagittal sinus pressure in children with head elevation, jugular venous compression, and PEEP. *J Neurosurg*. 1986;65(2):199-202.
20. Harris MM, Yemen TA, Davidson A, et al. Venous embolism during craniectomy in supine infants. *Anesthesiology*. 1987;67(5):816-819.
21. Faberowski LW, Black S, Mickle JP. Incidence of venous air embolism during craniectomy for craniosynostosis repair. *Anesthesiology*. 2000;92(1):20-23.
22. Prabhakar H, Singh GP, Anand V, Kalaivani M. Mannitol versus hypertonic saline for brain relaxation in patients undergoing craniotomy. *Cochrane Database Syst Rev*. 2014;(7):CD010026. doi(7):CD010026.
23. Kochanek PM, Carney N, Adelson PD, et al. Guidelines for the acute medical management of severe traumatic brain injury in infants, children, and adolescents—second edition. *Pediatr Crit Care Med*. 2012;13(suppl 1):S1-S82.
24. Piper BJ, Harrigan PW. Hypertonic saline in paediatric traumatic brain injury: a review of nine years' experience with 23.4% hypertonic saline as standard hyperosmolar therapy. *Anaesth Intensive Care*. 2015;43(2):204-210.
25. Hardesty DA, Sanborn MR, Parker WE, Storm PB. Perioperative seizure incidence and risk factors in 223 pediatric brain tumor patients without prior seizures. *J Neurosurg Pediatr*. 2011;7(6):609-615.
26. Geiduschek JM, Haberkern CM, McLaughlin JF. Pain management for children following selective dorsal rhizotomy. *Can J Anaesth*. 1997; 41:492-496.
27. Elredge EA, Rockoff MA, Medlock MA, Scott RM, Millis MB. Postoperative cerebral edema occurring in children with slit ventricles. *Pediatrics*. 1997;99:625-630.
28. Eldredge A, Soriano SG, Rockoff MA. Neuroanesthesia. *Neurosurg Clin N Am*. 1995;6:505-520.
29. Soriano SG, Martyn JA. Antiepileptic-induced resistance to neuromuscular blockers: mechanisms and clinical significance. *Clin Pharmacokinet*. 2004;43(2):71-81.
30. Sarang A, Dinsmore J. Anaesthesia for awake craniotomy—evolution of a technique that facilitates awake neurological testing. *Br J Anaesth*. 2003;90(2):161-165.
31. Jimenez DF, Barone CM. Endoscopic craniectomy for early surgical correction of sagittal craniosynostosis. *J Neurosurg*. 1998;88(1):77-81.
32. Jimenez DF, Barone CM, Cartwright CC, Baker L. Early management of craniosynostosis using endoscopic-assisted strip craniectomies and cranial orthotic molding therapy. *Pediatrics*. 2002;110(1 pt 1):97-104.

33. Burrows PE, Robertson RL. Neonatal central nervous system vascular disorders. *Neurosurg Clin N Am*. 1998;9(1):155-180.

34. Ashida Y, Miyahara H, Sawada H, Mitani Y, Maruyama K. Anesthetic management of a neonate with vein of Galen aneurysmal malformations and severe pulmonary hypertension. *Paediatr Anaesth*. 2005;15(6):525-528.

35. Baykan N, Ozgen S, Ustalar ZS, Dagcinar A, Ozek MM. Moyamoya disease and anesthesia. *Paediatr Anaesth*. 2005;15(12):1111-1115.

36. Parray T, Martin TW, Siddiqui S. Moyamoya disease: a review of the disease and anesthetic management. *J Neurosurg Anesthesiol*. 2011;23(2):100-109.

37. Robertson RL, Chavali RV, Robson CD, et al. Neurologic complications of cerebral angiography in childhood moyamoya syndrome. *Pediatr Radiol*. 1998;28(11):824-829.

38. Vavilala MS, Kernic MA, Wang J. Acute care clinical indictors associated with discharge outcomes in children with severe traumatic brain injury. Pediatric guideline adherence and outcomes study. *Critical Care Medicine*. 2014;42(10):2258-2266.

39. Sulton C, McCracken C, Simon HK, et al. Pediatric procedural sedation using dexmedetomidine: a report from the Pediatric Sedation Research Consortium. *Hosp Pediatr*. 2016;6(9):536-544.

Anesthesia for Ophthalmic Procedures

Kristen Labovsky

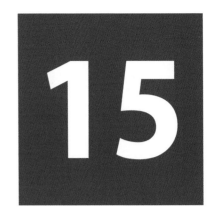

ANATOMY OF THE EYE

The maximum growth of a child's eyeball occurs during the first two years of life with an infant's eyeball volume increasing by 40%.[1] The outer transparent mucous membrane that covers the inner surface of the lids and the sclera is the **conjunctiva** (Figure 15-1). The conjunctiva is continuous with the skin at the margin of the lid. The **sclera** is a collagen containing outer fibrous layer of the eye. The **cornea** is an avascular, transparent layer that acts as the glass of a watch. The ophthalmic division of the trigeminal nerve supplies the sensory nerves to the cornea. The **iris** divides the anterior chamber from the posterior chamber and the round aperture in the center is the pupil. The iris, using a balance between parasympathetic mediated constriction and sympathetic mediated dilation, controls the amount of light entering the eye. The **ciliary body** contains the ciliary process that produces aqueous humor and the ciliary muscle, which allows a variable focus of the lens by altering the tension on the lens capsule. The lens is an avascular, transparent structure that separates the aqueous anteriorly from the vitreous posteriorly. It is suspended behind the iris by zonules that connect to the ciliary muscle. The **retina** is a thin multilayer neural membrane that lines the inner posterior two-thirds of the globe. Images are focused on the retina with signals sent to the brain. The **optic nerve** contains approximately 1 million axons that arise from the ganglion cells of the retina and exits the posterior portion of the globe. The blood supply for the optic nerve consists of branches of the central retinal artery, ophthalmic artery, and other internal carotid branches. The extraocular muscles consist of two oblique muscles which primarily control torsion movements and four rectus muscles that depress, elevate, adduct, and abduct the globe. Cranial nerve VI (abducens) innervates the lateral rectus muscle, cranial nerve IV (trochlear) innervates the superior oblique, and cranial nerve III (oculomotor) innervates the inferior oblique and superior, medial, and inferior rectus.[2]

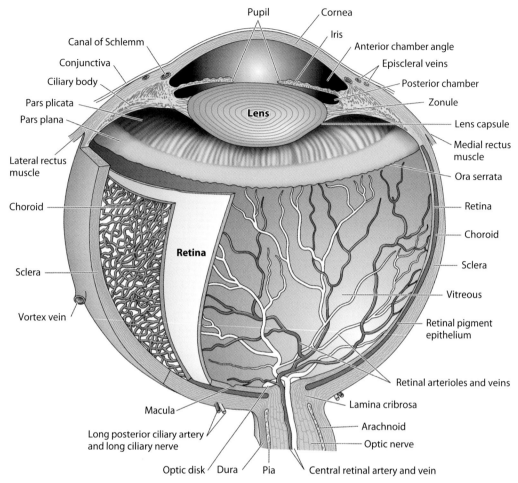

▲ **Figure 15-1.** Anatomy of the eye. (Reproduced with permission, from Riordan-Eva P, Augsburger JJ. *Vaughan & Asbury's General Ophthalmology*. 19th ed. 2018. https://accessmedicine.mhmedical.com. Copyright © McGraw Hill LLC. All rights reserved.)

PHYSIOLOGY OF THE EYE

Careful consideration and understanding of intraocular pressure (IOP) is important in managing anesthesia for eye surgeries. Normal IOP is reached by age 5 and is 10 to 20 mm Hg.[3] It is determined by changes in intraocular volume, external pressure, and venous congestion. Aqueous humor, produced by the ciliary bodies, is regulated to maintain normal IOP. Aqueous humor drainage is decreased with mydriasis and can lead to increased IOP.[4] Elevated IOP can lead to decreased arterial perfusion and optic nerve ischemia.[8] Physiologic factors that affect IOP are listed in Table 15-1. Anesthetic agents can also have an effect on IOP and this is important to consider when caring for patients with increased IOP (Table 15-2).

Table 15-1. Effect of Physiologic Factors on IOP

Factors	Effect on IOP
Elevated venous pressure	Increase
Cough, valsalva, vomiting	Increase (up to 40 mm Hg)
Hypoxia	Increase
Hyperoxia	Decrease
Metabolic alkalosis, respiratory acidosis	Increase
Metabolic acidosis, respiratory alkalosis	Decrease
Elevated systemic arterial pressure	Minimal effect, autoregulated

Table 15-2. Effect of anesthetic agents on IOP[4]

Agent	Effect
CNS depressants (barbiturates, benzodiazepines, opioids)	Decrease
Thiopental, propofol, etomidate	Decrease
Ketamine	No consensus, associated with blepharospasm and nystagmus
Volatile anesthetics	Decrease
Succinylcholine	Increase (may be able to attenuate change with opioids, propofol, and precurarization with rocuronium)

Source: Reproduced with permission, from Davis P, Cladis F, eds. *Smith's Anesthesia for Infants and Children.* 9th ed. 2017. Copyright © Elsevier. All rights reserved.

The oculocardiac reflex (OCR) (Figure 15-2) is also important to consider in the anesthetic management of ophthalmologic procedures. The occurrence is as high as 65% to 79% during pediatric cases where no prophylaxis was given.[5–7] The afferent pathway is via the ophthalmic division of the trigeminal nerve and the efferent pathway involves the vagal nerve. The reflex is triggered by pressure on the eye or traction on the extraocular muscles and usually results in sinus bradycardia. More significant rhythm disturbances can include ventricular bigeminy, ventricular tachycardia, atrioventricular block, and asystole. Effects of the OCR usually end once the stimulus is removed.[4]

COMMONLY USED OPHTHALMIC MEDICATIONS

Ophthalmologists will often use topical medications to alter IOP or to achieve optimal conditions for exam and surgery. Table 15-3 lists the common topical medications employed and side effects seen.[8]

OCULAR DISEASES AND PROCEDURES

Strabismus

Strabismus is defined as misalignment of the eyes, either by turning out (exotropia), being crossed (esotropia), or vertical misalignment (hypertropia, hypotropia). Repair of strabismus involves manipulation of the eye muscles to realign the eyes. The surgical repair involves moving, strengthening, or weakening the eye muscles.

Table 15-4 shows common strabismus procedures to achieve alignment.

Nasolacrimal Duct Surgeries

The nasolacrimal duct is not open distally in 60% of newborns.[9] It is most spontaneously opened or opened with conservative treatment (massaging) during the first year of life, with studies showing a resolution rate of 96%.[10] Surgery involves nasolacrimal duct probing where a metal probe is passed into the canaliculi to the lacrimal sac and down into the nose.[9] In recurrent cases, a silicone tube may be placed to function as a stent. If the nasolacrimal duct does not function, a drainage path from the eye through the lacrimal sac to the nose can be created during a dacryocystorhinostomy.

Glaucoma

Increased intraocular pressure that results in an optic neuropathy is referred to as glaucoma. Treatment can be surgical or medical. Common medications used to decrease intraocular pressure in children include beta-blockers, alpha agonists, and carbonic anhydrase inhibitors. If intraocular pressure remains elevated after topical medications, oral and intravenous agents, such as acetazolamide, may be used. Surgery is indicated if medical management does not decrease intraocular pressure. Laser or cyrotherapy is used to destroy ciliary processes and decrease aqueous humor production.

Retinoblastoma

Retinoblastoma is the most common form of intraocular cancer in children and is generally diagnosed by age 3. The prevalence is 1:20,000 and half of the cases are due to a mutation in the retinoblastoma gene. Treatment for retinoblastoma has included enucleation, external beam radiation, and chemotherapy.[11] There is a risk of secondary cancers in the field of external beam radiation, so currently patients with bilateral disease that require enucleation or diffuse vitreous and subretinal seeding are considered candidates for this radiation treatment. Patients with less advanced disease may be managed with chemoreduction and focal ablation.[4] There has been a shift in treatment toward chemotherapy, delivered either intravenously, intra-arterially, intravitreally, or periocularly.[12]

Retinopathy of Prematurity

The incidence of retinopathy of prematurity reported from a multicenter U.S. study was 68% in infants less than 1251 g.[13] Retinopathy of prematurity (ROP) is classified by the zone of the retina involved (Figure 15-3), the severity of disease, and the degree of venous congestion.[14] Zone 1 is central (and more likely to progress to severe) and zone 3 is most peripheral, while severity is divided into five stages. "Plus disease" indicates a significant amount of venous congestion or arteriolar tortuosity. Treatment should be performed within 72 hours of diagnosis in patients with high-risk pre-threshold disease:

OCULOCARDIAC REFLEX
(The Complete Arc)

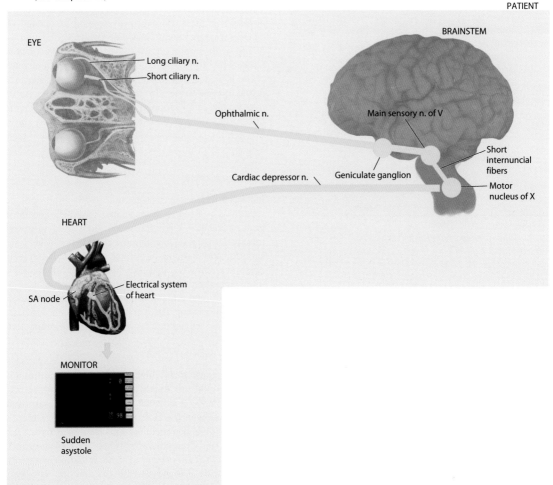

PATIENT

▲ **Figure 15-2.** Oculocardiac reflex (Reproduced with permission, from Hadzic A. *Hadzic's Textbook of Regional Anesthesia and Acute Pain Management*. 2nd ed. 2017. https://accessanesthesiology.mhmedical.com. Copyright © McGraw Hill LLC. All rights reserved.)

- Any stage ROP with plus disease in zone I
- Stage 3 ROP without plus disease in zone I
- Stage 2 or 3 ROP with plus disease in zone II[15,16]

Earlier treatment of high-risk threshold ROP has been shown to reduce unfavorable structural outcomes, such as retinal folds involving the macula or retinal detachment involving the macula later in life.[17] Treatment involves laser therapy or anti-VEGF (vascular endothelial growth factor) therapy.

▷ **Trauma**

A child with a ruptured globe is an emergency and must undergo surgical repair within several hours of the injury.

An important consideration is avoiding increases in IOP that may occur with anxiety provoking for IV placement and induction. Premedication with oral midazolam and use of topical anesthetics may be useful for IV placement and a modified rapid sequence induction using a nondepolarizing neuromuscular blocker can be used for induction in the emergent case that is not NPO.[4] Succinylcholine may also be used with precurarization to prevent fasciculations and subsequent increase in IOP.

ANESTHESIA FOR EYE PROCEDURES

Premedication of children prior to eye surgery can include oral midazolam (usually 0.25–0.5 mg/kg, max 10–15 mg) with effect reached between 10 to 20 minutes.[18] Other options include oral valium, intranasal midazolam (0.2 mg kg, max

Table 15-3. Common Topical Medications

Drug Class	Drug Names	Uses	Side Effects
Beta-blockers	Timolol Betaxolol Levobunolol	Decrease IOP by decreased aqueous humor production	Caution in children with asthma
Carbonic anhydrase inhibitors	Dorzolamide brinzolamide	Decrease IOP by decreased aqueous humor production	No systemic side effects, metallic taste
Alpha agonists	Brimonidine, apraclonidine	Decrease IOP by decreased aqueous humor production and increased outflow from eye	Brimonidine (crosses blood-brain barrier)–bradycardia, respiratory depression, hypothermia, lethargy in infants
Beta agonists	Dipivefrin	Decrease IOP	No side effects–least potent
Parasympathomimetics	Pilocarpine	Decrease IOP by increased outflow from eye	Pain with use, headaches, blurry vision
Alpha 1 agonist	Phenylephrine 2.5%	Mydriasis	Increased blood pressure
Anticholinergic	Atropine 0.5%	Cycloplegia, mydriasis	Tachycardia, fever, flushing, delirium
Anticholinergic	Cyclopentolate 0.5%	Cycloplegia, mydriasis	Inhibits cholinesterase in vitro, caution with succinylcholine
Anticholinergic	Tropicamide 0.5%	Cycloplegia, mydriasis	No side effects

Table 15-4. Strabismus Surgical Procedures

Resection	Strengthening muscle by tightening
Recession	Weakening muscle by transection or moving insertion posteriorly
Transposition	Changing action of muscle by moving insertion site

10 mg), or intranasal dexmedetomidine (1–2 mcg/kg). Preoperative assessment should include a thorough airway assessment as ocular problems can be associated with diseases that may involve difficult airways, such as Pierre Robin syndrome, Treacher Collins syndrome, Apert syndrome, Crouzon disease, mucopolysaccharidosis, and glycogen storage disease.[8]

Pediatric patients mostly require general anesthesia for ophthalmologic procedures and commonly will have a mask induction with nitrous oxide and sevoflurane. Depending on the patient, duration of procedure, and comorbidities, a supraglottic device or intubation with an endotracheal tube may be used. Frequently, the pediatric ophthalmologist will measure the IOP prior to any further procedure. This can be accomplished immediately after general anesthesia has been induced and when adequate deep state has been established. General anesthesia is then maintained with volatile anesthetics, opioids, and neuromuscular blockade, if needed. As described earlier, the OCR frequently occurs in pediatric patients undergoing eye surgery and protection against this can be accomplished with pretreatment with atropine 0.02 mg/kg up to 0.6 mg or glycopyrrolate 0.01mg/kg.[8] If a patient does have bradycardia from the OCR, the inciting stimulus should be stopped and then atropine 0.01 to 0.02 mg/kg can be administered. If inert gas (sulfur hexafluoride, SF_6) is inserted into the eye after a retinal procedure, nitrous oxide should be avoided.

Premature infants needing therapy for ROP are a distinct population with unique considerations. Numerous anesthetic techniques have been employed including topical anesthesia, sedation, and general anesthesia. A study of 97 treatments comparing topical anesthesia, general anesthesia (GA), and fentanyl infusion showed greater cardiorespiratory instability in patients treated with topical anesthesia.[19] Intubation allows for less movement, more stability, and improved ability to complete the treatment with good pain relief.[20] However, this may result in prolonged intubation, especially in the setting of chronic lung disease, and has led some to utilize sedation with nasopharyngeal long prongs.[21] Patient history and comorbidities, individual center personnel availability (neonatologist, pediatric anesthesiologist), procedure location (neonatal intensive care unit, operating room), and coordination with ophthalmologist all must be taken into consideration when planning for these patients.

Caution should be used at the end of the operation to avoid coughing. To prevent this challenge, deep extubation

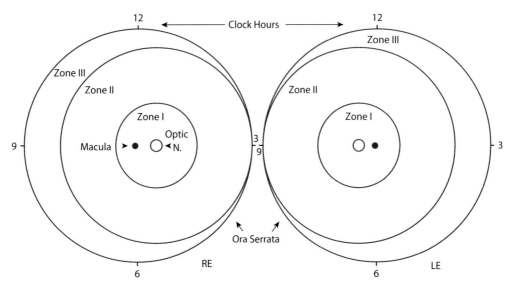

▲ **Figure 15-3.** Zones of the retina. (Reproduced with permission, from Kline MW, ed. *Rudolph's Pediatrics*, 23rd ed. 2018. https://accesspediatrics.mhmedical.com. Copyright © McGraw Hill LLC. All rights reserved.)

with spontaneous breathing and stage 3 anesthesia has been utilized by many pediatric anesthesiologists. Others have used lidocaine at 1.5 mg/kg intravenously prior to extubation.

A significant postoperative consideration for ophthalmic procedures includes prophylaxis for postoperative nausea and vomiting (PONV). Pediatric patients undergoing strabismus surgery have a high rate of PONV, ranging from 40% to 90%.[22,23] Ondansetron has been shown to decrease rates of PONV.[24-27] Combination therapies such as ondansetron and dexamethasone are also effective.[28] Other agents such as scopolamine patch, diphenhydramine, and droperidol also decrease PONV but can have side effects such as sedation.[8,24,28] Combination prophylaxis therapy of dexamethasone and ondansetron has also been shown to decrease the risk of PONV compared to either agent alone.[29]

REFERENCES

1. Moeller H. Milestones and normative data. In: Lambert S, Lyons C, eds. *Pediatr Ophthalmol.* London: Blackwell Scientific; 2017:40-49.
2. Riordan-Eva P. Anatomy and embryology of the eye. In: Riordan-Eva P, Augsburger JJ, eds. *Vaughan & Asbury's General Ophthalmology.* 19th ed. New York: McGraw-Hill.
3. Pensiero, Da Pozzo S, Perissutti P. Normal intraocular pressure in child. *J Pediatr Ophthalmol Strabismus.* 1992;29:79.
4. Ricketts K, Valley RD, Bailey AG, Justice LT. Smith's Anesthesia for Infants and Children, 2017; 34: 892-912
5. Ruta U, Möllhoff T, Markodimitrakis H, Brodner G. Attenuation of the oculocardiac reflex after topically applied lignocaine during surgery for strabismus in children. *Eur J Anaesthesiol.* 1996;11.
6. Allen LE, Sudesh S, Sandramouli S, Cooper G. The association between the oculocardiac reflex and post-operative vomiting in children undergoing strabismus surgery. *Eye.* 1998;12:193.
7. Ducloyer J, Couret C, Magne C, et al. Prospective evaluation of anesthetic protocols during pediatric ophthalmic surgery. *Eur J Ophthalmol.* 2019;29(6):606-614.
8. Bissonette, Anderson BJ. *Pediatric Anesthesia: Basic Principles–State of Art-Future.* Shelton, CT: People's Medical Publishing House; 2011.
9. Hurwitz J. *The Lacrimal System.* Philadelphia, PA: Lippincott-Raven; 1996.
10. MacEwen CJ, Young JD. Epiphora during the first year of life. *Eye (Lond).* 1991;5(pt 5):596-600.
11. Abramson DH. Retinoblastoma: saving life with vision. *Annu Rev Med.* 2014;65:171-184.
12. Kaliki S, Shields CL. Retinoblastoma: achieving new standards with methods of chemotherapy. *Indian J Ophthalmol.* 2015;63(2):103-109.
13. Good WV, Hardy RJ, Dobson V, et al. The incidence and course of retinopathy of prematurity: findings from the early treatment for retinopathy of prematurity study. *Pediatrics.* 2005;116(1):15.
14. Screening examination of premature infants for retinopathy of prematurity. A joint statement of the American Academy of Pediatrics, the American Association for Pediatric Ophthalmology and Strabismus, and the American Academy of Ophthalmology. *Ophthalmology.* 1997;104:888.
15. The Committee for the Classification of Retinopathy of Prematurity. An international classification of retinopathy of prematurity. *Arch Ophthalmol.* 1984;102:1130-1134.
16. International Committee for the Classification of Retinopathy of Prematurity. The international classification of retinopathy of prematurity revisited. *Arch Ophthalmol.* 2005;123:991-999.

17. Good WV. The early treatment for retinopathy of prematurity study; structural findings at age 2 years. *Br J Ophthalmol.* 2006;90:1378-1382.
18. Cote CJ, Cohen IT, Suresh S, et al. A comparison of three doses of a commercially prepared oral midazolam syrup in children. *Anesth Analg.* 2002;94(1):37-43, table of contents.
19. Jiang JB, Strauss R, Luo XQ, et al. Anaesthesia modalities during laser photocoagulation for retinopathy of prematurity: a retrospective, longitudinal study. *BMJ Open.* 2017;7(1):7e013344.
20. Sato, et al. Multicenter observational study comparing sedation/analgesia protocols for laser photocoagulation treatment of retinopathy of prematurity. *J Perinatol.* 2015;35:965-969.
21. Woodhead DD, Lambert DK, Molloy DA, et al. Avoiding endotracheal intubation of neonates undergoing laser therapy for retinopathy of prematurity. *J Perinatol.* 2007;27(4):209-213.
22. Baines D. Postoperative nausea and vomiting in children. *Paediatr Anaesth.* 1996;6:7-14.
23. Kuhn I, Sheiffler G, Wissing H. Incidence of nausea and vomiting in children after strabismus surgery and postoperative vomiting in children after strabismus surgery following desflurane anesthesia. *Paediatr Anaesth.* 1999;9:521-526.
24. Tramér M, Moore A, McQuay H. Prevention of vomiting after paediatric strabismus surgery: a systemic review using the numbers to treat method. *Br J Anaesth.* 1995;75:556-561.
25. Patel RI, et al. Single-dose ondansetron prevents postoperative emesis in children. *Anesthesiology.* 1996;85:270-276.
26. Lawhorn CD, Stewart FC, Stoner JM, Shirey R, Volpe P, et al. Ondansetron dose response curve in high-risk pediatric patients. *J Clin Anesth.* 1997;9:637-642.
27. Patel RI, Davis PJ, Orr RJ, et al. Single-dose ondansetron prevents postoperative vomiting in pediatric outpatients. *Anesth Analg.* 1997;85:538-545.
28. Horimoto Y, Tomie H, Hanzawa K, Nishida Y. Scopolamine patch reduces postoperative emesis in paediatric patients following strabismus surgery. *Can J Anaesth.* 1991;38:441-444.
29. Shen YD, Chen CY, Wu CH, Cherng YG, Tam KW. Dexamethasone, ondansetron and their combination and postoperative nausea and vomiting in children undergoing strabismus surgery: a meta-analysis of randomized controlled trials. *Pediatric Anesthesia.* 2014;24:490-498.

Anesthesia for Otolaryngologic Procedures

Joseph Sisk

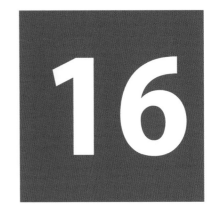

MYRINGOTOMY TUBES

FOCUS POINTS

1. Bilateral myringotomy tube placement is frequently a short case. Rapid turnover is usually expected.
2. Children presenting for bilateral myringotomy tube (BMT) placement may have an active or recent URTI. The risks and benefits of proceeding should be evaluated and discussed with the caregivers and surgeon.
3. Bilateral myringotomy tube placement is frequently done under inhalational anesthesia with mask ventilation. Peripheral IV access is not mandatory for otherwise healthy patients.
4. Nitrous oxide may be used to distend the tympanic membrane.
5. Children with trisomy 21 may have narrow ear canals, which increases the operative time. IV and laryngeal mask airway (LMA) placement may be appropriate.
6. Pain control may be achieved with nasal and IM medications supplemented by acetaminophen and/or ibuprofen.

INTRODUCTION

Ear, nose, and throat (ENT) surgery encompasses a wide variety of procedures, frequently short, taking as little as 5 minutes for uncomplicated myringotomy tubes. Given the brief nature of many pediatric ENT procedures, multiple surgeries are routinely scheduled in an operating room (OR), and a rapid turnover is often expected. ENT procedures carry a high incidence of airway complications, and a balance must be achieved between safety and efficiency. The anesthesia team must remain vigilant and be prepared to manage perioperative complications such as laryngospasm and bronchospasm. A factor that increases the risk of airway complications is that children presenting for ENT surgery are frequently experiencing or recovering from an upper respiratory tract infection (URTI). ENT procedures also vary in the amount of pain the patient may experience, from unstimulating brainstem auditory evoked response (BAER) evaluations to tonsillectomy and adenoidectomy surgeries. A wide variety of anesthesia techniques may be safely utilized for ENT procedures; however, there is no one "recipe" for each case and an anesthetic plan must be individualized to each patient and procedure.

As with any anesthetic, preoperative evaluation and physical examination should be performed, and any comorbid conditions should be medically optimized prior to proceeding with elective surgery. Preparation of the anesthesia workstation should include rescue medications and emergency airway management equipment.

Case

A 14-month-old girl presents for BMTs, 6 days after being diagnosed with acute otitis media, and has been taking antibiotics as prescribed by her pediatrician. The patient had been referred to an ENT surgeon for BMT placement after being treated for multiple episodes of acute otitis media in the preceding months. Discussion with the patient's family reveals that she was born at term and is otherwise healthy. The parents state that she has had multiple "ear infections" over the past several months, and it seems like she is "always fighting one." Physical exam reveals a playful, well-developed 14-month-old child with dried mucus in her bilateral nares. Cardiac and pulmonary auscultation are unremarkable and her vital signs are age-appropriate.

Background

Indications

Bilateral myringotomy tube placement is one of the most common surgical procedures performed in the United States. It may be performed for indications such as recurrent acute otitis media or chronic ear effusions.

Patient Considerations

Children presenting for bilateral myringotomy tube placement frequently present with an active case of acute otitis media or have recovered from such an infection within the past month. While all patients should be evaluated and medically optimized prior to proceeding with an anesthetic, it is also common for patients to present having recently experienced a URTI. Recent URTI increases the risk of laryngospasm, bronchospasm, and oxygen desaturation. A discussion of risks and benefits of proceeding should be held between the surgeon and the patient's parents or guardian. If it is unlikely that the patient will experience complete URTI recovery prior to onset of another URTI, consideration should be given to proceeding while taking actions to minimize the risk of airway reactivity intraoperatively.[1,2] Tait and Malviya have proposed an algorithm for assessment and management of a child with a URTI, which may be useful in determining whether to proceed with an anesthetic (Figure 16-1).

Specific consideration should also be given to the patient's comorbid conditions. Children with trisomy 21 may have atlantoaxial instability, and care should be taken when manipulating the patient's head for surgical exposure. Some surgeons and anesthesiologists opt to brace the patient's head in place while tilting the entire surgical table to facilitate exposure. Additionally, children with trisomy 21 commonly have narrow ear canals, leading to a technically difficult procedure. If a prolonged procedure is expected, consideration should be given to obtaining intravenous access and placing a LMA.[3]

Anesthetic Management

While it is common to defer IV access during this brief procedure, IV access equipment should be readily available.

Children less than 10 months of age are unlikely to experience separation anxiety and do not routinely require anxiolysis. Above this age, preoperative anxiolysis may be achieved using a variety of means. Distraction is an effective means of managing some children. The use of toys, videos, or pretend-plays, such as having the child breathe into the mask to "blow up the balloon," may be enough to ensure a smooth induction. Alternatively, consideration may be given to having a parent present at induction. The benefit to the child should be weighed against the risk of the parent becoming distressed or disruptive during induction of anesthesia. Parents should be briefed on the physical signs of the excitement stage and reassured that these

signs are normal for the child's age. Sedative medications may also be employed. Oral midazolam (0.3–0.5 mg/kg) is appropriate for anxious or combative children but may result in delayed emergence and an extended PACU stay following a brief procedure.[4]

Standard American Society of Anesthesiologists (ASA) monitors should be utilized. An inhalational induction with a mixture of nitrous oxide, oxygen, and gradually increased sevoflurane is the most commonly used combination, although preoperative IV placement and IV induction may be considered for larger children. After the child passes through the excitement stage (Table 16-1), the patient may be maintained with sevoflurane volatile anesthetic administered via a facemask. The surgeon may request the use of nitrous oxide to cause the tympanic membranes to bulge, allowing for easier tympanostomy. The procedure is most commonly performed in the supine position with the bed unturned. Tympanostomy requires a still surgical field; if mask ventilation is difficult or there is a need to switch hands, clear communication with the surgeon is required to avoid accidental movement of the field as the surgeon incises the tympanic membrane. There are no procedure-specific hemodynamic or physiologic goals and blood loss is usually negligible.

Postoperative pain may be managed using a number of options. Administration of fentanyl (1–2 mcg/kg) via a nasal atomizer is common. Additionally, intramuscular (IM) injections of morphine (0.1 mg/kg) and/or ketorolac (0.5 mg/kg) may be used. Oral acetaminophen (10–15 mg/kg) or ibuprofen (10 mg/kg) may be given preoperatively or in the recovery room. Most patients do not have postoperative pain significant enough to require IV narcotics in the post-anesthesia care unit (PACU). Older children, or those with a history of postoperative nausea and vomiting (PONV), may benefit from post-induction peripheral IV placement and the administration of PONV prophylactic medications such as dexamethasone (0.3–0.5 mg/kg) and ondansetron (0.1–0.15 mg/kg).

Appropriately selected patients may be taken to the PACU in a deep plane of anesthesia while breathing spontaneously. Recovery room staff must be familiar with the management of an emerging patient, and be trained in the identification and management of airway obstruction if emergence is to occur in the PACU. Patients experiencing signs of increased airway reactivity or airway obstruction should be emerged from anesthesia under care of an anesthesia provider skilled in airway management with emergency airway equipment readily available.

Common complications during BMT placement are primarily airway related, such as upper airway obstruction, bronchospasm, and laryngospasm. Upper airway obstruction may be secondary to large, obstructing tonsils, abnormal airway anatomy, or excessive soft tissue secondary to obesity. Jaw thrust and oral airway placement are first-line management techniques, although placement of an LMA or endotracheal tube (ETT) may be necessary.

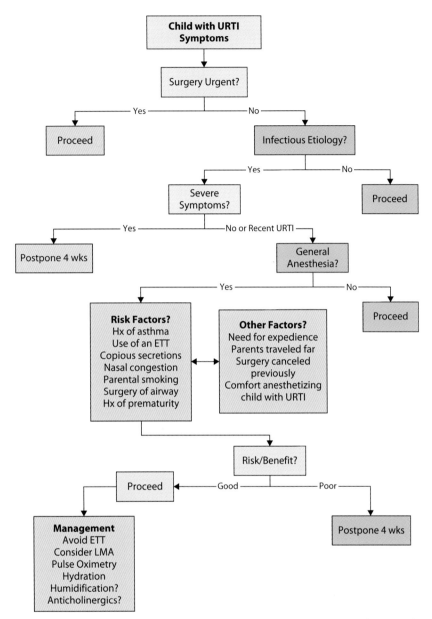

▲ **Figure 16-1.** Algorithm for assessment and management of a child with URTI. (Reproduced with permission, from Tait AR, Malviya S. Anesthesia for the Child with an Upper Respiratory Tract Infection: Still a Dilemma? *Anesthesia & Analgesia.* 2005;100(1), 59-65. https://journals.lww.com/anesthesia-analgesia.)

Partial laryngospasm may present with signs such as stridor and neck retraction, while complete laryngospasm may present with absent air movement with or without signs of respiratory effort. This most commonly occurs during the second stage of anesthesia when airway reflexes are the most disinhibited. Continuous positive airway pressure (CPAP) delivered via facemask is frequently enough to break laryngospasm and is considered first-line.

Care should be taken to avoid high CPAP pressures as gastric insufflation may occur with continuous pressures greater than 12-cm H_2O.[5] Intramuscular succinylcholine (2–4 mg/kg) may be given to break laryngospasm if it is unresponsive to nonpharmacologic management. Given the high parasympathetic tone in young children, it is common to co-administer IM atropine (0.02 mg/kg) if IM succinylcholine is given. If IV access is present, IV

Table 16-1. Classic Stages and Planes of Inhalational Anesthesia

- **Stage 1** is defined as the time between the normal waking state and the loss of consciousness (**hypnosis**) caused by an anesthetic agent. There is also mild **analgesia** in stage 1 anesthesia.
- **Stage 2** is associated with loss of awareness and recall (**amnesia**). Stage 2 is associated with the undesired effects of cardiovascular instability, excitation, dysconjugate ocular movements, and emesis.
- **Stage 3** is defined as surgical anesthesia, a state during which **movement in response to pain is suppressed**. Various planes of anesthesia were described by Guedel[*] based on additional physiological signs:
  - o **Plane 1** is associated with deep respiration, coordinated thoracic and diaphragmatic muscular activity, and pupillary constriction.
  - o **Plane 2** is associated with diminished respiration, as well as fixed midline and dilated pupils.
  - o **Plane 3** is associated with continued diaphragmatic movement, diminished thoracic movement, and further pupillary dilation.
  - o **Plane 4** is associated with thoracic immobility and diminished diaphragmatic movement.
- **Stage 4** is associated with cessation of spontaneous respiration and medullary cardiac reflexes and may lead to death.

[*]Guedel A. *Inhalation Anaesthesia: A Fundamental Guide.* New York: Macmillan; 1937.
Source: Reproduced with permission, from Longnecker DE, Mackey SC, Newman MF, et al. eds. *Anesthesiology.* 3rd ed. 2018. https://accessanesthesiology.mhmedical.com. Copyright © McGraw Hill LLC. All rights reserved.

succinylcholine (0.25–1 mg/kg) may be administered. An IV bolus of an induction agent such as propofol (1–2 mg/kg) may also break laryngospasm; however, this requires enough induction agent to move the nearly emerged patient to a deeper plane of anesthesia and will require the patient to reenter stage 2 of anesthesia, with a possible recurrence of laryngospasm as he emerges a second time.[6]

Bronchospasm should also be considered on the differential when the patient experiences airway obstruction. It may be identified by a "shark fin" appearance of the end-tidal carbon dioxide ($EtCO_2$) waveform. Auscultation of the chest may demonstrate wheezing or absent air entry in the setting of severe bronchospasm. A recent URTI increases the predisposition to airway reactivity including both bronchospasm and laryngospasm. Avoiding airway instrumentation may decrease these risks.[1] Bronchospasm may be treated with deepening the inhaled anesthetic and administration of inhaled albuterol if air movement is not significantly impaired. Severe bronchospasm may impair the delivery of volatile anesthetic and inhaled albuterol. In this situation, a bolus of IV epinephrine (0.5–1 mcg/kg) is appropriate and may be repeated until symptoms improve.[7]

Emergence delirium is common with short procedures involving a rapid emergence from anesthesia. This disassociated state may present as an incoherent, screaming, and thrashing child who refuses to make eye contact. Movement is non-purposeful but may be violent. In addition to causing distress among caregivers, violent thrashing may result in the child inadvertently injuring himself or dislodging IV lines.[8] Allowing the patient to recover from a deep plane of anesthesia in PACU decreases this incidence. Intraoperative IV placement and prophylactic IV dexmedetomidine (0.5 mcg/kg bolus) should be considered for high-risk patients. Nasal fentanyl has been shown to effectively treat emergence delirium in patients without peripheral IV access.[8–10]

Our Case

The child is brought to the OR and standard ASA monitors are placed. A mask induction is performed using nitrous oxide and progressively increased sevoflurane. Upon achieving an adequate depth of anesthesia, fentanyl (1 mcg/kg) is administered nasally using an atomizer and ketorolac (0.5 mg/kg) is administered intramuscularly to the left deltoid. An oral airway is placed, and the airway is maintained with mask ventilation throughout the procedure. Upon completion of the procedure, the patient is placed in the left lateral decubitus position. She is then taken to the recovery room in a deep plane of anesthesia while breathing spontaneously, where she emerges from her anesthetic without issue. Her recovery stay is uneventful, and she is discharged after receiving oral acetaminophen and tolerating a popsicle.

BRAINSTEM AUDITORY EVOKED RESPONSE (BAER)

FOCUS POINTS

1. BAER evaluation is performed in patients with suspected hearing impairment.
2. An ear examination under anesthesia (EUA) and BMT may precede the BAER study.
3. BAER evaluation is not painful, and the lack of stimulation may lead to relative hypotension.
4. Patients with recent meningitis or recurrent ear infections may display URTI symptoms with increased airway reactivity during the BAER study.
5. While volatile anesthesia does not affect the quality of the study, OR noise can have a negative impact on the results.

Case

A 3-year-old boy presents for a BAER evaluation under general anesthesia. He has a past medical history significant for being unvaccinated and he experienced haemophilus influenzae type B meningitis approximately 6 weeks ago with full symptom resolution 4 weeks prior to presentation. A BAER evaluation has been ordered due to concerns of hearing loss secondary to meningitis. Preoperative vital signs are appropriate for the patient's age and physical exam demonstrates an anxious child who appears fearful of medical staff but is otherwise unremarkable. The parents say that the child developed a fear of medical staff during his hospital stay.

Background

Indications

A BAER evaluation is a common study when there is concern for hearing impairment. Patients presenting for BAER have frequently failed an initial hearing screen or may have suffered a neurological insult, such as meningitis, that is suspected to have damaged the patient's hearing. BAER may also be performed to accurately assess hearing impairment in anticipation of cochlear implant placement.[11]

Patient Considerations

Patients presenting for BAER evaluation under general anesthesia are unable to participate in traditional hearing exams. This may be due to young age or other intellectual disabilities. Of note, patients presenting for BAER evaluation following meningitis may have active or recent URTI symptoms which can increase airway reactivity. BAER is frequently combined with an ear EUA. If an effusion is noted at the time of ear EUA, myringotomy tubes may be placed prior to the exam to ensure the accuracy of the results.

Anesthetic Management

If needed, anxiolytic premedication may be given without impacting the quality of the study.

Anesthesia may be induced with volatile anesthetic followed by peripheral IV placement. The airway can be maintained using a LMA for most patients. Anesthesia may be maintained with volatile anesthetic without impacting the quality of the study. Alternatively, total intravenous anesthesia (TIVA) with propofol infusion may be administered with either a natural airway or an LMA.

Of note, auditory-evoked responses are less susceptible to the effects of volatile anesthesia when compared to sensory or motor-evoked responses. Electrode placement may be stimulating, but the procedure itself has minimal postoperative pain. PONV and emergence delirium prophylaxis should be considered in appropriate patients.

As with most procedures, standard ASA monitors should be employed during the anesthetic. While BAER evaluation results are resistant to the effects of volatile anesthesia, noises in the OR can impact the quality of the study. Monitor volume should be minimized, and the OR should remain quiet while the procedure is in progress. As the procedure is not painful, relative hypotension may occur due to deep anesthesia. This frequently resolves with IV fluid administration and a decreased depth of anesthesia. Blood products are generally not indicated. Upon completion of the study, appropriate patients may be extubated and taken to PACU in a deep plane of anesthesia. Most patients are discharged to home the same day as the procedure.

Our Case

Given the patient's anxiety, oral midazolam (0.5 mg/kg) is administered and the patient is observed until effective anxiolysis is achieved (about 10–20 minutes). The patient is brought to the OR and anesthesia is induced using nitrous oxide and slowly increasing concentrations of sevoflurane. A peripheral IV is obtained and an LMA is placed successfully. Monitor volume is decreased to minimal levels, and the audiologist performs the BAER evaluation. Relative hypotension is noted during the case, but this resolves with IV fluid administration and decreased inspired sevoflurane concentrations. Upon completion of the exam, the patient's LMA is removed under deep anesthesia with spontaneous ventilation and the patient is taken to the recovery room where he emerges uneventfully.

TONSILLECTOMY AND ADENOIDECTOMY

FOCUS POINTS

1. Tonsillectomy and adenoidectomy (T&A) surgery is frequently a short case with a rapid turnover expected.
2. Children with recurrent tonsillitis may have recently recovered from a URTI and are at increased risk of airway reactivity.
3. Children with severe obstructive sleep apnea (OSA) are prone to postoperative airway obstruction and are very susceptible to the respiratory suppressant effects of narcotic medications. Adjuvant analgesics should be maximized in this population. If utilized, long-acting narcotics should be dosed with caution.
4. Any airway surgery involving electrocautery or laser carries a risk of airway fire.
5. Deep extubation helps prevent coughing and may decrease bronchospasm during emergence and emergence delirium postoperatively. It should be avoided in patients with moderate to severe OSA and in those with difficult mask ventilation or intubation.

Case

A 4-year-old girl with history of loud snoring presents for T&A surgery. Overnight polysomnography demonstrated an apnea hypopnea index (AHI) of 25 with a minimum oxygen saturation (SpO_2) of 74%. Discussion with the patient's family reveals that she was born at term and is otherwise healthy. They affirm that the child snores loudly on a nightly basis. She has been observed having apneic episodes which resolve spontaneously, and the family observes that she regularly experiences daytime somnolence. Airway examination reveals grade 4 "kissing" tonsils. Physical exam reveals a well-developed 4-year-old. Cardiac and pulmonary auscultations are unremarkable, and her vital signs are age appropriate.

Background

Indications

Tonsillectomy and adenoidectomy is one of the most common surgical procedures performed on children. It may be performed as a treatment for recurrent tonsillitis or for the management of obstructive sleep apnea (OSA) in children. Children presenting for T&A due to recurrent tonsillitis may have recently experienced a URTI, which entails an increase in airway reactivity. Children presenting for T&A due to obstructive sleep apnea have increased incidence of airway obstruction during mask ventilation and often demonstrate increased sensitivity to the respiratory suppressant effects of narcotic medications. If performed, a polysomnography study allows quantification and stratification of this risk:

	Apnea Hypopnea Index (AHI)	Oxygen Saturation (%)
Mild OSA	2–5	88–92
Moderate OSA	5–10	80–88
Severe OSA	>10	<80

Children with severe OSA are at particular risk of postoperative airway obstruction and apnea. It is policy at many centers to observe children with severe OSA or children under the age of 2 years overnight prior to discharge home.[12-15]

Anesthetic Management

Preoperative anxiolysis may be managed as described in the myringotomy tubes section; however, sedative premedications should be used with caution in children with severe OSA. Standard ASA monitors should be used. IV induction or inhalational induction followed by peripheral IV placement may be performed as clinically indicated. Endotracheal intubation is commonly performed with a cuffed endotracheal tube (either straight or RAE) taped midline down the chin. Care should be taken to ensure that the endotracheal tube follows this midline course in the mouth and does not deviate to the side as retractor placement may then lead to unintentional extubation.

Anesthesia may be maintained with volatile anesthesia; however, nitrous oxide should be used with caution and the FiO_2 should be kept below 30%, as both gases support oxidation which increases the risk of airway fire. Airway fire is a potential hazard of any oral surgery involving electrocautery or laser. The "Fire Triad" describes the three sources required to allow a fire:

1. An oxidizing agent: Both oxygen and nitrous oxide may serve as oxidizing agents allowing the propagation of an OR fire.
2. An ignition source: Surgical electrocautery or laser can ignite an OR fire.
3. A fuel source: Endotracheal tubes, pledgets, and surgical drapes may all act as fuel for an OR fire.

The anesthesia team should notify the surgical team of the FiO_2 in use prior to the activation of electrocautery or a laser in proximity to the airway. A "surgical fire" checklist (Figure 16-2) should be discussed with the OR team prior to starting such a case.

Airway fire is an emergency and should be managed with swift action. The surgeon should flood the field with saline or water, gas flow should be immediately disconnected, and the endotracheal tube should be immediately removed. Termination of gas flow may be accomplished by disconnecting the anesthesia circuit from the anesthesia machine ensuring that a "blowtorch" effect is avoided as the trachea is extubated. Once the fire has been extinguished, the airway should be reintubated and evaluated with fiberoptic bronchoscope to ensure that the trauma of the burn does not result in complete airway obstruction.[16]

During T&A procedures, the patient is frequently positioned supine with the table rotated 90 degrees. To allow surgical exposure, the patient is then placed in suspension for the procedure. There are no procedure-specific hemodynamic goals for T&A surgery. Blood loss is usually minimal during T&A surgery; however, patients with known coagulopathies should be evaluated and optimized in consultation with a hematologist prior to T&A surgery.

It is common to give intraoperative dexamethasone (0.2–0.5 mg/kg), although doses vary significantly by institution and surgeon. The steroid serves to decrease airway edema following surgery while simultaneously acting as an antiemetic. T&A surgery has a high incidence of PONV. Opioid pain medications, volatile anesthetics, and swallowed blood all increase the risk of nausea and vomiting. Additionally, surgical stimulation of the glossopharyngeal nerve acts as a potent stimulus of nausea and vomiting. Ondansetron (0.1–0.15 mg/kg) is frequently given in combination with dexamethasone to minimize PONV.[17]

Start Here

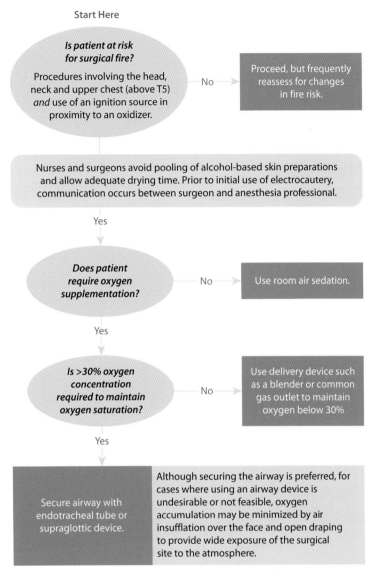

Figure 16-2. Operating room fire prevention algorithm. (Reproduced with permission, from Anesthesia Patient Safety Foundation. 2014. www.apsf.org. Copyright © Anesthesia Patient Safety Foundation. All rights reserved.)

Narcotic pain medications are a mainstay of intraoperative pain control, but should be used with caution in children with severe OSA. While children presenting for T&A for the management of recurrent tonsillitis may benefit from long-acting narcotics such as morphine (0.1 mg/kg) or hydromorphone (0.02 mg/kg), children with severe obstructive sleep apnea may be at risk for prolonged apnea and airway obstruction following administration of those drugs. In addition to short-acting narcotics such as fentanyl (1–2 mcg/kg), a multimodal pain medication regimen should be employed. Acetaminophen (10–15 mg/

kg oral or IV), surgical administration of local anesthetic, and ketorolac (0.5 mg/kg), if not surgically contraindicated, are some of the more commonly utilized adjuvants. IV dexmedetomidine (0.5 mcg/kg bolus) decreases opioid requirements but may also delay emergence and extubation. Consideration should be given to reserving dexmedetomidine administration for selected cases.

Tonsillectomy does not immediately cure the patient of OSA symptoms. Edema at the surgical site may duplicate or surpass the degree of obstruction caused by the enlarged tonsils. Additionally, surgical alleviation of the chronic airway obstruction does not immediately reduce the increased sensitivity to narcotics caused by chronic CO_2 retention.

The brief nature of T&A surgery, along with the associated pain, makes emergence delirium very common. Deep extubation for appropriately selected patients, along with boluses of IV dexmedetomidine (0.5 mcg/kg) or propofol (1 mg/kg at the end of the procedure), is the mainstay of emergence delirium prophylaxis. IV dexmedetomidine (0.5–1 mcg/kg) may also be utilized as a rescue agent in PACU if emergence delirium is suspected.[8–10]

The decision to extubate deep versus after complete emergence from anesthesia should be based on several factors. Patients with difficult mask ventilation or intubation should not be extubated deep, as rescue of the airway may be challenging. Consideration should be given to performing an awake extubation on children with documented moderate to severe OSA. Children at risk for bronchospasm, such as those suffering from a recent or active URTI, asthma, or bronchopulmonary dysplasia, may benefit from deep extubation. If there is high concern for a post-extubation airway event in a child that would benefit from deep extubation, consideration should be given to a deep extubation followed by emergence from anesthesia in the OR with mask ventilation.

Children undergoing T&A surgery should be observed in the PACU until they have recovered from the acute effects of general anesthesia. During this time, they should be observed for signs of acute postoperative tonsillar bleeding. Pain medication should be titrated to patient comfort and the child observed for signs of airway obstruction and apnea. Children should also be evaluated for tolerance of oral liquid intake prior to discharge home. Children under the age of 2 and those suffering from severe OSA should be admitted for observation and apnea monitoring overnight.[12–15]

Tonsillectomy and adenoidectomy surgery has a large number of potentially serious complications. In addition to laryngospasm and bronchospasm, which are discussed in greater detail earlier in this chapter, post-extubation stridor is a concern. The proximity of the surgical site to the airway increases the risk of edema impairing air movement following extubation. Smaller children are more likely to experience stridor related to airway edema. The Hagen-Poiseuille equation describes how the resistance to flow in the airway is inversely proportional to the radius of the airway raised to the fourth power. The implication is that a small decrease in the airway radius raises resistance to flow exponentially. IV dexamethasone may limit airway edema when given prophylactically but takes time to effect (minimum 1–2 hours). Nebulized racemic epinephrine causes local vasoconstriction, making it an excellent rescue medication if airway edema causes symptomatic stridor.[5]

Surgical encroachment on the airway is a common pitfall of T&A surgeries. When the patient is placed in suspension, the endotracheal tube may become kinked or dislodged. Evaluation of a sudden change in ventilation or loss of ETO_2 should entail a systematic evaluation beginning with the patient and leading to the anesthesia machine. Concerns should be immediately communicated to the surgeon and prompt action taken once the source of the problem is identified.

Our Case

The child is brought to the OR and standard ASA monitors are placed. A mask induction is performed using nitrous oxide and progressively increasing sevoflurane. The patient is noted to be obstructing as mask ventilation is attempted. Placement of an oral airway alleviates the obstruction, and a peripheral IV is placed. Fentanyl (1 mcg/kg) and propofol (3 mg/kg) are administered intravenously and the airway is secured with a 4.5 oral endotracheal tube which is taped midline down the patient's chin. The table is then rotated 90 degrees and the surgeon places the patient in suspension for the procedure. Local anesthetic is injected to the surgical site prior to completion. Dexamethasone (0.25 mg/kg) and ondansetron (0.1 mg/kg) are then administered intravenously. Upon completion of the surgery, the volatile anesthetic is discontinued, and the patient is placed on 100% oxygen. Following several minutes of controlled ventilation, the patient emerges from anesthesia and is extubated. She then proceeds to scream and thrash wildly. During this time, she fails to make eye contact with the OR staff and does not verbalize any identifiable words. Dexmedetomidine (0.5 mcg/kg) is given as an IV bolus and the patient calms. She is taken to PACU on supplemental oxygen via facemask and SpO_2 monitoring. Upon arrival to PACU, she is snoring gently. During her recovery, she receives two doses of fentanyl (0.5 mcg/kg per dose) and oral acetaminophen (15 mg/kg). She is admitted to the hospital for observation and is discharged to home the following morning following an uneventful night.

DIRECT LARYNGOSCOPY/RIGID BRONCHOSCOPY

FOCUS POINTS

1. Direct laryngoscopy/bronchoscopy may entail anything from a brief diagnostic evaluation to a lengthy surgical intervention on the airway.
2. The "shared airway" requires constant and clear communication with the surgical team.
3. Direct laryngoscopy/rigid bronchoscopy is a very stimulating procedure, but postoperative pain is frequently minimal. The anesthetic plan should account for periods of brief, intense stimulation followed by abrupt absence of stimulation.

4. Procedures involving laser treatment of the airway require careful balance of the risk of airway fire with adequate oxygenation of the patient.
5. Beware of postoperative edema and airway obstruction in these cases.

Case

A 3-year-old boy presents for direct laryngoscopy and bronchoscopy to evaluate and treat subglottic stenosis. The patient has a medical history of prematurity, having been born at 27 weeks' gestation. He had a 12-week stay in the neonatal intensive care unit, spending the first eight weeks after birth on mechanical ventilation via an endotracheal tube. The patient was diagnosed with bronchopulmonary dysplasia and discharged on oxygen via nasal cannula. He was weaned off of oxygen in the subsequent months. The patient's parents note that he seems to have less airway reactivity as he has grown, but they are concerned about persistent stridor. Physical exam reveals a well-developed 3-year-old. Cardiac and pulmonary auscultation are unremarkable, but auscultation over the patient's neck reveals biphasic stridor.

Background

Indications

Direct laryngoscopy and bronchoscopy may be performed for a variety of indications. It may be used for diagnostic evaluation of the airway to diagnose laryngotracheomalacia, subglottic stenosis, and vascular rings, or to identify a tracheoesophageal fistula. Surgical interventions may also be performed during direct laryngoscopy/bronchoscopy. These interventions include supraglottoplasty for laryngomalacia, laser treatment of subglottic stenosis or papilloma, injection of laryngeal cleft, and/or removal of an airway foreign body.[5,12,18]

Patient Considerations

Patients presenting for direct laryngoscopy and bronchoscopy may have a high degree of airway obstruction at baseline. A detailed history of obstructive symptoms should be obtained prior to induction of general anesthesia. Additionally, patients frequently have comorbid conditions such as bronchopulmonary dysplasia. This increases airway reactivity and decreases the patient's tolerance of apnea.

Anesthetic Management

Induction of anesthesia should be performed in a way that maintains spontaneous ventilation. A mask induction with volatile anesthetic followed by peripheral IV placement frequently accomplishes this goal. Direct laryngoscopy/bronchoscopy procedures are frequently performed without endotracheal intubation and an open airway that is shared with the surgeon. The surgeon or anesthetist, prior to relinquishing the airway, will typically apply local anesthetic to the vocal cords using a laryngotracheal atomizer to help minimize the risk of laryngospasm. Direct laryngoscopy and bronchoscopy are both very stimulating. Anesthetic depth should be deep enough to prevent laryngospasm and bronchospasm, while accounting for the possibility that removal of stimulation may lead to apnea caused by the depth of anesthesia without the mitigating influence of stimulation.

There are many safe and effective options for maintenance of anesthesia, most relying on a combination of medications. As the surgeon evaluates the airway, volatile anesthesia may be insufflated through the rigid bronchoscope. Alternatively, a 4.0 to 5.0 uncuffed endotracheal tube placed into the posterior pharynx can be used to passively deliver oxygen and volatile anesthetic. As the airway is open to the room, consistent delivery of volatile anesthetic may be difficult to achieve, and intravenous anesthetic agents may be needed to supplement. Intravenous infusions of propofol, dexmedetomidine, or remifentanil may be titrated to reach an adequate depth of anesthesia. Boluses of ketamine, dexmedetomidine, and fentanyl have also been utilized effectively. Caution should be used when bolusing opioids, as this may trigger apnea. Boluses or infusions of dexmedetomidine have the added benefit of minimizing emergence delirium. Steroids such as dexamethasone should be considered to minimize airway edema and postoperative nausea and vomiting prophylaxis may be accomplished by administering ondansetron.

Standard ASA monitors should be utilized during direct laryngoscopy/bronchoscopy. End-tidal CO_2 monitoring may be unreliable with an open airway, and alternative means must be used to ensure adequate oxygenation and ventilation. Adequate ventilation can be confirmed by observation of chest rise or by use of a precordial stethoscope. Pulse oximetry may be used to verify adequacy of oxygenation.

As may be inferred by the nature of the surgery, airway obstruction is the most commonly encountered complication of direct laryngoscopy/bronchoscopy. Laryngospasm may occur due to light anesthesia or surgical manipulation of the vocal cords. An adequate depth of anesthesia and surgical topicalization of the vocal cords may help prevent this. Treatment of laryngospasm should involve deepening the anesthetic and positive pressure via mask ventilation if needed. Muscle relaxation may be considered in refractory cases, but this prevents the spontaneous ventilation required to facilitate the surgery.[5,12,18]

Bronchospasm during direct laryngoscopy and bronchoscopy arises most commonly in children predisposed to airway reactivity, such as those with asthma, bronchopulmonary dysplasia (BPD), or a recent URTI.

Surgical stimulation in the setting of light anesthesia may precipitate bronchospasm. Prevention of bronchospasm relies on optimization of conditions that predispose to it. Asthma and BPD should be well controlled prior to proceeding with elective surgery, and elective airway procedures should be delayed several weeks following the resolution of URTI symptoms. Bronchospasm may be challenging to treat in the setting of a shared airway. Use of inhaled bronchodilators such as albuterol is likely to be ineffective and should not delay the use of bolus IV epinephrine (0.5–1 mcg/kg) to treat bronchospasm.[7]

Direct surgical intervention on the airway increases the risk of edema impairing air movement during or after the procedure. Smaller children are more likely to experience stridor related to airway edema. The Hagen-Poiseuille equation dictates that the resistance to flow in the airway is inversely proportional to the radius raised to the fourth power. The implication is that a small decrease in the airway radius raises resistance to air flow exponentially. IV dexamethasone may limit airway edema when given prophylactically. Nebulized racemic epinephrine causes local vasoconstriction, making it an excellent rescue medication if airway edema causes symptomatic stridor. Patients should be observed for recurrence of stridor after racemic epinephrine administration. Inhaled helium-oxygen (Heliox) when available has less resistance to air-flow through edematous areas of the trachea and may be required as a supportive measure until airway edema resolves.[5,12]

Direct laryngoscopy/bronchoscopy entails uncommon stressors to the patient's physiology. Effective ventilation may be decreased as the patient hypoventilates during the procedure. Apneic oxygenation using passively insufflated 100% oxygen may serve to delay desaturation; however, removal of carbon dioxide is impaired during this process, and $PaCO_2$ will continue to rise until effective ventilation is restored. Decreased PaO_2 and increased $PaCO_2$ both serve to increase pulmonary vascular resistance. Children with existing pulmonary hypertension may experience a pulmonary hypertensive crisis in the setting of these physiologic derangements. The anesthetic plan should aim to minimize decreases in PaO_2 and increases in $PaCO_2$.

The nature of a "shared airway" anesthetic requires constant communication with the surgical team. As the surgeon is manipulating the airway, it is the responsibility of the anesthetic team to facilitate the operative intervention while balancing this against the physiologic stresses the surgery entails. As the patient becomes hypoxic and hypercarbic, it is the responsibility of the anesthesia team to notify the surgeon when surgical intervention must be paused to allow mask ventilation or temporary intubation to restore oxygenation and ventilation.

Airway surgical interventions may involve the use of a laser. In these situations, inspired oxygen and nitrous oxide concentrations should be minimized to decrease the risk of an airway fire (see the section "Tonsillectomy and Adenoidectomy").

Concern for postoperative airway obstruction should dictate the plans for postoperative disposition. Patients undergoing diagnostic bronchoscopy may be eligible for same-day surgery and discharge to home following their procedure, whereas prolonged procedures, and those with surgical intervention that may result in significant postoperative edema (such as supraglottoplasty), may require admission to the pediatric intensive care unit (PICU) for observation.

Our Case

The patient is taken to the OR and standard ASA monitors are placed. Anesthesia is induced with nitrous oxide and sevoflurane. The patient is transitioned to 100% oxygen and sevoflurane. Spontaneous ventilation is maintained. A peripheral IV is obtained with some difficulty, as the patient is noted to have significant scarring at previous IV sites. A propofol infusion is started at 100 mcg/kg/min. Dexmedetomidine (0.5 mcg/kg) is administered, along with dexamethasone (0.5 mg/kg). Once the patient achieves a stable plane of anesthesia, the bed is turned 90 degrees and the surgeon assumes mask ventilation. As the surgeon begins evaluating the airway, an uncuffed endotracheal tube is placed in the side of the mouth and oxygen and sevoflurane are insufflated into the open airway using 5 L/min fresh gas flows. End-tidal carbon dioxide ($EtCO_2$) is not reliably captured at this time, so ventilation and oxygenation are confirmed by visualization of open vocal cords during bronchoscopy, chest movement, and SpO_2 monitoring. The surgeon notes subglottic stenosis and decides to perform a laser excision of the scar tissue. The FiO_2 is decreased to 25% and the surgeon begins resection. Several times during the resection, the patient's SpO_2 falls into the mid-80s. Laser excision is paused, and the patient is assisted with mask ventilation and 100% FiO_2 until return of optimal oxygen saturation. The FiO_2 is then lowered and the resection resumed. This process is repeated several times before completion of the procedure. At that time, the patient is placed on 100% FiO_2 and emerged from anesthesia in the OR. He is taken to the recovery room where he is noted to have worsening stridor. Nebulized racemic epinephrine is administered and the patient is observed in the recovery room for 2 hours following resolution of the stridor. The patient is then admitted overnight for observation prior to discharge home.

AIRWAY FOREIGN BODY

FOCUS POINTS

1. The "shared airway" requires constant and clear communication with the surgical team.
2. Foreign bodies can traumatize the local airway and lead to persistent obstruction at the site of the foreign body.

3. Foreign bodies that have been in place for prolonged periods may lead to accumulation of purulent material that can contaminate the contralateral lung upon foreign body removal.
4. Direct laryngoscopy/bronchoscopy is a very stimulating procedure, but postoperative pain is frequently minimal. The anesthetic plan should account for periods of brief, intense stimulation followed by abrupt absence of stimulation.
5. Beware of postoperative edema and airway obstruction.

Case

An 18-month-old girl presents to the OR for emergent removal of an airway foreign body. Three hours prior, her parents noted that she was running with what appeared to be an almond in her mouth when she tripped and fell. After falling, the child immediately began to have increased work of breathing and was found to be wheezing audibly. The patient was taken to the emergency department, where a chest radiograph demonstrated a foreign body in the right mainstem bronchus with hyperinflation of the right lung. The patient has no significant medical or surgical history. The child was eating almonds at the time of the incident and has been NPO since then. Cardiac auscultation is unremarkable. Pulmonary auscultation demonstrates decreased air movement and wheezing on the right side. The patient appears tachypneic with increased work of breathing. Vital signs are significant for tachypnea and tachycardia with an oxygen saturation of 91% on pulse oximetry on room air. A 22-g peripheral IV is in place in the patient's right hand.

Background

An airway foreign body is typically the result of aspiration of food or other household items. Aspirated items may be found in the trachea, mainstem, or distal bronchi. In addition to mechanical obstruction, airway foreign bodies may cause physical or chemical trauma to the airway epithelium. Sharp or jagged objects may puncture the airway, and foods with oils, such as unroasted nuts, may cause significant inflammation and edema at the site. Sharp or irregularly shaped foreign bodies may also wedge themselves in the airway, making extraction particularly challenging.

While patients with stable respiratory symptoms may be observed and delayed to allow an appropriate NPO status, airway foreign body removals are frequently emergent. Large, obstructing objects can impair oxygenation and ventilation and serve as a "ball valve," trapping air and leading to hyperinflation of the affected lung and subsequent barotrauma. Urgent removal may be necessitated to prevent patient decompensation. Unfortunately, these patients frequently do not meet NPO criteria, which creates a dilemma for the anesthesia team.

Airway foreign body extraction frequently requires rigid bronchoscopy which cannot be accomplished with an endotracheal tube in situ. While most emergency surgeries on non-NPO patients allow for a rapid sequence induction (RSI), emergent airway foreign body removal frequently does not allow for rapid securing of the airway via endotracheal intubation. The risks and benefits of proceeding must be discussed and understood by the anesthesia team, surgeon, and patient's guardian. Fatal gastric content aspiration events have not been reported during airway foreign body removal, while progression of partial airway obstruction to total airway obstruction and acute decompensation of the patient has been reported. If all parties agree that the benefits of proceeding outweigh the risks, this discussion should be documented in the patient's medical record and the removal performed emergently.[12,18-22]

Anesthetic Management

A preoperative discussion should occur between the anesthesia team and the surgeon. This should include discussion of the surgical plan and an agreement on how this may best be facilitated by the anesthesia team. While endotracheal intubation may be optimal for protection against aspiration contents, this may prevent successful extraction of the foreign body and an open airway approach may be required. In this situation, emergency and contingency plans should be discussed, and any necessary equipment prepared. Suction should be readily available and the anesthesia team or surgeon should be prepared to rapidly secure the airway should reflux of gastric contents occur.

While the anesthetic management of a shared-airway procedure is discussed in the section "Direct Laryngoscopy/Rigid Bronchoscopy," this section will highlight the differences and considerations unique to airway foreign body removal.

When preparing for rigid bronchoscopy to facilitate airway foreign body removal, induction of anesthesia should be titrated to ensure maintenance of spontaneous respiration. An inhalational induction may be performed; however, the use of nitrous oxide should be limited, as nitrous oxide may accumulate behind the foreign body and worsen air trapping. Anesthesia maintenance may be accomplished using the same techniques described in the section "Direct Laryngoscopy/Rigid Bronchoscopy."

To facilitate removal of the foreign body, the surgeon may manipulate the head and neck to create a straight line from the oropharynx to the foreign body and allow easier extraction with rigid bronchoscopy. If the foreign body is wedged or in a distal bronchus, the extraction may be prolonged. Prolonged or traumatic extractions increase the risk of airway edema and subsequent airway obstruction.

Several complications are more common during airway foreign body removal. When NPO time has not been adequate, anesthesia personnel should constantly observe for reflux of gastric contents, and be prepared to immediately suction and secure the airway if any gastric contents are identified. Upon successful extraction of the foreign body, the airway may then be intubated and the patient extubated after fully emerging from anesthesia.

As the surgeon performs the extraction, total airway obstruction may occur if the foreign body lodges in the trachea and cannot be quickly removed. If ventilation becomes impossible and the foreign body cannot be immediately extracted, the surgeon should push the foreign body back down into a distal airway allowing ventilation of the contralateral lung.[21]

If air trapping is severe, or if the foreign body has punctured the airway, pneumothorax may occur. Preoperative anesthesia planning should include a discussion of how a possible pneumothorax will be decompressed intraoperatively. Foreign bodies may also cause tracheoesophageal fistulae via mechanical pressure, puncture, or caustic trauma. On rare occasions, a foreign body may erode into the adjacent pulmonary vasculature, resulting in catastrophic hemorrhage and exsanguination.

Finally, a prolonged obstruction of distal airways may cause pneumonia and allow the accumulation of purulent material distal to the obstruction. Upon removal of the foreign body, this purulent material may contaminate the contralateral lung and significantly impair oxygenation/ventilation.[22]

Patients with significant airway edema, gastric content aspiration, or pneumothorax may require observation in the PICU postoperatively, and severe cases may warrant postoperative ventilation. Generous steroid administration (dexamethasone 0.5 mg/kg) may help prevent post-extraction airway edema.

Our Case

Following a detailed discussion of the risks, benefits, and alternatives to proceeding emergently, the patient is given IV midazolam (0.1 mg/kg) and taken to the OR. A mask induction is performed using 100% oxygen and gradually increasing concentrations of sevoflurane. A propofol infusion is started through the existing Peripheral IV, and the patient reaches a stable plane of anesthesia. The bed is rotated 90 degrees, and the surgeon assumes control of the airway. IV dexamethasone (0.5 mg/kg) is administered prior to the start of the procedure. The surgeon performs a brief direct laryngoscopy and topically anesthetizes the vocal cords using lidocaine. The patient's heart rate is noted to increase during laryngoscopy and the patient's breathing becomes erratic. An IV bolus of dexmedetomidine (0.5 mcg/kg) is administered, and the patient returns to a stable plane of anesthesia. The patient is briefly masked, and the surgeon then places the patient in suspension. The anesthesia circuit is attached to the ventilating port of the rigid bronchoscope and the surgeon begins the procedure.

One-hundred percent oxygen and sevoflurane are administered via the bronchoscope as the surgeon examines the airway. An end-tidal CO_2 waveform is visible on the anesthesia monitor. Chest rise is observed, and the vocal cords are seen to be patent on the bronchoscope's video feed. Oxygen saturation via pulse oximetry measures 100%. Using the rigid bronchoscope, the surgeon identifies the almond in the right mainstem bronchus. The surgeon attempts to remove the foreign body using forceps but the almond slips from her grasp as it passes the carina. At this point, the end-tidal CO_2 waveform is lost, and the patient begins to desaturate. The surgeon immediately uses the bronchoscope to push the foreign body back into the right mainstem bronchus, resulting in return of adequate oxygenation and ventilation leading to the stabilization of the patient's vital signs. The subsequent attempt to remove the foreign body is successful. A post-extraction evaluation of the airway demonstrates edema at the site of the foreign body but no residual foreign body fragments or purulent material. Control of the patient's airway is returned to the anesthesia team, sevoflurane and propofol delivery are terminated, and the patient is emerged from general anesthesia in the OR and taken to the recovery room in stable condition. The patient is observed in a monitored bed overnight prior to being discharged to home the following day.

TRACHEOSTOMY

FOCUS POINTS

1. Surgical dissection with electrocautery necessitates lowering the FiO_2 to prevent airway fire.
2. Patients presenting for tracheostomy frequently have pulmonary hypertension. Hypoxia and hypercarbia may exacerbate this leading to a pulmonary hypertensive crisis.
3. Pulmonary hypertensive crisis may require inhaled nitric oxide to treat.
4. As the surgeon enters the airway, clear communication is essential to ensure a safe transition from ventilation through an endotracheal tube to ventilation through the new tracheostomy.
5. Adequate sedation should be utilized postoperatively to minimize risk of tracheostomy dislodgement.
6. In an emergency, reintubate from above.

Case

A 2-year-old, former 26-week-premature male infant is scheduled to come to the OR for tracheostomy. In addition to prematurity, the patient has a medical history significant for bronchopulmonary dysplasia (BPD) and a small ventricular septal defect (VSD), which the patient's cardiologist has been observing. The patient contracted respiratory syncytial virus (RSV) and experienced respiratory distress, requiring intubation and mechanical ventilation 3 weeks prior. The patient has failed to wean from the vent multiple times, and has been scheduled for a tracheostomy to facilitate long-term mechanical ventilation. An echocardiogram performed in the PICU demonstrated a small VSD with bidirectional flow across it, as well as evidence of moderate-to-severe pulmonary hypertension. Vital signs have been stable without vasopressor support, and ventilation parameters have remained stable for several days. Physical exam shows an underweight toddler who is sedated on mechanical ventilation. Cardiac auscultation demonstrates a grade 3 holosystolic murmur. Pulmonary auscultation demonstrates coarse breath sounds in the setting of mechanical ventilation. The patient is receiving intravenous fentanyl and midazolam infusions for sedation via a peripherally inserted central venous catheter line.

Background

Indications

Tracheostomy may be indicated for prolonged intubation with failure to extubate, chronic ventilator requirement secondary to neuromuscular disease or injury, and refractory airway obstruction, such as those seen in patients with some craniofacial syndromes. Tracheostomy may also be performed emergently in the setting of failed intubation with difficult mask ventilation or severe facial trauma.[12]

Patient Considerations

The indication for the tracheostomy frequently dictates the anesthetic course. Patients presenting for tracheostomy may have severe pulmonary disease with associated pulmonary hypertension, or they may have obstructive sleep apnea symptoms. The anesthetic plan should be tailored to account for the patient's comorbid conditions.

Severe lung disease is frequently associated with pulmonary hypertension secondary to chronic hypoxic pulmonary vasoconstriction, leading to pulmonary vasculature remodeling. Patients with severe pulmonary disease and pulmonary hypertension are less likely to tolerate the low inspired oxygen concentrations and the interrupted ventilation required for tracheostomy placement. In patients with pulmonary hypertension, the presence of an intracardiac shunt determines the observable signs of a pulmonary hypertensive crisis. A patient with a baseline intracardiac left-to-right or bidirectional shunt may demonstrate reversal of flow through the shunt as pulmonary vascular resistance rises. The new right-to-left shunt may be identified as systemic oxygen desaturation on pulse oximetry. This "pop-off" mechanism prevents increased pressure

being transmitted to the right heart and may prevent the right heart from failing while maintaining forward-flow through the systemic circulation. If no shunt exists, acute right heart failure and hemodynamic collapse may be the presenting signs of a pulmonary hypertensive crisis.

Anesthetic Management

As with any anesthetic, preoperative evaluation and physical exam should be performed and any comorbid conditions should be medically optimized prior to proceeding with elective surgery. Preparation of the anesthesia workstation should include rescue medications and emergency airway management equipment. If the patient has a known difficult airway, difficult airway management equipment should be present in the OR to allow management of a lost airway during the procedure. Patients presenting for tracheostomy are frequently already intubated and require transport from the PICU to the OR. Full transport monitoring, including end-tidal CO_2, should be employed and adequate assistance should be available to help manage any emergencies that arise during transport. Emergency airway equipment should accompany the patient and a plan for managing airway loss during transport should be considered. An emergency airway plan may involve reintubation, temporary placement of an LMA, or mask ventilation of the patient until the patient can be reintubated in a controlled environment.

Consideration should be given to administration of a nondepolarizing muscle relaxant prior to transport or prior to surgical incision. IV narcotics and supplemental volatile anesthetic may be used to attenuate the physiologic stress of the surgery. Patients receiving sedative or opioid medications in the PICU over prolonged periods may demonstrate tolerance and require increased doses of these medications intraoperatively.

Standard ASA monitors, including capnography, should be used during transport and the surgical procedure. Invasive monitors such as arterial blood pressure or CVP monitoring may be indicated if the patient's comorbid conditions dictate their use. Blood products are not routinely required for tracheostomy, but may be indicated if the patient has anemia or coagulopathy at baseline. Inhaled nitric oxide should be available for patients with preexisting pulmonary hypertension, as the stress of tracheostomy placement may precipitate a pulmonary hypertensive crisis.

Anesthesia may be induced with volatile anesthetic delivered through the patient's existing endotracheal tube. This may be supplemented by nondepolarizing muscle relaxants, benzodiazepine, opioids, and other sedative/hypnotic agents. Maintenance of anesthesia should avoid nitrous oxide as this increases the risk of airway fire.

The patient will be positioned supine for the procedure with a shoulder-roll in place to extend the neck and optimize surgical exposure. Inspired oxygen concentration should be limited during surgical dissection to limit the risk of airway fire. Close communication with the surgical team is essential throughout the procedure. As the surgeon enters the airway, the endotracheal tube will be retracted so the tip is proximal to the tracheal incision. A large air leak will develop at this time, and achieving adequate tidal volume ventilation may be challenging. The surgeon will then place the tracheostomy tube and the anesthesia circuit will be handed over the drapes and connected to the tracheostomy tube by the surgeon. A flexible "accordion" extension attached to the anesthesia circuit may be used to decrease the tension on the new tracheostomy. Ventilation should be immediately resumed, and confirmation of end-tidal CO_2 should be communicated to the surgeon prior to proceeding. If ventilation cannot be established via the new tracheostomy, oral endotracheal reintubation should be emergently performed as emergent tracheostomy replacement can result in intubation of a false passage.

Following completion of the surgical procedure, the patient should be returned to the PICU. Dislodgement of a fresh tracheostomy may be fatal; therefore, generous sedation with muscle relaxation is indicated.

Tracheostomy placement may involve several complications that the anesthesia team should be prepared to manage. Hypoxia may occur due to inadequate oxygen delivery during dissection, or it may be related to existing pulmonary disease. Patients with an underlying pulmonary infectious process that lead to chronic ventilator dependence may have residual airway hyperreactivity, and are more likely to experience bronchospasm. Hypoxia and hypercarbia increase pulmonary vascular resistance which may worsen pulmonary hypertension and trigger a pulmonary hypertensive crisis. Intraoperatively, this may require inhaled nitric oxide to treat. Airway loss during the procedure or during transport is a potentially fatal event. Attempting to blindly replace a fresh tracheostomy may result in intubation of a false passage and fiberoptic guidance is unlikely to be successful in the presence of bleeding. In the setting of dislodgement of a recently placed tracheostomy, oral endotracheal intubation should be urgently performed.[12]

Our Case

The patient is evaluated in the PICU and given a bolus of rocuronium (1 mg/kg) in preparation for transport. The patient is then transported to the OR with AMBU bag assist on full ASA monitors including capnography. Upon arrival to the OR, the patient is transferred to the anesthesia machine ventilator and connected to the standard ASA monitors, also on the anesthesia machine. Inhaled nitric oxide had been ordered and is connected to the anesthesia circuit. The patient's sedation infusions are continued, and sevoflurane is administered via the existing endotracheal tube. The inspired oxygen concentration is decreased to 30% and the patient's oxygen saturation via pulse oximetry stabilizes at 96%.

The patient is prepped and draped, and a surgical time-out is performed. The patient receives a bolus of fentanyl (1 mcg/kg) and the procedure begins. As the surgeon prepares to enter the trachea, the inspired oxygen concentration (FiO_2) is reduced to 21%. The surgeon enters the trachea and notes the endotracheal tube cuff distal to the tracheotomy. The endotracheal tube is retracted until the end of the tube is proximal to the surgical site. A large air leak is noted at this time, and the patient begins to desaturate. The surgeon places the tracheostomy tube and the anesthesia ventilator circuit is transferred from the endotracheal tube to the new tracheostomy. Ventilation is resumed and end-tidal CO_2 is noted to be present with tidal volumes similar to those achieved through the oral endotracheal tube. Oxygen saturation nadired at 82% but has failed to recover following return of ventilation despite increasing the FiO_2 to 100%, and despite adequate ventilation noted upon auscultation of breath sounds. At this point, a diagnosis of pulmonary hypertensive crisis with right-to-left shunting across the patient's VSD is considered. Inhaled nitric oxide is initiated at 20 ppm, and oxygen saturation returns to baseline shortly thereafter. The procedure finishes uneventfully. Prior to transport, an additional bolus of rocuronium (1 mg/kg) is administered and the patient is returned to the PICU using full monitors including capnography. The patient remains stable and the nitric oxide is successfully weaned off that evening.

REFERENCES

1. Tait AR, Malviya S. Anesthesia for the child with an upper respiratory tract infection: still a dilemma? *Anesth Analg.* 2005;100(1):59-65.
2. Tait A, Malviya S, Voepel-Lewis T, Munro HM, Seiwert M, Pandit UA. Risk factors for perioperative adverse respiratory events in children with upper respiratory tract infections. *Anesthesiology.* 2001;95(2):299-306.
3. Rosenfeld RM, Schwartz SR, Pynnonen MA, et al. Clinical practice guideline: tympanostomy tubes in children. *Otolaryngol Head Neck Surg.* 2013;149(1 suppl):S1-S35.
4. Sola C, Lefauconnier A, Bringuier S, Raux O, Capdevila X, Dadure C. Childhood preoperative anxiolysis: is sedation and distraction better than either alone? A prospective randomized study. *Pediatr Anesth.* 2017;27(8):827-834.
5. Holzman R. Airway management. In: PJ Davis and FP Cladis, eds. *Smith's Anesthesia for Infants and Children.* 8th ed. Philadelphia, PA: Elsevier; 2011:344-364.
6. Larson PC. Laryngospasm–the best treatment. *Anesthesiology.* 1998;89(5):1293-1294.
7. Woods BD, Sladen RN. Perioperative considerations for the patient with asthma and bronchospasm. *Brit J Anaesth.* 2009;103(suppl 1):i57-i65.
8. Malarbi S, Stargatt R, Howard K, Davidson A. Characterizing the behavior of children emerging with delirium from general anesthesia. *Pediatr Anesth.* 2011;21(9):942-950.
9. Rosen HD, Mervitz D, Cravero JP. Pediatric emergence delirium: Canadian pediatric anesthesiologists experience. *Pediatr Anesth.* 2015;26(2):207-212.

10. Zhu M, Wang H, Zhu A, Niu K, Wang G. Meta-analysis of dexmedetomidine on emergence agitation and recovery profiles in children after sevoflurane anesthesia: different administration and different dosage. *Plos One.* 2015;10(4):e0123728.

11. Litman R, Cohen D, Sclabassi R, et al. Monitoring. In: PJ Davis and FP Cladis, eds. *Smith's Anesthesia for Infants and Children.* 8th ed. Philadelphia, PA: Elsevier; 2011:341-342.

12. Landsman I, Werkhaven J, Motoyama E. Anesthesia for pediatric otorhinolaryngologic surgery. In: PJ Davis and FP Cladis, eds. *Smith's Anesthesia for Infants and Children.* 8th ed. Philadelphia, PA: Elsevier; 2011:786-820.

13. Clinical practice guideline: diagnosis and management of childhood obstructive sleep apnea syndrome. *Pediatrics.* 2002;109(4):704-712.

14. Brown K, Laferrière A, Lakheeram I, Moss IR. Recurrent hypoxemia in children is associated with increased analgesic sensitivity to opiates. *Anesthesiology.* 2006;105(4):665-669.

15. Schechter MS. Technical report: diagnosis and management of childhood obstructive sleep apnea syndrome. *Pediatrics.* 2002;109(4):e69.

16. Apfelbaum JL, Caplan RA, Barker SJ, et al. Practice advisory for the prevention and management of operating room fires. *Anesthesiology.* 2013;118(2):271-290.

17. Development and validation of a risk score to predict the probability of postoperative vomiting in pediatric patients: the VPOP score. *Pediatr Anesth.* 2015;25(3):330-330.

18. Nicolai T. Pediatric bronchoscopy. *Pediatr Pulmonol.* 2001;31(2):150-164.

19. Mani N, Soma M, Massey S, Albert D, Bailey CM. Removal of inhaled foreign bodies—middle of the night or the next morning? *Int J Pediatr Otorhinolaryngol.* 2009;73(8):1085-1089.

20. Fidkowski CW, Zheng H, Firth PG. The anesthetic considerations of tracheobronchial foreign bodies in children: a literature review of 12,979 cases. *Anesth Analg.* 2010;111:1016.

21. Kendigelen P. The anaesthetic consideration of tracheobronchial foreign body aspiration in children. *J Thorac Dis.* 2016;8(12):3803-3807.

22. Tomaske M, Gerber AC, Weiss M. Anesthesia and periinterventional morbidity of rigid bronchoscopy for tracheobronchial foreign body diagnosis and removal. *Pediatr Anesthes.* 2006;16(2):123-129.

Anesthesia for Cardiovascular Procedures

Katherine L. Zaleski, Maricarmen Roche Rodriguez, and Viviane G. Nasr

17

FOCUS POINTS

1. Fetal cardiac development begins at approximately 22 days of gestation. The fetal circulation allows for preferential shunting of oxygenated blood to the brain and heart.
2. Beginning at birth, the cardiovascular system undergoes drastic physiological changes as it transitions from a parallel to a series circulation. In the transitional circulation, the fetal shunts (ductus arteriosus, ductus venosus, and foramen ovale) close functionally and eventually, anatomically.
3. Normal vital signs value change with age, reaching adult values in adolescence.
4. Congenital heart disease is the most common form of birth defect with an incidence of between 4 and 7 per 1000 live births. Patients with congenital heart disease may have associated extracardiac anomalies and genetic syndromes.
5. Congenital heart disease (CHD) can be classified as cyanotic or acyanotic, depending on the presence or absence of right-to-left shunting.
6. The magnitude of shunting and its hemodynamic significance depends on the location and size of the shunt as well as the pressure gradient across the shunt and the relative compliances of the downstream chambers or resistances of the downstream vessels.
7. Pediatric heart failure can be related to volume- or pressure-overload. It can occur in structurally normal heart with primary cardiomyopathy (dilated, hypertrophic, or restrictive) or secondary cardiomyopathy due to arrythmia, ischemic, toxicity, infection, or infiltrative diseases.
8. The approach to the patient with CHD undergoing noncardiac surgery should be systematic and team-based.

INTRODUCTION

A thorough understanding of cardiovascular physiology and pathophysiology is an unequivocally essential component of the practice of anesthesiology. Pediatric anesthesiologists must be cognizant of the normal physiologic changes that the cardiovascular system undergoes during growth and development, from fetal through adult life. They must be familiar with the broad spectrum of pathophysiology that accompanies congenital, and, to a lesser extent, acquired heart disease and its management. In this chapter, we will review the most salient aspects of this expansive subject and provide a basic framework for the clinical management of the patient with cardiac disease presenting for noncardiac surgery.

DEVELOPMENTAL PHYSIOLOGY

Fetal cardiac development begins at approximately 22 days' gestational age. Several intrauterine shunts form to divert blood away from the fetal lungs, which do not participate in gas exchange. These shunts also help optimize oxygen delivery to the developing brain and heart. Blood that has been oxygenated in the maternal circulation crosses the placenta and enters the fetal circulation via the umbilical vein with an oxygen saturation of 70% to 80%. The umbilical vein enters at the level of the liver, where a portion of the blood provides perfusion to the hepatic circulation and the rest is shunted across the **ductus venosus** toward the heart. This blood travels toward the right atrium (RA) independently from inferior vena cava (IVC) blood. The blood from the ductus venosus enters the RA and is shunted across the **foramen ovale** to the left atrium (LA), where it mixes with the small amount of blood that made it through the lungs and into the pulmonary veins. This mixture of blood (oxygen saturation about 65%) is ejected into the ascending aorta to preferentially supply oxygenated blood to the brain and heart. Deoxygenated blood from the superior vena cava (SVC) and IVC enters the RA and the right ventricle (RV) and exits via the pulmonary arteries, with a portion of this blood perfusing the lungs but the majority shunted right-to-left across the **ductus arteriosus** to the descending aorta. This blood has an approximate oxygen saturation of 60%.[1–3] In the fetal circulation, the branch pulmonary arteries are small, because the lungs only receive approximately 15% of combined ventricular output. The RV handles 55% of the combined ventricular output, and the LV handles the other 45%; thus, the RV is larger and more dominant than the left ventricle (LV). The pressure in the RV is identical to that in the LV, which is not the case in adult circulation.[4]

The transitional circulation consists of changes to the fetal circulation to accommodate extrauterine life. Once the fetus takes its first breath, the pulmonary vascular resistance (PVR) decreases secondary to the increased oxygen saturation, and ventilation and expansion of the fetal lungs. In addition, the neonate's systemic vascular resistance (SVR) increases due to clamping of the umbilical cord, which disconnects the low-resistance placenta from neonatal circulation. The increased SVR and increased pulmonary blood flow lead to increased left atrial pressures and functional closure of the foramen ovale.[1,3] The decrease in PVR also creates a shift to left-to-right blood flow across the ductus arteriosus with an increase in pulmonary blood flow, which increases left ventricular output and stroke volume. Decreases in intraluminal flow and circulating prostaglandins coupled with increases in vasoactive catecholamines and oxygen tension lead to the functional closure of the ductus arteriosus within the first 10 to 15 minutes of life.[1] Normal anatomic closure via vascular remodeling does not occur until 2 to 3 weeks of age. If PVR exceeds SVR before this occurs, blood flow via the ductus arteriosus can reverse (to become right-to-left) leading to differential cyanosis.

Throughout the first weeks of life, the neonatal heart is noncompliant and functions at close to maximum cardiac output with a fixed stroke volume. For this reason, cardiac output is heart rate–dependent. Increases in afterload result in a decrease in cardiac output.[5] Additionally, the immature heart has a significant parasympathetic tone, so infants and young children are prone to bradycardia with vagal stimulation, such as during tracheal intubation.

As the neonate grows, additional changes take place. The pediatric heart rate reaches a maximum rate at approximately 1 month of life, and then steadily declines to reach adult levels at 10 to 12 years of age. In contrast, there is a decline in respiratory rate from birth to early adolescence, with the steepest decline occurring in infants under 2 years of age. Blood pressure increases through childhood and adult values are usually reached in adolescence.[5] The average normal values for heart rate, respiratory rate, and blood pressure are included in Table 17-1.

CONGENITAL HEART DISEASE

Congenital heart disease (CHD) is the most common form of birth defect with a reported incidence of between 4 and 75 per 1000 live births.[6] Since Dr. Gross performed the first pediatric heart surgery in 1938, advances in surgical techniques, anesthesia management, the conduct of cardiopulmonary bypass, and perioperative medical management, especially neonatal critical care, have led to dramatic increases in survival for even the most complex lesions. Pediatric, and increasingly adult, anesthesiologists

Table 17-1. Normal Vital Signs by Age

Age	Heart Rate (beats/min)	Respiratory Rate (breaths/min)	Blood Pressure (mm Hg) (90th percentile BP for 50th percentile height)	
			Boys	Girls
Newborn	120–170	30–80	87/68	76/68
1 year	80–160	20–40	98/53	100/58
3 years	80–120	20–30	105/61	103/62
6 years	75–115	16–22	110/70	107/69
10 years	70–110	16–20	115/75	115/74
17 years	60–110	12–20	133/83	125/80

Source: Reproduced with permission, from Johns Hopkins Hospital, Kahl L, Hughes HK. *The Harriet Lane Handbook*, 21st ed. 2018. Copyright © Elsevier. All rights reserved.

will encounter patients at various stages of palliation and/or repair. In this section, we present the most commonly encountered lesions and their physiological implications.

Left-to-Right Shunts

Left-to-right shunts are the result of an aberrant anatomical connection between the systemic and pulmonary circulations. This group represents the most common group of congenital cardiac anomalies and encompasses a number of lesions including patent ductus arteriosus (PDA), atrial septal defect (ASD), ventricular septal defect (VSD), atrioventricular canal (AVC) defects, double-outlet right ventricle (DORV), aortopulmonary (AP) window, and partial anomalous pulmonary venous connection (PAPVC). Despite the various locations of the shunts and potential sidedness of cardiac structures, left-to-right shunts are defined by the physiologic direction of blood flow, that is, from the systemic to the pulmonary circulation. The magnitude of the shunt and its hemodynamic significance are secondary to the location and size of the shunt as well as the pressure gradient across the shunt and the relative compliances of the downstream chambers or resistances of the downstream vessels.

PDA

A PDA occurs when the ductus arteriosus fails to undergo normal anatomical closure. The estimated incidence is 1 per 500 to 2000 live births, which represents roughly 5% to 10% of all CHDs.[7] There is an increasing incidence of PDA with decreasing gestational age, likely reflecting a developmentally immature response to the changing flow dynamics and biochemical milieu of the transitional circulation. In term neonates, most cases of PDA are sporadic; however, genetic disorders and environmental factors such as high altitude, neonatal sepsis, and in utero exposures (eg, rubella, phenytoin, alcohol, amphetamine) have all been implicated as predisposing factors.[7] Because systemic vascular resistance (SVR) is generally greater than pulmonary vascular resistance (PVR), blood is primarily shunted from the descending aorta through the PDA into the pulmonary circulation with the degree of shunting determined by the dimensions of the duct and the relative difference in PVR and SVR. Increased pulmonary artery blood flow leads to pulmonary "overcirculation." Lung compliance is decreased and over time, microvascular injury leads to small vessel pulmonary vascular occlusive disease (PVOD; intimal proliferation, arteriolar medial hypertrophy) and pulmonary artery hypertension (PAH). As the pulmonary circulation is overperfused, the systemic circulation is underperfused, especially during diastole. The left heart, meanwhile, experiences greater blood return via the pulmonary veins causing left-sided volume overload—left atrial enlargement leads to arrhythmias, increased left ventricular end-diastolic pressure leads to hypertrophy, and increased catecholamine levels lead to tachycardia,

increased oxygen demand, decreased diastolic time, and worsened coronary artery steal. Neonates with PDA may present with signs of pulmonary overcirculation (eg, failure to extubate, respiratory distress syndrome, pulmonary hemorrhage) or poor systemic perfusion (eg, necrotizing enterocolitis, renal insufficiency, intraventricular hemorrhage). Infants and children may present with failure to thrive, exercise intolerance, and/or recurrent pneumonias, while adults may present with the same symptoms or with more advanced sequalae such as atrial arrhythmias, infective endocarditis, pulmonary artery hypertension with Eisenmenger physiology, and/or congestive heart failure (CHF).

In the neonate, conservative PDA management consists of protective lung ventilation, permissive hypercapnia, fluid restriction $\pm$ diuretics, and inotropic support $\pm$ afterload reducing agents. Definitive treatment for PDA is ductal closure approached with pharmacological (nonsteroidal anti-inflammatory drugs [NSAIDs] or acetaminophen), catheter-based devices, and/or surgical intervention. No consensus exists among providers at United States children hospitals regarding the use of indomethacin prophylaxis or NSAID and/or surgical PDA treatment; practice preferences vary between and within hospitals.[8] The relative effectiveness of the various treatment options and their risks, both short- and long-term, has been the subject of numerous studies and Cochrane reviews.[9–18]

ASD

ASDs are common, accounting for 7% to 10% of CHD. There are four types of atrial level shunts:

1. Primum ASD (ASD1), caused by failure of the septum primum to fuse with the developing endocardial cushions;

2. Secundum ASD (ASD2), caused by a relative deficiency of the septum primum following tissue resorption in the region of the ostium secundum;

3. Sinus venosus defect, an unroofed pulmonary vein at the junction of the right atrium (RA) with either the superior vena cava (SVC) or the inferior vena cava (IVC); and

4. Unroofed coronary sinus, the absence of the wall between the coronary sinus and the left ventricle.

ASD2 is the most common type, representing 50% to 70% of atrial-level shunts. Shunt magnitude is determined by the size of the defect and the relative compliances of the ventricles. The left-to-right shunting becomes more prominent with increasing age as the compliance of the left ventricle (LV) decreases. Atrial level shunts cause right-sided volume overload and increased pulmonary blood flow. There is the potential for paradoxical emboli, cerebral abscess formation, and the development of pulmonary artery hypertension.

ASD2 with diameters <3 mm and ≥3 to 8 mm spontaneously close before 18 months of age in 100% and >80% of cases, respectively, while those with diameters ≥8 mm rarely do.[19] ASD1, sinus venosus defects, and unroofed coronary artery sinus do not spontaneously resolve. ASD closure is indicated in symptomatic patients without pulmonary hypertension and in asymptomatic patients when the shunt is large (pulmonary blood flow: systemic blood flow ratio [Q_p:Q_s] ≥ 1.5:1). This can be done in the cardiac catheterization lab provided that the anatomy is favorable and the patient is of adequate size, or in the operating room with cardiopulmonary bypass, generally around 2 years of age. Postoperatively, these patients are at risk for atrial and nodal arrhythmias and more rarely, sick sinus syndrome.

VSD

Isolated VSDs are the most common congenital heart lesions, accounting for 15% to 20% of all CHDs, or up to 50%, if VSD in setting of complex CHD is included. There are four types of VSDs:

1. Membranous (aka perimembranous, subaortic, conoventricular);
2. Subpulmonic (aka infundibular, conoseptal, outlet, supracristal, subarterial);
3. AV canal (aka inlet); and
4. Muscular (aka trabecular).

Membranous VSDs represent the large majority of VSDs and are frequently associated with a PDA and coarctation of the aorta (CoA), whereas subpulmonic VSDs may be associated with aortic regurgitation in the setting of aortic valve leaflet prolapse into the VSD. The amount of shunting is dependent upon the size and pressure gradient across the defect. In small to moderate shunts, the LA and LV experience volume overload while the RV is relatively spared. In large shunts, the RV is subjected to both increased volume and pressure load, while the LA and RV are volume overloaded to an even greater extent. The increase in Q_p is variable and dependent upon the size of the defect and PVR. Small VSDs may remain asymptomatic, while large VSDs may present with failure to thrive (FTT), recurrent lung infections, and signs of CHF. Heart failure and PVOD occur earlier than in patients with ASD. PVOD is accelerated in patients with trisomy 21. The reported rate of spontaneous closure varies widely, from 8% to 83%, depending on the location and size of the defect with the highest rates of spontaneous closure occurring during the first year of life and for small, muscular lesions.[20]

A Q_p:Q_s > 2:1 is an indication for VSD closure. The timing of repair depends on the severity of symptoms. Asymptomatic patients typically undergo surgical repair between 2 and 4 years of age. Larger patients with favorable anatomy may be candidates for transcatheter device closure. During the first year of life, symptomatic VSDs are managed with diuretics, afterload reducers, and/or digoxin. Those that

respond to medical management undergo repair at 12 to 24 months, while those that are unresponsive to treatment and those with signs of rising PVR undergo semi-urgent repair regardless of age. If the surgical approach is dependent on a patient's size, pulmonary artery banding may be considered as a temporary palliation allowing for patient growth. Postoperative considerations include residual shunts and conduction abnormalities including right bundle branch block and complete heart block.

AVC Defects

AVC defects result from failure of the endocardial cushions to fuse with the developing atrial and ventricular septums. In a partial AVC defect, there is a primum ASD and a cleft in the anterior leaflet of the mitral valve (MV). Intermediate AVC defects are characterized by a primum ASD, an unrestrictive inlet VSD, and a divided common atrioventricular valve (AVV) with two distinct orifices. Transitional AVC defects consist of a primum ASD, a restrictive VSD, and a common AVV with single orifice. Finally, complete AVC defects (CAVCs) are composed of a primum ASD, a large unrestrictive VSD, and a common AVV with a single orifice. CAVCs can be further subdivided into three types according to the Rastelli classification based on valve morphology.[21] The presentation and clinical course of AVC defects depend on the magnitude and location of shunting (atrial, ventricular, AVV levels), the degree of ventricular imbalance and AVV regurgitation, as well as the presence of additional cardiac lesions.[22,23] In complete AVC, shunting at the level of the atria and ventricles leads to dilation of all four heart chambers, right greater than left. The degree of pulmonary blood flow is dependent on the relationship between PVR and SVR. Failure to thrive, recurrent pneumonias, and signs of CHF with or without pulmonary hypertension develop early in infancy in patients with CAVC and later with intermediate, transitional, and partial AVCs. Just as with isolated VSDs, PVOD occurs earlier and with greater severity in infants with trisomy 21. Airway obstruction at the level of the left mainstem bronchus may occur in the setting of severe left atrial dilation.

Primary surgical repair of CAVC is generally undertaken between 1 and 6 months of age. When CAVC is associated with other intracardiac lesions precluding repair at this age, pulmonary artery banding may be performed as a temporary palliation in order to limit pulmonary overcirculation and allow for patient growth. Postoperative considerations include residual shunts, AVV stenosis, and/or regurgitation, as well as sinoatrial and/or atrioventricular node conduction abnormalities. A total of 2.4% of patients status post CAVC repair require the placement of a permanent pacemaker.[24]

Obstructive Lesions

There are a number of congenital lesions that cause obstruction of flow to either the pulmonary or systemic circulations. Right-sided lesions include pulmonary stenosis (PS), pulmonary artery stenosis (PAS), tricuspid stenosis (TS), and double-chamber right ventricle (RV). Left-sided lesions include aortic stenosis (AS), coarctation of the aorta (CoA), interrupted aortic arch (IAA), hypoplastic left heart syndrome (HLHS), and mitral stenosis (MS). Given the relative rarity of many of these lesions, only the most common lesions will be discussed here.

Pulmonary Stenosis

Pulmonary stenosis may occur at the valvar, supravalvar, and/or subvalvar (infundibular) levels. Supravalvar PS is often associated with other cardiac and extra-cardiac anomalies and is seen in the setting of congenital rubella as well as several syndromes including Williams-Beuren, Alagille, and DiGeorge syndromes.[25] Subvalvar PS is generally accompanied by a large VSD as in tetralogy of Fallot. In valvar PS, the most common (about 90%) variant, the valve is thickened with fused or absent commisures and there is post-stenotic dilation of the main pulmonary artery (MPA). A variable degree of RV hypertension and hypertrophy with diastolic dysfunction will develop depending on the degree of stenosis present, although the RV may be hypoplastic in neonates with critical PS. Mild stenosis is typically not progressive, however, moderate and severe stenosis generally are. Neonates with critical PS will be maintained on IV prostaglandins in order to maintain pulmonary blood flow via the ductus arteriosus until a balloon valvotomy can be performed in the cardiac catheterization lab. Echocardiographic evidence of moderate or severe disease as well as symptoms of inadequate pulmonary blood flow such as angina, syncope, or pre-syncope regardless of Doppler gradient are also indications for pulmonary valvotomy. Surgery for isolated PS is rarely performed.[26] Long-term considerations in patients who have undergone valvotomy include re-stenosis and/or pulmonary regurgitation.

Aortic Stenosis

Left ventricular outflow tract obstruction (LVOTO) accounts for roughly 10% of CHD. As in PS, AS may occur at the valvar, supravalvar, and/or subvalvar levels. Valvar AS is most frequently caused by a bicuspid aortic valve, although a unicuspid valve is also possible.[27] In critical neonatal AS, the valve is myxomatous with a pinhole opening and the left-sided structures are varyingly hypoplastic.[28] Supravalvar aortic stenosis occurs at the upper margin of the sinuses of Valsalva and is frequently associated with Williams syndrome.[29,30] Subvalvar stenosis may be either tunnel-like or discrete. Discrete lesions such as a simple membrane or fibromuscular ridge are more common, and are in the majority of cases associated with other cardiac defects.[31] The LV is subjected to an increased pressure load leading to LV hypertrophy, the degree of which is dependent upon the severity of stenosis. Aortic

root dilation and aortic valve regurgitation may develop in valvar and subvalvar stenosis, respectively. Neonates with critical AS will be maintained on IV prostaglandins in order to maintain systemic blood flow via the ductus arteriosus until a balloon valvotomy can be performed in the cardiac catheterization lab. Balloon valvuloplasty is the primary treatment of choice for isolated valvar AS beyond the neonatal period, provided that there are adequate annular dimensions. Valvar AS with annular hypoplasia, valvar AS with aortic regurgitation (AR) status post balloon dilation, subvalvar AS, and supravalvar AS are all managed surgically. Long-term considerations for these patients include the development of AR, mitral regurgitation (MR), and recurrent AS (especially in subvalvar AS).

CoA

CoA represents 8% to 10% of CHDs, is associated with other lesions (most commonly bicuspid aortic valve), and is commonly seen in association with Turner and Williams syndromes. Less commonly, it may be acquired, as with Takayasu arteritis. Anatomically, there is segmental juxta-ductal stenosis of the descending thoracic aorta. Histologically, there is abnormal smooth muscle cell (SMC) migration and differentiation, such that the subendothelial layer more closely resembles that of the ductus arteriosus than normal aortic tissue.[32] Patients with CoA may be symptomatic or asymptomatic. With ductal closure, neonates and infants with severe CoA will present with signs of CHF (tachypnea, sweating, irritability), signs of poor perfusion (necrotizing enterocolitis [NEC], acute kidney injury [AKI], hepatic failure, seizures), and/or cardiogenic shock. In conjunction with medical optimization, including reopening the ductus arteriosus with prostaglandins, urgent surgical (or less commonly interventional) treatment is indicated in these patients. Less severe coarctation may remain largely asymptomatic throughout childhood and adolescence with patients complaining of rare leg pain and/or mild exercise intolerance. On exam these patients may be hypertensive with an upper-to-lower extremity blood pressure gradient, although the gradient is not a reliable indicator of the severity of stenosis in the setting of collateralization. Their chest x-ray may be notable for the stereotypical findings of a "figure 3 sign" (pre- and post-stenotic dilation of the thoracic aorta) and/or Roesler's sign (inferior notching of the 3rd-9th posterior ribs). Symptoms unresponsive to medical management, aortic diameter loss of more than 50%, and/or trans-CoA gradient more than 20 to 30 mm Hg are indications for interventional or surgical management. Although interventional management is the gold standard for recoarctation, its use for primary intervention remains controversial as the risk of short-term coarctation is higher.[33,34] Although CoA is anatomically a seemingly simple lesion, patients have life-long cardiovascular sequalae secondary to diastolic dysfunction and abnormal aortic elasticity predisposing them to hypertension, coronary artery disease, cerebral vascular accidents, CHF, and ruptured aortic and/or cerebral aneurysms. Additionally, these patients should be regularly screened for the development of recoarctation, AS (valvar and subvalvar), and MR.

Transposition of the Great Arteries

In transposition of the great arteries (TGA), there is discordance of the ventriculoarterial (VA) connections. There are two main types, denoted as dextro-TGA (d-TGA) and levo-TGA (l-TGA), so named for their ventricular looping patterns, with d-TGA being the more common anatomic form.

d-TGA

In d-TGA, the systemic and pulmonary systems are arranged in parallel—systemic blood returns from the systemic venous circulation and enters the right atrium and then passes through the tricuspid valve into the right ventricle which then pumps it into the aorta. Pulmonary venous blood is returned to the left atrium where it passes through the mitral valve into the left ventricle and then pumped back into the pulmonary circulation. This arrangement is uniformly fatal if there is not a communication (ASD, VSD, PDA) at which intracirculatory mixing can occur. d-TGA is the most common cause of cyanotic heart disease in the neonatal period and most neonates with d-TGA will present with cyanosis. Those with inadequate mixing will present with severe hypoxemia, progressive acidosis, and ultimately cardiovascular collapse. Prostaglandins are started at birth or at the time of diagnosis in order to maintain ductal patency; pulmonary blood flow is maintained with volume repletion and the maintenance of normal cardiac function. If an unacceptable degree of hypoxemia persists, a balloon atrial septostomy can be performed to create a second, unrestrictive communication.[35] Historically, d-TGA was palliated with an atrial level switch (Senning, Mustard); however, the current surgical approach is full anatomic repair via the arterial switch operation (ASO) performed during the neonatal period.[36-38] Long-term outcomes following aortic switch are favorable with neoaortic root dilation, neoaortic valve regurgitation, and coronary artery anomalies being the most common late complications.[39-41]

l-TGA

In l-TGA (also known as congenitally corrected or cc-TGA), there is both ventriculoarterial (VA) and atrioventricular (AV) discordance which result in a series circulation, albeit with a systemic RV. Blood returns from the systemic venous circulation and enters the right atrium and then passes through the mitral valve into the left ventricle which then pumps it into the pulmonary artery. Pulmonary venous blood is returned to the left atrium where it passes through the tricuspid valve into the right

ventricle and then pumped into the aorta. Patients with isolated l-TGA will be fully saturated and may not present until later in life when the systemic RV begins to fail. The overwhelming majority of l-TGA patients, however, will have concomitant lesions, most commonly VSD, multilevel LVOTO, tricuspid valve anomalies, and/or conduction abnormalities, which make presentation variable.[42] Traditionally, l-TGA was palliated with a physiological repair, that is, repair of the concomitant lesions but with maintenance of VA and AV discordance; however currently, an anatomic repair in which atrial and arterial switches ("double-switch procedure") convert the LV to the systemic ventricle is favored.[43] Long-term considerations in these patients include progressive AV conduction disturbances, arrhythmias, baffle obstruction, tricuspid valve regurgitation, and residual VSDs.

Cyanotic CHD

Cyanotic CHD involves right-to-left shunting of deoxygenated blood into the systemic circulation. There are three groups of lesions as follows:

1. Those with decreased pulmonary blood flow—tetralogy of Fallot (TOF), pulmonary atresia with intact ventricular septum, critical PS, and tricuspid valve abnormalities (tricuspid atresia, tricuspid stenosis with hypoplastic RV, Ebstein anomaly);

2. Those with increased pulmonary blood flow—truncus arteriosus, d-TGA, and total anomalous pulmonary venous return (TAPVR); and

3. Those associated with severe heart failure—HLHS, critical AS, critical CoA, and IAA.

TOF

Tetralogy of Fallot is comprised of the following four lesions:

1. A large, non-restrictive VSD,
2. RV outflow tract obstruction (RVOTO),
3. RV hypertrophy, and
4. An overriding aorta.

The pulmonary arteries may be hypoplastic. TOF accounts for roughly 10% of congenital heart disease and is the most common cause of cyanotic heart disease beyond the neonatal period. Several anatomic variants exist (TOF with PS, TOF with pulmonary atresia and major aortopulmonary collaterals, and TOF with absent pulmonary valve) with TOF with PA being the most common. For the sake of simplicity, only TOF with PS will be discussed further here.

Patients with TOF will have variable presentations depending on the anatomic level (infundibular, valvar, or both), severity and nature (dynamic, fixed, or both) of RVOTO. In patients with minimal RVOTO (acyanotic or "pink" TOF), the shunt across the VSD will be primarily left-to-right and the presentation will be similar to that of a large VSD with signs of congestive heart failure and a normal saturation. In patients with more significant RVOTO (cyanotic or "blue" TOF), the shunt will be bidirectional or primarily right-to-left and there will be some degree of cyanosis at baseline. During infancy, some patients with TOF will experience hypoxic (aka hypercyanotic or "tet") spells that are characterized by uncontrollable irritability, rapid shallow breathing, and severe cyanosis. If left untreated, these spells can progress to syncope, seizures, CVA, or death. They are most commonly seen in the early morning but can also be seen before/after eating and/or be precipitated by noxious stimuli, dehydration, prolonged episodes of agitation, or in relation to things which are known to decrease SVR (bathing, exercise, fever). Pathophysiologically, decreased SVR and/or infundibular spasm lead to increased right-to-left shunting across the VSD, which in turn leads to hypoxemia, hypercarbia, and acidosis. Activation of the respiratory center of the brain leads to hyperpnea. The altered breathing pattern, in turn, increases systemic venous return, further increasing the shunt volume and perpetuating the feed-forward loop. Treatment includes increasing SVR via femoral artery compression or holding the infant in a knee-to-chest position along with the administration of opioids (SC, IM, IV), vasopressors (IV), sodium bicarbonate, and supplemental oxygen. If unsuccessful, ketamine and beta-blockade can also be considered. TOF repair is generally performed in the first year of life, preferably after 3 to 4 months of age. The complete surgical repair entails VSD closure, and RV outflow tract reconstruction (valve-sparing vs transannular patch). Intervention in the neonatal period is reserved for those neonates with severe cyanosis or uncontrollable hypoxic spells and may either be palliative (RVOT stent vs surgical shunt) or a complete repair.[44-46] Post-repair considerations in these patients include residual lesions (VSD, PA stenosis, pulmonary regurgitation), residual RVOTO, arrhythmias, and conduction abnormalities.

HLHS

HLHS is a rare form of CHD characterized by a hypoplastic LV, mitral and aortic stenosis or atresia, and a hypoplastic aortic root and ascending aorta. The RV is functionally a single ventricle that must supply both the pulmonary and systemic circulations. Although a small amount of blood may pass anterograde through the left heart in the case of stenotic left-sided valves, the majority of pulmonary venous return will shunt left-to-right across an ASD; the flow to the coronary circulation and the head and neck vessels is supplied in a retrograde fashion by right-to-left shunting across the PDA. Without intervention, ductal closure will lead to metabolic acidosis and cardiovascular collapse. Neonates with HLHS are maintained on prostaglandin infusions in order to prevent this from happening.

As PVR drops during the first few days of life, the single RV will provide progressively more blood flow to the lungs and less to the body. Balancing the perfusion to the lungs and the body requires maintenance of cardiac output and avoidance of excessive drops in PVR or increases in SVR.

The complete repair of HLHS is comprised of three stages:

1. There are two main palliative techniques for neonates with HLHS—the Stage 1 palliation (Norwood) and the hybrid approach. The Stage 1 palliation is composed of an atrial septostomy (BAS), main pulmonary artery ligation, PDA ligation, creation of a neoaortic root comprised of the proximal PA and the hypoplastic aortic root and ascending aorta, and establishment of a stable source of pulmonary blood flow with either a modified Blalock-Taussig shunt (mBTS) or an RV-PA conduit (Sano). In the hybrid approach, done without cardiopulmonary bypass, the PDA is stented, bilateral PA bands are placed, and a BAS is performed to prevent left atrial hypertension; the aorta is reconstructed during the Stage 2 palliation. Physiologically, the circulation is relatively unchanged after this palliation, with $Q_p:Q_s$ dependent upon the ratio of PVR to SVR.

2. During the Stage 2 palliation, the bidirectional Glenn (BDG) procedure, the superior vena cava (SVC) is attached end-to-side to the ipsilateral PA and the mBTS or Sano conduit is taken down so that the entirety of PA blood blow is provided by venous return via the SVC. The single ventricle is partially volume off-loaded and the pulmonary blood flow is then dependent upon PVR, intrathoracic pressure, and the dynamics of the cerebral circulation.

3. In the third and final stage, the Fontan procedure, the inferior vena cava (IVC) blood flow is redirected to the ipsilateral PA, creating a single ventricle series circulation. A small fenestration between the systemic venous blood flow and the common atrium may be created at the time of the surgery in order to serve as a pop-off valve in the setting of systemic venous hypertension, preserving cardiac output at the expense of cyanosis. This fenestration has been shown to decrease immediate postoperative morbidity and shorten intensive care unit (ICU) stay.[47] It may close spontaneously or be closed at a later time with a mechanical device in the catheterization laboratory.

The Fontan circulation is inherently inefficient. It is a single ventricle series circulation with near-normal oxygen levels, but with both inherently decreased ventricular preload and increased systemic vascular resistance (SVR).[48] Ventricular preload is limited by the low-pressure, nonpulsatile driving pressure through the lungs as well as the limited recruitability of the pulmonary vascular bed. The elevation in SVR is due to the fact that the single ventricle must pump blood through three resistance beds (systemic vascular bed, cavopulmonary system, and the pulmonary vascular bed) as compared to the one resistance bed encountered by each ventricle in a biventricular circulation. The altered ventricular loading conditions result in the decreased mechanical efficiency of the Fontan circulation. Cardiac index (CI) and fractional shortening (FS) are lower both at rest and during stress in patients with Fontan physiology as compared with healthy controls.[48] Although the majority of contemporary Fontan patients have a normal ejection fraction (EF), only around a third have normal diastolic function.[49] Fontan patients have obligatory systemic venous hypertension and diminished venous capacitance at baseline. Pulmonary artery flow (ie, systemic venous return) is more dependent upon respiratory mechanics (negative inspiratory pressure and downward displacement of the diaphragm) than the healthy biventricular patient (30% vs 15% contribution) due to the absence of a subpulmonary ventricle and normal interventricular interaction.[48] This lack of interventricular dependence is the reason why Fontan patients do not develop pulsus paradoxus in the setting of cardiac tamponade. The altered hemodynamics of the Fontan circulation predispose these patients to end-organ dysfunction (renal failure, Fontan-associated liver disease, plastic bronchitis, Fontan-associated protein-losing enteropathy), progressive cardiac failure, thrombosis, and increased functional impairment.[50]

HEART FAILURE: ETIOLOGY, PATHOPHYSIOLOGY, AND MANAGEMENT

Heart failure (HF) in the pediatric population is a major public health concern. Although pediatric HF is uncommon compared to the adult population, an increasing number of these patients are reaching adulthood, secondary to the successes in the medical and surgical management of HF. Children whose hospitalization is complicated by HF have a more than 20-fold increase in the risk of death.[51] The most common cause of HF in the United States is congenital heart disease (CHD), while primary cardiomyopathies are the most common cause of HF in children with structurally normal hearts. The incidence of HF in children with CHD is 6% to 24%.[52] The incidence of new-onset HF is 0.87 per 100,000 children under 16 year of age with cardiomyopathies. The highest incidence occurred within the first year of life and more than half were due to dilated cardiomyopathy.[53]

HF is a clinical diagnosis with signs and symptoms that result from a structural or functional impairment of ventricular filling or ejection of blood. This could be secondary to ventricular dysfunction with or without volume or pressure overload. HF may lead to a combination of circulatory, neurohormonal, and molecular abnormalities. In children, these may manifest as poor growth, feeding difficulties, respiratory distress, exercise intolerance, and fatigue.[54,55] The cardiac causes of pediatric HF are listed in Table 17-2.

Cardiomyopathies in children are characterized by functional abnormalities of cardiac muscle in the absence of coronary, valvular, or congenital heart disease. The most common causes are idiopathic, familial, metabolic, or toxic. Pediatric cardiomyopathy may also be associated with metabolic, myopathic, hematologic, or neurologic diseases. For example, Duchenne's and Becker's muscular dystrophy are associated with high rates of cardiomyopathy.[56]

Determining the severity of HF is important in monitoring disease progression. This presents challenges in the pediatric population. The New York Heart Association (NYHA) Heart Failure Classification, which is widely used in adults, uses functional limitation to quantify severity and may only be useful in adolescents. Thus, the Ross Classification was created and recently modified for the assessment of infants in HF. It incorporates feeding difficulties, growth problems, and symptoms of exercise intolerance into a numeric score comparable with the NYHA classification (Table 17-3).[52]

The diagnosis of HF in children is based on a combination of clinical, radiographic, echocardiographic, and laboratory findings. These are discussed in Table 17-4.[56,57]

HF patients are managed based on the etiology of HF and the disease severity. It is important to understand the implications of the different modalities used in the management of these patients prior to providing anesthetic care. Many patients will be on several pharmacologic agents to provide symptomatic relief of HF symptoms. These include diuretics, digoxin, angiotensin-converting enzyme (ACE) inhibitors, and angiotensin II receptor blockers (ARBs). Patients with severe, decompensated HF that are in an inpatient setting may present to the operating room on intravenous diuretics and/or inotropes such as dopamine and epinephrine, which are used to improve cardiac output. These patients may also present on intravenous milrinone, a phosphodiesterase III inhibitor, which increases contractility and reduces afterload. Patients in severe heart failure may no longer respond to pharmacologic therapies and may require positive pressure ventilation, mechanical circulatory support or ultimately, heart transplantation. Positive pressure ventilation can be effective in relieving respiratory distress from cardiogenic pulmonary edema as well as providing alveolar recruitment, improved lung compliance, and decreased left ventricular preload and afterload. This improves cardiac output. Some patients that do not respond to medical therapy will benefit from cardiac resynchronization therapy (CRT). These are usually patients with reduced EF (ie, <35%) and a left bundle branch block (LBBB) pattern on electrocardiogram (ECG). The intraventricular conduction delay or LBBB may worsen HF by causing ventricular dyssynchrony. CRT uses biventricular pacing to decrease ventricular dyssynchrony.[58] HF patients may also suffer from arrhythmias and sudden cardiac death. These patients may require an implantable cardioverter defibrillator (ICD) and management of these devices will be required with the assistance of an electrophysiology specialist in the perioperative period.

Table 17-2. Causes of Pediatric Heart Failure

Congenital cardiac malformations	Volume overload	Left to right shunting	Ventricular septal defect
			Patent ductus arteriosus
		AV or semilunar valve insufficiency	Aortic regurgitation in bicommissural aortic valve
			Pulmonary regurgitation after tetralogy of Fallot repair
	Pressure overload	Left-sided obstruction	Severe aortic stenosis
			Aortic coarctation
		Right-sided obstruction	Severe pulmonary stenosis
	Complex CHD	Single ventricle	Hypoplastic left heart syndrome
			Unbalanced AV septal defect
		Systemic right ventricle	L-transposition of the great arteries
Structurally normal heart	Primary cardiomyopathy	Dilated	
		Hypertrophic	
		Restrictive	
	Secondary cardiomyopathy	Arrhythmogenic	-
		Ischemic	
		Toxic	
		Infiltrative	
		Infectious	

Table 17-3. Modified Ross Heart Failure Classification for Children

Class I	Asymptomatic
Class II	Mild tachypnea or diaphoresis with feeding in infants
	Dyspnea on exertion in older children
Class III	Marked tachypnea or diaphoresis with feeding in infants
	Marked dyspnea on exertion
	Prolonged feeding times with growth failure
Class IV	Symptoms such as tachypnea, retractions, grunting, or diaphoresis at rest

Children with decompensated HF and low cardiac output unresponsive to medical therapy could require mechanical circulatory support (MCS) to maintain end-organ function. MCS devices include extracorporeal membrane oxygenation (ECMO) or a ventricular assist device (VAD). MCS may be used as short-term support for reversible causes of HF, for long-term support as a bridge to cardiac transplantation, or less commonly in this population, as destination therapy. The choice of device depends on the size of the patient and the type of support required (cardiopulmonary vs cardiac). ECMO is capable of providing full cardiopulmonary support, while VADs are indicated for isolated ventricular dysfunction. ECMO may be used in the setting of imminent or actual cardiac arrest, during low cardiac output states, or electively in the setting of high-risk procedures.[59] Cannulation can be performed percutaneously, and ECMO can provide full cardiopulmonary support for days to weeks. Venous blood is drained from the patient and circulated through a membrane for gas exchange. Oxygenated blood is then returned to the patient through a large vein (venovenous or VV ECMO) or artery (venoarterial or VA ECMO). VV ECMO is used in patients that only require respiratory support, while VA ECMO can provide both respiratory and cardiac support. The goal of ECMO is to provide adequate gas exchange and oxygen delivery to allow time for the underlying disease process to resolve. The parameters that are monitored include the hemodynamics, acidosis, lactate, venous saturations, urine output, perfusion, and end-organ function. These patients commonly experience hypertension. The decrease in cardiac filling pressures from decompression of the atria by the ECMO circuit causes tachycardia and thus, hypertension. These patients may

Table 17-4. Modalities Used in the Preoperative Assessment of Children with Heart Failure

Modality	Findings	Additional Notes
Chest X-ray	Cardiomegaly, pulmonary edema/effusions	-
Electrocardiogram	ST segment or T wave changes, ventricular hypertrophy, axis deviations, bundle branch or AV block, arrhythmias	-
Echocardiography	Ventricular dilation, systolic dysfunction, AV valve regurgitation, pericardial effusion	-
Point of care ultrasound (U/S)	B-lines on lung U/S, diminished EF	
Laboratory studies	Elevated BNP, NT-BNP	May be useful to monitor trends
	Elevated troponin	May be elevated in myocarditis
	Elevated transaminases, creatinine	May indicate poor end-organ perfusion
Endomyocardial biopsy	Determines etiology of myocarditis	Examples: infectious, immune-mediated, storage diseases etc.

Abbreviations: AV:, atrioventricular; BNP:, B-type natriuretic peptide; EF, ejection fraction; NT-BNP, N-terminal probrain natriuretic peptide.

be treated with antihypertensives, but with caution as they can exacerbate the hypertension/tachycardia by further decreasing preload and filling pressures. Ventilation strategies should be aimed at lung protection and minimizing ventilator-associated lung injury.

VADs can offer either univentricular or biventricular support. Typically, for left ventricular support, blood is drained from the left atrium or left ventricular apex to the pump and returned to the ascending aorta. For right ventricular (RV) support, blood is drained from the right atrium or RV to the pump and returned to the main pulmonary artery. The choice of device depends on the patient's size, anticipated duration, goal of support, device availability, and diagnosis. Devices differ by flow design (pulsatile, centrifugal, or axial), pump location relative to patient (implantable, paracorporeal, or extracorporeal), and delivery system (percutaneous or central). The Berlin Heart EXCOR is the most popular pediatric long-term support device and is the only FDA-approved device for neonates and infants.[60]

There are a number of perioperative physiologic considerations for the patient managed with MCS. First, they are very sensitive to changes in venous and arterial capacitance and may require fluid and/or vasopressor support in the setting of anesthesia-induced vasodilation. Second, given the risk for thromboembolism, these patients are chronically anticoagulated. In the case of ECMO, unfractionated heparin is the most commonly used anticoagulant drug, although direct thrombin inhibitors such as bivalirudin or argatroban are used in the setting of heparin-induced thrombocytopenia (HIT) or heparin resistance. Patients with VADs are usually anticoagulated using heparin and transitioned to warfarin with the addition of antiplatelet

agents for long-term anticoagulation. The decision to lower the level of anticoagulation prior to surgery should be a discussion between the anesthesiologist, surgeon, and physician managing the MCS. Third is pharmacokinetics, which is concerned with how the patient's body processes drugs—absorption, distribution, metabolism, and excretion. Fourth, MSC support may alter the pharmacodynamics of administered drugs due to altered clearance, sequestration of drugs in the circuitry components, and an increase in volume of distribution. In patients supported with ECMO, lipophilic and protein-bound drugs are more likely to be sequestered.[61-66] Lastly, the patient with a VAD should be considered a full stomach because of the placement of the device (upper abdomen) even when appropriately nil per os (NPO).

The complications related to MCS devices include bleeding, thromboembolism, seizures, and infection. Bleeding can occur at the site of the cannulas, at the surgical site, from gastrointestinal hemorrhage, in the pericardium, or in the brain. In addition, there are potential sources of mechanical complications leading to pump failure. Due to these serious complications, weaning from support should be considered once the underlying disease process is reversed. However, prolonged support may be a bridge to transplantation.[67]

THE CARDIAC PATIENT FOR NONCARDIAC SURGERY: ANESTHETIC MANAGEMENT

A systematic approach to patients with CHD undergoing noncardiac procedures begins with an understanding of the anatomical and physiological implications of the patient's lesion and prior palliations/repairs as well as an

Table 17-5. Preoperative Evaluation

History	Signs and symptoms of congestive heart failure (eg, failure to thrive) Palpitations or syncope Additional congenital anomalies (eg, airway, genitourinary) Recent and current medications (eg, diuretics, digoxin, ACE inhibitors) Past surgical and intervwentional history Last follow-up
Physical examination	Heart murmur, thrill, arrhythmias Tachypnea, increased work of breathing, rales Poor peripheral perfusion, delayed capillary refill, bounding or diminished pulses Cool extremities, mottled skin, sweating. Hepatomegaly Edema.
Laboratory studies	CBC: erythrocytosis (secondary to cyanosis), anemia (secondary to malnutrition, iron deficiency) Electrolytes: hypokalemia, hyponatremia (secondary to diuretic therapy) Coagulation profile
Additional tests	Echocardiography: function and anatomy ECG: rhythm, signs of atrial or ventricular hypertrophy Chest X-ray: cardiomegaly, pulmonary edema, or infiltrates
Specific studies	Cardiac catheterization: anatomy, pressure gradients, saturations, shunts, resistances Cardiac MRI: anatomy, pulmonary blood flow, RV and LV function

Source: Reproduced with permission, from Nasr VG, DiNardo JA. *The Pediatric Cardiac Anesthesia Handbook*. 2017. Copyright © Wiley Blackwell. All rights reserved.

appreciation of the patient's current functional status. It allows for the formulation of intraoperative hemodynamic and respiratory management goals, and directs planning for postoperative disposition. One such approach includes the following seven steps: preoperative assessment, endocarditis prophylaxis, prevention of paradoxical embolization, monitoring devices and intravenous access special considerations, fluid management, hemodynamic and respiratory management, and preoperative planning and postoperative disposition.

Preoperative Assessment

A thorough preoperative assessment includes an understanding of the anatomy and pathophysiology of the underlying defect or disease as well as the evaluation of the current functional status and medications (Table 17-5).[68] Pediatric heart disease is often associated with genetic syndromes that have anesthetic implications of their own, as is shown in Table 17-6.[69] Performance of age-appropriate activities is a surrogate of patient's cardiac function and reserve. Physical examination may reveal cyanosis, clubbing, and signs of congestive heart failure (tachypnea, hepatomegaly, ascites, and edema). Access and airway need to be carefully evaluated. Patients with CHD may have congenital and/or acquired airway abnormalities. They may also have limited venous and arterial access due to multiple palliative procedures. While evaluating a pediatric CHD patient, the anesthesiologist must be mindful of the age of

the patient and the impact of multiple previous surgical and anesthetic experiences on the patient and the family.

Endocarditis Prophylaxis

Based on the 2007 AHA guidelines, for all dental procedures involving manipulations of gingival tissue or oral mucosa, endocarditis prophylaxis is recommended for patients with the following conditions:[70]

- Prosthetic cardiac valve or prosthetic material used for cardiac valve repair.
- Previous endocarditis.
- Congenital heart disease (CHD):
  - Unrepaired cyanotic CHD, including palliative shunts and conduits.
  - Completely repaired CHD with prosthetic material or device, whether placed by surgery or catheter intervention, during the first 6 months after the repair.
  - Repaired CHD with residual defects in the site or adjacent to the site of a prosthetic patch or prosthetic device (which inhibits endothelialization).
- Cardiac transplantation recipients who develop cardiac valvulopathy.

Endocarditis prophylaxis is not recommended for routine gastrointestinal or genitourinary procedures.[70]

Table 17-6. Common Syndromes, Associated Congenital Heart Diseases, and Anesthetic Implications

Syndrome	Commonly Associated CHD	Other Anesthetic Implications
CHARGE association (**C**oloboma, congenital **H**eart defects, choanal **A**tresia, **r**enal abnormalities, **G**enital hypoplasia, **E**ar deformities)	65% conotruncal anomalies, aortic arch anomalies	Difficult airway and intubation, renal dysfunction
DiGeorge syndrome (chromosome 22 deletion, catch 22)	Interrupted aortic arch, truncus arteriosus, VSD, PDA, TOF	Hypocalcemia, immunodeficiency, need for irradiated blood products
Duchenne muscular dystrophy	Cardiomyopathy	Hyperkalemic cardiac arrest with succinylcholine, rhabdomyolysis with inhalational agents
Ehler-Danlos syndrome	Aneurysm of aorta and carotid artery	Difficult intravenous access, increased bleeding risk
Ellis-van Creveld syndrome (chondroectodermal dysplasia)	50% common atrium	Possible difficult intubation
Fetal alcohol syndrome	25%–30% VSD, PDA, ASD, TOF	Difficult airway, renal disease
Friedreich's ataxia	Cardiomyopathy	Progressive neurological degeneration, glucose intolerance
Glycogen storage disease II (Pompe)	Cardiomyopathy	
Holt-Oram syndrome	ASD, VSD	Upper limb abnormalities
Leopard syndrome (cardiocutaneous syndrome)	PS, long PR interval, cardiomyopathy	Growth retardation, possible difficult intubation
Long QT syndromes: • Jervell and Lange Nielsen • Romano-Ward	Long QT interval, ventricular tachyarrhythmia	Congenital deafness
Marfan syndrome	Aortic aneurysm, AR, and/or MR	Spontaneous pneumothorax, cervical spine instability
Mucopolysaccharidosis: • Hurler (type I) • Hunter (type II) • Morquio (type III)	AR and/or MR, coronary artery disease, cardiomyopathy	Difficult airway, atlantoaxial instability, kyphoscoliosis
Noonan syndrome	PS (dystrophic valve), LVH, septal hypertrophy	Possible difficult intubation, platelet dysfunction, renal dysfunction
Tuberous sclerosis	Myocardial rhabdomyoma	Seizure disorder, renal dysfunction
Shprintzen syndrome (velocardiofacial, 22q deletion)	Conotruncal anomalies, TOF	Difficult airway
VACTERL association	**C**=CHD, VSD, conotruncal anomalies (TOF, truncus arteriosus)	**V**ertebral anomalies, **A**nal atresia, **T**racheoesophageal fistula, **E**sophageal atresia, **R**enal anomalies, **L**imb defects
Williams syndrome	Supravalvular AS, PA stenosis	Developmental delay, difficult airway, renal dysfunction
Zellweger syndrome (cerebrohepatorenal syndrome)	PDA, VSD, ASD	Neonatal jaundice, kidney and liver dysfunction, coagulopathy, hypotonia

Prevention of Paradoxical Embolization

Multiple CHD lesions including simple (ASD, VSD, CAVC) or complex (single ventricle lesions) have an intracardiac communication at the atrial or ventricular levels and repaired cardiac lesions may have a fenestrated patch closure. These intracardiac communications can allow air or thrombotic material to migrate from the venous circulation to the arterial circulation to the brain, gastrointestinal tract, or kidneys. Hence, careful administration of fluid and medications and the use of in-line air filters to prevent air emboli are important to decrease the risk of paradoxical embolization.

Monitoring and Intravenous Access

Standard ASA monitoring including noninvasive blood pressure, electrocardiogram (ECG), and pulse oximetry is recommended for all patients. A 5-lead ECG is recommended in patients at risk of arrhythmia or coronary ischemia such as patients with aortopulmonary shunts or long QT syndrome. Invasive monitoring of blood pressure (arterial line) and central venous pressure should be considered based on the type of procedure (eg, spinal fusion) and patient's cardiac condition and functional status. The location of blood pressure monitoring also depends on the cardiac lesion and prior/planned interventions. Patients with aortic coarctation will have higher blood pressure in the upper extremities compared to lower extremities. Patients with history of a classic BT shunt (subclavian to PA end-to-side anastomosis) may not have a measurable blood pressure in the ipsilateral arm while those with a current modified Blalock-Taussig (BT) shunt may have lower blood pressure on the ipsilateral side of the BT shunt due to steal. It is important to note that peripheral intravenous (IV) access may be difficult.

Management of Fluid Status

The NPO times are similar to other cases with 2 hours for clear fluids, 4 hours for breast milk, 6 hours for formula, and 6 to 8 hours for solid food. Some patients do not tolerate prolonged NPO times and preoperative hydration is required to prevent hemodynamic instability at induction. These patients include patients with Williams-Beuren syndrome, patients on chronic diuretic therapy, and preload-dependent patients such as those with bidirectional Glenn or Fontan physiology. In addition, dehydration in cyanotic patients may worsen blood hyperviscosity leading to thrombosis. If prehydration is not possible, a fluid bolus 5 to 10 mL/kg following induction and IV placement is recommended. Fluid administration should be judicious in patients with pulmonary vein stenosis, mitral stenosis, or diastolic dysfunction to avoid the development of pulmonary edema.

Hemodynamic and Respiratory Management

The anesthesiologist needs to understand the underlying pathophysiology, the hemodynamic goals, and potential risks of hemodynamic instability inherent to a patient's underlying CHD. Beta-blockers are usually continued prior to the procedure while ACE inhibitors are withheld for 24 hours prior to the procedure, and diuretics are either held or continued depending on the nature of the procedure and its intended fluid requirements.

Premedication is individualized based on the patient's and the family's prior experience. Midazolam 1 mg/kg (maximum 20 mg) combined with oral ketamine (3–5 mg/kg for infants and 5–10 mg/kg for children) can be used as an oral premedication. In children who cannot take oral premedication, intramuscular premedication is an option.

In addition to the routine anesthesia setup, it is important to be ready for hemodynamic instability and discuss the intraoperative management with the patient's cardiologist and surgeon. If the patient is at risk of arrhythmia, appropriate antiarrhythmic medications and equipment such as a defibrillator and pacing equipment need to be available. Pacemakers and ICDs should be interrogated prior to the procedure to ensure that they are properly functioning and to inform intraoperative device management. For example, pacemaker-dependent patients undergoing procedures where electrocautery will be used will likely require a setting change to an asynchronous pacing mode in order to ensure continuous pacing, while those with an ICD will require the ICD functionality to be suspended in order to prevent inappropriate shocks. If the patient's functional status requires inotropic support during the procedure, dopamine and epinephrine should be readily available. Table 17-7 lists the most common inotropic and antiarrhythmic drugs.

Preoperative Planning and Postoperative Disposition

Planning on the timing, location (surgery center, satellite hospital, tertiary main hospital campus), and staffing is an important component of preoperative planning. The patient should be medically optimized, NPO times should be minimized, and the location and staff capable of providing the necessary resources and expertise are required. The ability to escalate care and obtain cardiology support should always be considered even for seemingly simple procedures. Based on the patient's cardiac condition and planned procedure (diagnostic imaging, spine, dental rehabilitation), the postoperative course can range from recovery in the post-anesthesia care unit with discharge home, observation for 24 hours, admission as inpatient to the cardiac floor, to admission to the cardiac intensive care unit.

Table 17-7. Commonly Used Vasoactive Drugs and Antiarrhythmics

Drugs	Bolus	Infusion Rate	Comments
Adenosine 6 mg in 2 mL (3 mg mL^{-1})	100 μg kg^{-1} rapid IV bolus and flush (maximum 6 mg); second dose 200 μg kg^{-1} (max. 12 mg)		Reduce by half for patients who have had a heart transplant. Give as close to IV site followed by a flush
Atropine 8 mg in 20 mL (0.4 mg mL^{-1})	20 μcg kg^{-1} IV		Maximum dose 1 mg for child and 3 mg for adolescent
Amiodarone 150 mg in 3 mL (50 mg mL^{-1})	5 mg kg^{-1} IV slowly over 15–30 min	5–15 μg kg^{-1} min^{-1}	Adult max. bolus 300 mg for Vfib and/or VTach
Calcium gluconate 100 mg mL^{-1}	30–60 mg kg^{-1} IV		
Dopamine 400 mg in 10 mL (40 mg mL^{-1})		3–10 μg kg^{-1} min^{-1}	Titrate to effect
Epinephrine 1 mg mL^{-1}	1 μg kg^{-1} to treat hypotension IV; 10 μg kg^{-1} IV for cardiac arrest; repeat every 3–5 min as needed	0.02–0.1 μg kg^{-1} min^{-1}	Titrate to effect
Isoproterenol 1 mg in 5 mL (0.2 mg mL^{-1})		0.01–0.1 μg kg^{-1} min^{-1}	Tachycardia, palpitations, angina, pulmonary edema, hypertension, hypotension, ventricular arrhythmias, tachyarrhythmias
Lidocaine 20 mg in 2 mL (10 mg mL^{-1})	1 mg kg^{-1} IV	20–50 μg kg^{-1} min^{-1}	
Magnesium 50% 1 in 2 mL (0.5 g mL^{-1})	25–50 mg kg^{-1} IV		For torsades de pointes (max. 2 g)
Norepinephrine 4 mg in 4 mL (1 mg mL^{-1})		0.05 μg kg^{-1} min^{-1}	Titrate to effect
Phenylephrine 10 mg mL^{-1} vial	0.5 μg kg^{-1}	0.1 μg kg^{-1} min^{-1}	Titrate to effect
Procainamide 500 mg mL^{-1} 100 mg mL^{-1}	5–15 mg kg^{-1} IV loading dose over 30–60 min	20–80 μg kg^{-1} min^{-1}	ECG monitoring required Caution: hypotension and prolonged QT, widening of QRS
Vasopressin 20 units mL^{-1}	In children 0.1 unit In adults 1 unit	6–30 mU kg^{-1} min^{-1}	Titrate to effect
Ephedrine 5 mg mL^{-1}	0.05–0.1 mg kg^{-1}		

REFERENCES

1. Morton SU, Brodsky D. Fetal physiology and the transition to extrauterine life. *Clin Perinatol*. 2016;43:395-407.
2. Finnemore A, Groves A. Physiology of the fetal and transitional circulation. *Semin Fetal Neonatal Med*. 2015;20:210-216.
3. Hines MH. Neonatal cardiovascular physiology. *Semin Pediatr Surg*. 2013;22:174-178.
4. Park MK. *Park's The Pediatric Cardiology Handbook*. 5th ed. Philadelphia, PA: Elsevier/Saunders; 2016.
5. Johns Hopkins Hospital, Kahl L, Hughes HK. *The Harriet Lane Handbook E-Book*. Philadelphia, PA: Elsevier; 2017.

6. Hoffman JI, Kaplan S. The incidence of congenital heart disease. *J Am Coll Cardiol.* 2002;39(12):1890-1900.

7. Schneider DJ, Moore JW. Patent ductus arteriosus. *Circulation.* 2006;114(17):1873-1882.

8. Slaughter JL, Reagan PB, Bapat RV, Newman TB, Klebanoff MA. Nonsteroidal anti-inflammatory administration and patent ductus arteriosus ligation: a survey of practice preferences at US Children's Hospitals. *Eur J Pediatr.* 2016;175(6):775-783.

9. Jaillard S, Larrue B, Rakza, et al. Consequences of delayed surgical closure of patent ductus arteriosus in very premature infants. *Ann Thorac Surg.* 2006;81(1):231-234.

10. Fowlie PW, Davis PG, McGuire W. Prophylactic intravenous indomethacin for preventing mortality and mobidity in preterm infants. *Cochrane Database Syst Rev.* 2010;7(7):CD000174.

11. Ohlsson A, Walia R, Shah AA. Ibuprofen for the treatment of patent ductus arteriosus in preterm or low birth weight (or both) infants. *Cochrane Database Syst Rev.* 2015;18(2):CD003481.

12. Ohlsson A, Shah AA. Paracetamol (acetaminophen) for patent ductus arteriosus in preterm or low birth weight infants. *Cochrane Database Syst Rev.* 2015;11(3):CD010061.

13. Malviya MN, Ohlsson A, Shah SS. Surgical versus medical treatment with cyclooxygenase inhibitors for symptomatic patent ductus arteriosus in preterm infants. *Cochrane Database Syst Rev.* 2013;3:CD003951.

14. Ngo S, Profit J, Gould J, Lee H. Trends in patent ductus arteriosus diagnosis and management for very low birth weight infants. *Pediatrics.* 2017;139(4):1-9.

15. Barikbin P, Sallmon H, Wilitzki S, et al. Lung function in very low birth weight infants after pharmacological and surgical treatment of patent ductus arteriosus. *BMC Pediatrics.* 2017;17:5.

16. Weisz DE, More K, McNamara PJ, Shah PS. PDA ligation and health outcomes: a meta-analysis. *Pediatrics.* 2014;133(4):e1024-e1046.

17. Weisz DE, Mirea L, Rosenberg E, et al. Association of patent ductus arteriosus ligation with death or neurodevelopmental impairment among extremely preterm infants. *JAMA Pediatr.* 2017;171(5):443-449.

18. Backes CH, Cheatham SL, Deyo GM, et al. Percutaneous patent ductus arteriosus (PDA) closure in very preterm infants: feasibility and complications. *Cardiovasc Cerebrovasc Dis.* 2016;5(2):e002923.

19. Radzik D, Davignon A, van Doesburg N, Fournier A, Marchand T, Ducharme G. Predictive factors for spontaneous closure of atrial septal defects diagnosed in the first 3 months of life. *J Am Coll Cardiol.* 1993;22(3):851-853.

20. Zhang J, Ko JM, Guileyardo JM, Roberts WC. A review of spontaneous closure of ventricular septal defect. *Proc (Bayl Univ Med Cent).* 2015;28(4):516-520.

21. Rastelli JC, Kirklin JW, Titus JL. Anatomic observations on complete form of persistent common atrioventricular canal with special reference to atrioventricular valves. *Mayo Clin Proced.* 1966;41:296-308.

22. Ebels T, Elzenga N, Anderson RH. Atrioventricular septal defects. In: Anderson RH, Baker EJ, Penny D, Reddington AN, Rigby ML, Wernovsky G, eds. *Paediatric Cardiology.* 3rd ed. Philadelphia, PA: Churchill Livingstone; 2010:553-589.

23. Kaza AK, Minich LL, Tani LY. Atrioventricular septal defects. In: Da Cruz EM, Dunbar I, Jaggers J, eds. *Pediatric and Congenital Cardiology, Cardiac Surgery and Intensive Care.* London: Springer-Verlag; 2014:1479-1491.

24. Romer AJ, Tabbutt S, Etheridge SP, et al. Atrioventricular block after congenital heart surgery: analysis from the Pediatric Cardiac Critical Care Consortium. *J Thorac Cardiovasc Surg.* 2019;157(3):1168-1177.e2.

25. Cuypers JA, Witsenburg M, van der Linde D, Roos-Hesselink JW. Pulmonary stenosis: update on diagnosis and therapeutic options. *Heart.* 2013;99(5):339-347.

26. Jonas RA. Valve repair and replacement. In: Jonas RA, ed. *Comprehensive Surgical Management of Congenital Heart Disease.* 2nd ed. Boca Raton, FL: CRC Press; 2014:395-420.

27. Singh S, Ghayal P, Mathur A, et al. Unicuspid unicommissural aortic valve: an extremely rare congenital anomaly. *Tex Heart Inst J.* 2015;42(3):273-276.

28. Kaza AK, Pigula FA. Surgical approaches to critical aortic stenosis with unicommissural valve in neonates. *Expert Rev Cardiovasc Ther.* 2014;12(12):1401-1405.

29. Collins RT II. Cardiovascular disease in Williams syndrome. *Circulation.* 2013;127(21):2125-2134.

30. Flaker G, Teske D, Kilman J, Hosier D, Wooley C. Supravalvular aortic stenosis. A 20-year clinical perspective and experience with patch aortoplasty. *Am J Cardiol.* 1983;51(2):256-260.

31. Etnel JR, Takkenberg JJ, Spaans LG, Bogers AJ, Helbing WA. Paediatric subvalvular aortic stenosis: a systematic review and meta-analysis of natural history and surgical outcome. *Eur J Cardiothorac Surg.* 2015;48(2):212-220.

32. Jimenez M, Daret D, Choussat A, Bonnet J. Immunohistological and ultrastructural analysis of the intimal thickening in coarctation of human aorta. *Cardiovasc Res.* 1999;41(3):737-745.

33. Hu ZP, Wang ZW, Dai XF, et al. Outcomes of surgical versus balloon angioplasty treatment for native coarctation of the aorta: a meta-analysis. *Ann Vasc Surg.* 2014;28(2):394-403.

34. Dijkema EJ, Sieswerda GT, Takken T, et al. Long-term results of balloon angioplasty for native coarctation of the aorta in childhood in comparison with surgery. *Eur J Cardiothorac Surg.* 2018;53(1):262-268.

35. Boehm W, Emmel M, Sreeram N. Balloon atrial septostomy: history and technique. *Images Paediatr Cardiol.* 2006;8(1):8-14.

36. Senning A. Surgical correction of transposition of the great vessels. *Surgery.* 1959;45(6):966-980.

37. Mustard WT. Successful two-stage correction of transposition of the great vessels. *Surgery.* 1964;55:469-472.

38. Jatene AD, Fontes VF, Paulista PP, et al. Anatomic correction of transposition of the great vessels. *J Thorac Cardiovasc Surg.* 1976;72(3):364-370.

39. Lim HG, Kim WH, Lee JR, Kim YJ. Long-term results of the arterial switch operation for ventriculo-arterial discordance. *Eur J Cardiothorac Surg.* 2013;43(2):325-334.

40. Schwartz ML, Gauvreau K, del Nido P, Mayer JE, Colan SD. Long-term predictors of aortic root dilation and aortic regurgitation after arterial switch operation. *Circulation.* 2004;110(11 suppl 1):II128-II132.

41. McMahon CJ, Ravekes WJ, Smith EO, et al. Risk factors for neo-aortic root enlargement and aortic regurgitation following arterial switch operation. *Pediatr Cardiol.* 2004;25(4):329-335.

42. Karl TR. The role of the Fontan operation in the treatment of congenitally corrected transposition of the great arteries. *Ann Pediatr Cardiol.* 2011;4(2):103-110.

43. Spigel Z, Binsalamah ZM, Caldarone C. Congenitally corrected transposition of the great arteries: anatomic, physiologic repair, and palliation. *Semin Thorac Cardiovasc Surg Pediatr Card Surg Annu.* 2019;22:32-42.

44. Loomba RS, Buelow MW, Woods RK. Complete repair of tetralogy of Fallot in the neonatal versus non-neonatal period: a meta-analysis. *Pediatr Cardiol.* 2017;38(5):893-901.

45. Wilder TJ, Van Arsdell GS, Benson L, et al. Young infants with severe tetralogy of Fallot: early primary surgery versus transcatheter palliation. *J Thorac Cardiovasc Surg.* 2017;154(5):1692-1700.e2.

46. Quandt D, Ramchandani B, Stickley J, et al. Stenting of the right ventricular outflow tract promotes better pulmonary arterial growth compared with modified Blalock-Taussig shunt palliation in tetralogy of Fallot-type lesions. *JACC Cardiovasc Interv.* 2017;10(17):1774-1784.

47. Lemler MS, Scott WA, Leonard SR, Stromberg D, Ramaciotti C. Fenestration improves clinical outcome of the fontan procedure: a prospective, randomized study. *Circulation.* 2002;105(2):207-212.

48. Jolley M, Colan SD, Rhodes J, DiNardo J. Fontan physiology revisited. *Anesth Analg.* 2015;121(1):172-182.

49. Anderson PA, Sleeper LA, Mahony L, et al. Contemporary outcomes after the Fontan procedure: a Pediatric Heart Network multicenter study. *J Am Coll Cardiol.* 2008;52(2):85-98.

50. Gewillig M, Goldberg DJ. Failure of the fontan circulation. *Heart Fail Clin.* 2014;10(1):105-116.

51. Rossano JW, Kim JJ, Decker JA, et al. Prevalence, morbidity, and mortality of heart failure-related hospitalizations in children in the United States: a population-based study. *J Card Fail.* 2012;18:459-470.

52. Hsu DT, Pearson GD. Heart failure in children: part I: history, etiology, and pathophysiology. *Circ Heart Fail.* 2009;2:63-70.

53. Andrews RE, Fenton MJ, Dominguez T, Burch M. Heart failure from heart muscle disease in childhood: a 5-10 year follow-up study in the UK and Ireland. *ESC Heart Failure.* 2016;3:107-114.

54. Rossano JW, Shaddy RE. Heart failure in children: etiology and treatment. *J Pediatr.* 2014;165:228-233.

55. Kirk R, Dipchand AI, Rosenthal DN, et al. The International Society for Heart and Lung Transplantation Guidelines for the management of pediatric heart failure: executive summary. [Corrected]. *J Heart Lung Transplant.* 2014;33:888-909.

56. Romer AJ, Rajagopal SK, Kameny RJ. Initial presentation and management of pediatric heart failure. *Curr Opin Pediatr.* 2018;30:319-325.

57. Jefferies JL, Towbin JA. Dilated cardiomyopathy. *Lancet.* 2010;375:752-762.

58. Hinton RB, Ware SM. Heart failure in pediatric patients with congenital heart disease. *Circulation Research.* 2017;120:978-994.

59. Zaleski KL, Scholl RL, Thiagarajan RR, et al. Elective extracorporeal membrane oxygenation support for high-risk pediatric cardiac catheterization. *J Cardiothorac Vasc Anesth.* 2019;33(7):1932-1938.

60. Dipchand AI, Kirk R, Naftel DC, et al. Ventricular assist device support as a bridge to transplantation in pediatric patients. *J Am College Cardiol.* 2018;72:402-415.

61. Nasr VG, Meserve J, Pereira LM, et al. Sedative and analgesic drug sequestration after a single bolus injection in an ex vivo extracorporeal membrane oxygenation infant circuit. *ASAIO J.* 2019;65(2):187-191.

62. Harthan AA, Buckley KW, Heger ML, Fortuna RS, Mays K. Medication adsorption into contemporary extracorporeal membrane oxygenator circuits. *J Pediatr Pharmacol Ther.* 2014;19(4):288-295.

63. Yang S, Noh H, Hahn J, et al. Population pharmacokinetics of remifentanil in critically ill patients receiving extracorporeal membrane oxygenation. *Sci Rep.* 2017;7(1):16276.

64. Kleiber N, Mathôt RAA, Ahsman MJ, Wildschut ED, Tibboel D, de Wildt SN. Population pharmacokinetics of intravenous clonidine for sedation during paediatric extracorporeal membrane oxygenation and continuous venovenous hemofiltration. *Br J Clin Pharmacol.* 2017;83(6):1227-1239.

65. Ahsman MJ, Hanekamp M, Wildschut ED, Tibboel D, Mathot RA. Population pharmacokinetics of midazolam and its metabolites during venoarterial extracorporeal membrane oxygenation in neonates. *Clin Pharmacokinet.* 2010;49(6):407-419.

66. Mulla H, McCormack P, Lawson G, Firmin RK, Upton DR. Pharmacokinetics of midazolam in neonates undergoing extracorporeal membrane oxygenation. *Anesthesiology.* 2003;99(2):275-282.

67. Jenks CL, Raman L, Dalton HJ. Pediatric extracorporeal membrane oxygenation. *Crit Care Clin.* 2017;33:825-841.

68. Nasr VG, DiNardo JA. Preoperative evaluation. In: *The Pediatric Cardiac Anesthesia Handbook.* Hoboken, NJ: Wiley Blackwell; 2017:23-30.

69. Schure AY. Noncardiac surgery in neonates and infants with cardiac disease. In: McCann ME, Greco C, Matthes K. *Essentials of Anesthesia in Infants and Neonates.* Cambridge, UK: Cambridge University Press; 2018:302-320.

70. Wilson W, Taubert KA, Gewitz M, et al. Prevention of infective endocarditis: guidelines from the American Heart Association: a guideline from the American Heart Association Rheumatic Fever, Endocarditis, and Kawasaki Disease Committee, Council on Cardiovascular Disease in the Young, and the Council on Clinical Cardiology, Council on Cardiovascular Surgery and Anesthesia, and the Quality of Care and Outcomes Research Interdisciplinary Working Group. *Circulation.* 2007;116(15):1736-1754.

Anesthesia for Thoracic Procedures

Anne E. Cossu and Doris M. Hardacker

18

FOCUS POINTS

1. Type II pneumocytes develop at 24 to 26 weeks of gestation and begin producing surfactant. Eight to ten percent of the number of adult alveoli are present at birth

2. Infants and children have reduced functional residual capacity (FRC) and higher oxygen consumption (6 to 8 ml/kg/min) rendering them susceptible to faster oxygen desaturation.

3. Etiologies for increased ventilation to perfusion (V/Q) mismatch during thoracic surgery include lateral positioning, general anesthesia and blunting of hypoxic pulmonary vasoconstriction, mechanical ventilation and surgical manipulation or single-lung ventilation.

4. One-lung ventilation (OLV) can be achieved utilizing single lumen endotracheal tubes inserted into the main stem bronchus, endobronchial blockers, Univent tubes or double lumen tubes dependent on the size of the patient.

5. Management of hypoxemia during OLV includes 100% oxygen, continuous positive airway pressure (CPAP) to the nondependent lung, positive end-expiratory pressure (PEEP) to the dependent lung, double lung ventilation and in extremis occlusion of the pulmonary artery to the operative lung.

   Thoracic and mediastinal masses are lesions that may cause airway compromise prior to or during a procedure under anesthesia. Thorough preoperative evaluation that includes review of echocardiogram, available imaging, and

symptoms allow for a safer anesthetic. Spontaneous ventilation with min sedation may be the anesthetic of choice.

DEVELOPMENT OF THE RESPIRATORY SYSTEM

The morphological development of the lung begins several weeks after conception and continues well into the first decade of life. Four stages of lung development and maturation were described initially by Dubreuil,[1] which was then updated in 1988 by Thurlbeck.[2] The first stage, called the embryonic stage, spans from 2–3 to 7–8 weeks of gestation and begins as an outgrowth of endoderm, surrounded by mesenchymal tissue, from the ventral foregut. This outgrowth extends into the pleuroperitoneal cavity and eventually forms lung buds.[3] A concurrent event is the development of the tracheoesophageal ridge. Incomplete separation of this ridge may lead to formation of a tracheoesophageal fistula.[4] The next phase, the pseudoglandular stage, extends from 7 to 16 weeks postconception and is punctuated by the formation of the conducting airways and pulmonary vasculature. Therefore, a fetus cannot survive if born at this stage of development.[5] The diaphragm forms during this time frame and consequently, any disruption may lead to herniation of abdominal organs into the thorax and hypoplasia of the lung, that is, congenital diaphragmatic hernia.[6] The canalicular phase, extending from 17 to 28 weeks postconception, is characterized by the development of acini and adjacent vascular growth. During this stage, bronchi and bronchioles increase in luminal diameter.[7] Type II pneumocytes develop by 24 to 26 weeks' gestation and potentially as early as 20 weeks.[8,9] These cells produce surfactant, which acts to reduce surface tension and stabilize airspaces.[10] Capillary networks surrounding the acini proliferate and allow for sufficient respiratory exchange by 26 to 28 weeks.[11] Premature infants can survive if born at 24 weeks; however, exogenous surfactant may be required to reduce pulmonary morbidity at this point. From 29 to 36 weeks of gestation, lung development enters the saccular phase at which time acini mature into saccules and there is formation of an extensive capillary network.[12] The last stage called the alveolar stage may begin as early as 32 weeks in some fetuses but is not consistently present until 36 weeks and extends well beyond birth. At this point, alveoli begin to develop from saccules.[13,14]

There are approximately 20 to 50 million terminal air sacs (mostly saccules) present at birth in the neonatal lung, approximately 8% to 10% of that present in the adult lung. During the next 12 to 18 months of postnatal life, the remaining saccules mature into alveoli and there is further development of alveolar ducts connecting to new alveoli.[15] By age 9, there is an estimated 280 million alveoli, which closely approximates adult levels. As the chest wall increases in size from childhood to adulthood, there is a matched expansion of lung surface area due to an increase in size of alveoli and the conducting airways.[16]

NORMAL RESPIRATORY PHYSIOLOGY

▶ Perinatal Adaption to Respiration

Rapid removal of liquid from the fetal lungs is essential to the establishment of pulmonary gas exchange at birth. With the initial gasps of air after birth, there is generation of a negative inspiratory force of up to −70 to −100 cm of H_2O that fills the lungs with air.[17] Residual amniotic fluid is removed from the lungs over days through lymphatic channels and pulmonary capillaries. Rhythmic breathing, which begins during fetal life and hypothetically may be necessary for normal pulmonary development, is maintained after birth due to interrupted umbilical blood flow and hyperoxia relative to the hypoxic fetal environment.[18]

▶ Control of Respiration

After birth, control of respiration is mediated by a complex interplay of the brainstem, stretch receptors in the airways and lung via the vagal nerve, peripheral and central chemoreceptors, and spinal reflexes.[19] The dorsal respiratory group (DRG) of neurons, located in the dorsomedial medulla, contains inspiratory neurons. The ventral respiratory group (VRG), in the ventrolateral medulla, contains both inspiratory and expiratory neurons.[20–22] Rhythmic breathing in humans is thought to be due to the pre-Botzinger complex, a small cluster of pacemaker neurons, which acts to initiate and maintain breathing in neonates and fetuses.[23]

The upper airways, trachea, bronchi, and chest wall contain mechanoreceptors and chemoreceptors, which function to affect respiration. Stimulation of receptors in the nose produce sneezing, apnea, and alter bronchomotor tone.[24] Infants, neonates, and premature neonates have highly sensitive upper airway reflexes, which may be directly stimulated with inhalational induction. Receptors in the pharynx are involved with swallowing, which coordinate the inhibition of breathing, closure of the larynx, and contraction of the pharyngeal muscles. When pharyngeal reflexes have been blunted, accumulating secretions can stimulate laryngeal receptors leading to prolonged breath holding, apnea, and laryngospasm via the superior laryngeal nerve.[25,26] Hypocapnia and hyperthermia are both known to worsen this response, whereas hypoventilation with hypercapnia, positive end-expiratory pressure, and deep anesthesia can suppress this response.[27]

Tracheobronchial and pulmonary receptors have been classified into three types: the slowly adapting (pulmonary) stretch receptors, the rapidly adapting (irritant or deflation) receptors, and the unmyelinated C-fiber endings (J receptors). Both the slowly adapting and rapidly adapting receptors lead to vagal afferent fibers.[28–31] Slowly adapting receptors (SARs) are located in the smooth muscle of the trachea and central airways.[32] SARs are activated by distension during inhalation and cause inhibition of inspiratory neurons, which is also called the Hering-Breuer inflation reflex. Rapidly adapting receptors (RARs) are located in epithelial cells lining the carina and large bronchi.[30,33] They respond to mechanical and chemical stimuli, such as smoke, inhalation anesthetics, and other irritating gases. RAR stimulation may cause coughing, mucus production, and bronchospasm.[34] J receptors are located near the pulmonary or capillary walls and are stimulated by pulmonary edema and congestion, pulmonary emboli, and inhaled irritants such as inhaled anesthetics. Stimulation may lead to rapid breathing, mucus production, bronchospasm, decreased tidal volume, hypotension, and bradycardia.[35] The muscles of the thorax, including the diaphragm and intercostal muscles, contain various types of mechanoreceptors, such as muscle spindles and Golgi tendon organs.[36,37] Muscle spindles are located in intercostal muscles and are a type of slowly adapting mechanoreceptor that detect stretch. Golgi tendon organs, a type of slowly adapting mechanoreceptor, are located at the point of insertion of muscle fiber into tendon.[22]

The main function of the peripheral and central chemoreceptors is the maintenance of normal pH, PaO_2 and $PaCO_2$ (P and a, respectively, are abbreviations for partial pressure and arterial).[38] The central chemoreceptors, which are located in the ventrolateral medulla, are sensitive to hydrogen ion concentration in the adjacent cerebrospinal fluid. The blood-brain barrier is highly permeable to CO_2 and it easily diffuses into the surrounding cerebrospinal fluid (CSF), which has poor buffering capacity. For this reason, respiratory acidemia readily stimulates respiration via the central chemoreceptors.[39] Conversely, with acute metabolic acidemia or alkalemia, alterations in hydrogen ion concentration in the blood are not transferred to the CSF as rapidly. With chronic metabolic acid-base disturbances, pH of the CSF remains rather close to 7.3 regardless of blood pH. Consequently, ventilation in these circumstances is dependent on the response of the peripheral chemoreceptors.[40]

The peripheral chemoreceptors, called the carotid bodies (located at the bifurcation of the common carotid artery), are sensitive to changes in pH, $PaCO_2$ and the PaO_2. The main role of the carotid bodies is to detect changes in PaO_2.[41] In adults, acute hypoxemia stimulates carotid bodies to increase ventilatory rate, which is partially opposed by hypocapnia due to suppression of central chemoreceptors.[42] Chronic hypoxemia, occurring over years, may cause the carotid bodies to lose their hypoxic response.[43] Neonates exhibit a biphasic response to hypoxemia and hyperoxia in the first several weeks of life.[44] Moderate hypoxemia produces a transient increase in respiratory rate followed by sustained respiratory depression, whereas 100% O_2 causes a transient decrease in respiratory rate, which is then followed by a sustained increase in respiratory rate.[45,46] This biphasic response to hypoxemia is lost by 3 weeks after birth, and conversely hypoxemia produces a sustained increase in ventilation.[46] Premature infants, on the other hand, continue to have this biphasic response to hypoxemia for a longer amount of time. Thus, the proper response to hypoxemia may occur only when the respiratory system has matured on a time course consistent with postconceptual age rather than postnatal age.[47]

In normal adults, ventilation increases linearly with increasing concentration of inspired CO_2 but only to a point, after which ventilation starts to decrease.[48] Hypoxemia potentiates the CO_2 response through carotid body stimulation, which shifts the CO_2 response curve to the left and increases the slope of the curve.[49] Anesthetics, opioids, and barbiturates suppress the medullary chemoreceptors, decrease the slope, and shift the CO_2 response curve to the right. Thus, with increasing concentration of anesthetics, there is a decrease in ventilatory response to an increasing concentration of CO_2.[50] Neonates increase ventilatory rate in response to hypercapnia but to a lesser extent than older infants. With increased gestational age and postnatal age, the slope of the CO_2 response curve increases, which may be due to increased sensitivity of the chemoreceptors and/or maturing mechanics of the thorax. In contrast to adults, hypoxemia in newborn infants decreases the slope and shifts the CO_2 response curve to the right, whereas hyperoxemia has the opposite effect.[51]

Lung Volumes

In normal children and adolescents, lung volumes are proportional to body size and height. In the early stages of lung development after birth, the total lung capacity of neonates and infants is disproportionately small in relation to body size. Additionally, due to high infantile metabolic rate per kilogram of body weight, ventilation per unit of lung volume is much higher versus older children and adults. In sum, the infant has less reserve in lung surface area for oxygen exchange.[52]

Total lung capacity (TLC) is the maximal volume allowed during inspiration and is divided into a number of subsets. Residual volume is the volume of air in the lungs after maximal expiration. Functional residual capacity (FRC) results from the balance between outward distention of the thorax and inward elastic recoil of the lungs. FRC is typically 50% of the total lung capacity in healthy children in upright position but decreases to 40% while supine.[52]

Infants have a smaller FRC, a factor that causes a greater and more rapid decrease in oxygen saturation with hypoventilation versus adults.[53] However, dynamic FRC is maintained in awake infants and young children by several mechanisms to prevent lung collapse. These mechanisms include sustained tonic activities of the inspiratory muscles throughout the respiratory cycle, narrowing of the glottis during expiration, inspiration starting at mid-expiration, and rapid respiratory rate in relation to the expiratory time rate.[52] Under the age of 6 years, closing capacity is greater than the FRC when supine.[53] Elevated closing capacity can lead to small airway collapse and decreased arterial oxygen saturation while in the supine position. Positive end expiratory pressure (PEEP) is important in restoring FRC. Infants and children under the age of 3 greatly benefit from PEEP because it is thought to improve compliance by 75%.[52] General anesthesia, surgery, abdominal distention, and lung disease may all negatively affect lung volumes. When in supine or prone position versus sitting or standing, infants and children experience a reduction in FRC due to the cephalic shift of abdominal contents. The reduction in FRC is more profound in young infants and greatly reduces oxygen reserve.[54]

Ventilation Mechanics

The elastic properties of the lung and thorax are measured in terms of compliance which is expressed in units of volume change per units of pressure change. Expansion of the lung and chest wall by the inspiratory muscles is counteracted by elastic recoil of the lungs and thoracic cage. In general, pediatric patients have decreased lung compliance.[52] As a whole, compliance of the respiratory system increases in the first 12 months of life due primarily to an increase in lung compliance.[55] The infant chest wall, conversely, is highly compliant at birth and decreases over time. As such it provides minimal support to the noncompliant lungs at birth. Conversely, chest wall elastic recoil is low at birth and increases with age primarily due to ossification of the cartilaginous structures and development of intrathoracic muscles.[56] The combination of a highly compliant chest wall and poorly compliant lungs leads to increased work of breathing and decreased FRC. Therefore, neonates and infants are even more prone to atelectasis while under general anesthesia compared to children and adolescents.[57] Muscle relaxation due to general anesthesia and paralytic medications decreases FRC further.

Ventilation

Ventilation is the movement of air in and out of the lungs. The intercostal and accessory inspiratory muscles are utilized with maximum inspiratory effort, but the diaphragm is the most important muscle for normal, "quiet" inspiration. Expiration is considered passive and is due to diaphragm relaxation and elastic recoil of the lungs and chest wall.[52] However, expiration in the newborn is an active process, and involves use of the intercostal and particularly the abdominal muscles.[58] Tidal volume (V_t) is the amount of air moved in and out of the lungs with each breath. Minute ventilation (V_e) is the amount of air moved in and out of the lungs per minute of time. The frequency of quiet breathing decreases with increasing age.[52] Humans may adjust respiratory rate to minimize work, although the exact mechanism for this adjustment is unknown.[59]

Only part of the minute ventilation is used in effective gas exchange, referred to as alveolar ventilation (V_a). The rest is referred to as noneffective, dead space ventilation (V_d). Airway obstruction can increase dead space. Physiological dead space is influenced by the relative quality of gas distribution. Therefore, when gas exchange is uneven as it is, eg, in patients with cystic fibrosis, physiological dead space will increase. This is also the case when blood supply to an area or areas of the lung decreases; physiological dead space will increase as well.[52]

Anatomic dead space serves to warm and humidify air as it enters the lung. Both endotracheal intubation and tracheostomy negate these functions. The dead space in children and at adolescence mirrors body height. The dead space to tidal volume (V_d/V_t) in normal lungs is consistent from infancy to adulthood at 0.3. However, increased dead space is much more detrimental to infants than adults, and this is because an infant has a much smaller tidal volume and a much larger proportional increase in dead space.[52]

Ventilation is variably distributed to the lung from apex to base. At the end of expiration, alveolar pressure is zero (atmospheric). Intrapleural pressure is negative and increases from apex to base (more negative at the apex and less negative at the base). Due to this, transmural pressure is higher and regional FRC is larger at the apex than at the base. Consequently, at the end of inspiration a larger proportion of the inspired air will be distributed to the lung base.[52] Similarly, with adults in the lateral decubitus position, the dependent lung receives a greater proportion of the tidal volume.[60] The opposite is true of infants such that oxygenation and ventilation are improved in the upper or nondependent lung when in the lateral decubitus position.[61,62] In infants up

to 27 months of age with or without lung disease, krypton-81m ventilation scans have shown that ventilation is preferential to the uppermost or apical portion of the lung.[61] This distribution of ventilation may be explained by premature airway closure at the lung base and due to the fact that the infant's chest is more compliant, creating near atmospheric intrapleural pressure rather than negative intrapleural pressure.[62] In this situation, airway closure occurs and when in the lateral decubitus position, oxygenation and ventilation preferentially shift to the upper, nondependent lung.[63] When adults are paralyzed and mechanically ventilated, tidal ventilation is shifted to the uppermost part of the lung presumably due to similar reasons.[64]

For the pediatric anesthesiologist, it is important to be mindful that general anesthesia causes decreased FRC, contributes to uneven ventilation, and increases physiological dead space. Other factors to consider are the dead space and internal compliance of the anesthesia circuit, both of which increase dead space. This necessitates an increase in tidal volume with mechanical ventilation, perhaps using 10 to 12 mL/kg. An inspiratory to expiratory ratio of 1:2 is typical for pediatric patients. Respiratory rate should be set to 10 to 14 for adolescents, 14 to 20 for children, and 20 to 30 for infants as a starting point. Further refinement can be accomplished with capnography or arterial blood gas monitoring. The addition of low-level PEEP at 5 to 7 cm of H_2O should be used to restore FRC.[52,65]

Perfusion

In adults, perfusion is nonuniform from the apex to the base due to the effect of gravity on pulmonary blood flow. The same is true of ventilation in adults; the result is well-matched ventilation and perfusion. As mentioned previously, ventilation in infants is normally distributed to nondependent regions of the lung. Perfusion is more evenly distributed in the infant due to high pulmonary arterial pressure and also because the effect of gravity is lessened.[65,66]

West divided properties of upright lung perfusion into four zones.[67-69] The interrelationship of three pressures, alveolar pressure, pulmonary arterial pressure, and pulmonary venous pressure, determines the distribution of perfusion. In zone I, alveolar pressure exceeds both pulmonary arterial and pulmonary venous pressure. Therefore, alveolar capillary blood flow is absent and ventilation is wasted here. High PEEP can increase zone I and create excessive dead space ventilation. In zone II, pulmonary arterial pressure exceeds alveolar pressure and is referred to as the waterfall zone. Perfusion pressure in this zone is the difference between pulmonary arterial pressure and alveolar pressure, which then determines blood flow. Blood flow increases linearly toward the lung base, until the pulmonary venous pressure exceeds the alveolar pressure, as it does in zone III. Similarly, perfusion pressure in zone III is the difference between pulmonary arterial pressure and pulmonary venous pressure. Typically, perfusion pressure remains constant in zone III, but flow increases toward the base due to increases in both pulmonary arterial and venous pressures. In zone IV, blood flow decreases toward the base due to increased interstitial pressure surrounding the extraalveolar vessels. Zone IV increases in size with reduction in total lung volume near residual volume.[67-69]

Ventilation and Perfusion

Normal alveolar gas exchange depends on the balance between regional ventilation and perfusion. A normal relationship of ventilation to perfusion (V/Q) is 0.8.[68] With a patient in upright position, both blood flow and ventilation is less at the apex and greater at the base. The difference in blood flow from apex to base is greater than the ventilation difference such that the V/Q ratio decreases from apex to base. In supine position, there is a similar but smaller change in ventilation and perfusion between anterior and posterior lung. In infants, ventilation is normally distributed to the nondependent areas of the lung and perfusion is more evenly distributed for reasons mentioned previously, resulting in higher V/Q.[69]

With pulmonary disease, V/Q mismatch occurs due to uneven ventilation, uneven perfusion, or both. Pulmonary embolism, reduced pulmonary capillary bed, and intrapulmonary/anatomic right to left shunting may all cause V/Q mismatch. In congenital heart disease (CHD) with increased pulmonary blood flow due to left to right shunting, V/Q is decreased. In CHD with decreased pulmonary blood flow due to right to left shunting V/Q is increased.[52]

There is an intrinsic mechanism in the lungs that functions to preserve V/Q matching. In areas of high V/Q and low pCO_2, the airways constrict and the vessels dilate. The opposite occurs in areas of low V/Q with high pCO_2. In addition, hypoxic pulmonary vasoconstriction (HPV) works to further constrict blood flow thereby increasing V/Q. Certain drugs themselves can diminish or abolish HPV including nitroprusside, nitroglycerin, isoproteronol, and inhaled anesthetics.[70–73]

PERIOPERATIVE CONSIDERATIONS FOR THORACIC SURGERY

A detail-oriented and complete preoperative evaluation is essential for the neonate, infant, or child who is undergoing thoracic surgery. Choice of the type of induction, that is, inhalational versus intravenous induction, should be carefully considered depending on the potential for difficult intubation and the presence of intrathoracic lesions that may cause compression of the trachea or major vascular structures. Inhalational induction with maintenance of spontaneous respiration is preferred when there is concern for compression of the airway and major vascular structures by large intrathoracic masses. In this instance, availability of a rigid bronchoscope may also be useful if the trachea becomes compressed by an intrathoracic mass and

if there is an inability to ventilate either before or after intubation. Intravenous induction may be preferred if there is concern for lung contamination. Placement of adequate intravenous access, possibly a central line, and an arterial catheter should be weighed in light of the type of procedure to be performed, that is, thoracoscopy versus thoracotomy, potential for blood loss, and the need to monitor hemodynamics and arterial blood gases during one lung ventilation and manipulation of the thoracic structures.[74]

Inhalational anesthetics are commonly used for the maintenance of anesthesia in thoracic surgery, but have the disadvantage of attenuating hypoxic pulmonary vasoconstriction. In general, nitrous oxide should be avoided due to risk of pneumothorax after thoracoscopy or thoracotomy. Total intravenous anesthesia can also be utilized and thereby one can avoid the potential deleterious effects of inhaled anesthetics on hypoxic pulmonary vasoconstriction. A variety of techniques to treat postoperative pain can be utilized after thoracoscopy or thoracotomy. Bupivacaine infiltration of incision sites is one approach. A variety of regional anesthetic techniques can be utilized, including paravertebral and intercostal nerve blocks and caudal or epidural catheter placement.[74]

THORACOSCOPIC PROCEDURES

Video-assisted thoracoscopic surgery (VATS) has become more common in infants and children due to the advantage of smaller incisions, reduced pain, and shortened hospitalization with faster recovery.[75,76] With this may come the expectation of one lung ventilation (OLV) and the likelihood should be discussed between surgeon and anesthesiologist on a case by case basis, including risks, benefits, and indications. OLV is desirable during thoracoscopy as lung deflation leads to better visualization of the thoracic cavity and potentially reduces the risk of damage to surrounding structures by retraction. Thoracoscopic procedures in infants and children include diagnostic inspection, lung biopsy, lobectomy, sequestration removal, lung decortication, thymectomy, esophageal atresia repair, aortopexy, mediastinal mass resection, patent ductus arteriosus ligation, and sympathectomy.[74] The absolute indications for OLV in adults and adolescents include the following:

1. Prevention of contamination of healthy lung by bleeding or infection
2. Control of ventilation in patients with bronchopleural fistula, unilateral bullae, or tracheobronchial disruption
3. Bronchoalveolar lavage such as with alveolar proteinosis

Relative indications include the following:

1. Surgical exposure—high importance
   a. Thoracic aortic aneurysm
   b. Pneumonectomy
   c. Upper lobectomy

2. Surgical exposure—low importance
   a. Middle and lower lobectomies
   b. Esophageal resection
   c. Thoracoscopy
   d. Anterior thoracic spine surgery

TECHNIQUES FOR SINGLE LUNG VENTILATION IN INFANTS AND CHILDREN

▶ Single-Lumen Endotracheal Tube

The simplest method to provide OLV in children is to purposefully intubate the mainstream bronchus with a single-lumen endotracheal tube (ETT).[77] Several approaches can be used when the goal is to intubate the left mainstem bronchus. One method is to rotate the bevel of the ETT 180 degrees to the left and turn the child's head to the right.[78] The ETT is advanced until breath sounds are no longer heard on the right side. Placement is confirmed with a fiberoptic bronchoscope (FOB).[74] Another approach is to use fluoroscopic guidance.[79]

Several problems can occur with the use of single lumen ETTs for OLV. First, an uncuffed ETT can lead to significant leak if there is not an adequate seal with the bronchial wall. This can cause lack of collapse of the operative lung and possible contamination with blood or infectious material to the healthy, ventilated lung. Placement of a cuffed ETT in the main bronchus may result in obstruction of the right upper lobe orifice if the distance from the proximal cuff to the tip of the ETT is longer than the length of the right main stem bronchus. Hypoxemia can then occur due to obstruction of the upper lobe. This is more likely to occur on the right due to the short distance from the carina to the right upper lobe bronchus.[74]

▶ Balloon-Tipped Bronchial Blockers

Bronchial blockade and OLV can be provided with a Fogarty embolectomy catheter or an end-hole, balloon wedge catheter.[80,81] The distal tip of a Fogarty catheter has a bendable tip which facilitates placement into the mainstem bronchus on the operative side. The FOB can be used to confirm and facilitate placement of the Fogarty catheter. There are a variety of ways to place the Fogarty catheter outside the ETT. One approach is to intubate a mainstem bronchus with a single lumen ETT and then place a guide wire inside the ETT. The ETT would then be removed and the Fogarty catheter could be threaded over the guide wire. A single lumen ETT could be reinserted into the trachea alongside the Fogarty catheter. The Fogarty catheter balloon would then be positioned in the proximal mainstem bronchus using the FOB for visualization.[80]

There is risk of dislodgment and occlusion of the trachea, which could prevent ventilation of the lungs bilaterally or prevent collapse of the operative lung. The

Table 18-1. Single-Lumen Uncuffed Tracheal Tube Diameters

Inner Diameter (mm)	Outer Diameter (mm)
3.0	4.3
3.5	4.9
4.0	5.5
4.5	6.2
5.0	6.8
5.5	7.5
6.0	8.2
6.5	8.9
7.0	9.6
7.5	10.2
8.0	10.8

balloons of most bronchial blockers are low compliance with low volume and high pressure. As such, overdistention of the balloon can lead to mucosal ischemia or airway rupture.[82] When the blocker is placed outside the ETT, it is important to be cognizant of the total airway diameter and injury that could be caused by compression of the tracheal mucosa by the ETT and bronchial blocker together. Therefore, the combined diameter of the bronchial blocker and outer diameter of the ETT should not exceed the expected tracheal diameter. Table 18-1 lists the diameters of pediatric sized uncuffed ETTs. These numbers estimate tracheal diameter, which is the predicted size of an uncuffed ETT that should produce a seal with the tracheal wall.[74] Cuffed tubes have an additional 0.5 mm outer diameter.

▶ Combination ETT and Bronchial Blockers

The Univent tube is an endotracheal tube with a second internal lumen housing a bronchial blocker. The blocker can be advanced into a mainstem bronchus.[83] A FOB must be used to facilitate placement. The bronchial blocker has an internal lumen and a balloon at the distal tip. Therefore, ventilation, suction, and continuous positive airway pressure (CPAP) can be applied to the operative lung. The blocker position within the outer ETT is very stable and dislodgment is rather unlikely.[74]

The Univent tube is available with lumen diameters as small as 3.5 and 4.5 mm for patients as young as approximately 6 years.[84] The internal area occupied by the bronchial blocker is rather high and consequently the outer diameter is quite large. For example, a Univent tube with a 3.5 mm internal luminal diameter corresponds to a 7.5/8.0 mm outer diameter (Table 18-2). As with the Fogarty catheter,

Table 18-2. Univent Tube Diameters

Inner Diameter (mm)	Outer Diameter (mm)
3.5	7.5
4.5	8.5
6.0	10.0
6.5	10.5
7.0	11.0
7.5	11.5
8.0	12.0
8.5	12.5
9.0	13.0

Table 18-3. Double-Lumen Tube Diameters

Size (French)	Main Body Outer Diameter (mm)
26	8.7
28	9.4
32	10.6
35	11.7
37	12.4
39	13.1
41	13.7

the Univent balloon has low volume and high pressure such that overinflation can cause mucosal ischemia.[74]

Double-Lumen Tubes

The double-lumen tube (DLT) consists of two unequal length tubes molded together as one. The shorter tube is designed to occupy the trachea while the longer tube should reside in a mainstem bronchus. Each tube has a balloon at the distal tip. Typically, the endobronchial balloon resides on the distal tip of the bronchial lumen and is blue colored for easy identification with the FOB. DLTs have balloons with high compliance and low pressure, which minimizes pressure on the bronchial and tracheal wall.[74] With the endobronchial balloon inflated in the mainstem bronchus, ventilation of either lung in isolation or at the same time is possible. There are right- and left-sided DLTs. The right-sided DLT has a long tube designed to go into the right mainstem bronchus, whereas the long tube of the left-sided DLT should occupy the left mainstem. The right DLT endobronchial balloon has a donut shape designed to allow right upper lobe ventilation. However, the right upper lobe orifice may still become occluded by the endobronchial balloon despite it altered design.[85] The smallest DLT size available in the United States is 26F, which is designed for children 8 years of age. There are also 28F and 32F DLTs that accommodate children 10 years and older. Adults' sizes range from 35 to 41F.[74] Table 18-3 lists the outer diameters of the various sizes of DLTs.

The same method used to insert a DLT into an adult can be used for a child. The tip of the tube is inserted just past the vocal cords and the tube is then rotated 90 degrees to the operative side and advanced in the trachea. Breath sounds should then be auscultated to confirm placement. With the tracheal cuff inflated, breath sounds should be auscultated on both sides. With the bronchial cuff inflated, breath sounds should be heard on both sides to ensure the bronchial cuff has not herniated across the trachea.

Fiberoptic bronchoscopy can also be performed through the tracheal lumen to confirm placement of the bronchial cuff in the right or left mainstem bronchus. Additionally, the tracheal lumen can be clamped and breath sounds auscultated. When a left-sided DLT has been properly positioned, breath sounds should be heard on the left only when the tracheal lumen clamped. The opposite holds true for a right-sided DLT.[74]

One major disadvantage of the DLT is the possibility of the need for continued controlled ventilation in the postoperative period. Therefore, exchange to a single lumen endotracheal tube is necessary. This is of particular concern when the initial intubation was challenging. Further, reintubation may become challenging after surgery due to swelling, secretions, and blood in the airway or trauma from the first intubation. An exchange catheter may facilitate the exchange for a single lumen tube.[86] An additional advantage is that exchange catheters can be used for oxygen insufflation and jet ventilation.

MANAGEMENT OF SINGLE-LUNG VENTILATION

Once proper position of a SLT, bronchial blocker or DLT is confirmed, it is necessary to determine the peak airway pressures required for OLV. In general, peak airway pressures should be minimized and not exceed 40 cm of water (H_2O) during OLV. Once lateral decubitus positioning is obtained, position of the bronchial blocker, SLT, or DLT should be reconfirmed with fiber-optic bronchoscope as the position can be disrupted with patient positioning. After transition to OLV, an inspired oxygen concentration of 100% is typically necessary. The goal partial pressure of oxygen (PaO_2) should be approximately 100 to 200. Tidal volumes should be 8 to 10 mL/kg and respiratory rate should be adjusted to maintain a partial pressure of carbon dioxide ($PaCO_2$) at a range of 45 to 60, unless the patient's physiology cannot tolerate hypercapnia.[87]

If hypoxemia occurs during OLV, several steps can be undertaken. First the patient can be manually ventilated

Table 18-4. Recommended Tube Sizes for One Lung Ventilation in Pediatric Patients

Age (yr)	Endotracheal Tube Inner Diameter (mm)	Bronchial Blocker (French)	Univent (mm)	Double-Lumen Tube (French)
0.5–1	3.5–4.0	2		
1–2	4.0–4.5	3		
2–4	4.5–5.0	5		
4–6	5.0–5.5	5		
6–8	5.5–6.0	5	3.5	
8–10	6.0	5	3.5	26
10–12	6.5	5	4.5	26–28
12–14	6.5-7.0	5	4.5	32
14–16	7.0	5, 7	6.0	35
16–18	7.0–8.0	7, 9	7.0	35, 37

Source: Reproduced with permission, from Cote CJ, Lerman J, Anderson BJ, eds. *A Practice of Anesthesia for Infants and Children.* 5th ed. 2013. Copyright © Elsevier Saunders. All rights reserved.

and placed on 100% oxygen. To determine if the tube or endobronchial blocker is in correct position, FOB may then be undertaken. Several measures that may improve oxygenation include application of continuous positive airway pressure to the nondependent lung if this is tolerable to the surgeon and use of PEEP to the dependent lung. One further option is to occlude the pulmonary artery to the operative lung to decrease shunt. If there is persistent hypoxemia despite these measures, return to two-lung ventilation is imperative.

Appropriate tube selection for OLV in children can be predicted using Table 18-4. There is great variability in size among the different age groups in the pediatric population and these recommendations are based upon average airway dimensions.

SURGICAL LESIONS OF THE THORAX

▶ Neonates and Infants

Congenital Cystic Lesions

Congenital cystic lesions encompass various thoracic lesions that can be further subdivided into four groups: bronchogenic cysts, cystic adenomatoid malformations, congenital lobar emphysema, and bronchopulmonary sequestration. The presentation of these lesions may vary. Each lesion can be prenatally diagnosed and treated with fetal surgery. Though the rate of occurrence is only 5 per 10,000 fetuses, there is significant morbidity and mortality associated with these lesions.[88]

Bronchogenic cysts are also known as foregut duplications with 85% occurring in the mediastinum and 15% intrapulmonary. They can be filled with air or fluid and can be central or peripheral. Most are asymptomatic.[89]

Congenital cystic adenomatous malformations (CCAM) are intrapulmonary lesions that result from abnormal lung development of the terminal bronchioles. They are characterized by multicystic areas of overproliferation and dilation of terminal respiratory bronchioles that lack normal alveoli.[90] They are unilobar, unilateral, and account for 25% of all congenital lung malformations. Almost all are detected on antenatal ultrasound by 20 weeks.

Congenital lobar emphysema results from weakened or absent bronchial cartilage that permits focal bronchial collapse. This results in a ball-valve phenomenon which traps air, causing hyperinflation of the affected lobe. Causes of ball-valve phenomenon can be intrinsic (dysplastic bronchial cartilage, intraluminal obstruction) or extrinsic from vascular abnormalities such as anomalous pulmonary vascular return or pulmonary artery sling. This can result in contralateral mediastinal shift, decreased cardiac output, and ensuing hypoxia and hypotension. It occurs 1 in 20,000 births with a 3:1 ratio in males versus females. Fifty percent of the cases involve the upper lobe of the left lung. Although less severe cases may not initially present until childhood, most cases are encountered in the neonatal period. The neonatal cases may present with acute respiratory distress that necessitates surgical intervention and resection of the affected lobe. A total of 15% to 20% of neonates have concurrent congenital heart lesions involving atrial or ventricular septal defects or pulmonary hypertension.[91]

Surgical resection is recommended for congenital cystic lesions to avoid potential infection, hemorrhage, and respiratory complications. Induction and intubation are critical events and should be planned to avoid Valsalva maneuver that would increase air trapping. An inhalation induction and maintenance of anesthesia that preserves spontaneous ventilation until thoracotomy is preferred. Gentle manual ventilation with inspiratory pressures less than 20 cm H_2O may be required to maintain oxygenation. Nitrous oxide is contraindicated. Selective endobronchial intubation and high-frequency ventilation are additional options for ventilation until thoracotomy is achieved. Due to the possibility of lung overinflation on induction, a surgeon should be present in the event a thoracotomy is needed to relieve the overdistention.[90,92]

Bronchopulmonary sequestration is an embryonic mass of lung tissue that is isolated from neighboring lung tissue and has no connection to the bronchial tree and is nonfunctioning: 75% intralobar with the remaining 25% being extralobar. It receives its blood supply from an aberrant branch of the descending aorta and should be resected since heart failure can result from its large blood flow.[93]

Childhood

Anterior Mediastinal Masses

While the occurrence of anterior mediastinal masses is uncommon in children, anesthesia for such cases can be very challenging and fraught with hazard. The anesthetic plan will be dependent on the pathology, specific location, procedure, and age of the patient. Information obtained from the patient's history, exam, and radiological workup will guide and determine the anesthetic plan.

The anterior mediastinal space is defined by the sternum anteriorly, sternomanubrial junction superiorly, pericardium posteriorly and diaphragm inferiorly, and the parietal pleura laterally. Masses of the mediastinum encompass tumors that are both benign and malignant. While anterior mediastinal masses are predominantly lymphomas in origin, other less common lesions include thymomas, teratomas, lipomas, and cystic lymphatic malformations.[94]

A retrospective chart review by Garey et al demonstrated that a mean age of 11 years had poor correlation of symptoms with anatomical airway obstruction or complications.[95] Large masses can present without any airway compression.[96] King et al reported no statistically significant association between degree of compression/clinical symptoms and size of tumor.[97] Treatment plans rely on tissue diagnosis and therefore patients will present for various procedures including CT-guided needle biopsy, superficial lymph node biopsy, VATS, or mediastinoscopy. Any one of these procedures could require either sedation or a general anesthetic.

Any anesthetic should be well-planned in advance and undoubtedly will involve the expertise of the multiple care teams. In published studies, the overall complication rate in patients with mediastinal masses was 20%, and 5% of patients had a serious complication related to anesthesia.[98] There are numerous reports of sudden refractory cardiorespiratory collapse during induction or maintenance of anesthesia in both symptomatic and asymptomatic patients.[99] As such, multiple backup plans must be established prior to induction and appropriate equipment must be readily available along with adequate support staff.

Since pulmonary and cardiac symptoms may significantly contribute to or help predict complications, proceeding forward with an anesthetic is best guided by the patient's history, physical exam, and radiological/diagnostic information. Any preoperative evaluation should include a review of the patient's symptoms. Important factors for consideration include the effect of position on signs and symptoms such as dyspnea, stridor, dysphagia, chest pain/fullness, cough, or syncope.[94] Of the aforementioned symptoms, stridor was the only sign that predicted an anesthetic complication in a published study.[98] Imaging such as a chest x-ray and computed tomography (CT) will also provide useful information. CT imaging can provide adequate images in approximately 20 seconds. The patient's head may be elevated during a CT scan to 30 degrees without compromising scan quality.[100] A greater than 50% decrease in the diameter of the tracheobronchial lumen may be associated with complete airway obstruction during the induction or emergence from general anesthesia.[101] Echocardiography may be used to evaluate cardiovascular compromise. In addition, awake bronchoscopy and flow-volume studies can provide information regarding airway dynamics and compression.

Mediastinal tissue biopsy can be performed with the application of EMLA cream, local anesthetics, and sedation with ketamine (0.5–1 mg/kg). Antisialagogue agents are useful to decrease salivation caused by ketamine. Ketamine is particularly useful for sedation in patients with hemodynamic compromise. Dexmedetomidine may also provide analgesia and amnesia while maintaining spontaneous respirations. Sedative agents such as benzodiazepines and opioids can cause undesired muscle relaxation and respiratory depression, respectively.[98] If a general anesthetic is required for either tissue biopsy or definitive surgery, induction of anesthesia may be accomplished with inhalational agents, etomidate, propofol, and/or ketamine. Spontaneous ventilation is the safest strategy to prevent complete airway collapse with institution of positive pressure ventilation. Muscle relaxants should be utilized only when positive pressure ventilation has been documented with the current airway in place. One approach to intubation would be an awake fiberoptic intubation with subsequent use of an armored endotracheal tube placed distal to the compression or a double lumen tube where the bronchial lumen is placed distal to the obstruction. If during the operative procedure ventilation is severely compromised, the anesthetic can be reversed to awaken the patient. Alternatively, the patient can be repositioned to either the prone or lateral position. Finally, the airway can be splinted with a rigid bronchoscope to ventilate distal to the obstruction. Sternotomy or thoracotomy with retraction of the mass from the airway and great vessels has also been utilized as an option. While cardiopulmonary bypass has been described as an option prior to the start of any procedure in a patient with an anterior mediastinal mass,[102] the logistics of instituting bypass once compromise has occurred may result in prolonged hypoxia and subsequent cardiac arrest.

REFERENCES

1. Dubreuil G. Observations sur le developpement du poumon humain. *Bull Histol Technol Physiol.* 1936;13:235.
2. Thurlbeck W. *Lung Growth.* New York: Thieme; 1988.
3. Emery JL. *The Anatomy of the Developing Lung.* London: Heinemann Medical Books; 1969.

4. Smith EI. The early development of the trachea and esophagus in relation to atresia of the esophagus and tracheoesophageal fistula. *Contrib Embryol Carnegie Inst Wash.* 1957;36:41.

5. Boyden EA. *Development of the Human Lung.* New York: Harper and Row; 1972.

6. Areechon W, Eid L. Hypoplasia of lung with congenital diaphragmatic hernia. *Br Med J.* 1963;1(5325):230-233.

7. Boyden EA. The mode of origin of pulmonary acini and respiratory bronchioles in the fetal lung. *Am J Anat.* 1974;141(3):317-328.

8. Spear GS, Vaeusorn O, Avery ME, et al. Inclusions in terminal air spaces of fetal and neonatal lung. *Biol Neonate.* 1969;14:344.

9. Lauweryns JM. "Hyaline membrane disease" in newborn infants: macroscopic, radiographic and light and electron microscopic studies. *Hum Pathol.* 1970;1:175.

10. Brumley GW, Hodson WA, Avery ME. Lung phospholipids and surface tension correlations in infants with and with hyaline membrane disease and in adults. *Pediatrics.* 1967;40(1):13-19.

11. Potter EL. *Pathology of the Fetus and Infant.* Chicago, IL: Year Book Medical Publishers; 1961.

12. Justin Lockman Book 3.

13. Langston C, Kida K, Reed M, Thurlbeck WM. Human lung browth in late gestation and in the neonate. *Am Rev Respir Dis.* 1984;129(4):607-613.

14. Weibel ER. *Morphometry of the Human Lung.* Berlin: Springer-Verlag; 1963.

15. Langston D, Kida K, Reed M, et al. Human lung growth in late gestation and in the neonate. *Am Rev Respir Dis.* 1984;129:607.

16. Hislop A, Reid L. Development of the acinus in the human lung. *Thorax.* 1974;29(1):90-94.

17. Karlberg P, Cherry RB, Escardo FE, et al. Respiratory studies in newborn infants. II. Pulmonary ventilation and mechanics of breathing in the first minutes of life, including onset of respiration. *Acta Paediatr Scand.* 1962;51:121.

18. Cook CD, Drinker PA, Jacobson HN, Levison H, Strang LB. Control of pulmonary blood flow in the foetal and newly born lamb. *J Physiol.* 1963;169:10-29.

19. Cherniack NS, Pack AI. *Control of Ventilation.* 3rd ed. New York: McGraw-Hill; 1998.

20. von Euler C. Brainstem mechanisms for generation and control of breathing pattern. In: Cherniack NS, Widdicombe JG, eds. *Handbook of Physiology. Section 3. The Respiratory System. Control of Breathing,* Part 1, Vol 2. Bethesda, MD: American Physiology Society; 1986.

21. Tabatabai M, Behnia R. Neurochemical regulation of respiration. In: Collins JV, ed. *Physiological and Pharmacological Basis of Anesthesia.* Philadelphia, PA: Williams & Wilkins; 1995.

22. Berger AJ. Control of breathing. In: Murray JF, Nadel JA, eds. *Textbook of Respiratory Medicine.* Philadelphia, PA: WB Saunders; 2000.

23. Smith JC, Ellenberger HH, Ballanyi K, Richter DW, Feldman JL. Pre-Botzinger complex; a brainstem region that may generate respiratory rhythm in mammals. *Science.* 1991;254(5032):726-729.

24. Widdicombe JG. Reflexes from the upper respiratory tract. In: Cherniak NS, Widdicombe JG, eds. *Handbook of Physiology. Section 3. The Respiratory System. Control of Breathing,* Part 1. Vol. 2. Bethesda, MD: American Physiological Society; 1985.

25. Pickens DL, Schefft GL, Thach BT. Pharyngeal fluid clearance and aspiration preventive mechanisms in sleeping infants. *J Appl Physiol.* 1989;66(3):1164-1167.

26. Sasaki CT, Suzuki M. Laryngeal spasm: a neurophysiologic redefinition. *Ann Otol Rhinol Laryngol.* 1977;86(2):150-157.

27. Motoyama E, Finder JD. Respiratory Physiology in Infants and Children. In David PJ, Cladis FP, Motyama EK, eds. *Smith's Anesthesia for Infants and Children.* 8th ed. Pittsburg, PA: Elsevier; 2011.

28. Pack AI. Senosry inputs to the medulla. *Annu Rev Physiol.* 1981;43:73.

29. Widdicome JG. Nervous receptors in the respiratory tract and lungs. In: Hornbein TF, ed. *Regulation in Breathing, Part I.* New York: Marcel Dekker; 1981.

30. Sant'Ambrogio G. Information arising from the tracheobronchial tree of mammals. *Physiol Rev.* 1982;62:531.

31. Coleridge JCG, Coleridge HMG. Afferent vagal C fiber innervation of the lungs and airways and its functional significance. *Rev Physiol Biochem Pharmacol.* 1984;99:1.

32. Bartlett D Jr, Jeffrey P, Sant'Ambrogio G, et al. Location of stretch receptors in the trachea and bronchi of the dog. *J Phsiol (Lond).* 1976;258:409.

33. Pack AI. Sensory inputs to the medulla. *Annu Rev Physiol.* 1981;43:73.

34. Sampson SR, Virdruk EH. Properties of "irritant" receptors in canine lung. *Respir Physiol.* 1975;25:9.

35. Paintal AS. Vagal sensory recpetors and their reflex effects. *Physiol Rev.* 1973;53:159.

36. Newsom-Davis J. Control of the muscles of breathing. In: Widdicombe JG, ed. *Respiratory Physiology.* Vol 2. Baltimore, MD: University Park Press; 1974.

37. Duron B. Intercostal and diaphragmatic muscle endings and afferents. In: Hornbein TF, ed. *Regulation of Breathing, Part I.* New York: Marcel Dekker; 1981.

38. Leusen I. Regulation of cerebrospinal fluid composition with reference to breathing. *Physiol Rev.* 1972;52:1.

39. Papperheimer JR, Fenci V, Heisey SR, et al. Role of cerebral fluids in control of respiration as studied in unanesthetized goats. *Am J Physiol.* 1965;208:436.

40. Mitchell RA, Carman CT, Severinghaus JW, et al. Stability of cerebrospinal fluid pH in chronic acid-base disturbances in blood. *J Appl Physiol.* 1965;20:443.

41. Severinghaus JW. Hypoxic respiratory drive and its loss during chronic hypoxia. *Clin Physiol.* 1972;2:57.

42. Severinghaus JW, Mitchell RA, Richardson BW, et al. Respiratory control of high altitude suggesting active transport regulation of CSF pH. *J Appl Physiol.* 1963;18:1155.

43. Sorensen SC, Severinghaus JW. Irreversible respiratory insensitivity to acute hypoxia in man born at high altitude. *J Appl Physiol.* 1968;25:217.

44. Martin RJ, Abu-Shaweesh JM. Control of breathing and neonatal apnea. *Biol Neonate.* 2005;87(4):288-295.

45. Rigatto H, Brady JP, de la Torre Verduzco R. Chemoreceptor reflexes in preterm infants: II. The effect of gestational and postnatal age on the ventilatory response to inhaled carbon dioxide. *Pediatrics.* 1975;55(5):614-620.

46. Dripps RD, Comroe JH Jr. The respiratory and circulatory response of normal man to inhalation of 7.6 and 10.4 percent CO_2 with a comparison of the maximal ventilation produced by severe muscular exercise, inhalation of CO_2 and maximal voluntary hyperventilation. *Am J Physiol.* 1947;149(1):43-51.

47. Rigatto H. Apnea. In: Thibeault DW, Gregory GA, eds. *Neonatal Pulmonary Care.* Norwalk, CT: Appleton-Century-Crofts; 1986.

48. Dripps RD, Comroe JH Jr. The respiratory and circulatory response of normal man to inhalation of 7.6 and 10.4 percent CO_2 with a comparison of the maximal ventilation produced by severe muscular exercise, hyperventilation. *Am J Physiol.* 1947;149:43.

49. Nielsen M, Smith H. Studies on the regulation of respiration in acute hypoxia. *Acta Physio Scand.* 1951;24:293.

50. Munson ES, Larson CP, Babad AA, et al. The effects of halothane, fluroxene and cyclopropane on ventilation: a comparative study in man. *Anesthesiology.* 1966;27:716.

51. Rigatto H, Brady JP, Chir B, et al. Chemoreceptor reflexes in preterm infants. II. The effect of gestational and postnatal age on the ventilator response to inhaled carbon dioxide. *Pediatrics.* 1975;55:614.

52. Motoyama EK. Respiratory physiology in infants and children. In: Davis PJ, Cladis FP, Motoyama EK, eds. *Smith's Anesthesia for Infants and Children.* 8th ed. Philadelphia, PA: Elsevier Mosby; 2011.

53. Mansell A, Bryan C, Levison H. Airway closure in children. *J Appl Physiol.* 1972;33(6):711-714.

54. Westbrook PR, Stubbs SE, Sessler AD, et al. Effects of anesthesia and muscle paralysis on respiratory mechanics in normal man. *J Appl Physiol.* 1973;34:81.

55. Marchal F, Crance JP. Measurement of ventilator system compliance in infants and young children. *Respir Physiol.* 1987;68(3):311-318.

56. Halfaer MA, Nicols DG, Rogers MC. *Developmental Physiology of the Respiratory System.* 3rd ed. Baltimore, MD: Williams & Wilkins; 1996.

57. Guslits BG, Gaston SE, Bryan MH, England SJ, Bryan AC. Diaphragmatic work of breathing in premature human infants. *J Appl Physiol.* 1987;62(4):1410-1415.

58. Freund F, Roos A, Dood RB. Expiratory activity of the abdominal muslces in man during general anesthesia. *J Appl Physiol.* 1964;19:963.

59. McIlroy MB, Marshall R, Christie RV. The work of breathing in normal human subjects. *Clin Sci.* 1954;13:127.

60. Kaneko K, Milic-Emili J, Dolovich MB, et al. Regional distribution of ventilation and perfusion as a function of body position. *J Appl Physiol.* 1966;21:767.

61. Haef DP, Helms P, Gordon I, et al. Postural effects on gas exchange in infants. *N Engl J Med.* 1983;308:1505.

62. Davies H, Kitchman R, Gordon I, et al. Regional ventilation in infancy: reversal of adult pattern. *N Engl J Med.* 1985;313:1626.

63. Milic-Emili J, Henderson JAM, Dolovich MB, et al. Regional distribution of gas in the lung. *J Appl Physiol.* 1966;21:749.

64. Rehder K, Hatch DJ, Sessler AD, et al. The function of each lung of anesthetized and paralyzed man during mechanical ventilation. *Anesthesiology.* 1972;37:16.

65. Morman A, Chidambaran V. Pediatric anesthesiology review topics. In: Lockman JL, ed. *Book 3: The Pediatric Airway and Thoracic Surgery.* Philadelphia, PA: Naerthwyn Press; 2013.

66. Hughes JMB, Glazier JB, Maloney JE, et al. Effect of lung volume on the distribution of pulmonary blood flow in man. *Respir Physio.* 1968;4:58.

67. West JB. Blood flow to the lung and gas exchange. *Anesthesiology.* 1974;41:124.

68. West JB. Topographical distribution of blood flow in the lung. In: Fenn WO, Rahn H, eds. *Handbook of Physiology. Section 3. Respiration.* Vol 2. Washington, DC: American Physiological Society; 1965.

69. West JB. *Ventilation/Blood Flow and Gas Exchange.* 2nd ed. Oxford: Blackwell Scientific; 1970.

70. Goldzimer EL, Konopka RG, Moser KM. Reversal of perfusion defect in experimental canine labor pneumococcal pneumonia. *J Appl Physiol.* 1974;37:85.

71. Colley PS, Cheney FW Jr, Hlasta MP. Ventilation-perfusion and gas exchange effects of sodium nitroprusside in dogs with normal edematous lungs. *Anesthesiology.* 1979;30:489.

72. Hill AB, Chir B, Sykes MK, et al. A hypoxic pulmonary vasoconstrictor response in dogs during and after infusion of sodium nitroprusside. *Anesthesiology.* 1979;50:484.

73. Benumof JL. Respiratory physiology and respiratory function during anesthesia. In: Miller RD, ed. *Anesthesia.* 4th ed. New York: Churchill Livingstone; 1994.

74. Hammer G. Anesthesia for thoracic surgery. In: Cote CJ, Lerman J, Anderson BJ, eds. *A Practice of Anesthesia for Infants and Children.* 5th ed. Philadelphia, PA: Elsevier Saunders; 2013.

75. Mouroux J, Clary-Meinesz C, Padovani B. Efficacy and safety of videothoracosopic lung biopsy in the diagnosis of interstitial lung disease. *Eur J Cardiothorac Surg.* 1997;11:22-26.

76. Mackinlay TA, Lyons GA, Chimondeguy DJ, et al. VATS debridement versus thoracotomy in the treatment of loculated postpneumonia empyema. *Ann Thorac Surg.* 1996;61:1626-1630.

77. Rowe R, Andropoulos D, Heard M, et al. Anesthetic management of pediatric patients undergoing thoracoscopy. *J Cardiothorac Vas Anesth.* 1994;8:563-566.

78. Kubota H, Kubota Y, Toyoda Y, et al. Selective blind endobronchial intubation in children and adults. *Anesthesiology.* 1987;67:587-589.

79. Cohen DE, McCloskey JJ, Motas D, Archer J, Flake AW. Fluoroscopic-assisted endobronchial intubation for single lung ventilation in infants. *Pediatr Anesth.* 2011;21:681-684.

80. Hammer GB, Manos SJ, Smith BM, et al. Single lung ventilation in pediatric patients. *Anesthesiology.* 1996;84:1503-1506.

81. Ginsberg RJM. New technique for one-lung anesthesia using a bronchial blocker. *J Thorac Cardiovasc Surg.* 1981;82:542-546.

82. Borchardt RA, LaQuaglia MP, McDowall RH, Wilson RS. Bronchial injury isolation in a pediatric patient. *Anesth Analg.* 1998;87:324-325.

83. Kamaya H, Krishna RP. New endotracheal tube (Univent tube) for selective blockade of one lung. *Anesthesiology.* 1985;63:342-343.

84. Hammer GB, Brodsky JB, Redpath J, Cannon WB. The Univent tube for single lung ventilation in children. *Pediatr Anesth.* 1998;8:55-57.

85. Cohen E. Con: right-sided double lumen tubes should not be used routinely in thoracic surgery. *J Cardiothorac Vasc Anesth.* 2002;16:249-252.

86. Ho AC, Chung HS, Lu PP, et al. Facilitation of alternative one-lung and two-lung ventilation by use of an endotracheal tube exchanger for pediatric empyema during video-assisted thoracoscopy. *Surg Endosc.* 2004;18:1752-1756.

87. Cohen E. Oxygenation and hemodynamic changes during one-lung ventilation. *J Cardiothorac Anesth.* 1988;2:134-140.

88. Barikbin P, Roche C, Wilitzki S, et al. Postnatal lung function in congenital cystic adenomatoid malformation of the lung. *Ann Thorac Surg.* 2015;99:1164-1169.

89. Kamal K. Congenital lung malformations. Medscape. Available at http://emedicine.medscape.com/article/905596-overview. Acessed January 31, 2020.

90. Durell J, Lakhoo K. Congenital cystic lesions of the lung. *Early Human Development.* 2014;90:935-939.

91. Parray T, Apuya J, Abraham E, Ashanti F, Professor S. Anesthesiologist's dilemma in a patient with congenital lobar emphysema. *Internet J Anesthesiol.* 2009;24(2).

92. Gogia AR, Baja JK, Husain F, Mehta V. An Anesthetic management of a case of congenital lobar emphysema. J Anaesthesiology Clin Pharmacol. 2011;27(1):106-108.

93. Hertzenber C, Daon E, Kramer J. Intralobar pulmonary sequestration in adults: three case reports. *J Thorac Dis*. 2012;4(5):516-519.

94. Hanna AM, VanderWel B. Thoracoscopic approach to pediatric ediastinal masses. In: Walsh D, Ponsky T, Bruns N, eds. The SAGES Manual of Pediatric Minimally Invasive Surgery. Cham, Switzerland: Springer; 2017.

95. Garey CL, Laituri CA, Valusek PA, St. Peter SD, Snyder CL. Management of anterior mediastinal masses in children. *Eur J Pediatr Surg*. 2011;21:310-313.

96. Bray RJ, Fernandez FJ. Mediastinal tumors causing airway obstruction in anaesthetized children. *Anaesthesia*. 1982;37:571-575.

97. King DR, Patrick LE, Ginn-Pease ME, et al. Pulmonary function is compromised in children with mediastinal lymphoma. *J Pediatr Surg*. 1997;32(2):294-299.

98. Hack HA, Wright NB, Wynn RF. The anaesthetic management of children with anterior mediastinal masses. *Anesthesia*. 2008;63:837-846.

99. Datt V, Tempe D. Airway management in patients with mediastinal masses. *Indian J. Anaesth*. 2005;49(4):344-352.

100. Slinger P, Karsli C. Management of the patient with a large anterior mediastinal mass: recurring myths. *Curr Opin Anaesthesiol*. 2007;20:1-3.

101. Azizkhan RG, Dudgeon DL, Buck Jr, et al. Life threatening airway obstruction as a complication to the management of mediastinal masses in children. *J Ped Surg*. 1985;20:816-822.

102. Uljancic B, Pirtovsek S, Berger J. Anaesthetic management of children with anterior mediastinal mass—clinical case. Posted in Abstracts, Book of Abstracts, Vol 13, Suppl 2; April 10, 2017. Available at http://www.signavitae.com/2017/04/anaesthetic-management-of-children-with-anterior-mediastinal-mass-clinical-case/. Accessed January 31, 2020.

Anesthesia for Gastrointestinal Procedures

Kallol Chaudhuri

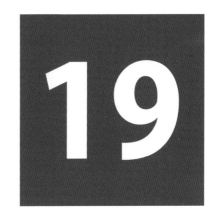

FOCUS POINTS

1. Pyloric stenosis is a medical and not a surgical emergency managed first by volume repletion. Hypochloremic, hypokalemic metabolic alkalosis is the classic derangement and once corrected, pyloromyotomy is the surgical intervention of choice.
2. An international randomized multicenter trial did not find any strong evidence that infants exposed to general anesthesia for 1 hour during inguinal herniorrhaphy had any measurable neurocognitive or behavioral deficits at 5 years of age.
3. Insufflation of the peritoneum with CO_2 for laparoscopic procedures leads to increased intra-abdominal pressure (IAP) with sometimes clinically significant cardiorespiratory, neuro, and renal physiological changes.
4. Intussusception is the most common abdominal emergency in patients less than 2 years of age with classic presentation of abdominal pain, and bloody (currant jelly) stool.
5. Gastroschisis is usually an isolated abdominal defect, whereas omphaloceles are usually associated with a wide variety of abnormalities (cardiac defects, congenital diaphragmatic hernia, chromosomal anomalies).
6. Congenital diaphragmatic hernia (CDH) presents at birth with respiratory distress-tachypnea, grunting, use of accessory muscles, and cyanosis. Prognostic indicators include the degree of lung hypoplasia and the presence of pulmonary hypertension.
7. The classic presentation of appendicitis includes periumbilical abdominal pain with anorexia, nausea, and vomiting. Leukocytosis and fever may be present. Transabdominal ultrasound (US) is the most common diagnostic modality.
8. Hirschsprung disease or congenital intestinal agangliosis is the most common cause of intestinal obstruction in neonates. Neonates who fail to pass meconium within 48 hours of life should be assessed for this disorder.

INTRODUCTION

A wide variety of gastrointestinal surgeries for various types of clinical disorders are performed in pediatric patients. Since the majority of disorders involve neonates and young infants, a general understanding of the embryological development would be helpful to appreciate the pathology and the clinical presentations of those disorders.

In this chapter, we will provide clinical presentations and treatment options, and brief descriptions of the anesthetic management of several pediatric diseases related to the gastrointestinal system: pyloric stenosis, inguinal hernia, umbilical hernia, laparoscopic surgery, intussusception, gastroschisis, omphalocele, congenital diaphragmatic hernia, appendicitis, aganglionic megacolon (Hirschsprung disease).

PYLORIC STENOSIS

Hypertrophic pyloric stenosis is the most common gastrointestinal surgical disorder in neonates. This disorder was first reported in 1717 by Patrick Blair, but a complete description with autopsy findings was then described by

Harald Hirschsprung in 1887. The operative procedure of pyloromyotomy for pyloric stenosis was first described by Ramstedt in 1912.

The incidence of pyloric stenosis (PS) is 0.9 to 5.1 per 1000 live births[1] and is more common in first born male infants. It usually presents at 3 to 8 weeks of age. The primary pathology is segmental hypertrophy of circular muscle fibers of the pyloric region of the stomach, resulting in gastric outlet obstruction. No definite inheritance pattern is noted, but the possibility of polygenic mode of inheritance pattern influenced by environmental factors has been suggested. Erythromycin, a motilin antagonist,[2] and maternal smoking[3] have also been implicated to play a role in the development of PS.

Symptoms of PS begin in an otherwise healthy infant with nonbilious projectile vomiting that starts immediately following feeding. As vomiting continues, the progressive loss of gastric acid (hydrogen and chloride ion) and fluid leads to hypochloremic metabolic alkalosis. Loss of intravascular fluid initiates increased absorption of sodium in exchange for potassium at the renal tubules, stimulated by aldosterone. The classic metabolic abnormality is hypochloremic, hypokalemic metabolic alkalosis. Urine may be alkaline due to systemic alkalosis. However, due to persistent hypokalemia, H^+ is exchanged in renal tubules for Na^+ to preserve K^+. The loss of H^+ causes paradoxical acidic urine with a systemic alkalosis. At later stages, persistent dehydration may lead to poor tissue perfusion, lactic acidosis, and metabolic acidosis. The classic finding of "olive," an olive-sized mass at the upper abdomen, is occasionally missing in PS patients. Confirmation of diagnosis is commonly done by ultrasound examination which has replaced the traditionally performed gastrointestinal barium study.

Management

Pyloric stenosis is a medical and not a surgical emergency. Replacement of intravascular volume and correction of electrolyte abnormalities (hypochloremia, hypokalemia, alkalosis) are essential prior to surgical correction. A tentative target of laboratory values includes serum bicarbonate >30 mEq/L, serum chloride >100 mEq/L, serum sodium >132 mEq/L, serum potassium >3.2 mEq/L, and serum pH 7.30 to 7.45.

Surgical correction of choice for PS patients is pyloromyotomy which includes incising the muscles of pylorus up to the layer of submucosa, leaving the mucosa intact. Currently, laparoscopic pyloromyotomy is preferred over open pyloromyotomy. The laparoscopic approach, compared to open approach, allows early initiation of postoperative feeding and shorter hospital stay.

Anesthetic Management

1. Standard ASA monitors should be placed prior to induction.

2. Patency of existing IV access should be confirmed.

3. A large orogastric catheter should be placed for decompression of stomach (four quadrant suctioning) prior to induction of anesthesia.

4. Glycopyrrolate (10 mcg/kg) may be considered to prevent reflex bradycardia during laryngoscopy.

5. Induction:

Inhalation induction: Although these patients are at high risk for pulmonary aspiration, inhalation induction with oxygen and inhalation agent (sevoflurane) has been reported to be a safe technique.[4]

Intravenous induction: Modified rapid sequence induction with low airway pressure ventilation is a popular method. The drugs used are propofol (2–3 mg/kg) or a combination of propofol (1–2 mg/kg) and ketamine (0.5–1 mg/kg). Ketamine by itself, at a dose of 1 to 2 mg/kg, has been shown to be an effective induction agent with minimum hemodynamic changes. Succinylcholine (2 mg/kg) or rocuronium (0.5–1 mg/kg) is commonly used as muscle relaxant. Rapid sequence induction with propofol (2.5–3 mg/kg) and remifentanil (2.5–3 mcg/kg) without any muscle relaxant was also used[5] for induction in pediatric patients, but hemodynamic changes, especially hypotension, are a concern in neonates.

6. Maintenance of anesthesia is achieved by using sevoflurane or desflurane in combination with oxygen and air. Nitrous oxide and remifentanil (2 mcg/kg/min) without any inhalation agent were also used without any significant hemodynamic alteration in open pyloromyotomy.[6] Nitrous is usually avoided in laparoscopic pyloromyotomy as it may cause distension of bowel. Intraoperative opioids (fentanyl) are also avoided because they may prolong emergence. Opioids can also increase the risk of postoperative apnea, a unique complication in these patients, thought to be related to persistent elevation of CSF pH, a determinant of respiratory drive.[7]

Relative intraoperative hypotension (systolic blood pressure <20% below baseline) was reported to be routine (in more than 70% patients less than 2 months old) and absolute intraoperative hypotension (mean arterial BP <35 mm Hg) was also reported to be common (12–21% in babies less than 2 months) during general anesthesia in patients undergoing laparoscopic pyloromyotomy.[8] This is of significant concern as these group of patients are most vulnerable to cerebral hypoperfusion.

Spinal anesthesia has been used successfully in laparoscopic pyloromyotomy. The advantages include avoidance of airway manipulations and related complications, avoidance of the debatable role of general anesthesia as neurotoxin in neonates, better hemodynamic profile with higher intraoperative blood pressure, and rapid recovery after surgery.[9,10] The technique was performed at L3-L4 level with a 22-gauge needle using hyperbaric bupivacaine (1 mg/kg).[9]

Postoperative analgesia is usually provided by

1. Infiltration of surgical wound by local anesthetic
2. Intravenous acetaminophen (15–20 mg/kg) preferable or rectal administration (30 mg/kg, variable absorption)

Opioids, such as morphine or fentanyl, are rarely needed for postoperative analgesia. Most patients tolerate oral feedings within a few hours after surgery.

INGUINAL HERNIA

Inguinal hernia is one of the commonest clinical conditions which requires surgical correction in pediatric patients. The overall incidence varies between 3.5% and 5% in term infants but is higher (13%) among the preterm infants.[11] It is more common in boys.

The majority of pediatric hernias are indirect in nature and result from failure of obliteration of the processus vaginalis. Processus vaginalis is a peritoneal diverticulum which precedes the testis in its journey to relocate from retroperitoneum to the scrotum at 25 to 33 weeks of gestation. The processus vaginalis normally fuses at 36th weeks of gestation and closes the internal ring. In cases where the processus vaginalis does not involute and remains patent, fluid or intraabdominal contents can migrate through the sac creating a hydrocele or indirect hernia, respectively.

The hallmark presentation for an inguinal hernia is a swelling at the groin or in the scrotum, the size of which increases with increased intraabdominal pressure (with crying, coughing). If the hernia becomes incarcerated, it presents with an irreducible tender erythematous swelling with symptoms of irritability, abdominal pain, and vomiting. The incarceration of intestines may lead to intestinal obstruction with worsening of previous symptoms along with abdominal distension, fever, and leukocytosis.

Because inguinal hernia usually does not resolve spontaneously and carries the risk of incarceration of bowel and testicular atrophy, all inguinal hernias in pediatric patients, especially in infants, are recommended to undergo surgical repair. However, the decision and timing of operative repair must be balanced against the overall medical condition of the child and potential anesthetic complications. Prematurity, which is associated in a number of these patients, can make the operative procedure more challenging. Early elective herniorrhaphy is also recommended in these patients; delaying the repair 1 week after diagnosis[12] or performing surgery beyond 40 weeks of conceptual age[13] significantly increases the risk of incarceration, strangulation, and intestinal obstruction.

In most cases, the surgical repair is carried out by laparoscopy; the advantages of laparoscopic repair include smaller incision and scar, shorter postoperative stay, and lesser need for postoperative analgesia. Laparoscopic approach also offers an option to assess the contralateral side without any significant injury to vas deferens and related blood vessels.

Anesthetic Management

Both general anesthesia and regional anesthesia have been used successfully for inguinal hernia repair.

General Anesthesia

General anesthesia with both endotracheal tube and laryngeal mask airway has been successfully used for repair of uncomplicated inguinal hernia. Endotracheal tubes are commonly used in laparoscopic procedures to provide adequate muscle relaxation and effective ventilation and in complicated hernia repair. LMA (Proseal) has been successfully used in laparoscopic hernia repair of short duration, with average surgical time of 15 minutes and average total anesthesia time of half an hour.[14]

Premedication: Midazolam (oral 0.5 mg/kg; IV 0.05 mg/kg) as indicated

Standard ASA monitors

Induction: Inhalation induction with oxygen/nitrous/sevoflurane; intravenous induction with propofol (2–3 mg/kg) or combination of ketamine (0.5–1 mg/kg) and propofol (1–2 mg/kg) may consider supplementing with lidocaine (0.5 mg/kg) and fentanyl (1 mcg/kg) or remifentanil (2 mcg/kg)

Muscle relaxation with rocuronium (0.6–0.8 mg/kg)

Maintenance of anesthesia with oxygen/air/sevoflurane or isoflurane

Ondansetron (50–200 mcg/kg IV) and dexamethasone 0.15–1 mg/kg IV as antiemetics

May consider dexmedetomidine (0.5 mcg/kg IV) and/or ketorolac (1 mg/kg IV) for postoperative analgesia given prior to completion of surgery

Postoperative Analgesia

1. Local wound infiltration with local anesthetics (bupivacaine or lidocaine)
2. Acetaminophen (20 mg/kg IV)
3. Ilioinguinal nerve block with 0.2% ropivacaine[15]
4. Caudal block (prior to surgery): ropivacaine 0.2% at 1 mL/kg. Clonidine (1–2 mcg/kg) or dexmedetomidine (1–2 mcg/kg) is a common adjunct drug.

It is suggested that all formerly preterm infants of less than 60 weeks postconceptual age should be monitored until they are apnea free for 12 hours.

Awake Regional Anesthesia

Spinal anesthesia has been reported to be effective in a wide variety of pediatric surgeries including inguinal hernia repair, circumcision, pyloromyotomy, and orthopedic procedures. The technique was also found to be effective in infants undergoing inguinal hernia repair using laparoscopic approach.[16]

There are some distinct advantages of spinal anesthesia over general anesthesia in infants and neonates:

1. Decreased respiratory complications including hypoxemia (oxygen desaturation <90%).[17]

2. Better hemodynamic stability. Compared to sevoflurane anesthesia, the incidence of hypotension (MAP <35 mm Hg) was reported to be significantly lower in infants (less than 60 weeks of postconceptual age) who underwent inguinal hernia repair under spinal anesthesia.[18]

3. Decreased apnea in the first 30 minutes postoperatively in infants (60 weeks or younger postconceptual age) undergoing inguinal herniorrhaphy, though there was no difference between spinal and general anesthesia groups in the first 12 postoperative hours.[19]

4. Spinal anesthesia is usually performed in the sitting or lateral decubitus position at L4-L5 level using a 22- (1.5 in.) or 25-gauge spinal needle. Standard ASA monitors are placed, and IV access is confirmed. Currently recommended drugs for spinal anesthesia are isobaric bupivacaine (0.5%) or isobaric ropivacaine (0.5%) at 1 mg/kg. Bupivacaine 0.75% in 8.25% dextrose is also used at a dose of 0.75 to 1 mg/kg.

The success rate of spinal anesthesia in neonates and infants primarily depends on the experience of the anesthesiologist; failure rate could be as high as 20%.[19] Total spinal anesthesia may occur especially during lifting the legs for placement of electrocautery pads in the back of the patient immediately after spinal. Respiratory support should be provided immediately with continuous monitoring of pulse, oxygen saturation, and blood pressure. Bradycardia and hypotension should be treated promptly. Post-dural-puncture headache is thought to be rare, but difficult to diagnose in these group of patients.

Of note, although there have been concerns regarding neurotoxicity and long-term neurocognitive effects of younger patients undergoing general anesthesia, an international randomized multicenter trial did not find any strong evidence that infants exposed to general anesthesia for 1 hour during inguinal herniorrhaphy had any measurable neurocognitive or behavioral deficits at 5 years of age.[20]

UMBILICAL HERNIA

Umbilical hernia is the protrusion of bowel or omentum due to weakness or defective closure of the umbilical ring where umbilical vessels enter the umbilical cord. The condition is common in low–birth-weight infants and in African Americans. The hernia usually presents as a swelling during straining but does not cause any painful symptoms unless strangulated. The umbilical hernia may be associated with congenital hypothyroidism, Down syndrome, and mucopolysaccharide storage disease.

Majority of the umbilical hernias close spontaneously by 5 to 6 years of age. Surgery is indicated in cases of strangulation, in hernias causing symptoms, or ones that persist after 4 to 5 years of age.

▶ Anesthetic Management

Usually provided by general anesthesia. Airway management with LMA can safely be provided in otherwise healthy child with a small to medium-sized uncomplicated hernia. For a large defect and in strangulated hernias, endotracheal intubation with inhalation or IV induction with propofol and rocuronium is recommended. Maintenance of anesthesia is usually provided with oxygen, air, and sevoflurane or desflurane.

LAPAROSCOPIC SURGERY

Minimally invasive approach surgeries, such as laparoscopic and robot-assisted laparoscopic procedures, have become increasingly popular in the last 10 to 15 years. The magnified image of the surgical field offered by advanced endoscopic instruments and improved laser technology allow the surgeons to perform precise dissection in several commonly performed pediatric surgeries. The advantages of minimally invasive surgeries include smaller surgical scars, less blood loss, fewer intraabdominal adhesions, shorter postoperative hospital stay, and decreased postoperative pain.

Pneumoperitoneum is created during laparoscopic surgery by insufflating carbon dioxide inside the peritoneal cavity, which allows better visualization. This process can potentially produce significant pathophysiological changes and complications:

- *Cardiovascular:* The increased intraabdominal pressure (IAP) causes a decrease in venous return, leading to a decrease in left ventricular preload, in cardiac output and in blood pressure. IAP may also cause significant reflex bradycardia by stimulation of the vagus nerve due to peritoneal stretching during needle placement.

  An increase in peripheral vascular resistance due to an increase in plasma norepinephrine during pneumoperitoneum may counterbalance the reduction in blood pressure.[21]

  Positioning of patient in the Trendelenburg position during robot-assisted surgery significantly increases cardiac filling pressures and cardiac workload.

  Due to the aforementioned negative cardiac effects, increased IAP may not be well tolerated by patients with hypovolemia, anemia, or significant cardiac disease.

  Pneumopericardium may occur when CO_2 passes via the membranous diaphragm or to the mediastinum via IVC. Serious injury to major vessels may happen due to accidental insertion of trocar into the vascular channels.

- *Respiratory:* Increased IAP from pneumoperitoneum pushes the diaphragm cephalad which increases peak inspiratory pressure, reduces compliance of the respiratory system (mainly chest wall compliance in neonates and infants), functional residual capacity (FRC), and total lung capacity. Loss of FRC may cause atelectasis and hypoxemia which get exaggerated in the head-down position. Depressed cardiac function during laparoscopy along with the pulmonary atelectasis increases V/Q mismatch. Pneumothorax may complicate the laparoscopy by entry of gas into the pleural cavity during dissection around esophagus, a diaphragmatic defect, tear in the visceral peritoneum, or rupture of an emphysematous bulla.[22]

Higher solubility of CO_2 leads to higher absorption of the gas and hypercarbia; the solubility is age dependent, more in neonates due to the relatively larger peritoneal surface area.[23]

- *Renal:* Pneumoperitoneum may decrease urine output by reducing renal blood flow and glomerular filtration rate. Urine output may also be decreased by stimulation of ADH secretion, a result of the direct compression of renal parenchyma.[24] Oliguria may continue for several hours after surgery.[25]

- *Intracranial pressure:* Intracranial pressure may increase in laparoscopy. Head-down position, hypercapnia, and increased IAP are possible contributory factors. Increase in ICP with low cardiac output and increased intrathoracic pressure may compromise cerebral perfusion pressure.[26]

- *Carbon dioxide embolism:* This is a rare but serious complication of pneumoperitoneum, which can occur due to direct placement of needle in the vessels. CO_2 embolism may present as sudden onset of hypotension, hypoxemia, increased end-tidal CO_2, and arrhythmia, which can progress to pulmonary edema.

Because increased IAP is related to these wide range of physiological changes and potential complications, it is suggested to keep the insufflation pressure low (8–12 mm Hg) in neonates and infants. Insufflation should begin at lowest flow rate, which may be increased as it attains the target pressure.[27] The IAP in older children should be limited to less than 15 mm Hg.

Low-pressure pneumoperitoneum with IAPs not exceeding 5 mm Hg in infants and children did not reduce cardiac index.[28]

Anesthetic Management

There are several important issues to remember regarding anesthetic management of patients for minimally invasive surgeries. Since access to the patient gets limited after surgical draping and docking of robots (in robot-assisted cases), standard monitors should be properly secured. Placement of a precordial stethoscope over left chest is helpful in small babies to quickly diagnose endobronchial migration of ET tube. A second IV access should be considered in long procedures. As end-tidal CO_2 concentration may not represent the arterial pCO$_2$ accurately in very small children, placement of an arterial line may be considered in selected cases of long duration. Inaccurate end-tidal CO_2 may lead to incorrect ventilator strategies in small babies.[26] Proper positioning and padding are important for infants due to their high vulnerability to positional injuries. An orogastric tube is helpful for gastric decompression.

General anesthesia with placement of endotracheal tube is commonly employed in laparoscopic cases. The cuffed endotracheal tube should be properly secured at correct mid-tracheal point, since downward displacement during steep Trendelenburg position may cause hypoxia or bronchospasm. Inhalational agents with opioids (as indicated) are used for maintenance of anesthesia. Nitrous should be avoided to limit bowel distension. Muscle relaxation is necessary for effective ventilation and pneumoperitoneum. Proper monitoring of temperature and urine output is mandatory.

INTUSSUSCEPTION

Intussusception is the telescopic invagination of a proximal segment of intestine, usually in the ileocolic region (intussusceptum), into an adjacent segment. The incidence peaks in children between 4 and 7 months, higher in fall and winter, and is the most common abdominal emergency in patients less than 2 years of age. Incidence is approximately 1 to 4 per 1000 live births and more common in males. In 90% cases it is idiopathic, but a prior respiratory infection, viral gastroenteritis, intestinal lymphoid hyperplasia, and Henoch-Schonlein purpura have been associated with intussusception. In some patients, a lead point such as Meckel's diverticulum, intestinal polyp, appendix, lymphoma, or hemangioma are recognized. Interruption of venous drainage of the mesentery associated with intussusceptum leads to edema and mucosal bleeding and if not relieved may lead to strangulation, gangrene, and shock.

The classic presentation of intussusception in children is abdominal pain, palpable abdominal mass, and bloody (currant jelly) stool. Typically, the initial symptom is a paroxysm of abdominal pain with intermittent crying with flexed knees and hips. Progressively, the pain becomes more frequent, the child vomits, becomes lethargic, and bloody diarrhea ensues.

Ultrasound is commonly used for diagnostic purposes, which has sensitivity and specificity of 98%. The patient with typical presentation should begin receiving intravenous fluid boluses and transported to the radiology suite for emergent hydrostatic reduction under fluoroscopy, which is both diagnostic and therapeutic. Success rate of hydrostatic reduction is approximately 80%. The patient with suspected peritonitis, bowel perforation, shock, and multiple recurrences should be taken to the operating room for surgical reduction.

Anesthetic Management

1. Review patient's history, vital signs, associated medical issues, laboratory results (glucose, electrolytes, H/H)
2. Confirm patency of intravenous access, premedication if appropriate
3. In the operating room: placement of ASA monitors
4. Rapid sequence IV induction with propofol (2–3 mg/kg) or ketamine (1–2 mg/kg), fentanyl (1 mcg/kg) and rocuronium (1 mg/kg), and endotracheal intubation with appropriate sized cuffed tube
5. Placement of large intravenous catheter and arterial line if indicated
6. Placement of nasogastric tube to evacuate the stomach
7. Aggressive fluid replacement with normal saline, lactated ringers, 5% human albumin in patients with intravascular volume deficits (shock, peritonitis, perforation, etc.)
8. Appropriate antibiotics, antiemetics (ondansetron and dexamethasone)
9. Maintenance of anesthesia with air/oxygen/sevoflurane or desflurane with fentanyl boluses, if appropriate
10. Extubate when awake
11. Acetaminophen (20 mg/kg IV), morphine (0.05–0.1 mg/kg IV), and/or dexmedetomidine (0.5 mcg/kg IV) for postoperative analgesia

GASTROSCHISIS AND OMPHALOCELE

Gastroschisis and omphalocele are two most common congenital abdominal wall defects observed in pediatric patients.

Gastroschisis

Gastroschisis, where the intraperitoneal contents protrude through an inborn defect of the ventral abdominal wall, appears like a "ruptured physiological hernia" and was first accurately described by Bernstein in a left-sided case which he named "epigastro-schisis."[29] An increase in incidence of gastroschisis has been noted in recent years from 3.6 per 10,000 births during 1995 to 2005 to a current report of 4.9 per 10,000 births during 2006 to 2012.[30]

The defect in the abdominal wall in gastroschisis is a full thickness paraumbilical opening with evisceration of intestines without any covering membrane. It is approximately 3 to 5 cm in diameter and is commonly present to the right of the umbilical cord insertion. Herniated bowel usually contains jejunum or ileum, and often appears thickened, edematous, or covered with fibrinous exudate.

Maternal factors implicated in gastroschisis include younger age, use of vasoconstrictive agents (nicotine, cocaine), and maternal infections.[30] Gastroschisis is divided into simple and complex cases. Complex cases are associated with other pathologies, eg, intestinal atresia,

volvulus, perforation, intestinal obstruction, and necrotizing enterocolitis. Neonatal mortality in complex cases is more than sevenfold higher than those with simple gastroschisis.[31] Pregnancy with gastroschisis babies also has a higher incidence of preterm birth, intrauterine growth retardation,[32] and stillbirth.[33] Prenatal diagnosis of gastroschisis is commonly done by ultrasonography, usually diagnosed during the second trimester. It is important to differentiate gastroschisis from omphalocele, which is covered by a membranous sac. The umbilical cord is inserted into the membranous sac in omphalocele, unlike in gastroschisis where it is inserted into the abdominal wall.

Several etiological factors are proposed to explain the development of gastroschisis:

1. Result of failure of the body wall to close, primarily involving right lateral fold being unable to meet the left one in the midline
2. Vascular accident causing atresia of midgut either due to early involution of the right umbilical vein or intrauterine interruption of the right omphalomesenteric artery leading to infarction of the abdominal wall
3. Failure of the yolk sac to insert into the body stalk and thus forming an extra opening in the amniotic cavity through which intestine will develop

Embryological abnormalities are also thought to be perpetuated by some environmental factors, eg, tobacco smoking, exposure to pesticides, Chlamydia infection.[29]

Compared to spontaneous vaginal delivery, planned cesarean delivery (CD) did not show any decreased risk of complications related to bowel ischemia, bowel injury, and necrotizing enterocolitis.[34] Yet, the rate of CD is higher in the United States (60.9%) perhaps due to planned cesarean deliveries or unexpected fetal distress.[35]

Surgical treatment depends on the condition of the eviscerated bowel and the ability to reduce the eviscerated intestine inside the abdomen. Primary reduction and immediate closure without causing abnormally high abdominal pressure are helpful as they reduce the evaporation of fluid and exposure to infection. Staged reduction involves creating a silo to keep the bowel inside the bag and then gradually reducing the size of silo to allow the eviscerated bowel to enter into the abdominal cavity. The abdominal defect is closed with suture after completion of reduction. The complex gastroschisis cases, patients with atresia, perforation, volvulus are managed depending on the status of the intestine and overall clinical status of the patient.[36]

Omphalocele

Omphalocele, the other common congenital abdominal wall defect, presents with a midline protrusion of herniated intraabdominal organs through the umbilicus into the umbilical cord. Umbilical cord is inserted into the membrane which is composed of peritoneum, Wharton's jelly, and amnion. The herniated organs include midgut and occasionally spleen and gonads. The incidence of omphalocele is estimated to be 1.9 per 10,000 live births.[37] A fetus with omphalocele is at high risk for associated chromosomal abnormalities, intrauterine growth restriction (IUGR), premature delivery, and fetal death.[38] The infant mortality rate is reported to be around 28% and significantly higher in neonates born with chromosomal abnormalities.[37] The other factors associated with mortality are pulmonary hypertension and respiratory insufficiency at birth, large omphalocele containing 75% liver, and rupture of sac.[39]

Unlike gastroschisis, omphalocele is associated with a wide variety of malformations:

1. Beckwith-Wiedemann syndrome: omphalocele, macrosomia, and hypoglycemia

2. Pentalogy of Cantrell: omphalocele, anterior diaphragmatic hernia, sternal cleft, ectopia cordis, intracardiac defect (VSD, ASD, tetralogy of Fallot, etc.)

3. Chromosomal defect: trisomy 18, 13, 21. Chromosomal defects may occur up to 49% of fetuses diagnosed with omphalocele[40]

4. Congenital heart defect (ASD, PDA, VSD, tricuspid valve anomaly, VACTERL): 18% to 24% incidence of cardiac anomalies[41]

5. Genitourinary system: exstrophy of bladder or cloaca

6. Central nervous system defect: spina bifida, anencephaly

7. OEIS complex (omphalocele, exstrophy of bladder, imperforate anus, spinal defect)

8. Donnai-Barrow syndrome (omphalocele, congenital diaphragmatic hernia, corpus callosum agenesis)

Embryology

The embryo develops to a three-layered flat disc of ectoderm, mesoderm, and endoderm with amniotic cavity dorsally and yolk sac ventrally. Around the fourth to fifth week of gestation, due to increased growth of neural tube, the embryonic disc is folded toward the ventral surface and a fetal configuration develops. The four body folds (cranial, caudal, and two lateral) converge toward the umbilicus to form the umbilical ring which separates the developing body wall from the amnion. The gastrointestinal tract, which develops more rapidly in relation to the abdominal cavity, herniates through the umbilical ring into the umbilical cord. At around 10 to 12 weeks of gestation, the bowel returns to the abdominal cavity and fixes to its final position. The omphalocele probably develops due to malformations of the embryonic folding process which interferes with the physiological reentry of abdominal organs from the umbilical cord.[42]

Prenatal diagnosis of omphalocele is made reliably after the first trimester with ultrasonography and the detection of high maternal serum AFP levels and prenatal ultrasound. An omphalocele may be classified as small (<5 cm), giant (>5cm) with a sac containing liver, and ruptured. Karyotyping using chorionic villi sampling may be useful to rule out any associated major chromosomal abnormalities.[43]

Although controversy exists whether outcome is improved with CD,[44] surgical delivery is indicated in cases of giant omphalocele in order to prevent injury to the liver or disruption of the sac.

The small to medium-sized omphalocele in an otherwise stable neonate is closed by primary closure of the skin and fascia after reduction of the herniated organs and excision or inversion of the sac. In large omphaloceles, the ultimate goal is to provide complete reduction with closure of the defect without causing excessive intraabdominal pressure. The increased intraabdominal pressure may cause cardiorespiratory compromises such as the ones mentioned in minimally invasive procedures above. Intraabdominal hypertension (usually >20 mm Hg) can progress to abdominal compartment syndrome (ACS) with potentially devastating complications, eg, renal failure, gut ischemia, necrotizing enterocolitis, wound dehiscence, sepsis, and enterocutaneous fistula.

Central venous pressure monitoring has been reported as a useful guide to assess IAP; an increase of more than 4 mm Hg during placement of silo in delayed closure or fascia closure during primary repair correlated with a decrease in cardiac index.[45]

A giant omphalocele is surgically repaired with a staged closure initially placing a silicone plastic "silo" and gradually reduced it in size returning the herniated organs to the abdominal cavity over few days. Silastic silo closure is associated with wound infection and wound dehiscence. Staged closure has also been reported using intraabdominal tissue expander placement, component separation, and bipedicle skin flap technique. Escharotic therapy with topical application of silver sulfadiazine results in gradual epithelialization of the omphalocele sac. After completion of epithelialization, the ventral hernia is repaired using prosthetic mesh and skin flap.

Anesthetic Management of Gastroschisis and Omphalocele

Preoperative Management

1. Genetic evaluation to diagnose any coexisting chromosomal anomalies (eg, trisomy 13, 18, 21 in 30–40% cases).

2. Echocardiography for patients with omphaloceles to rule out congenital heart disease and pulmonary hypertension.

3. Abdominal ultrasound to look for any associated renal abnormality.

4. Blood sugar levels in premature patients and in patients with omphalocele and possible Beckwith-Wiedemann syndrome (12% cases).

5. Gastric decompression with NG tube in both gastroschisis and omphalocele to prevent intestinal distension.

6. Adequate intravenous access to ensure fluid resuscitation to replace evaporative fluid loss from herniated intestines.

7. Prevention of heat loss by increasing the ambient temperature. Also, the herniated bowel and omphalocele should be wrapped in warm saline soaked gauge to reduce evaporative loss. In case of gastroschisis, care should be taken to avoid kinking of the mesentery.

Intraoperative Management

1. Standard ASA monitors. Intraarterial catheter can be helpful to monitor continuous blood pressure, laboratory studies (glucose, electrolytes, arterial blood gases), fluid status. Pulse oximeter in right upper extremity (preductal) and in toes/feet (to assess lower extremity perfusion during closure of abdomen).

2. Central venous line to monitor the effect of increased abdominal pressure and as additional access for vasopressors and volume infusion.

3. Nasogastric tube placement and aspiration prior to induction.

4. Urinary catheter to measure urine output and intravesical pressure.

5. Temperature probe either rectal or esophageal.

Induction: Rapid sequence intravenous induction after adequate preoxygenation. Propofol (2–4 mg/kg) or ketamine (1–2 mg/kg) or a combination of lower doses of ketamine and propofol may be used for hypnosis. Rocuronium at 0.8 to 1 mg/kg produces intubating condition in 30 seconds. Glycopyrrolate (10 mcg/kg) to prevent vagal-mediated bradycardia during intubation and fentanyl (1 mcg/kg) may also be used as supplemental agents.

In patients with possible difficult airway (such as macroglossia in Beckwith-Wiedemann syndrome) a video laryngoscope (CMAC) with appropriate blade should be available.

Fluid management should be continued with D5 or D10 with 0.2% NaCl solution. In cases of neonatal hypoglycemia (serum glucose less than 40 mg/dL in term or preterm infant) D5 to D12.5W at 4 to 8 mg/kg/min should be used. For intravenous fluid replacement of surgical or evaporative/insensible fluid loss, replace with 5 to 15 mL/kg/h of lactated ringer's solution and/or normal saline, or 5% human albumin (50 mg/mL; 0.5 g/kg/dose).

Hypothermia (body temperature <36°C) should be prevented by increasing the OR temperature (78–80°F), by adding warming blanket on the operating table to reduce conductive heat loss, by placing overhead heat lamps to reduce radiant heat loss, and by transporting in a thermoneutral incubator or a bed with overhead heater.

Anesthesia is maintained with inhalation anesthesia (oxygen/sevoflurane or desflurane) and narcotics (fentanyl) boluses. Nitrous oxide should be avoided to reduce bowel distension.

Intraabdominal pressure is closely monitored during abdominal closure, and for serial approximation of Silo by intravesical pressure, intragastric pressure, or CVP. Other surrogate indicators of increased IAP include high ventilation pressure (peak pressure >30 mm Hg), high end-tidal pCO_2, significant drop in MAP not responsive to fluid boluses, and low pulse oximetry reading in lower extremities.

CONGENITAL DIAPHRAGMATIC HERNIA

Congenital diaphragmatic hernia (CDH) is a complex clinical syndrome represented by a development defect in the diaphragm and herniation of abdominal organs into the thoracic cavity, which can interfere with development of the lung. At birth, the pulmonary hypoplasia and pulmonary hypertension present a major threat to survival of the neonate. CDH commonly occurs in 1 in 3000 live births.[46] Majority of the hernia is left sided and the commonest defect is in posterolateral diaphragm (Bochdalek type). The other forms are anterior (Morgagni type) and central.

Approximately 30% to 40% of CDH cases are reported to have associated congenital malformations, eg, cardiovascular (VSD, ASD, tetralogy of Fallot), central nervous system abnormalities (neural tube defects, hydrocephalus), and limb abnormalities (polydactyly, syndactyly, reduction defects). Regarding associated chromosomal abnormalities, trisomy 18 is the most common one.[47]

▶ Embryology

The diaphragm is developed from the following embryonic components: (1) septum transversum, which forms the central tendon of the diaphragm, and (2) pleuroperitoneal membrane: the primary source of the future diaphragm. Failure or defect in the fusion of the pleuroperitoneal membrane with other components of the developing diaphragm about the 10th week of gestation is the main embryological pathology in the formation of CDH. As the right pleuroperitoneal canal closes before the left one, left-sided CDH is more common than the right-sided CDH.[48]

Herniation of abdominal contents in the lung cavity and shift of mediastinal structures to the contralateral side contribute to the pulmonary hypoplasia. An abnormal genetic expression, which regulates the development of both diaphragm and lungs may also be involved in causing pulmonary hypoplasia. Hypoplasia affects the total surface area of the lung involved with gas exchange. Developmental arrest of the pulmonary vasculature with increased thickness of the arterial wall decreases cross-sectional area of the pulmonary vascular bed and increases pulmonary vascular resistance.[49]

Diagnosis is usually made by ultrasonography during routine prenatal screening. The fluid-filled intestines with or without the liver, and displacement of the heart are seen in the thorax. Fetal lung-to-head ratio (LHR), as measured by ultrasound, helps to assess the lung hypoplasia. Lung size could also be assessed by MRI or 3D ultrasound. Herniation of the liver and stomach has been associated with poor outcome. Diagnosis in early pregnancy helps in prenatal counseling, referral to a tertiary center for advanced tests, fetal interventions, and termination of pregnancy, in selected cases.

Clinical Presentation and Management

Respiratory distress, characterized by tachypnea, grunting, use of accessory muscles, and cyanosis, is the cardinal feature of babies with CDH. Scaphoid abdomen may also be present. Auscultation of the chest may reveal bowel sounds on the left side of the chest, and rightward shift of the point of maximal cardiac impulse may be heard. A chest X-ray will confirm the diagnosis with bowel gas pattern in the chest and mediastinal shift.

Historically, CDH used to be considered a surgical emergency, and prompt surgical exploration to reduce the herniated organs back to the abdominal cavity was thought to be the primary treatment. Mortality though continued to remain high is primarily due to persistent pulmonary hypertension. Today, the key principle of management following birth is to optimize the respiratory status, deteriorated by the combination of lung hypoplasia, increased PVR, and right-to-left shunt. Initial management should include quick evaluation of the cardiorespiratory status, endotracheal intubation without prolonged mask and bag ventilation, establishment of IV access, and decompression of gut by nasogastric tube. Aggressive bag and mask ventilation should be avoided as it affects oxygenation by enlarging the stomach and compressing the lungs. Factors which worsen pulmonary hypertension, eg, hypoxia, acidosis, and hypothermia, should be avoided.

Proper ventilator strategies are important for newborns with CDH. Initial approach to resolve pulmonary hypertension and right to left shunt by inducing with aggressive hyperoxia and hyperventilation produced several significant complications, including barotrauma (pneumothoraces, pulmonary hemorrhage) and residual lung disease.[50]

The advent of the concept of "permissive hypercapnia" by gentle ventilation in the management of infant pulmonary hypertension reduced ventilator-induced lung injury and improved survival.

The current recommendations suggest keeping the ventilator mode as intermittent mandatory ventilation (IMV) with PIP <25 cm H_2O: PEEP 3 to 5 cm H_2O, keeping preductal SaO_2 $>85\%$ and pCO_2 <60 mm Hg. If the goals for oxygenation and ventilation are not accomplished by this method, high-frequency oscillatory ventilation (HFOV) may be used to optimize alveolar recruitment with mean airway pressure of 13 to 15 cm H_2O with a pressure delta ranging from 30 to 40 cm H_2O.[51] Use of HFOV as an early intervention strategy rather than rescue mode, keeping

$PaCO_2$ around 40 to 55 mm Hg and pressure delta of 35 to 45 cm H_2O, has been reported to improve survival.[52]

The general medical management of persistent pulmonary hypertension in CDH includes administration of adequate intravascular volume, maintenance of hemoglobin and glucose at normal levels, and maintenance of normal temperature. Although high-frequency ventilation with inhaled nitric oxide (iNO) is considered for selected patients, iNO has not been shown to reduce risk of death or ECMO use. Use of other potential agents, eg, sildenafil, milrinone, prostaglandin analogues (prostacyclins, PGE1), and Bosentan, has not gained sufficient evidence for clinical use.

ECMO (Extracorporeal Membrane Oxygenation)

ECMO has been used in many centers to stabilize the infant prior to surgery. In ECMO, the blood is oxygenated outside the body, so the need for gas exchange in the lung is not needed. The following criteria have been considered by Scottish Congenital Diaphragmatic Hernia Network for ECMO.[53]

1. Inability to maintain preductal saturation $>85\%$ despite optimal ventilation and management of pulmonary hypertension

2. Arterial pCO_2 above target range with respiratory acidosis (pH 7.15) despite optimum ventilation

3. PIP consistently above 25 cm H_2O to achieve ventilator goals or failure to convert after HFOV

4. Metabolic acidosis (pH <7.15) and lactate >5 mmol/L

5. Systemic hypotension resistant to fluid and inotropes with a urine output <0.5 mL/kg/h over 12 to 24 hours

Contraindications of ECMO therapy are as follows:

1. Gestational age less than approximately 34 weeks

2. Weight less than approximately 2 kg

3. Ongoing bleeding disorder or uncorrectable coagulopathy

4. Intraventricular hemorrhage.

The outcome benefit of the ECMO procedure in patients with CDH has not been well established. A two-center study in two cities (Boston and Toronto) concluded that the overall survival rate with HFOV as rescue was equivalent to the overall survival rate in patients with ECMO as rescue. In both groups, permissive hypercapnia significantly increased survival. The leading cause of mortality was pulmonary hypoplasia and associated anomalies.[54,55]

There appears to be no difference in survival benefit between the two modes of ECMO (VV [venovenous] and VA [venoarterial]) in CDH patients. The optimal timing of repair while on ECMO has not been identified yet, but early repair may improve survival as it decreases complications.

In recent years, a fetal therapy for CDH, named fetoscopic endoluminal tracheal occlusion (FETO), has been practiced. The procedure prevents egress of fluid from the lung and thus increases pulmonary pressure. The increased pressure promotes proliferation of pulmonary tissue, increases the total alveolar surface area, and helps to mature the pulmonary vasculature.

Surgical Management

Surgical repair of CDH is deferred until the pulmonary status is stabilized, since mortality rate in these infants is primarily related to pulmonary hypoplasia and persistent pulmonary hypertension. Despite generalized agreement in the benefits of delayed surgery, specific parameters of cardiorespiratory stability and timing of surgery remain unconfirmed. The usual practice is to control the pulmonary hypertension, thus requiring lower ventilator settings with low PIP, minimal shunting, and low FiO_2.

The CDH-EURO consortium states that surgical repair should be performed when the following criteria are met:[56]

- Mean arterial blood pressure normal for gestational age
- Preductal saturation levels between 85% and 95% with a fractional inspired oxygen <50%
- Serum lactate <3 mmol/L
- Urine production >2 mL/kg/h

Other set of recently reported parameters include the following:[57]

- Oxygen saturation >92% (FiO_2 <0.5)
- Mean arterial pressure >45 mm Hg
- Pulmonary artery pressure less than two-thirds of the systemic pressure
- Weaning iNO (<10 ppm)
- Hemoglobin >10 g/dL

Surgical approaches to repair CDH include minimally invasive approach (thoracoscopy) and open repair. Thoracoscopic approach has the advantages of better visualization of the defect and mobilization of herniated contents to the abdomen, which happens due to thoracic insufflation with CO_2. Disadvantages of thoracoscopic repair are a higher 1-year recurrence rate, longer operative time, and need to adjust ventilatory parameters due to absorbed CO_2. The defect is repaired with prosthetic material (Gore-Tex) or muscle flap (abdominal wall muscles).

In many centers, surgical repair of CDH is performed in the neonatal ICU to avoid accidental disconnection of different lines and significant changes in ventilatory support.

Anesthetic Management

Two important goals of anesthetic management in CDH patients: avoiding volutrauma and preventing worsening pulmonary hypertension

Standard ASA monitors

Pulse oximetry in right upper extremity (preductal)

Arterial line (right radial artery; preductal)

Position of ETT tube to be checked

NG tube placement

Central venous line access or an extra-large gauge intravenous line placement for volume replacement.

Maintenance fluid with glucose-containing solution continuation

ICU ventilator use for continuation of ventilation during surgery; pressure control ventilation with PIP <25 cm H_2O

Maintenance of anesthesia with fentanyl (10–30 mcg/kg) and inhalational agent as tolerated; in case of ventilation with NICU ventilator, propofol infusion (100–150 mcg/kg/min) and fentanyl infusion (2 mcg/kg/h)

Neuromuscular blocking agent (rocuronium) use to keep the patient paralyzed

Nitrous oxide avoidance

Avoidance of hypothermia, acidosis, and hypoxia (triggers of pulmonary hypertension)

At the end of surgery, patient to be kept intubated and sedated, and transferred to the neonatal intensive care unit

APPENDICITIS

Acute appendicitis is the most common surgical urgency/emergency in children, with approximately 70,000 pediatric cases each year in the United States.[58] It occurs in approximately 1 to 4 per 1000 children per year.[59] The estimated life risk is reported to be 7% to 8%.[60] Appendicitis is more common in children aged 12 to 18 years, and less common in children less than 5 years of age.

The pathogenesis of appendicitis is thought to be due to direct luminal obstruction by a fecalith, lymphoid hyperplasia, or tumor, which leads to a series of pathological changes including distension of lumen, venous congestion, edema, bacterial infections, reduced blood supply, ischemia, necrosis, and gangrene. Recent studies suggest genetic factors, and environmental factors also might play a role.[60] Bacterial infections with agents such as *Escherichia coli*, *Salmonella*, *Shigella*, and Bacteroides might play an important role in initiating the development of appendicitis in some cases.

The classic presentation of appendicitis includes abdominal pain with anorexia, nausea, and vomiting. Abdominal pain begins as a dull periumbilical pain, shifting to the right lower quadrant of the abdomen. The classic presentation is noted in less than 50% of patients. In other children, it may start with some flu-like symptoms, eg, anorexia and malaise, and then rapidly progressing to abdominal pain and fever. Continuation of these symptoms may lead to perforation of appendix within 36 to 48 hours after initial presentation of the illness. Due to initial absence of typical symptoms along with difficulty in elicitation of definitive signs in pediatric patients, the incidence of complications such as perforation, abscess, and gangrene are high. The signs of appendicitis include localized tenderness, rebound tenderness, and guarding in the right lower quadrant. The point of tenderness in patients with appendicitis is classically described as McBurney's point, at the junction of the lateral one-third and medial two-thirds of the line joining the umbilicus and right anterior superior iliac spine. A scoring system (Pediatric Appendicitis Scores) has been developed to assist in the diagnosis of appendicitis in pediatric patients; components of the system include eight relevant clinical and laboratory data such as fever >38°C, anorexia, nausea/vomiting, migration of pain, right lower quadrant tenderness, cough/percussion/hopping tenderness, leukocytosis >10,000 cells/µL, and polymorphonuclear neutrophilia >7500 cells/µL. Transabdominal ultrasound is the most common diagnostic modality for appendicitis, because it does not expose the patient to radiation and is less expensive than computed tomography (CT). In some centers, there is increasing reliance on CT scan, and it has become the most accepted diagnostic strategy.

In the majority of cases, appendectomy is the standard management. Preoperative antibiotics with broad coverage of gram-negative bacteria, IV fluids, analgesics, and antipyretics are usually started after diagnosis. Laparoscopic appendectomy over open appendectomy is the preferred surgical approach.

Anesthetic Management

1. Preoperative evaluation should include assessment of vital signs, BMI, associated comorbidities (obesity, obstructive sleep apnea, symptoms of gastroesophageal reflux), current medications, and NPO status.
2. Standard American Society of Anesthesiologists (ASA) monitors: Arterial line may be considered in patients with abdominal sepsis and peritonitis.
3. Rapid sequence induction with propofol (2–3 mg/kg), and succinylcholine (1.5–2 mg/kg) or rocuronium (1 mg/kg)
4. Endotracheal intubation: Video laryngoscopy and other airway management equipment should be accessible in patients with anticipated difficult airway.
5. Nasogastric tube is used to decompress the stomach.
6. Inhalational agents (sevoflurane or desflurane) with oxygen/air are used for maintenance of anesthesia. Nitrous oxide should be avoided.
7. Intraoperative narcotics (fentanyl 1–2 mcg/kg, morphine 0.05–0.1 mg/kg) and antiemetics (dexamethasone 0.2–0.5 mg/kg and ondansetron 0.1–0.15 mg/kg) should be considered.
8. Postoperative analgesia:
   - Infiltration of surgical wound with local anesthetics at the completion of surgery
   - Acetaminophen (15 mg /kg IV)
   - Dexmedetomidine (0.5–1 mcg/kg IV) at the completion of surgery
   - Ketorolac (0.5 mg/kg IV)
   - Morphine (0.05–0.1 mg/IV)
   - Regional anesthesia: TAP block; rectus sheath block may be considered at selected cases
   - Patient-controlled analgesia (PCA) with opioids for ruptured cases

AGANGLIONIC MEGACOLON (HIRSCHSPRUNG DISEASE)

Hirschsprung disease or congenital intestinal aangliosis, named after Dr. Harold Hirschsprung, is the most common cause of intestinal obstruction in neonates. The disease occurs in 1 in 5000 live births and is more common in males. It may be associated with other congenital anomalies including Down syndrome, tumors of neural crest origin (neurofibromatosis), microcephaly, mental retardation, multiple endocrine neoplasia type 2 (MEN 2) syndrome, DiGeorge syndrome, and congenital hypoventilation syndrome.[61] The malformation primarily occurs to the structures which are embryologically derived from the neural crest.

Hirschsprung disease is characterized by the absence of ganglionic cells in the myenteric and submucosal plexuses of the bowel wall. The myenteric plexus is formed from the vagal neural crest cells which migrate in a craniocaudal direction at 5th to 12th weeks of gestation. Failure of migration of the precursor cells to the distal gut is thought to be the primary etiology of Hirschsprung disease. The short segment variety of the disease, where the aganglionic segment primarily involves the rectosigmoid region, accounts for 80% of the cases. Peristalsis cannot propagate through this aganglionic segment, causing distension of the bowel proximal to the segment. The other 10% to 15% of patients have long-segment disease which involves the area proximal to the sigmoid colon.

Healthy full-term infants pass meconium within 48 hours after birth. Any baby that fails to pass meconium within this timeframe should be investigated for Hirschsprung disease. Progressive intestinal obstruction causes abdominal distension, failure to feed, and vomiting. The intestinal obstruction may lead to stasis and bacterial overgrowth with *Clostridium difficile*, *Staphylococcus aureus*, and coliforms, leading to enterocolitis and diarrhea with foul smelling and bloody stools, fever, obstruction, and sepsis. Enterocolitis is the major cause of death in Hirschsprung disease and the mortality rate may be as high as 30% in patients with enterocolitis. Failure to thrive, constipation, episodes of obstruction, and blood-flecked diarrhea (suggestive of enterocolitis) are common symptoms.

Diagnosis of Hirschsprung disease is confirmed by histological and histochemical tests of the specimen obtained from a rectal biopsy. Initial treatment is decompression of the gastrointestinal tract, fluid resuscitation, and administration of broad-spectrum antibiotics. Decompression of the colon may be carried out by rectal catheter (with irrigation) and temporary ostomy.

Definitive surgery is a single-stage pull-through procedure which is usually performed after a few months. The aganglionic bowel with the transitional zone is resected, and the normal functioning bowel is moved down and connected to the dentate line of the anal canal. Functions of the anal sphincter are preserved. Laparoscopy is used for definitive repair in pull-through procedures.

Anesthetic Management

1. Preoperative evaluation: Presence of any other coexisting disease (Down syndrome, neurofibromatosis, etc.) should be ruled out. Vital signs, airway, IV access, hydration (fontanelles, capillary refill), and oxygenation should be assessed. Premedication with midazolam if appropriate.

2. Anesthetic management depends on the clinical status of the patient (hypovolemic, in shock state) or nature of surgery (initial ostomy for decompression or primary pull through).

3. A single-shot spinal anesthesia may be considered if it is a short procedure for biopsy and colostomy in selected patients.

4. General anesthesia is the most common modality for anesthesia management.

5. Standard ASA monitors: Arterial line may be considered in patients for fluid resuscitation, support vasopressor infusion, and continuous monitoring of electrolytes or other laboratory values.

6. A single-shot caudal block may be considered for postoperative analgesia. Caudal catheters are sometimes difficult to maintain because of the area of surgery involved.

7. Glycopyrrolate (10 mcg/kg to prevent reflex bradycardia during intubation) and fentanyl (1 mcg/kg)

8. Induction: Rapid sequence induction should be considered with propofol or ketamine (in volume-deficient patient) with succinylcholine (1.5–2 mg/kg) or rocuronium (1 mg/kg) in patients with obstruction, or perforation of intestines.

9. Oral endotracheal intubation with appropriate-sized cuffed endotracheal tube.

10. Additional intravenous access for hypovolemic patients.

11. Maintenance of anesthesia with sevoflurane/desflurane with oxygen and air. Nitrous oxide should be avoided.

12. Fluid resuscitation with normal saline, lactated ringer's solution, 5% albumin if warranted.

13. Vasopressor (phenylephrine, dopamine, norepinephrine, dobutamine) consideration to maintain hemodynamic stability.

14. Extubation at the completion of procedure.

15. Morphine (0.05–0.1 mg/kg), dexmedetomidine (0.5 mcg/kg IV), acetaminophen (15 mg/IV) for postoperative analgesia.

REFERENCES

1. Kamata M, Cartabuke RS, Tobias JD. Perioperative care of infants with pyloric stenosis. *Pediatr Anesth.* 2015;25:1193-1206.
2. Lund M, Pasternak B, Davidsen RD, et al. Use of macrolides in mother and child and risk of infantile hypertrophic pyloric stenosis. Nationwide cohort study. *BMJ.* 2014;348:g1908.
3. Sorensen HT, Norgard B, Pedersen L, et al. Maternal smoking and risk of hypertrophic infantile pyloric stenosis: 10 year population based cohort studies. *BMJ.* 2002;325(7371):1011-1012.
4. Scrimgeour GE, Leather NWF, Pery RS, et al. Gas induction for pyloromyotomy. *Pediatr Anesth.* 2015;25:677-680.
5. Dewhirst E, Tobias JD, Martin DP. Propofol and remifentanil for rapid sequence intubation in a pediatric patient at risk for aspiration with elevated intracranial pressure. *Pediatr Emerg Care.* 2013;29(11):1201-1203.
6. Davis PJ, Galinkin J, McGowan F. A randomized multicenter study of remifentanil compared with halothane in neonates and infants undergoing pyloromyotomy. I. Emergence and recovery profiles. *Anesth Analg.* 2001;93:1380-1386.
7. Andropoulos DB, Heard MB, Johnson KL, et al. Postanesthetic apnea in full term infants after pyloromyotomy. *Anesthesiology.* 1994;80:216-219.
8. Simpao AF, Ahumada LM, Galvez JA, et al. The timing and prevalence of intraoperative hypotension in infants undergoing laparoscopic pyloromyotomy at a tertiary pediatric hospital. *Pediatr Anesth.* 2017;27:66-76.
9. Islam S, Larson SD, Kays DW. Feasibility of laparoscopic pyloromyotomy under spinal anesthesia. *J Pediatr Surg.* 2014;49:1485-1487.
10. Ing C, Sun SL, Friend AF. Differences in intraoperative hemodynamics between spinal and general anesthesia in infants undergoing pyloromyotomy. *Pediatr Anesth.* 2017;27:733-741.
11. Grosfeld JL. Current concepts in inguinal hernia in infants and children. *World JSurg.* 1989;5:506-515.
12. Vaos G, Gardikis S, Kambouri K. Optimal timing for repair of an inguinal hernia in premature infants. *Pediatr Surg Int.* 2010;26:379-385.
13. Lautz TB, Raval MV, Reynolds M. Does timing matter? A national perspective on the risk of incarceration in premature neonates with inguinal hernia. *J Pediatr.* 2011;158:573-577.
14. Tulgar S, Boga I, Cakiroglu B, et al. Short-lasting pediatric laparoscopic surgery: are muscle relaxants necessary? Endotracheal intubation vs laryngeal mask airway. *J Pediatr Surg.* 2017;52:1705-1710.
15. Tsuchiya N, Ichizawa M, Yoshikawa Y, et al. Comparison of ropivacaine with bupivacaine and lidocaine for ilioinguinal block after ambulatory inguinal hernia repair in children. *Pediatr Anesth.* 2004;14:468-470.
16. Disma N, Withington D, McCann ME, et al. Surgical practice and outcome in 711 neonates and infants undergoing hernia

repair in a large multicenter RCT: secondary results from the GAS study. *J Pediatr Surg.* 2018;53:1643-1650.

17. Williams RK, Adams DC, Aladjem EV, et al. The safety and efficacy of spinal anesthesia for surgery in infants: the Vermont infant spinal registry. *Anesth Analg.* 2006;102:67-71.

18. Mccann ME, Withington BM, Arup SJ, et al. Differences in blood pressure in infants after general anesthesia compared to awake regional anesthesia (GAS study—a prospective randomized trial). *Anesth Analg.* 2017;125:837-845.

19. Davidson AJ, Morton NS, Arup SJ, et al. Apnea after awake regional and general anesthesia in infants. *Anesthesiology.* 2015;123:38-54.

20. McCann ME, de Graaff JC, Dorris L, et al. Neurodevelopmental outcome at 5 years of age after general anaesthesia or awake-regional anaesthesia in infancy (GAS): an international, multicenter, randomized, controlled equivalence trial. *Lancet.* 2019;393:664-677.

21. Myre K, Rostrup T, Buanes T. Plasma catecholamines and hemodynamic changes during pneumoperitoneum. *Acta Anaesthesiol Scand.* 1998;42:343-347.

22. Munoz CJ, Nguyen HT, Houck CS. Robotic surgery and anesthesia for pediatric urologic procedures. *Curr Opin Anesthesiol.* 2016;29:337-344.

23. McHoney M, Corizia I, Eaton S, et al. Carbon dioxide elimination during laparoscopy in children is age dependent. *J Pediatr Surg.* 2003;38:105-110.

24. Sodha S, Nazarian S, Adshed JM, et al. Effect of pneumoperitoneum on renal function and physiology in patients undergoing robotic renal surgery. *Curr Urol.* 2016;9:1-4.

25. Gomez BH, Karanik E, Gluer S. Anuria during pneumoperitoneum in infants and children: a prospective study. *J Pediatr Surg.* 2005;40:1454-1458.

26. Wedgewood J, Doyle E. Anaesthesia and laparoscopic surgery in children. *Paediatr Anaesth.* 2001;11:391-399.

27. Kim SJ, Barlog JS, Akhavan A. Robotic-assisted urologic surgery in infants: positioning, trocar placement and physiological considerations. *Front Pediatr.* 2019;6(article 211): 1-10.

28. Dewaal EEC, Kalkman CJ. Hemodynamic changes during low-pressure carbon dioxide pneumoperitoneum in young children. *Paediatr Anaesth.* 2003;13:18-25.

29. Beaudoin S. Insights into the etiology of gastroschisis. *Semin Pediatr Surg.* 2018;27:283-288.

30. Jones AM, Isenburg J, Salemi JL, et al. Increasing prevalence of gastroschisis—14 states,1995–2012. *Morb Mortal Wkly Rep.* 2016;65:23-26.

31. Bergholz R, Boettcher M, Reinshagen K, et al. Complex gastroschisis is a different entity to simple gastroschisis affecting morbidity and mortality: a systemic review and meta analysis. *J Pediatr Surg.* 2014;49:1527-1532.

32. Anteby EY, Sternhell KS, Dicke JM. The fetus with gastroschisis managed by a trial of labor: antepartum and intrapartum complications. *J Perinatol.* 1999;19(7):521-524.

33. Sparks TN, Shaffer BL, Page J, et al. Gastroschisis: mortality risks with each additional week of expectant management. *Am J Obstet Gynecol.* 2017;216(1):66.e1-7.

34. Segel SY, Marder SJ, Parry S, et al. Fetal abdominal wall defects and mode of delivery: a systematic review. *Obstet Gynecol.* 2001:98:867-873.

35. Youssef F, Cheong AHL, Emil S. Gastroschisis outcomes in North America: a comparison of Canada and the United States. *J Pediatr Surg.* 2016;51:891-895.

36. Petrosyan M, Sandler AD. Closure methods in gastroschisis. *Semin Pediatr Surg.* 2018;27:304-308.

37. Marshall J, Salemi JL, Tanner JP, et al. Prevalence, correlates, and outcomes of omphalocele in the United States, 1995–2005. *Obstet Gynecol.* 2015;126:284-293.

38. Fratelli N, Papageorghiou AT, Bhide A, et al. Outcome of antenatally diagnosed abdominal wall defects. *Ultrasound Obstet Gynecol.* 2007;30:266-270.

39. Baerg JE, Thorpe DL, Sharp NE, et al. Pulmonary hypertension predicts mortality in infants with omphalocele. *J Neonat-Perinat Med.* 2015;8:333-338.

40. Brantberg A, Blaas HG, Haugen SL, et al. Characteristics and outcome of 90 cases of fetal omphalocele. *Ultrasound Obstet Gynecol.* 2005;26:527.

41. Baird PA, McDonald EC. An epidemiology study of congenital malformation of anterior abdominal wall in more than half a million consecutive live births. *Am J Hum Genet.* 1981;33:470-478.

42. Khan FA, Hashmi A, Islam S. Insights into embryology and development of omphalocele. *Semin Pediatr Surg.* 2019;28:80-83.

43. Verla MA, Style C, Olutoye O. Prenatal diagnosis and management of omphalocele. *Semin Pediatr Surg.* 2019;28(2):84-88.

44. Segel SY, Marder SJ, Parry S, et al. Fetal abdominal wall defects and mode of delivery: a systemic review. *Obst Gynecol.* 2001;98:867-873.

45. Yaster M, Scherer TLR, Stone MM, et al. Prediction of successful primary closure of congenital abdominal wall defects using intraoperative measurements. *J Pediatr Surg.* 1989;24(12):1217-1220.

46. Langham MR, Kays DW, Ledbetter DJ. Congenital diaphragmatic hernia: epidemiology and outcome. *Clin Perinatol.* 1996;23:671-688.

47. Pober B. Overview of epidemiology, genetics, birth defects and chromosome abnormalities associated with CDH. *Am J Med Genet C.* 2007;145C:158-171.

48. Moore KL, Persaud TVN, Torchia MG. Body Cavities, Mesenteries, and Diaphragm. L. Keith, TVN (Vid)Persaud Moore, MG Torchia. *Before We Are Born.* 9th ed. Philadelphia, PA: Elsevier/Saunders; 2016, pp. 91-99.

49. Keller RL. Antenatal and postnatal lung and vascular anatomic and functional studies in congenital diaphragmatic hernia. *Am J Med Gene C.* 2007;145C:184-200.

50. Bernbaum JC, Rossell P, Sheridan PH, et al. Long-term follow up of newborns with persistent pulmonary hypertension. *Crit Care Med.* 1984;12(7):579-583.

51. Puligandla PS, Grabowski J, Austin M, et al. Management of congenital diaphragmatic hernia: a systematic review from the APSA outcomes and evidence-based practice committee. *J Pediatr Surgery.* 2015;50:1958-1970.

52. Bohn D. Congenital diaphragmatic hernia. *Am J Respir Crit Care Med.* 2002;166:911-915.

53. McHoney M, Hammond P. Role of ECMO in congenital diaphragmatic hernia. *Arch Dis Child Fetal Neonatal Ed.* 2018;103:F178-F181.

54. Wilson JM, Lund DP, Lillehoi CW. Congenital diaphragmatic hernia—a tale of two cities: the Boston experience. *J Pediatr Surg.* 1997;32(3):401-405.

55. Azarow K, Messineo A, Pearl R. Congenital diaphragmatic hernia—a tale of two cities: the Toronto Experience. *J Pediatr Surg.* 1997;32(3):395-400.

56. Sluiter I, van de Van CP, Wijnen RMH. Congenital diaphragmatic hernia: still a moving target. 2011. *Semin FetNeonat Med.* 2011;16:139-144.

57. Fennessy P, Crowe S, Lenihan M, Healy M. Anesthesia consensus on clinical parameters for the timing of surgical

repair in congenital diaphragmatic hernia. *Pediatr Anesth.* 2018;28(8):751-752.

58. Brennan GDG. Pediatric appendicitis: pathophysiology and appropriate use of diagnostic imaging. *CJEM.* 2006;8(6):425-432.

59. Kutasy B, Puri P. Appendicitis in obese children. *Pediatr Surg Int.* 2013;29:537-544.

60. Bhangu A, Soreide, Saverio S, et al. Acute appendicitis: modern understanding of pathogenesis, diagnosis and management. *Lancet.* 2015;386:1278-1287.

61. Chhabra S, Kenny SE. Hirschsprung's disease. *Surgery.* 2016;34(12)628-632.

Anesthetic Considerations for Endocrine Disorders

Galit Kastner

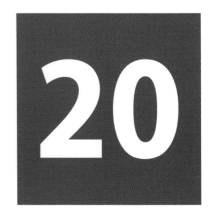

20

GLYCEMIC CONTROL

DIABETES MELLITUS

Diabetes mellitus (DM) is hallmarked by the dysregulation of glucose homeostasis leading to hyperglycemia. The causes may be attributed to absence of insulin, diminished insulin levels, or insensitivity of the peripheral tissues to insulin. Gluconeogenesis and lipolysis are affected and may result in lactic acidosis and ketosis. The incidence and prevalence of all diabetes types appear to be on the rise. According to Centers for Disease Control and Prevention (CDC) data, approximately 200,000 children and adolescents are affected across the United States.[1] The mortality rates from diabetes and its complications among young people appear to be stable at approximately 1/1,000,000. Diabetes may be divided into the following subtypes that define some of the pathophysiological processes.[2,3]

Type 1 diabetes mellitus (DM-1)

Type 2 diabetes mellitus (DM-2)

Genetic defect of β-cell function

 Mature onset diabetes of the young (MODY)[3,4]

 Mitochondrial disorders

Exocrine pancreas disease

 Cystic fibrosis

 Thalassemia

Congenital rubella

Insulin resistance

    Rabson-Mendenhall

Endocrinopathies

    Autoimmune polyglandular syndrome

    Cushing syndrome

Drug induced

Steroids

Chemotherapy agents

Genetic

    Down syndrome

    Klinefelter syndrome

    Myotonic dystrophy

    Prader-Willi syndrome

    Turner syndrome

    Werner syndrome

    Wolfram syndrome

DM-1 is characterized by autoimmune-mediated pancreatic insulin-secreting β-cell destruction, and an absolute deficiency of insulin. New theories on etiology link onset of autoimmune DM-1 (anti-pancreatic β-cell) to genetic susceptibility and to an infectious etiology, as diagnosis rates increase during autumn and winter months mirroring increased rates of viral infections in the pediatric population.[2] The prevalence of DM-1 in U.S. youth (0 to 19 years of age) is on the rise, and increased from 1.48 per 1,000 in 2001, to 1.93 per 1,000 in 2009.[5] The etiology of the increase is unclear.

DM-2 is hallmarked by insulin resistance and relative insulin deficiency. Previously, DM was thought to be a disorder of the aging and overweight adult population but with the increase in youth obesity rates, DM-2 has been rising in the pediatric population as well. DM-2 correlates with family history of diabetes, suggesting a genetic link.[5] In 2009, the prevalence of DM-2 in adolescents (ages 10 to 19) was 0.46 per 1,000, a 30% increase from 2001[5] and the incidence of diabetes in the adult population is expected to surpass 40% by 2025.[6]

MODY is a non-insulin-dependent DM that is inherited in an autosomal dominant manner and presents in childhood or early adolescence with mild hyperglycemia, and slowly progressive disease.[3,4] Patients are initially asymptomatic, and may be treated with diet and oral agents. Insulin is rarely required during initial phase, lasting 5 years, or longer. MODY can be further divided into subtypes 1 to 5 by the causative genetic defect and varying severity.

Other genetic conditions that are often associated with DM include cystic fibrosis, Prader-Willi syndrome, Down syndrome, Turner syndrome, Wolfram syndrome, Cushing syndrome, as well as some chronic steroid regimens and chemotherapy agents.

There are significant ethnic and racial disparities in the incidence, prevalence, and mortality rates related to diabetes. The incidence of DM-1 and prevalence of DM-2 among white children and adolescents is higher than among black children and adolescents. But the mortality rate among the black population was reportedly higher for the same time period.[7] The incidence of obesity, DM-2, and MODY with dyslipidemia has been rising in the Asian adolescence population as well.[8]

Preoperative Planning for Glycemic Control

Preoperative planning must be tailored to the patient's treatment regimen optimizing glycemic control perioperatively. Preoperative evaluation for elective surgery should include assessment of glycemic control, electrolyte status, and presence or absence of ketones, as well as any additional tests such as ECG and chest x-ray guided by clinical history and other comorbidities. Goals of glycemic control, as evaluated by hemoglobin A1c (HbA1C) are age dependent (Table 20-1). A diabetic patient case should be scheduled as first case of the day, if possible, to minimize duration of preoperative fasting. If metabolic studies are unacceptable, patients should be referred back to their endocrinologist for adjustment of therapy. Glycemic control goals and regimen should ideally be coordinated with the endocrinology service.[9]

Acceptable glycemic control for patients with DM-1 is most commonly achieved with "split-mixed" insulin regimen[9] (intermediate or long-acting baseline regimen, and rapid or short-acting boluses for meals). For those who use insulin pumps, adjustments to the pump infusion rate are to be made on the day of surgery.[10] For DM-2, similar workup is needed, and endocrinology should be consulted regarding adjustments to insulin or oral agents in preparation for surgery.[11]

Day of Surgery and Intraoperative Management

"Split-mixed" regimen plan requires adjustments to insulin dosing on the day of surgery. The recommended modifications are as follows:

1. Hold rapid/short-acting insulin [regular or lispro (Humalog®)].

Table 20-1. Glycemic Control by Age[9]

Age	HbA1c levels
<5 years	7–9%
5–13 years	6–8.5%
>13 years	6–8%

Data from Rhodes ET, Ferrari LR, Wolfsdorf JI. Periopertaive management of pediatric surgical patients with diabetes mellitus. *Anesth Analg*. 2005;101:986-999. https://journals.lww.com/anesthesia-analgesia.

2. Administer half (50%) of AM dose of intermediate (NPH or Lente) or long-acting (ultralente) insulin dose.

3. Skip breakfast and follow appropriate NPO guidelines for surgical/imaging procedures.

4. Recheck blood glucose, electrolytes, and ketones (blood or urine) upon arrival.

5. Proceed with case if patient is normoglycemic (glucose <250 mg/dL) and electrolytes are normal. If patient is hyperglycemic (glucose >250 mg/dL), correct glucose level with short-acting insulin dose subcutaneously, according to patient's usual sliding-scale insulin regimen. In the absence of a sliding-scale regimen, the appropriate dose of insulin may be calculated using the "1500 rule" (Box 20-1).

6. Follow blood glucose levels once hyperglycemia is treated to confirm normoglycemia.

7. For patients using electronic continuous glucose monitoring, correlating monitor with on-site lab is suggested.

When the patient is using an *insulin pump* to manage his or her diabetes, there are a number of issues to consider[10]: For short procedures (less than 2 hours) where the pump does not interfere with the procedure:

1. Eliminate preprandial bolus.

2. Maintain basal infusion rate with hourly glucose checks.

3. Know typical bolus rate required to decrease glucose 50 mg/dL, and use if necessary (learn sequence to program pump for bolus, or have a supplemental dose for SC administration available).

4. Resume preoperative diet schedule as soon as possible.

Procedures lasting more than 2 hours require conversion to insulin infusion with D101/2 NS at the maintenance fluids rate. Glucose levels should be followed intraoperatively at least hourly, and infusion rates adjusted accordingly. The goal of insulin therapy with insulin infusion is 150 mg/dL.[9]

To initiate an insulin infusion, initial rate should be at 1 unit per 5-g dextrose for children 12 or younger, and 1 unit per 3-g dextrose for patients older than 12. The insulin and dextrose should be administered via the same IV line, via Y-connector, if possible, minimizing the risk of unintended bolus or interruption of the

infusions. Interruption of either one without the other can be catastrophic, leading to severe hyperglycemia or hypoglycemia.[9]

Patients who use glargine (Lantus®) should take their full dose on the evening prior to surgery or the morning of surgery and omit their short- or rapid-acting insulin dose on the day of surgery. Rapid-acting insulin [Lispro (Humalog®)] should be used according to the child's "correction factor" to achieve glucose level of 150 mg/dL.

For children with DM-2 and MODY on oral regimen, the preoperative adjustments start prior to the day of surgery. Metformin (Glucophage®) should be held 24 hours prior to surgery; sulfonylureas [glipizide (Glucotrol®), glyburide (Micronase®)] and thiazolidinediones [rosiglitazone (Avandia®), pioglitazone (Actos®)] should be discontinued on the morning of surgery. Preoperative hyperglycemia should be treated with rapid-acting [Lispro (Humalog®)] insulin 0.1 U/kg SC and continue to monitor hourly.[9]

Postoperative Management

Insulin/dextrose infusion should be discontinued as soon as the patient is able to tolerate oral intake. Glucose levels should be monitored postoperatively. For those who are unable to resume oral intake, maintain dextrose-containing maintenance fluids, and consider intermittent insulin dosing instead of infusion for the duration of their postoperative fasting.

Associated Comorbidities

Overweight and obese patients with DM-2 exhibit signs of insulin resistance, including acanthosis nigricans, precocious puberty, hypertension, dyslipidemia, and polycystic ovary syndrome. Many of the advanced complications of diabetes are present long before they become symptomatic. Microangiopathy leads to nephropathy, renal insufficiency, and retinopathy. Dyslipidemia and hypertension lead to atherosclerotic vascular changes affecting both cardiac and peripheral vasculature. Autonomic dysfunction related to chronic hyperglycemia and hypertonicity may be present, and manifest as orthostatic hypotension, resting tachycardia, lack of respiratory variation of heart rate, and blunted or absent symptoms of hypoglycemia. Gastroparesis increases aspiration risk, and peripheral neuropathy can lead to perioperative injury.[12]

Hyperglycemia impairs wound healing, decreases chemotaxis and phagocytosis, and has been shown to increase rate of surgical infection.[13] Surgery and anesthesia are stressful, and as such can have profound effect on glucose metabolism. While minimally concerning in a healthy patient, derangement can be dramatic in the diabetic patient. Stress response encompasses catabolism with elevated cortisol, glucagon, catecholamine, and growth hormone levels, increased gluconeogenesis and lipolysis, and decreased insulin levels. The potent inhaled anesthetics can induce hyperglycemia due to fatty acid mobilization

---

BOX 20-1. INSULIN CORRECTION FACTOR CALCULATION[9]

The 1,500 rule calculates the anticipated reduction in glucose level per unit of insulin, based on the patient's daily dose of insulin. This "insulin correction factor" is obtained by dividing 1500 by the total units of insulin required daily to treat the child.

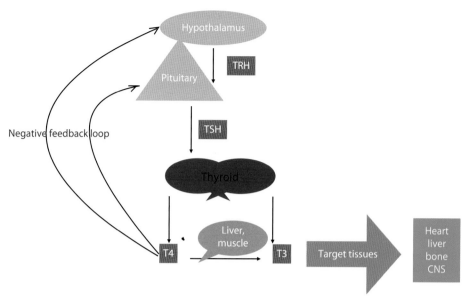

▲ **Figure 20-1.** Hypothalamic-pituitary-thyroid axis.

and inhibition of insulin secretion. Propofol may increase lipid load, benzodiazepines decrease ACTH levels, and opioids may block the hypothalamic-pituitary axis. While spinal and epidural anesthetic techniques may attenuate the metabolic changes associated with surgical stress, there is no evidence that neuraxial anesthesia affects morbidity or mortality in the diabetic patient.[2]

THYROID DISORDERS

Thyroid hormone production and release is autoregulated by a negative feedback loop involving the hypothalamic-pituitary-thyroid axis (Figure 20-1). The hypothalamus releases thyrotropin-releasing hormone (TRH), which stimulates the anterior pituitary to release thyroid-stimulating hormone (TSH), which, in turn, stimulates the thyroid gland to release thyroid hormone. Thyroid hormone inhibits the release of TRH and TSH, closing the feedback loop.[14]

Production of thyroid hormone depends on the hormonal controls and on availability of iodine in the diet. Iodine is easily absorbed by the gut, and as much as 90% of the body's iodine is stored in the thyroid gland. After iodine is taken up by the follicular cells in the thyroid gland, it is rapidly oxidized, and combined with tyrosyl residues within thyroglobulin to form monoiodotyrosine (MIT) and diiodotyrosine (DIT). MIT and DIT then combine to form T_3 (triiodothyroxine) and T_4 (thyroxine), and are subsequently stored bound to thyroglobulin in the colloid center of the follicular cells. Thyroid hormone in circulation is protein bound, attached to thyroxine-binding protein (TBG), albumin, and transthyretin. Once

dissociated from its protein, the lipophilic thyroid hormone rapidly diffuses into the cells, and acts as a prohormone in the cell's nucleus and mitochondria.[15]

▶ Hyperthyroidism (Box 20-2)

Hyperthyroidism is defined as the excess production and release of thyroid hormone, resulting in inappropriately high levels of serum thyroid hormone and a hypermetabolic state.[15] Thyroid hormone affects every organ system and can present with varied symptoms.[15] Symptoms of hyperthyroidism in the pediatric population are nonspecific, and easily overlooked.[16] They can range from nervousness, fatigue, sleep disturbances, and behavioral and learning disorders to congestive heart failure, altered mental status, and death.[15,16]

Graves disease, an autoimmune disease producing TSH-receptor stimulating antibodies resulting in excess production and release of T_3 and T_4, is the most common cause of hyperthyroidism in children and adolescents, with incidence of 0.02%.[13,17] As in the adult population, the treatment options range from antithyroid medication to radioactive iodine ablation (RIA) to thyroidectomy. In contrast to the adult population, RIA is controversial in the pediatric population, owing to concerns about radiation exposure during periods of growth, and potential long-term complication from exposure (although there is no data to support these concerns). Antithyroid medication is limited to methimazole, as propylthiouracil is contraindicated in children due to high incidence of liver injury and liver failure requiring liver transplantation.[16,18] Methimazole is associated with minor side effects, but does carry

BOX 20-2. CAUSES OF HYPERTHYROIDISM IN CHILDREN[15,17]

Graves disease (diffuse toxic goiter)
Toxic multinodular goiter
Toxic thyroid adenoma
TSH-secreting pituitary adenoma
Thyrotoxicosis
Hashimoto's chronic lymphocytic thyroiditis
DeQuervain's subacute granulomatous thyroiditis
Subacute lymphocytic thyroiditis
Thyroid storm
Malignancy (MEN-2A, MEN-2B)

Table 20-2. Thyrotoxicosis in Children[15,17]

Differential Diagnosis	Thyroid Storm
Acute pulmonary edema	Heat stroke
Malignant hyperthermia	Sepsis/septic shock
Sympathomimetic overdose	Seratonin syndrome
Tachyarrhythnia	

Data from Devereaux D, Toweled S. Hyperthyroidism and thyrotoxicosis. *Emerg Med Clin N Am.* 2014;32:277-292. https://www.sciencedirect.com/journal/emergency-medicine-clinics-of-north-america. Knollman PD, Giese A, Bhayani MK. Surgical intervention for medically refractory hyperthyroidism. *Pediatric Annals.* 2016;45(5):e171-e175. https://www.healio.com/pediatrics/journals/pedann.

more serious risks of agranulocytosis in a dose-dependent fashion—Stevens-Johnson syndrome, vasculitis, and lupus-like syndrome. Methimazole is not curative for Graves disease; it merely mitigates the symptoms until the disease goes into spontaneous remission.[17] Remission rates range from 20% to 30%, and are worse for patients with high antibody levels, very high free T_4 levels at diagnosis, and with large gland. Relapse rates range from 25% to 60% after withdrawal of medication.[17] Younger children have higher relapse rates and lower remission rates, necessitating definitive treatment.[16,19,20] The most common cause of treatment failure in the pediatric population remains noncompliance due to prolonged course of therapy (Table 20-2).[17]

Thyroid surgery for Graves disease and other thyrotoxic conditions can present numerous challenges perioperatively. Thyroid hormone level should be suppressed with antithyroid drugs (methimazole) preoperatively, and symptoms must be treated supportively (β-blockers). The gland is inflamed, and more vascular, and thus, more challenging to resect. In fact, several recent publications cite increased risk of complications in the pediatric population compared with adults after thyroidectomy.[16] Electromyogram (EMG) endotracheal tubes have been used successfully to detect proximity to the recurrent laryngeal nerve during thyroid resection and reduce risk of nerve injury. The possibility of a difficult intubation must be considered, although reports of difficult intubation correlate with advanced age, and have not been reported in the pediatric population.[21–24]

Intraoperative management of thyroidectomy for a secretory condition should avoid sympathomimetics and vagolytics, and include medications to treat a potential thyroid storm, such as β-blockers. The astute clinician must also consider a differential diagnosis in the event of a hypermetabolic crisis (malignant hyperthermia, sepsis, etc.) (Table 20-3).[13] If available, EMG endotracheal tube can be placed with the aid of a video laryngoscope to ensure proper placement and allow monitoring of pharyngeal/vocal cord innervation during thyroid resection.

Postoperative Considerations

Postoperative concerns include hypocalcemia from parathyroid trauma causing muscle weakness, respiratory insufficiency due to vocal cord paresis/paralysis, tracheomalacia from a large compressive tumor, and obstruction from surgical site hematoma.[23,25–27] Although the incidence of post-op hypocalcemia was similar in adults and children, children reported more symptoms of transient hypocalcemia (35% vs. 21% of adults) and were prescribed calcitriol more frequently and for a longer duration compared with adults.[16,27] The rate of parathyroid reimplantation was significantly higher in children who had a total thyroidectomy (10.9%) vs. partial thyroidectomy (3.1%).[25] The rate of transient nerve palsy was slightly higher in children (10%) than adults (5%) but not statistically significant except for patients <1 year old: incidence of >14%,[25] and the rate of permanent complications was low in both adults and children.[16] It is notable that children <6 years old, especially those <1 year of age having a total thyroidectomy, do carry a significantly higher risk of postoperative complications (Figure 20-2).[25]

Hypothyroidism

Hypothyroidism is the most common cause of preventable intellectual disability. Its incidence has been rising since the mid-1970s, with the advent of newborn screening and reduction of threshold to include milder cases.[18] At present, congenital hypothyroidism affects 1:2,500 live births in North America, with wide variations across demographics. Eighty-five percent of cases of congenital hypothyroidism are caused by gland dysgenesis, and approximately two-thirds of cases are related to ectopic location of the gland. Most cases of thyroid dysgenesis or agenesis are sporadic and idiopathic. Iatrogenic congenital hypothyroidism is seen in infants whose mothers received radioactive iodine after the tenth week of gestation. Transient hypothyroidism may be seen in newborns of mothers on thyroid suppression drugs, and mothers who are iodine deficient. Notably, newborns with large congenital hepatic hemangiomas may present with hypothyroidism as well.[18] Symptoms of hypothyroidism are varied (Table 20-5), from early decreased activity, prolonged jaundice, hypotonia, hypothermia,

Table 20-3. Treatment Strategies for Hyperthyroidism[15]

Drug Type and Name	Mechanism of Action	Neonatal Dose*	Pediatric Dose**	Adult Dosing	Thyroid Storm Dosing***
Antithyroid					
Propylthiouracil (PTU)	Prevents T_3/T_4 production in thyroid gland Blocks T_4 to T_3 conversion Maintenance: $1/3 - 2/3$ initial dose, divided in q8h dosing	5–10 mg/kg/day PO divided in q8h dosing	Initial: 5–7 mg/kg/day PO divided in q8h Maintenance: $1/3 - 2/3$ initial dose, divided in q8h dosing	Initial: 100–200 mg PO q6–8h Maintenance: 50–100 mg/d	500–1,000 mg loading dose 250 mg q4–6h PO/NG/OG
Methimazole (MMI)	Prevents production of thyroid hormone	N/A	Initial: 0.4–0.7 mg/kg/day PO divided in q8h dosing Max: 30 mg/day	Initial: 10–20 mg PO q8–12h Maintenance: 2.5–10 mg/day	60–80 mg/day POnNG/OG
Iodides					
Lugol solution	Blocks release of stored thyroid hormone from gland	1 drop PO q8h	N/A	4–8 drops q6h–q8h PO/NG/OG	10 drops q12h PO/NG/OG
			1–5 drops q8h PO/NG/OG	5–10 drops q6–8h PO/NG/OG	5–10 drops q6–8h one hour after PTU or MMI
Glucocorticoids					
Dexamethasone	Blocks conversion of T_4 to T_3			2 mg q6h PO	2 mg q6h IV/PO/NG/OG
Hydrocortisone			2 mg/kg q6h PO/IV		300 mg IV load, 100 mg IV q6–8h
Prednisone				40–60 mg PO daily ×1 week, then taper	
Beta-blockers					
Propranolol	Reduces symptoms of catecholamine response, blocks T_4 to T_3 conversion	2 mg/kg/day PO divided in q6–12h dosing	0.5–1 mg/kg/d divided q6–8h	10–40 mg PO q6–8h	1 mg/min IV as needed
Atenolol			0.5–1 mg/kg PO qd (up to 100 mg/day)	25–100 mg PO qd (up to 200 mg/day)	60–80 mg q4h PO/NG/OG
Esmolol		100–500 mcg/kg IV load, then 100 mcg/kg/min	100–500 mcg/kg IV load, then 25–100 mcg/kg/min		500 mcg/kg/min for one minute, then 50–100 mcg/kg/min

*Neonatal thyrotoxicosis is a result of maternal Graves disease, and transplacental passage of thyroid-stimulating antibodies. It is self-limited, as antibodies decline in 3–4 months.[15]

**PTU is associated with hepatotoxic reaction and fulminant liver failure in children, and is therefore contraindicated.[15,20]

***Avoid salicylates during thyroid storm, as they can increase free thyroxin level by decreasing thyroid-binding protein. Use acetaminophen and cooling devices for hyperthermia.[15]

Reproduced with permission, from Devereaux D, Toweled S. Hyperthyroidism and thyrotoxicosis. *Emerg Med Clin N Am.* 2014;32:277-292. https://www.sciencedirect.com/journal/emergency-medicine-clinics-of-north-america.

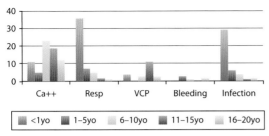

▲ Figure 20-2. Post-thyroidectomy complication rates by patients' age.[25] (Adapted from Hanba C, et al. Pediatric thyroidectomy: hospital course and perioperative complications. *Otolaryngol Head Neck Surg.* 2017;156(2): 360-367. https://journals.sagepub.com/home/oto.)

edema of the eyelids and extremities, and a protuberant abdomen, to late findings of poor sucking effort, developmental delay, poor growth, hoarse cry, decreased activity, and lethargy, to myxedema and coma.

Acquired primary hypothyroidism is most commonly a result of autoimmune (Hashimoto) thyroiditis but may also be a side effect of medication (Table 20-6).[32] It may present with a goiter, poor growth velocity, decreased energy, declining school performance, constipation, and in girls with precocious puberty and hyperprolactinemia. It may also coexist with Graves disease, and signs and symptoms may alternate between the two autoimmune conditions.[18] Secondary (central) hypothyroidism is a result of hypothalamic or pituitary dysfunction which can be congenital, neoplastic, or traumatic (Table 20-7).

Table 20-4. Familial Endocrine Neoplasia

Familial Neoplasm syndrome	MEN-1 (Wermer Syndrome) 2–3:100,000	MEN-2A (Sipple Syndrome)	MEN-I2B 1:200,000	Familial Medullary Thyroid Carcinoma (FMTC)
Genetics	Chr.11, *PYGM* gene, menin (11q13), autosomal dominant	RET proto-oncogene, (codone 634) Chr.10 autosomal dominant	RET proto-oncogene, (codone 918) Chr.10 autosomal dominant	RET proto-oncogene, Chr.10 (10q11) autosomal dominant
Endocrine manifestation	Parathyroid hyperplasia: hyperparathyroidism (100% by age 50)	Parathyroid hyperplasia (10–20%)		
		Medullary thyroid cancer (>90%)	Medullary thyroid cancer (>95%)	Medullary thyroid cancer (100%)
	Pituitary tumor: anterior pituitary adenoma (10–20%), prolactinoma/galactorrhea, acromegaly			
	Pancreatic islet cell tumor (pNET): gastrinoma (Zollinger-Ellison syndrome), insulinoma, VIPoma, carcinoid			
		Pheochromocytoma (40–50%)	Pheochromocytoma (50%)	
Cutaneous and connective tissue manifestations	Facial angiofibromas (88%)	Cutaneous lichen/amyloidosis	Marfanoid habitus (80%)	
	Facial collagenomas (>70%)		Mucosal neuromas (>95%), intestinal ganglio-neuromas, megacolon, chronic constipation	
	Lipomas (20–30%)			
	17% present before age 21; screening by age 11	Thyroidectomy by age 5 Screen for pheochromocytoma at age 11	Thyroidectomy ASAP Screen for pheochromocytoma at age 11	Screen by age 5

Sources: Data from Norton JA, Krampitz G, Jensen RT. Multiple endocrine neoplasia: genetics & clinical management. *Sure Once Clin N Am.* 2015;24(4):795-832. https://www.journals.elsevier.com/surgical-oncology-clinics-of-north-america. Wasserman JD, Tomlinson GE, et al. Multiple endocrine neoplasia and hyperparathyroid–jaw tumor syndromes: clinical features, genetics, and surveillance recommendations in childhood. *Clin Cancer Res.* 2017;23(13):e123-e132.https://clincancerres.aacrjournals.org/.

Table 20-5. Congenital Hypothyroidism Signs and Symptoms[18]

Onset	Signs and Symptoms
Early findings	Macrosomia
	Decreased activity
	Large anterior fontanelle
	Edema of eyelids, hands, and feet
	Prolonged jaundice
	Hypotonia
	Coarse facial features
	Hypothermia
	Pallor
	Goiter
	Protuberant abdomen
Late findings	Poor sucking
	Developmental delay
	Lethargy, decreased activity
	Poor growth trajectory
	Umbilical hernia
	Mottled, cool, dry skin
	Difficult breathing
	Macroglossia
	Myxedema (generalized swelling)
	Hoarse cry

Source: Reproduced with permission, from Diaz A, Lipman-Diaz EG. Hypothyroidism. *Pediatr Rev.* 35(8):336-347; quiz 348-9. Copyright © 2014 by the AAP. https://pedsinreview.aappublications.org/.

Table 20-6. Medication Effects on Native Thyroid Function[32]

Decreased TSH	Dopamine, glucocorticoids, octreotide, metformin, opiates, rexinoids, carbamazepine/oxcarbamazepine, metformin
Decreased thyroid hormone secretion	Lithium, iodine/iodinated contrast, amiodarone, aminoglutethimide
Increased thyroid hormone metabolism	Phenobarbital, rifampin, phenytoin, carbamazepine
Inhibition of T_4/T_3 synthesis	Propylthiouracil, methimazole
Thyroiditis	Interferon, interleukin-2, sunitinip, amiodarone

Source: Data from Haugen BR. Drugs that suppress TSH or cause central hypothyroidism. *Best Pract Res Clin Endocrinol Metab.* 2009;23(6):793-800. https://www.journals.elsevier.com/best-practice-and-research-clinical-endocrinology-and-metabolism.

Table 20-7. Syndromes and Disorders Associated with Hypothyroidism[14,18]

Down Syndrome	Turner Syndrome	Williams Syndrome
Costello syndrome	Septo-optic dysplasia	
Craniopharyngioma	Pituitary adenoma	Meningioma
Rathke's cleft cysts	Empty sella/ Sheehan syndrome	
Combined pituitary hormone deficiencies	Lymphocytic hypophysitis	Polyglandular autoimmune syndrome
Sarcoidosis— Langerhans histiocytosis	Infection (syphilis, tuberculosis)	
Head trauma	Head and neck irradiation	Surgery

Source: Data from Dubbs SB, Spangler R. Hypothyroidism: causes, killers, and life-saving treatments. *Emerg Med Clin N Am.* 2014;32:303-317. https://www.sciencedirect.com/journal/emergency-medicine-clinics-of-north-america. Diaz A, Lipman-Diaz EG. Hypothyroidism. *Pediatr Rev.* 2014;35(8):336-347; quiz 348-9. Copyright © 2014 by the AAP. https://pedsinreview.aappublications.org/.

Hypothyroid condition should be corrected, and patient should have laboratory testing to confirm euthyroidism prior to operative interventions. Since thyroid hormone is essential for all organ systems' appropriate function,[23] anesthesia in the setting of hypothyroid condition has an increased incidence of morbidity, and potential mortality. In the emergent situation, thyroid hormone replacement can be initiated in the perioperative setting.[31] Caution should be exercised in patients with heart disease. The need for replacement should be weighed against potential complications of increased myocardial contractility and myocardial oxygen demand. For those with undergoing procedures for ischemic and coronary heart disease, replacement of thyroid hormone may best be reserved for the postoperative period (Box 20-3).[18]

Thyroid Malignancy and Multiple Endocrine Neoplasia

Thyroid nodules are uncommon in children and adolescents, with an incidence of 1% to 2% of the pediatric population, and up to 13% in adolescents. The rate of malignancy can be as high as 20% to 26%, especially in larger nodules and those associated with lymphadenopathy.[28,29] Papillary thyroid cancer (PTC) is the most common malignancy of the thyroid in children. As many as 70% of pediatric patients have lymph node involvement at presentation, and 19% to 25% have pulmonary metastases. Even so, the prognosis for

BOX 20-3. KEY ANESTHETIC CONSIDERATIONS FOR THYROID DISORDERS.

Hyperthyroidism does not change minimum alveolar concentration of anesthesia. However, a deeper plane of anesthesia may be needed to blunt sympathetic response.

Caution/avoid sympathomimetics as they may cause exaggerated sympathetic response. Avoid salicylates, as they displace thyroid hormone from protein-binding sites.

Hypothyroidism does not reduce anesthetic requirement. Clinical observation suggests that increased sensitivity to anesthetics is likely due to decreased cardiac output and blunted physiological safeguards (baroreceptors, etc.).

Caution with airway due to edema or compressive mass.

PTC in children is favorable, with >95% survival rates at 15 years and 90% to 99% survival rate at 30 years.[28]

Surgical intervention requires total or near total thyroidectomy, given an increased incidence of bilateral and multifocal disease in pediatrics, and the increased risk of complications at reoperation.[28] Radioactive iodine (^{131}I) therapy for residual disease carries the risk of a secondary malignancy (1:112) at 8 years after treatment, and pulmonary fibrosis (1:11). This must be weighed against the low disease-specific mortality rate (2.68%).[28,29]

Medullary thyroid carcinoma (MTC) arises from the calcitonin-producing C-cells of the thyroid gland. Twenty-five percent of MTC are associated with germ-line mutation of chromosome 10 (10q11.2) RET proto-oncogene, encoding a transmembrane tyrosine kinase receptor. The mutation is inherited in an autosomal dominant fashion, and results in multiple endocrine neoplasia type 2 (MEN-2). MEN-2 is further divided into three subtypes: MEN-2A and MEN-2B, and familial medullary thyroid carcinoma (FMTC) (Table 20-4).[26]

MEN-2 is rare with an incidence in the population of 1:200,000. One hundred percent of patients with RET mutation will develop MTC. Survival depends on complete resection of MTC, and absence of metastatic disease at the time of resection.[30] MEN-2A is the most common of the three syndromes accounting for 55% of patients. FMTC accounts for 35%, whereas MEN-2B is the rarest and most virulent accounting for 5% to 10%.

With 100% of the patients with MEN-2 developing MTC, screening for malignancy should start as early as 5 years of age. Total thyroidectomy is recommended in cases where the gland is affected. MEN-2B commonly develops more aggressive tumors, and initiation of screening for MTC at the time of diagnosis of MEN-2B is indicated. A more radical thyroid resection with central lymph node resection is the surgery of choice. FMTC (the least virulent) screening should start at age 21, barring symptoms and surgical removal of the thyroid gland without central lymph node dissection are adequate, with serum levels of calcitonin and carcinoembryonic antigen (CEA) monitored starting at 6 months postoperatively. Normal levels at 5 years are considered a cure, and no further follow-up is needed.[30]

Half the patients with MEN-2A will develop pheochromocytoma (PCC). Mean age at presentation is 36 years, and most tumors are benign and confined to the adrenal gland. In 65% of patients, the tumors are bilateral, and those with unilateral tumor will develop a contralateral lesion within 10 years. Surgical excision of PCC takes precedence to thyroid resection due to the significant morbidity of untreated PCC. If patient requires bilateral adrenalectomy, they are at very high risk of Addisonian crisis, and should have the appropriate steroid and mineralocorticoid replacement postoperatively.[30]

MEN-1 is an autosomal dominant, germ-line mutation–driven syndrome, with several endocrine neoplastic conditions. Its prevalence in the population is 2–3:100,000. The mutation is on the long arm of chromosome 11 (11q13) tumor suppressor gene, encoding the protein menin (Table 20-4). The initial presenting disorder in patients with MEN-1 is hyperparathyroidism (>90%), followed by pancreatic neuroendocrine tumors (pNET) of which gastrinoma is the most frequent, pituitary adenomas, adrenal tumors, and thyroid adenomas (<10%).[30]

Hyperparathyroidism treatment is controversial. Some advocate complete removal, others removal only of the adenoma. Current recommendations settled on removing 3-1/2 of the parathyroid, leaving 50-g gland in the neck and marked with a hemoclip.[30]

Pituitary adenomas associated with MEN-1 secrete prolactin most frequently. Medical treatment with bromocriptine and cabergoline is recommended for prolactin-secreting adenomas, and octreotide and lanreotide for growth hormone–secreting adenomas <1 cm in size. Transsphenoidal surgery is recommended for discrete macroadenomas (>1 cm). Although surgery may offer a definitive cure, tumors have recurred on long-term follow-up. Surgery carries major morbidity, including permanent diabetes insipidus (DI).[30]

pNETs carry the greatest mortality risk for MEN-1 patients. They are typically multicentric and multifocal, spread throughout the pancreas and duodenum. Surgical resection of duodenal gastrinomas and nonfunctioning pancreatic tumors is controversial. Secretory pancreatic tumors should be removed. Malignant behavior pNET is the cause of death in >60% of patients, followed by thymic carcinoid (10% to 25%).[30]

Adrenal tumors are infrequent in MEN-1 and should be treated in similar manner to sporadic adrenal tumors. Most are discovered incidentally; they are small, nonfunctioning, benign, and asymptomatic.[30]

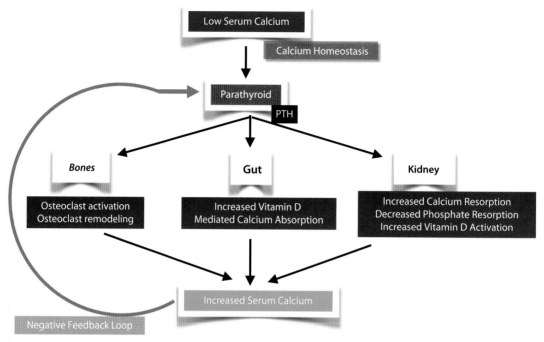

▲ **Figure 20-3.** Parathyroid hormone homeostasis.[43] (Data from Mannstadt M, Bilezikian JP, Thakker RV, et al. *Hypoparathyroidism. Nat Rev Dis Primers.* 2017;3:17055. https://www.nature.com/nrdp/.)

PARATHYROID DISORDERS

The parathyroid, like the thyroid and thymus, originates from the embryonic foregut, specifically from the third and fourth branchial pouches. Histologically, the gland is comprised of chief cells, oxyphil cells, fibrovascular stroma, and adipose tissue. Chief cells constitute almost the entirety of the gland's parenchyma. They are large (6 to 8 μm) clear cells and contain lipid and argyrophilic cytoplasmic granules. Oxyphilic cell content is small in children and increases with age. Oxyphil cells' function is unclear, but they do not seem to be degraded chief cells.[33,45]

Parathyroid hormone (PTH) is a large protein encoded by three exons of chromosome 11 (11p15). Its secretion is regulated by a direct negative feedback loop with serum calcium (Figure 20-3). The calcium sensor on chief cell membrane [calcium sensing receptor(CaSR)] is a 500-kD protein with a single-membrane spanning domain and is structurally related to the low-density lipoprotein receptor superfamily. The target tissues for PTH include bone, kidney, gut, smooth muscle cells, and fat cells (Figure 20-3). Serum half time for PTH is short, and it's degradation depends on hepatic Kupffer cells, GFR (reabsorption), and proteolysis.[34] PTH receptor (CaSR) is a large peptide with seven transmembrane domains and G-protein coupling. The receptor expression is sensitive to PTH level in a negative feedback loop. Parathormone is an 84 amino acid protein stored in secretory granules in the parathyroid gland and released when decreased calcium concentration results in decreased CaSR signaling.[43]

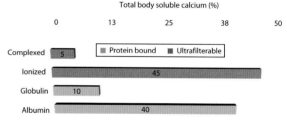

▲ **Figure 20-4.** Total body soluble calcium distribution.[35] (Data from Clark OH, Duh QY, Kebebew E, eds. *Textbook of Endocrine Surgery.* 2nd ed. 2005. Copyright © Elsevier Saunders. All rights reserved.)

Most of the body's calcium (98%) is in the insoluble hydroxyapatite crystal form, deposited in bones.

A little more than 1% of the total body's calcium is in its soluble form, and approximately 1% of it is in the extracellular fluid. Fifty percent of the soluble calcium is bound to protein (mostly albumin) and 50% is in an ultra-filterable form, mostly as ionized calcium (Figure 20-4).[35]

Hyperparathyroidism (Table 20-8)

Signs and symptoms of hypercalcemia and hyperparathyroidism include painful bones, kidney stones, abdominal discomfort, psychosis, cardiac conduction abnormalities, hypertension, and fatigue (Box 20-4)

Primary hyperparathyroidism (HPT) is common in adults (approx. 3 per 1,000) but infrequent in children (2 to

Table 20-8. Genetic and Metabolic Hyperparathyroid and Hypercalcemic Syndromes[38,39]

Syndrome (chromosome, gene)	Inheritance	PTH	Ca	Frequency	Presentation
Familial Hypocalciuric Hypercalcemia (FHH) FHH-1 (3q21.1, CaSR loss-of-function) FHH-2 (19p13, GNA11) FHH-2 (19q13.2-13.3, AP2S1 loss-of-function)	Autosomal Dominant (AD)	↑/nl	↑	~65% <5% ~20%	Asymptomatic Failure to thrive Learning disabilities
Familial Isolated Hyperparathyroidism (FIHP) (11q13, MEN1) (1q31.2, CDC73) (3q21.1, CaSR) (6p24.2, GMC2)		Nonsense mutation	nl	>100 families	Diagnosis of exclusion
Neonatal Severe HPT (NSHPT) (3q21.2, CaSR)	AD or AR		↑↑		Osteoclast hyperactivity. At birth: respiratory distress, hypotonia, bone demineralization, fatal by 3 months, if untreated
Non-Syndromic Primary HPT (nsPHPT) (11p15.3-15.1, PTH) (6p21.2, CDKN1A) (9p21, CDKN2B) (1p32, CDKN2C) (6p24.2, GMC2 activating mutation)	AD		↑		
Multiple Endocrine Neoplasia (MEN) MEN-1 (11q13, MEN1 menin) MEN-2 (10q11.2, RET proto-oncogene) MEN-3 (10a11.2, RET) MEN-4 (12p13, CDKN1B)	AD	↑ or nl	↑	>95% ~20% rare 100%	As early as 8 yrs old
Hyperparathyroid–Jaw Tumor (PHT_JT) (1q31.2, CDC73 aka HRPT2 parafibromin inactivation)	AD		↑		Brown tumor of the jaw, often recurrent

Source: Data from Stokes VJ, Nielsen MF, Hannan FM, Thakker RV. Hypercalcemic disorders in children. *J Bone Mineral Res.* 2017;32(11): 2157-2170. https://asbmr.onlinelibrary.wiley.com/journal/15234681.

BOX 20-4. STRESS STEROID CONSIDERATIONS[12]

Stress steroid replacement should not be necessary after a short (<2 week) course of steroids that ended >2 weeks ago, or treatment that lasted longer than 2 weeks, but has been discontinued >6 months ago.

5 per 100,000).[36] Most pediatric HPT is sporadic. Less than 5% of cases of pediatric HPT can be attributed to familial inherited genetic causes. Many patients with genetic HPT harbor an inherited or sporadic germ-line mutation.[37,38]

HPT most commonly presents as incidental finding of asymptomatic hypercalcemia. Other common presentations of primary HPT in children include rickets, osteomalacia, short stature, hypercalcemia, and hypercalciuria. Early investigation centers on exclusion of genetic malignancy syndromes[38] and on appropriate follow-up for other malignancies if familial or germ-line cause is discovered. The treatment of symptoms may include calcimimetic drugs, which have been used safely and effectively in adults, with minimal side effects (mostly nausea and vomiting). In the pediatric population, recent publications recommend calcimimetic medications be combined with calcitriol and thiazide diuretics[40] to prevent hypocalcemia and hypercalciuria.

Vitamin levels should be investigated, and if adequate, referral for surgical/oncological evaluation should follow. For secretory adenoma, parathyroidectomy is the only cure, and is frequently combined with thymectomy due to risk of supernumerary, intrathymic glands.[37] Such sporadic presentation and tertiary causes (chronic renal failure, hypophosphatemic rickets, etc.) of HPT are most common.[38] However, even sporadic presentation of HPT has >10% incidence of de novo germ-line mutations.

Hypercalcemia has been reported as a cause of acute pancreatitis at a rate of 2 to 5 per 100,000. Although much less frequent than the adult population, the resulting pancreatitis may be lethal.[36] Pathological fractures, and brown tumors, have also been reported in children.[41]

Hyperparathyroidism is the most common presenting endocrinopathy in MEN-1, with a penetrance of near 100% by age 50. In many young patients (20- to 25-year-olds), it may present concomitantly with Zollinger-Ellison syndrome (ZES) (gastrinoma). Parathyroid carcinomas are rare, occurring in 0.28% of all patients with MEN-1.[30]

In children with hyperparathyroid–jaw tumor syndrome (HPT-JT), presentation may include ossifying fibroma of the jaw (25% to 50%), parathyroid adenoma (70%), or rarely parathyroid carcinoma (15%). Children with known familial pathological genetics must begin surveillance as early as 5 years of age.[37,39]

Hypoparathyroidism

Hypoparathyroidism presents with hypocalcemia, hyperphosphatemia, and low or inappropriately normal PTH. Hypocalcemia manifests as fatigue, confusion, paresthesias, muscle cramps, twitching, bronchospasm, laryngospasm, seizures, congestive heart failure, and myocardial conduction abnormalities such as prolonged QT.[42,43] The etiologies of hypoparathyroidism with hypocalcemia range from iatrogenic to genetic (Table 20-9), and include hormone deficiency and hormone resistance.[41] The most common etiology is removal or injury to the parathyroid gland.[43] Fewer than 10% of all cases of hypoparathyroidism are of genetic etiology.[43] Of the more common genetic causes, DiGeorge syndrome and cardiovelofacial syndrome, with similar genetics owing to deletion of *TBX1* gene on chromosome 22q11, are commonly seen in pediatric hospitals. Hypocalcemia occurs in approximately 60% of patients with DiGeorge syndrome.[42] Hypocalcemia often resolves in the first 2 years of life, but may recur with stress (surgical, sepsis, etc.) or periods of accelerated growth (adolescence).[45,46] As such, preoperative laboratory studies and clinical evaluation are indicated, and careful calcium and electrolyte replacement is necessary to avoid complications related to cardiac conduction problems and generalized weakness.

HYPOTHALAMIC-PITUITARY-ADRENAL AXIS

The adrenal gland originates from embryonic mesoderm forming the adrenal cortex, and embryonic neural crest forming chromaffin cells of the adrenal medulla. The adrenal cortex (endocrine system), in conjunction with the hypothalamus and pituitary, controls mineralocorticoid, glucocorticoid, and androgen hormone homeostasis. The cortex is divided into three zones with different secretory functions. The zona glomerulosa regulates mineral balance and volume status by synthesizing and secreting the mineralocorticoid aldosterone. The zona fasciculata synthesizes

and secretes glucocorticoids (cortisol) regulating glucose homeostasis and metabolism. Lastly, the zona reticularis synthesizes and secretes androgens (Figure 20-5).[47] The adrenal medulla, part of the neuroendocrine system, secretes vasoactive stress hormones integral to the sympathetic nervous system.

ADRENAL DISORDERS: ADRENAL CORTEX

Mineralocorticoid Derangements (Zona Glomerulosa) (Figure 20-6)

Primary aldosteronism (*Conn's syndrome*) is a group of conditions of inappropriately high aldosterone secretion, independent of the renin-angiotensin system. Normally, aldosterone synthesis by the glomerulosa cells is stimulated by the renin-angiotensin system in response to hypovolemia or hyperkalemia. Pediatric patients with primary aldosteronism are rare, and in older case reports, many had bilateral adrenal hyperplasia. A more recent investigation describes a genetic mutation in a potassium channel gene $KCNJ_5(Kir_{3,4})$ that occurs in as many as 34% of patients with a unilateral adrenal gland and has been described in germ-line mutation of familial forms of the syndrome. The typical clinical presentation or primary aldosteronism is moderate to severe hypertension, headaches, polydipsia, polyuria, nocturia, and hypokalemic alkalosis. Muscle weakness, cramping, and intermittent paralysis (likely related to hypokalemia) have also been reported. Severe cases have also presented with cardiac symptoms, ophthalmological and neurological abnormalities, hepatic dysfunction, and renal dysfunction.[48,49,54]

Aldosterone hypersecretion is treated surgically when the source is a solitary adrenal adenoma, and medically for adrenal hyperplasia. Preoperative assessment and planning should be preceded by pharmacological control of hypertension and correction of electrolyte abnormalities. It should include evaluation of electrolytes, renal function, electrocardiogram (ECG) and possibly echocardiogram, aldosterone secretion suppression, and optimization of antihypertensive regimen.[50] The hallmark of medical treatment is spironolactone, a competitive aldosterone receptor antagonist and potassium sparing diuretic. Eplerenone, also a competitive aldosterone receptor antagonist, is a second choice, in the event that spironolactone's side effects (inhibition of testosterone and progesterone) become significant. This must be accompanied with sodium restriction and cautious potassium replacement. Intraoperative and postoperative monitoring of volume status, electrolytes, and renal function should be expected.

Hypoaldosteronism is usually tied to renin production. Both hyperreninemic and hyporeninemic conditions exist. The first condition, usually due to medications, can occur in the setting of adrenal crisis/Addisonian crisis or with aldosterone synthase deficiency due to CYP11B2 deficiency. The second condition is usually related to

Table 20-9. Hypoparathyroidism[41-43]

Causes	Associated Condition	Defective Function
Iatrogenic	Post-surgical Radiation	Post-thyroidectomy external radioactive iodine
Acquired	Autoimmune	Anti-CaSR antibodies Graves disease Adrenal insufficiency
Infiltrative	Metastatic/malignant deposition	Iron: Hemochromatosis Copper: Wilson disease
Congenital	DiGeorge syndrome Velocardiofacial syndrome	Chr. 22q11 deletion (*TBX1* gene)
	Hypoparathyroidism–deafness–renal dysplasia syndrome (RDS) Barakat syndrome	Reduced GATA3 transcription factor (autosomal dominant)
	Kenny-Caffey syndrome Sanjad-Sakati syndrome	AR loss of function mutation TBCE, bone dysplasia
	Isolated hypoparathyroidism	Germ-line missense mutation of PTH gene
	Autosomal hypoparathyroidism	Gain of function mutation CaSR
Genetic	Maternally inherited mitochondrial DNA defect (MELAS)	Mitochondrial DNA defect (maternal)
	Kearnes-Sayre syndrome	Mitochondrial DNA
	Mitochondrial trifunctional protein deficiency syndrome (MTPDA)	AR, fatty acid oxidation disorder, CMP, peripheral neuropathy, liver dysfunction, retinopathy
	Familial hypercalciuric hypocalcemia	Autosomal dominant gain–of-function mutation CaSR
	Familial hypoparathyroidism	
	Autoimmune polyglandular syndrome (APS)	AIRE autoimmune regulator gene mutation [thymic T-cell regulation (AR mostly)] Variants may also have Addison disease, DM-1, hypothyroidism, pernicious anemia, hepatitis, ovarian atrophy, keratitis, vitiligo, alopecia
Pseudohypoparathyroidism	Maternal GNAS mutation	Peripheral resistance to PTH (uncoupling of cAMP from PTH)
	Albright's hereditary osteodystrophy Blomstrand lethal chondrodysplasia	PTH/PTHrP receptor mutation (autosomal recessive, lethal)
	Pseudopseudohypoparathyroidism	Paternal GNAS mutation, normal labs

CaSR, Calcium Sensing Receptor Antibodies; TBX1, T-box transcription factor; GATA3, protein coding gene; PTH, parathyroid hormone; PTHrP, parathyroid hormone-related protein; AR, androgen receptor; TBCE, Tubulin folding Cofactor E; DNA, Deoxyribonucleic acid; AIRE, autoimmune regulator; GNAS, protein coding gene.

Sources: Data from Mitchell D, Rybak LP, Glatz FR. Hyperparathyroid risis in a pediatric patient. *Int J Pediatr Otorhinolaryngol.* 2004;68:237-241. Al-Azem H, Khan AA. Hyperparathyroidism. *Best Pract Res Clin Endocrinol Metabol.* 2012;26:517-522. Mannstadt M, Bilezikian JP, Thakker RV, et al. Hypoparathyroidism. *Nat Rev Dis Primers.* 2017;3:17055.

renal dysfunction from concomitant diseases, such as diabetes.[49]

Glucocorticoid Derangements (Zona Fasciculata) (Figure 20-7)

Primary adrenal insufficiency (PAI—Addison's disease) is defined by the inability of the adrenal cortex to produce appropriate quantities of glucocorticoids and mineralocorticoids. It may be precipitated by an acute illness, genetic factors, or adrenal suppression due to steroid therapy. Symptoms are nonspecific, and include volume depletion,

hypotension, hyponatremia, hyperkalemia, fever, abdominal pain, hyperpigmentation, and especially in the pediatric population, hypoglycemia.[44] Treatment for PAI in children should include hydrocortisone 8 mg/m^2 divided into three to four doses per day. The 2016 practice guidelines of the Endocrine Society on PAI also recommend avoiding synthetic long-acting glucocorticoids in children and adjusting the dosage of steroid replacement by clinical assessment of the child's growth velocity, body weight, blood pressure, and energy levels. If true aldosterone deficiency exists, fludrocortisone [Florinef (Teva Pharmaceuticals)] 100 µg/d should be prescribed, and in the newborn

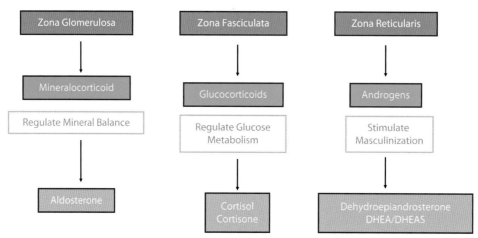

▲ **Figure 20-5.** Adrenal medulla.[47] (Data from Gallo-Payet N, Battista MC. Steroidogenesis—adrenal cell signal transduction. *Compr Physiol.* 2014;4(3):889-964. https://onlinelibrary.wiley.com/doi/book/10.1002/cphy.)

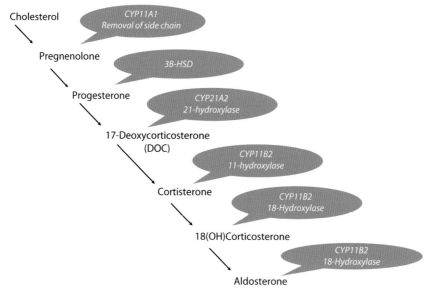

▲ **Figure 20-6.** Zona glomerulosa and mineralocorticoid production.[47] (Data from Gallo-Payet N, Battista MC. Steroidogenesis—adrenal cell signal transduction. *Compr Physiol.* 2014;4(3):889-964. https://onlinelibrary.wiley.com/doi/book/10.1002/cphy.)

and infant population, sodium chloride supplementation is also recommended.[51]

During times of physiological stress or illness, the adrenal gland increases the rate of cortisol secretion substantially but not so in patients with adrenal insufficiency. It is, therefore, incumbent on the clinician to adjust the steroid dose for the child during episodes of stress. "Stress steroids" dosing is controversial for mild stresses such as immunization and uncomplicated viral illness. "Stress" dosing is absolutely required for more severe illness such as febrile illness (fever >38°C), vomiting, diarrhea, inadequate oral intake, lethargy, dental work, and most

certainly for trauma, burns, and major surgery. Severe surgical and medical stresses are to be treated aggressively with doses of hydrocortisone up to 100 mg/m²/day IV divided into every 6 hours dosing. For elective surgical procedures, a preoperative dose of hydrocortisone 50 mg/m² IV 30 to 60 minutes before induction, and an additional 50 mg/m² divided into 6-hour dosing for the next 24 hours, is recommended.[52]

Addisonian crisis in children in shock should be treated with a rapid bolus of 20 to 60 mL/kg of normal saline over the first hour and then with hydrocortisone bolus of 50 to 100 mg/m², followed by 50- to 00 mg/m²/day divided in 6-hour

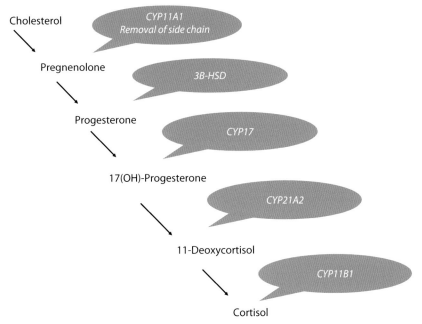

▲ **Figure 20-7.** Zona fasciculata and glucocorticoid production.[47] (Data from Gallo-Payet N, Battista MC. Steroidogenesis— adrenal cell signal transduction. *Compr Physiol.* 2014;4(3):889-964. https://onlinelibrary.wiley.com/doi/book/10.1002/cphy.)

dosing. Hypoglycemia should be treated with a dextrose-containing solution at 0.5 to 1 g/kg infused slowly at a rate of 2 to 3 mL/min, or D10W at a rate of 5 to 10 mL/kg (Box 20-4).[51]

Glucocorticoid derangement (Cushing syndrome) is a condition of pathological hypercortisolism with significant comorbidities and clinical symptoms, and significantly increased mortality. Major causes of mortality include cardiovascular disease, venous thrombosis, and infections. Major morbidities include obesity, arterial hypertension, insulin resistance, and glucose tolerance, dyslipidemia, osteoporosis, and diminished linear growth leading to short stature, as well as psychiatric and cognitive dysfunction.[53]

Causes of hypercortisolism (Cushing Disease) can be elucidated with appropriate laboratory testing and radiologic imaging. Secretory lesions include: primary adrenal secretory tumor, adrenal hyperplasia, secretory pituitary adenoma, or paraneoplastic syndrome with ACTH secretion. Surgical excision of malignancies, and medical management may be planned accordingly. Medical management may include ketoconazole (inhibits side-chain cleavage 17,20-lyase and 11β hydroxylase), metyrapone (inhibits 11β hydroxylase), mitotane (used for adrenal cancer, inhibits CYP11A1, and is directly cytotoxic to the adrenal cortex) or glucocorticoid receptor antagonist mifepristone, for nonsurgical disease, and etomidate IV for patients who are unable to tolerate oral medication. Cushing disease, an ACTH-secreting pituitary adenoma, is best treated surgically if possible. ACTH suppression may be achieved medically with cabergoline, a dopamine agonist, or pasireotide, a somatostatin receptor agonist.[53] Cushing syndrome and Cushing disease do not require any specific preanesthesia adjustment but normalized laboratory values (glucose and electrolytes) and symptomatic support (hypertension, obesity, potential for difficult airway, osteoporosis, wound healing, etc.).

DERANGEMENT OF THE ADRENAL CORTEX ZONA RETICULARIS

Derangement of Androgens/ Sex Hormones (Zona Reticularis) (Figure 20-8)

Congenital adrenal hyperplasia (CAH) due to 21-hydroxylase deficiency is an autosomal recessive genetic syndrome hallmarked by profound virilization in girls, and potential for life-threatening salt wasting in both genders if unrecognized in the newborn period.[55] The incidence of CAH is 1:10,000 to 1:20,000 live births, with 21-hydroxylase deficiency making up 95% of the patients. For these children, the synthesis of aldosterone and cortisol is compromised by the enzyme deficiency, and consequently, the steroid metabolic pathway diverts the excess progesterone and 17-(OH) progesterone to the androgen pathway. There are more than 100 described CYP21A2 mutations causing defective 21-hydroxylase.[56]

In order to suppress virilization, patients are treated with hydrocortisone, the preferred glucocorticoid, since it has some mineralocorticoid function. If salt wasting exists, and persists after initiation of hydrocortisone therapy, fludrocortisone must be added. These children will require "stress-dose" steroid regimen perioperatively.[55]

The newborn girls typically present between 2 and 6 months of age for surgical reconstruction of their external genitals, and vaginoplasty. Boys with feminization syndromes may present for removal of gonadal streak, or for staged hypospadias repair.[57] Earlier surgical urogenital surgery is now recommended. Tissues are softer and more pliable from in utero estrogen exposure, and allow for an easier, one-stage repair.[56]

Adrenal Medulla: Catecholamine Production

The adrenal medulla is a neuroendocrine organ responsible for the production of catecholamines (Figure 20-9). Catecholamine synthetic pathway starts with tyrosine

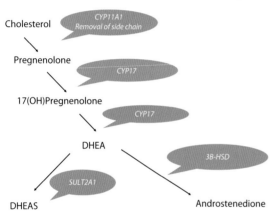

▲ **Figure 20-8.** Zona reticularis and androgens (sex hormones).[47] (Data from Gallo-Payet N, Battista MC. Steroidogenesis—adrenal cell signal transduction. *Compr Physiol.* 2014;4(3):889-964. https://onlinelibrary. wiley.com/doi/book/10.1002/cphy.)

conversion to dihydroxyphenylalanine (DOPA) by tyrosine hydroxylase. This is the rate-limiting step in catecholamine synthesis. DOPA is them transformed to dopamine by DOPA decarboxylase, then to norepinephrine (NE) by dopamine-β-hydroxylase, and finally to epinephrine by phenylethanolamine-N-methyltransferase (PNMT). The conversion of NE to epinephrine is dependent on exposure to high cortisol level. Epinephrine and NE breakdown takes place in the mitochondria, where monoamine oxidase breaks both down to dihydroxymandelic acid. Catechol-O-methyltransferase (COMT) then methylates catecholamines and their metabolites to their final metabolic waste products.

The prevalence of hypertension in the pediatric population has risen from 2% to 4.5%, much of which is attributed to increase in the rates of obesity-induced hypertension. Secondary hypertension in young children is more likely to be a result of renovascular or renal parenchymal disease (78% to 80%), endocrine disease (11%), cardiac disease (2%), etc. Only 0.5% to 2% of pediatric hypertension is caused by pheochromocytomas (PCC) and paragangliomas (PGL) (Table 20-10).[58]

Derangements of the Adrenal Medulla

Pheochromocytomas (PCC) are rare neuroendocrine, catecholamine-secreting tumors arising from chromaffin cells of the adrenal medulla (80% to 85%), while paragangliomas (PGL) are catecholamine-secreting tumors arising in extra-adrenal locations (15% to 20%). PGL can be further distinguished by their origins. Sympathetic PGL arise along the sympathetic ganglion chain in the spine, and parasympathetic PGLs from parasympathetic tissue of the head and neck, and rarely secrete catecholamines.[58] Ninety-five percent of PCC and PGL are intra-abdominal and pelvic, and 90% are benign. Other sites of presentation include the bladder and the organ of Zuckerkandl located at the aortic bifurcation.[59]

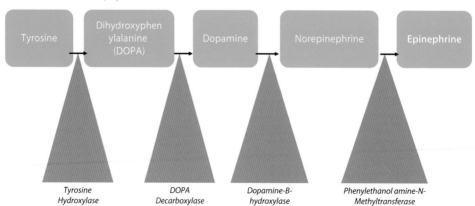

▲ **Figure 20-9.** Adrenal medulla catecholamine production. (Data from Gallo-Payet N, Battista MC. Steroidogenesis—adrenal cell signal transduction. *Compr Physiol.* 2014;4(3):889-964. https://onlinelibrary.wiley.com/doi/book/10.1002/cphy.) [47]

Table 20-10. Causes of Secondary Hypertension and Its Differential Diagnosis[37]

Organ System	Differential Diagnosis for Secondary Hypertension
Renal parenchyma	Glomerulonephritis
	Renal failure
	Congenital renal malformation
	Polycystic kidney disease
	Systemic vasculitis (SLE, ANCA, HSP, PAN)
	Parenchymal scar (pyelonephritis, VUR, HUS)
Renovascular	Renal vein thrombosis
	Renal artery stenosis
	Fibromuscular dysplasia
	Syndromes: Williams, Turner, NF-I
	Arteritis: Takayasu, Kawasaki, Moyamoya
	Renal transplant artery stenosis
	Tumor compression of renal vessels
Endocrine	catecholamine excess: PCC/PGL, neuroblastoma, sympathomimetic drugs
	Corticosteroids: Cushing syndrome, ACTH dependent and independent
	Mineralocorticoid excess: CAH, aldosterone-secreting tumor
	Thyroid disease: hyperthyroidism, hypothyroidism
	Hypercalcemia: primary or secondary to malignancy
	Hyperparathyroidism, vitamin D intoxication
Cardiac	Coarctation of the aorta, mid-aortic syndrome
Pulmonary	OSA, BPD
CNS	Intracranial hypertension, seizures
Medications	Steroids, immunosupressants (cyclosporine, tacrolimurs, sirolimus), oral contraceptives, ketamine, erythropoietin
Monogenic HTN	Liddle syndrome, Gordon syndrome (pseudohypoaldosteronism type 3), apparent mineralocorticoid excess, glucocorticoid remediable aldosteronism (familial hyperaldosteronism type 1)
Other	Post-ECMO, cyclical vomiting syndrome

SLE, systemic lupus erythematosus; ANCA, antineutrophil cytoplasmic antibody; HSP, Henoch-Schonlein-Purpura; PAN, Polyarteritis nodosa; VUR, vesicoureteral reflux; HUS, Hemolytic Uremic Syndrome; NF-1, Neurofibromatosis type 1; PCC, Pheochromocytoma; PGL, Paraganglioma; ACTH, adrenocorticotropic hormone; CAH, congenital adrenal hyperplasia; OSA, obstructive sleep apnea; BPD, bronchopulmonary dysplasia; ECMO, extracorporeal membrane oxygenation.
Source: Adapted with permission, from Bholah R, Bunchman TE. Review of pediatric pheochromocytoma and paraganglioma. *Front Pediatr.* 2017;5:155. https://www.frontiersin.org/journals/pediatrics#.

Pheochromocytomas and Paragangliomas[58]

The average age of presentation of PCC and PGL in pediatrics is 11 to 13 years, and males are affected at twice the rate of females. The clinical presentation is variable, with sustained hypertension noted in 60% to 90% of children compared with paroxysmal hypertension that affects 50% of adult PCC presentation. Other common symptoms of PCC and PGL in children include headaches (67%), and palpitations, sweating, pallor, nausea, and flushing in 47% to 57% of cases. Polyuria and polydipsia are rarer. Patients may also have retinopathy and cardiomyopathy at diagnosis. The presenting symptoms depend on the type of hormone being secreted. In addition to norepinephrine-secreting tumors' symptoms, patients with epinephrine-secreting tumors can present with hypoglycemia and hypotensive shock/circulatory collapse. Dopamine-secreting tumors may be asymptomatic, delaying diagnosis until mass effect of tumor causes symptoms (Table 20-11).[58] Approximately 80% of PCC/PGL tumors in the pediatric portion of the European-American-Pheochromocytoma-Paraganglioma-Registry (EAPPR) had a germ-line mutation in a known tumorigenic gene. The more common germ-line causes of PCC/PGL include *RET* gene associated with MEN-2, and succinate dehydrogenase gene (SDHA) that is common in neurofibromatosis type I (NF-I) and VonHipple-Lindau syndrome type 2 (VHL-2). Carney triad syndrome, Carney-Stratakis syndrome, and Pacak-Zhuang syndrome also present with germ-line mutations involving SDH complex.[58,59]

Those mutations have been divided into *Cluster 1*, mutations which reduce the oxidative response (VHL, SDHx, HIF), and *Cluster 2*, mutations which activate the kinase signaling pathways (RET, NF1, KIF1B, TMEM127, MAX). Cluster 1 tumors are more prevalent in children (76%) vs. Cluster 2 tumors (39%).

Preoperative Assessment and Preparation

Patients with catechol-secreting PCC and PGL are at risk of metabolic derangements as well as end-organ damage from excess circulating catecholamines. Patients are volume contracted, and may be hyperglycemic or hypoglycemic, depending on the catecholamine being secreted by the tumor. Assessing plasma catecholamine metabolites including plasma-free metanephrine (MN) and normetanephrine (NMN), and 24-hour urinary fractionated metanephrines are the new gold standard for diagnosis of PCC. For those with levels more than four times the upper limit of normal, imaging and genetic testing for localization should ensue. If levels are only slightly elevated, stop all interfering medications, avoid exercise for one day, and retest, drawing the blood in a supine

Table 20-11. Vasoactive Secretory Tumors: Genetics, Characteristics, and Presentation[58,59]

Syndrome	Mutation	Chromosome	Characteristics	Location
MEN-1	MEN-1 inactivation of tumor suppression gene	11q13		Adrenal
MEN-2A MEN-2B	RET (95%) RET (98%) Proto-oncogene		Adenoma, 2.9% malignancy rate	Adrenal Adrenal, Epinephrine/NE
Paraganglioma				
Type 1	Succinate dehydrogenase subunit D (SDHD)	11q23	Nonfunctional, parasympathetic 3.5% malignant	HNPGL (head & neck PGL)
Type 2	SDHAF2 loss-of-function	11q13.1	Nonfunctional, parasympathetic	HNPGL
Type 3	SDHC missense	1q21	Nonfunctional mostly (NE, rarely dopamine), parasympathetic	HNPGL, GIST (gastrointestinal stromal tumors)
Type 4	SDHB inactivation of tumor suppression gene	1p35-36	Increased malignancy rate (17–30.7%), association with renal cell carcinoma, papillary thyroid cancer	Abdomen, pelvis, mediastinum, skull base, neck
VonHippel Lindau (VHL)	VHL tumor suppressor gene regulates oxygen-sensing pathways, targets hypoxia-inducible factors (HIF) for degradation, nonhypoxia pathways regulation of angiogenesis, tumorigenesis.	3p25-26	Benign and malignant (3%) tumors	Bilateral PPC, PGL in mediastinum, abdomen, pelvis produces NE
Neurofibromatosis type 1	Inactivation of NF1 tumor suppressor gene coding neurofibromin that inhibits RAS activity	17q11.2	2% of patients develop catecholamine-secreting PCC/PGL, 9.3–33% malignancy rate	Mostly benign adrenal adenoma. Rarely bilateral. Rarely abdominal/periadrenal, produce epinephrine/NE
Carney triad	Unknown		47% will have PGL/PCC, 92% PGL	
Carney-Stratakis	SDHB, SDHC, SDHD		58% with PCC/PGL	
Pacak-Zhuang	HIF2		PCC/PGL	

NE, norepinephrine; MEN, multiple endocrine neoplasia; RET, proto-oncogene encoding a receptor tyrosine kinase; SDHAF2, succinate dehydrogenase complex assembly factor 2; RAS, reticular activating system proto-oncogene; HIF, hypoxia inducible factor
Source: Data from from Bholah R, Bunchman TE. Review of pediatric pheochromocytoma and paraganglioma. *Front Pediatr.* 2017;5:155. https://www.frontiersin.org/journals/pediatrics#.

position. If metabolite levels return at 2 to 4 upper limits of normal, consider suppression (Table 20-12). Patients with MN/NMN <2 are unlikely to have PCC/PGL.[58] Cardiac workup, including 12-lead ECG and echocardiogram, is a must. Unusual forms of cardiomyopathy (Takotsubo cardiomyopathy) and myocardial dysfunction in general have been described in PCC/PGL.[60–62]

Intraoperative Management of Pheochromocytoma and Paraganglioma Resection

A thoughtful regimen of antihypertensive polypharmacy and fluid and electrolyte resuscitation is required

in preparation for resection of catecholamine-secreting tumors to minimize risk of hemodynamic instability, which can increase morbidity and mortality. The first step is to initiate α-*blockade*, and fluid-resuscitation in the child, in order to control the hypertension. The choices of α-blockers are phenoxybenzamine, a long-acting agent, or doxazosin and prazosin, shorter acting drugs. All three agents are equally effective in controlling hypertension. Phenoxybenzamine-treated patients tend to have a longer period of hypotension postoperatively, requiring medication, likely due to phenoxybenzamine's long half-life. Metyrosine, a catecholamine synthesis inhibitor, has been

Table 20-12. Drugs Used in Preoperative Blockade for Pediatric Catecholamine-Secreting Tumors[58]

Drug Name/Class	Starting Dose	Maintenance Dose	Side Effects
Phenoxybenzamine Nonselective α-blocker	0.2 mg/kg/day (max 10 mg/dose)	Increase 0.2 mg/kg/day every 4 days in q6–q8 dosing, max 4 mg/kg/day	Orthostatic hypotension Tachycardia Nasal congestion
Doxazosin Selective α-1 blocker	1–2 mg/day	Increase to 4–16 daily, or in q12 dosing	Orthostatic hypotension Dizziness
Propranolol Nonselective β-blocker	1–2 mg/kg/day in 2–4 times daily dosing	4 mg/kg/day up to 640 mg/day ÷2–4 times daily	Dizziness, fatigue Asthma exacerbation
Atenolol Selective β-1 blocker	0.5–1 mg/kg/day daily or in 2 times daily dosing	2 mg/kg/day up to 100 mg/day	Edema, dizziness fatigue
Labetolol α- and β-Blocker	1–3 mg/kg/day in 2–3 times daily dosing	10–12 mg/kg/day up to 1,200 mg/day in 2–3 times daily dosing	Dizziness, fatigue Asthma exacerbation
Metyrosine *Tyrosine hydroxylase inhibitor*	20 mg/Kg/d ÷q6hr, or 125 mg/d	Increase up to 60 mg/kg/day in q6h dosing, or increase 125 mg/day every 4–5 days up to 2.5 g/day	Orthostatic hypotension Diarrhea, sedation, extrapyramidal symptoms, crystalluria

Source: Reproduced with permission, from Bholah R, Bunchman TE. Review of pediatric pheochromocytoma and paraganglioma. *Front Pediatr.* 2017;5:155. https://www.frontiersin.org/journals/pediatrics#.

used in adults in conjunction with phenoxybenzamine or prazosin, resulting in better BP control. The literature on the use of metyrosine in the pediatric population is limited and inconclusive. Once α-blockade is established, *β-blockade* can be added to suppress reflex tachycardia. It is also important to avoid all sympathomimetic medications during this time to avoid triggering a hypertensive crisis.[58]

In the immediate preoperative period, the challenges of preventing a hypertensive crisis continue. Anxiety is a significant factor in catecholamine-mediated preoperative hypertension. *Anxiolysis* is imperative in preparation for the operating room. Invasive hemodynamic monitoring is required, including a preinduction arterial catheter, and a central venous catheter for monitoring and for vasoactive drug infusion. The timing of the central venous catheter placement is at the discretion of the anesthesiologist. Placement of pulmonary artery catheter is rare in children, but transesophageal echocardiography (TEE) probe may be used in its place to assess cardiac function and volume status. In the adult population, whole-body bioimpedance cardiography may offer an alternative to PA catheters and TEE.[61,62]

Intravenous anesthetic agents without sympathomimetic characteristics, such as propofol and etomidate, are safe for the induction of general anesthesia. Dexmedetomidine, remifentanil, sufentanil, as well as a propofol infusion are appropriate for maintaining adequate depth of anesthesia and analgesia. Fentanyl and hydromorphone may be used as well, but morphine and meperidine should be avoided due to their sympathomimetic and histamine release profiles that may trigger a hypertensive episode. In fact, all agents with sympathomimetic properties (ephedrine, ketamine) or that may trigger hypertension (droperidol) should be avoided.

Neuromuscular blockade can be achieved with vecuronium, rocuronium, or cisatracurium. All three agents have few or no autonomic effects, and no histamine release. Atracurium with its histamine release and pancuronium with its vagolytic profile should be avoided.

Regional anesthesia should be utilized with caution. Neuraxial block can cause profound hypotension in the volume-depleted patient, and epinephrine-containing local anesthetics should not be used.

It is essential to maintain adequate depth of anesthesia to blunt response to noxious stimuli such as laryngoscopy, tracheal intubation, skin incision, and insufflation for laparoscopic procedure in order to avoid catecholamine release and a hypertensive crisis.

Inhalation agents sevoflurane, isoflurane, and nitrous oxide have all been used safely to maintain anesthesia in patients undergoing resection of PCC and PGL. Sevoflurane probably has the most hemodynamically favorable profile, lacking arrhythmogenic potential. Desflurane should be avoided, as it is known to have sympathomimetic properties, including tachycardia, hypertension, and bronchial irritation, which may exacerbate hemodynamic disturbance in patients with PCC and PGL.[62]

More severe hypertensive response can be elicited by catecholamine release from the tumor itself during manipulation and resection. Vasoactive drugs are used to attenuate the catecholamine response during this manipulation, and to treat the subsequent vasoplegic hypotension after tumor removal. *Magnesium* infusion acts as a vasodilator by inhibiting catecholamine release, antagonizing catecholamine receptors directly, and directly antagonizing endogenous calcium. In addition to its antihypertensive properties, magnesium is an antiarrhythmic, and it is readily available and cost-effective with a high therapeutic index.[63] *Nitric oxide modulators* such as sodium nitroprusside (SNP) and nitroglycerin (NTG) are commonly used to control intraoperative hypertension. SNP decreases both preload and afterload. Onset is immediate and duration of action is between 1 and 3 minutes. At high concentrations, and prolonged infusion, SNP's degradation products cyanide, thiocyanide, and methemoglobin can cause serious toxicity and side effects. Nitroglycerin has a similar immediate onset of action, but with 3 to 5 minutes duration of action. It mostly affects capacitance vessels, and preload. *β-Adrenergic antagonists* are used to manage tachycardia and tachyarrhythmias. Intraoperative infusion of esmolol is commonly used to control tachycardia. Esmolol is a selective β1-antagonist with fast (1 to 2 minutes) onset and short duration of action (9 minutes). In addition to its chronotropic actions, it works to reduce systolic blood pressure without affecting diastolic blood pressure. *Calcium channel blockers* (CCBs) are an alternative to SNP and NTG. CCBs reduce preload more gently, and therefore have fewer instances of hypotension, and no rebound hypertension or tachycardia on discontinuation of infusion, and no risk of cyanide toxicity. Nicardipine has a strong arterial vasodilatory effect. Its onset of action is between 1 and 5 minutes, but duration of action may last 3 to 6 hours, and can therefore result in prolonged hypotension. Clevidipine is an ultrashort-acting arterial vasodilator. It has fast onset of action (about 1 minute) and short half-life (approximately 1 minute), since it is metabolized by plasma esterases.[58,62]

After tumor removal, it is not uncommon to have sudden hypotension due to increase in venous capacitance and vasodilation, residual α-adrenergic and β-adrenergic blockade, absence of the tumor's catecholamine supporting vascular tone, all combined with inadequate intravascular volume. The hypotension may be resistant to catecholamine infusions due to adrenergic receptor downregulation response to the prolonged exposure in the preoperative period. If norepinephrine, phenylephrine, and dopamine are ineffective, *vasopressin* may be a better choice. Vasopressin acts on V_1 receptors on smooth muscle to increase vascular tone, independent of adrenergic

receptors. There are anecdotal reports of hemodynamic rescue with methylene blue in response to vasoplegia after tumor removal, but the efficacy has not been adequately validated at this time.

Postoperative Course

Profound hypotension has been described in the immediate postoperative period. If the hypotension is unresponsive to catecholamine infusion and vasopressin, ECMO has been described as a rescue for refractory shock. Additional perturbation may include hypoglycemia, hypertension, hypovolemia, and adrenal insufficiency requiring steroid replacement (when bilateral adrenalectomies were performed). Reduction in circulating catecholamines reduces the inhibitory effects on insulin secretions and gluconeogenesis. Hyperinsulinemia and increased peripheral glucose uptake follow the reduction in circulating catecholamine load and result in hypoglycemia that may last 24 to 48 hours postoperatively.[61]

REFERENCES

1. Centers for Disease Control and Prevention. *Childhood Obesity Facts 2014*. Atlanta, GA: CDC.
2. Chadwick V, Wilkinson KA. Diabetes mellitus and the pediatric anesthetist. *Pediatr Anesth*. 2004;14:716-723.
3. Seino Y, Nanjo K, Tajima N, et al. Report of the Committee on the Classification and Diagnostic Criteria of Diabetes Mellitus. *J Diabetes Investigat*. 2010;1(5):212-228.
4. Hattersley AT. Maturity-onset diabetes of the young: clinical heterogeneity explained by genetic heterogeneity. *Diabetic Med*. 1998;15:15-24.
5. Dabelea D, Mayer-Davis E, Saydah S, et al. Prevalence of type 1 and type 2 diabetes among children and adolescents from 2001 to 2009. *JAMA*. 2014;311(17):1778-1786.
6. Vann MA. Perioperative management of ambulatory surgical patients with diabetes mellitus. *Curr Opin Anaesthesiol*. 2009;22:718-724.
7. Saydah S, Imperatore G, et al. Disparities in diabetes deaths among children and adolescents—United States, 2000–2014. *MMWR Morb Mortal Wkly Rep*. 2017;66:502-505.
8. Kwon EB, Lee HS, Shim YS, Jeong HR, Hwang JS. The changes of subtypes in pediatric diabetes and their clinical and laboratory characteristics over the last 20 years. *Ann Pediatr Endocrinol Metal*. 2016;21:81-85.
9. Rhodes ET, Ferrari LR, Wolfsdorf JI. Perioperative management of pediatric surgical patients with diabetes mellitus. *Anesth Analg*. 2005;101:986-999.
10. Ahmed Z, Lockhart CH, et al. Advances in diabetic management: implications for anesthesia. *Anesthe Analg*. 2005;100:666-669,
11. Cornelius BW. Patients with type 2 diabetes: anesthetic management in the ambulatory setting: Part 2: pharmacology and guidelines for perioperative management. *Anesth Prog*. 2017;64:39-44.
12. Hannon TS, Rao G, Arslanian SA. Childhood obesity and type 2 diabetes mellitus. *Pediatrics*. 2005;116:473-480.
13. Kohl BA, Schwartz S. How to manage perioperative endocrine insufficiency. *Anesthesiol Clin*. 2010;28:139-155.

14. Dubbs SB, Spangler R. Hypothyroidism: causes, killers, and life-saving treatments. *Emerg Med Clin N Am.* 2014;32:303-317.

15. Devereaux D, Toweled S. Hyperthyroidism and thyrotoxicosis. *Emerg Med Clin N Am.* 2014;32:277-292.

16. Elfenbein DM, et al. Thyroidectomy for Graves' disease in children: indications and complications. *J Ped Sure.* 2016;51:1680-1683.

17. Knollman PD, Giese A, Bhayahi MK. Surgical intervention for medically refractory hyperthyroidism. *Pediatric Annals.* 2016;45(5):e171-e175.

18. Diaz A, Lipman-Diaz EG. Hypothyroidism. *Pediatr Rev.* 2014;35(8):336-347; quiz 348-9.

19. Bajwa SJS, Sehgal V. Anesthesia and thyroid surgery: the never ending challenges. *Indian J Endocrinol Metab.* 2013;17(2):228-234.

20. Bahn RS, et al. Hyperthyroidism and other causes of thyrotoxicosis: management guidelines of the American Thyroid Association and American Association of Clinical Endocrinologists. *Endoc Pract.* 2011;17(3):458-520.

21. Raval CB, Rahman SA. Difficult airway challenges—intubation and extubation matters in a case of large goiter with retrosternal extension. *Anesth Essays Res.* 2015;9(2):247-250.

22. Amathieu R, Smail N, Catineau J, Poloujadoff MP, Samii K, Adnet F. Difficult intubation in thyroid surgery: myth or reality? *Aneth Analg.* 2006;103(4):965-968.

23. Loftus PA, et al. Risk factors for perioperative airway difficulty and evaluation of intubation approaches among patients with benign goiter. *Ann Otol Rhinol Laryngol.* 2014;123(4):279-285.

24. Bouaggad A, et al. Prediction of difficult tracheal intubation in thyroid surgery. *Anesth Analg.* 2004;99:603-606.

25. Hanba C, et al. Pediatric thyroidectomy: hospital course and perioperative complications. *Ototlaryngol Head Neck Surg.* 2017;156(2):360-367.

26. Kluijfhout WP, et al. Postoperative complications after prophylactic thyroidectomy for very young patients with multiple endocrine neoplasia type 2. *Medicine.* 2015;94(29):e1108.

27. Yu YR, Fallon SC, Carpenter JL, et al. Perioperative determinants of transient hypocalcemia after pediatric total thyroidectomy. *Ped Surg.* 2017;52:684-688.

28. Tracy ET, Roman SA. Current management of pediatric thyroid disease and differentiated thyroid cancer. *Curr Opin Oncol.* 2016;28:37-42.

29. Francis GL, et al. Management guidelines for children with thyroid nodules and differentiated thyroid cancer. The American Thyroid Association Guidelines Task Force on Pediatric Thyroid Cancer. *Thyroid.* 2015;25(7):716-759.

30. Norton JA, Krampitz G, Jensen RT. Multiple endocrine neoplasia: genetics & clinical management. *Sure Once Clin N Am.* 2015;24(4):795-832.

31. Hannoush ZC, Weiss RE. Defects of thyroid hormone synthesis and action. *Endocrinol Metab Clin N Am.* 2017;46(2):375-388.

32. Haugen BR. Drugs that suppress TSH or cause central hypothyroidism. *Best Pract Res Clin Endocrinol Metab.* 2009;23(6):793-800.

33. Herrera MF, Gamboa-Dominguez A. Parathyroid embryology, anatomy, and pathology. In: Clark OH, Duh QY, Kebebew E, eds. *Textbook of Endocrine Surgery.* 2nd ed. Philadelphia, PA: Elsevier Saunders; 2005:365-371.

34. Tezelman ST, Siperstein AE. Signal transduction in thyroid neoplasms. In: Clark OH, Duh QY, Kebebew E, eds. *Textbook of Endocrine Surgery.* 2nd ed. Philadelphia, PA: Elsevier Saunders; 2005:265-279.

35. Monchick JM. Normocalcemic hyperparathyroidism. In: Clark OH, Duh QY, Kebebew E, eds. *Textbook of Endocrine Surgery.* 2nd ed. Philadelphia, PA: Elsevier Saunders; 2005:424-429.

36. Tsuboi K, Takamura M, Sato Y, et al. Severe acute pancreatitis as an initial manifestation of primary hyperparathyroid adenoma in a pediatric patient. *Pancreas.* 2007;35(1):100.

37. Wasserman JD, Tomlinson GE, et al. Multiple endocrine neoplasia and hyperparathyroid–jaw tumor syndromes: clinical features, genetics, and surveillance recommendations in childhood. *Clin Cancer Res.* 2017;23(13):e123-e132.

38. Stokes VJ, Nielsen MF, Hannan FM, Thakker RV. Hypercalcemic disorders in children. *J Bone Mineral Res.* 2017;32(11):2157-2170.

39. Kelly TG, et al. Surveillance for early detection of aggressive parathyroid disease: carcinoma and atypical adenoma in familial isolated hyperparathyroidism associated with a germline HRPT2 mutation. *J Bone Mineral Res.* 2006;21(10):1666-1671.

40. VanSickle JS, Srivastava T, Alon US. Use of calcimimetics in children with normal kidney function. *Pediatr Nephrol.* 2019;34:413-422.

41. Mitchell D, Rybak LP, Glatz FR. Hyperparathyroid risis in a pediatric patient. *Int J Pediatr Otorhinolaryngol.* 2004;68:237-241.

42. Al-Azem H, Khan AA. Hyperparathyroidism. *Best Pract Res Clin Endocrinol Metabol.* 2012;26:517-522.

43. Mannstadt M, Bilezikian JP, Thakker RV, et al. Hypoparathyroidism. *Nat Rev Dis Primers.* 2017;3:17055.

44. Clarke BL, Brown EM, Collins MT, et al. Epidemiology and diagnosis of hypoparathyroidism. *J Clin Endocrinol Metal.* 2016;101:2284-2299.

45. Mantovani G, Elli FM, Corbetta S, et al. Hypothyroidism associated with parathyroid disorders. *Best Pract Res Clin Endocrinol Metab.* 2017;31:161-173.

46. Levy-Shraga Y, Gothelf D, Goichberg Z, et al. Growth characteristics and endocrine abnormalities in 22q11.2 deletion syndrome. *Am J Med Genet Part A.* 2017;173A:1301-1308.

47. Gallo-Payet N, Battista MC. Steroidogenesis—adrenal cell signal transduction. *Compr Physiol.* 2014;4(3):889-964.

48. Oberfield SE, Levine LS, Firpo A, et al. Primary hyperaldosteronism in childhood due to unilateral macronodular hyperplasia. a case report. *Hypertension.* 1984;6:75-84.

49. Miller WL, Fluck CE. Adrenal cortex and its disorders. In: Sperling MA, ed. *Pediatric Endocrinology.* 4th ed. Philadelphia, PA: Elsevier Saunders; 2017:471-532.

50. Obara T, Ito Y, Iihara M. Hyperaldosteronism. In: Clark OH, Duh QY, Kebebew E, eds. *Textbook of Endocrine Surgery.* 2nd ed. Philadelphia, PA: Elsevier Saunders; 2005:595-603.

51. Bornstein SR, Allolio B, Arit W, Barthei A. Diagnosis and treatment of primary adrenal insufficiency: an Endocrine Society Clinical Practice guideline. *J Endocrinol Metab.* 2016;101(2):364-389.

52. Shulman DI, Palmert MR, Kemp SF; Lawson Wilkins Drug and Therapeutics Committee. Adrenal insufficiency: still a cause of morbidity and death in childhood. *Pediatrics.* 2007;119:e484-e494.

53. Nieman LK, et al. Treatment of Cushing's syndrome: an Endocrine Society clinical practice guideline. *J Clin Endocrinol Metab.* 2015;100(8):2807-2831.

54. Carey RM, Padia SH. Primary mineralocorticoid excess disorders and hypertension. In: Jameson JL. DeGroot LJ, eds. *Endocrinology: Adult and Pediatric.* 7th ed. Philadelphia, PA: Elsevier Saunders; 2016:1871-1891.

55. Clayton PE, et al. Consensus statement on 21-hydroxylase deficiency from The Lawson Wilkins Pediatric Endocrine Society and The European Society for Pediatric Endocrinology. *J Clin Endocrinol Metab*. 2002;87(9):4048-4053.

56. Speiser PW, et al. Congenital adrenal hyperplasia due to steroid 21-hydroxylase deficiency: an Endocrine Society Clinical Practice Guideline. *J Clin Endocrinol Metab*. 2010;95(9):4133-4160.

57. Schnitzer JJ, Donahue PK. Surgical treatment of congenital adrenal hyperplasia. *Endoc Metab Clin N Am*. 2001;30(1):137-154.

58. Bholah R, Bunchman TE. Review of pediatric pheochromocytoma and paraganglioma. *Front Pediatr*. 2017;5:155.

59. Tsirlin A, et al. Pheochromocytoma: a review. *Maturitas*. 2014;77:229-238.

60. Capel I, Tasa-Vinyals E, et al. Takotsubo cardiomyopathy in amiodarone-induced hyperthyroidism. *Endocrinol Diabetes Metab Case Rep*. 2017. pii: 16-0116.

61. Naranjo J, Dodd S, Martin YN. Perioperative management of pheochromocytoma. *J Cardiothoracic Vascular Anesth*. 2017;31:1427-1439.

62. Salinas FV. Contemporary perioperative and anesthetic management of pheochromocytoma and paraganglioma. *Advanc Anesth*. 2016;34:181-196.

63. Minami T, et al. An effective use of magnesium sulfate for intraoperative management of laparoscopic adrenalectomy for pheochromocytoma in a pediatric patient. *Anesth Analg*. 2002;5:1243-1244.

Anesthesia for Genitourinary Procedures

Swapna Chaudhuri

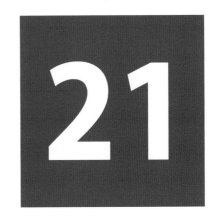

FOCUS POINTS

1. Pediatric patients undergo a wide variety of genitourinary procedures, which can range from isolated outpatient surgeries to complex reconstructions.
2. Most urological procedures are elective in nature, and majority of these patients are healthy or with stable chronic medical conditions.
3. Latex-free precautions during perioperative management are highly recommended in patients with chronic urological conditions due to concerns of hypersensitivity after repeated latex exposure.
4. Regional anesthesia and analgesia are excellent alternative/complementary techniques for genitourinary procedures with minimal risk when performed in asleep patients.
5. Perioperative medications should be reviewed in advance and administration or discontinuation discussed [chronic steroids or other immunosuppressants, antihypertensive medications such as angiotensin-converting enzyme inhibitors (ACEIs) or angiotensin II receptor blockers (ARBs)].
6. Renally excreted medications should be adjusted perioperatively to decrease the risk of further renal impairment.
7. End-stage renal disease (ESRD) patients on dialysis should be particularly reviewed for fluid status and symptoms between dialysis sessions.

INTRODUCTION

The genitourinary system has been described to have the highest percentage of congenital anomalies. A study of antenatal ultrasounds reported a frequency of 21% for urinary tract abnormalities;[1] this is supported by a review that estimated the screening sensitivity of urogenital anomalies to be almost 88%.[2] In the newborn period, ultrasonography is the preferable diagnostic tool for initial evaluation of abdominal masses; almost 55% of these have been shown to be of renal origin.[3] It is important to remember that nephrogenesis continues to progress until 36 weeks of postconceptual age. At birth, there is a significant decrease in renal vascular resistance with an associated increase in glomerular filtration rate.

Children undergoing urological procedures may be prone to emotional disturbances because of repeated interventions. In addition, patients with obstructive uropathy and chronic renal insufficiency are susceptible to frequent urinary tract infections (UTIs). Therefore, special attention to their psychological well-being and to the risk of septicemia is warranted in the perioperative period.[4]

This chapter highlights key surgical conditions involving the genitourinary system, and provides a brief overview of the anesthetic management for this diverse population of surgical patients.

KEY SURGICAL CONDITIONS

External Genitalia and Urethra

Circumcision

Circumcision, which involves surgical removal of foreskin of the penis, is a common outpatient operation in healthy male children. Besides religious and sociocultural reasons, medical indications include phimosis, balanitis, and urine outlet obstruction.

Neonatal circumcision has a low complication rate and is usually performed in the nursery under local anesthesia. In infants and children, circumcision is performed under general anesthesia, using face mask, laryngeal mask airway (LMA), or endotracheal tube.[5] While a caudal block may be performed for postoperative analgesia, a multimodal regimen using acetaminophen (10 to 15 mg/kg IV) and topical anesthesia (lidocaine-prilocaine) or a dorsal penile block is equally effective.

Two major complications of circumcision include infection and bleeding.

Hypospadius and Chordee

Hypospadius refers to malposition of the urethral meatus on the undersurface of the penis; 15% to 20% have an associated downward curvature of the penis (chordee), while 8% have an undescended testis.[4] Depending on the severity of the hypospadius, the operation may require a staged repair.

The procedure is usually performed at 6 to 18 months of age. Based on patient age, premedication may be needed (usually after age 6 months) to overcome separation anxiety. General anesthesia is usually initiated with an inhalation induction for outpatients without an existing IV, and maintenance accomplished with a balanced volatile agent–narcotic technique.

Regional anesthesia choice usually depends on preference of the surgeon as well as location of the hypospadius. For a distally located malposition, penile nerve block, together with nonsteroidal analgesics, can be quite effective. For more severe abnormalities and longer procedures, a caudal epidural block (0.2% ropivacaine or 0.25% bupivacaine, 0.8 to 1 mL/kg), with/without an indwelling catheter intraoperatively for supplementation, can reduce analgesic requirements, without delaying micturition.

Posterior Urethral Valves

Posterior urethral valves (PUVs) are a common etiology for congenital urethral obstruction that can produce a spectrum of urological and renal sequelae.[6] Antenatal diagnosis, proteinuria, and hydronephrosis have all been postulated as predictors of poor long-term renal function; nadir creatinine, the lowest creatinine during the first year after diagnosis, has been demonstrated as an independent prognostic indicator for poor renal outcomes.[6]

These patients are usually scheduled for elective surgery. Because they often present with various degrees of renal insufficiency, serum electrolytes and other renal function tests should be examined preoperatively. General anesthetic technique is usually required; close monitoring of urine output and of intravenous fluid administration is highly recommended.

Cystoscopy

Cystoscopy is performed for various diagnostic and therapeutic procedures, including assessment of urological anomalies, recurrent UTIs, correction of urethral strictures, as well as treatment of urolithiasis. Prophylactic antibiotics are usually needed (gentamicin 5 mg/kg or amoxicillin/clavulanic acid 30 mg/kg).

Anesthetic management involves preoperative medication for separation anxiety if needed, and general anesthesia with face mask or LMA. Postoperative care often includes dexmedetomidine (0.5 mcg/kg) and acetaminophen (IV or oral: 10 to 15 mg/kg) for pain management, and ondansetron (0.1 mg/kg) for prophylaxis against postoperative nausea and vomiting (PONV). Patients should be monitored for hemorrhage and hyponatremia (which could be caused by absorption of irrigation fluid).

Feminizing Genitoplasty

Feminizing genital surgery is performed to treat disorders of sexual development (DSD), and involves three surgical procedures—clitoroplasty, labioplasty, and vaginoplasty. The commonest cause for DSD is congenital adrenal hyperplasia (CAD), believed to result from exposure of a 46 XX female fetus to androgens before the 12th week of gestation.[7] CAD is an autosomal recessive disorder primarily caused by deficiency of 21-hydroxylase enzyme in the steroidogenic pathway; CAD patients have both glucocorticoid and mineralocorticoid deficiencies.

The first two reconstructive surgeries may be undertaken in infancy, while vaginoplasty is recommended around puberty. During general anesthetic management, key issues to address are metabolic disturbances and adequate steroid supplementation. Postoperative analgesia can be provided effectively via a caudal epidural catheter.

▶ Scrotum and Testes

Cryptorchidism and Orchiopexy

Approximately 33% of premature male infants are born with one undescended testis; if left untreated, cryptorchidism is associated with a tenfold greater risk of malignancy. Besides the higher incidence of prematurity, cryptorchidism is often associated with congenital conditions such as Noonan syndrome, Prader-Willi syndrome, and cloacal exstrophy.[4]

Orchiopexy involves mobilization of the testis from the inguinal canal, or less commonly, from the abdominal cavity. Surgical placement of the testis often requires a two-stage repair; both stages of the Fowler-Stephens approach (clipping and transecting the testicular vessels) may be performed with laparoscopic surgery.

Preoperative evaluation for residual complications of prematurity and oral premedication to manage separation anxiety are recommended. Anesthetic management involves general endotracheal anesthesia with muscle relaxation, especially if performed by laparoscopy. Traction and manipulation of the spermatic cord and testicle may cause bradycardia and laryngospasm; relieving traction, deepening of anesthesia, administering anticholinergic medications (atropine, glycopyrrolate), and intraoperative blocks can alleviate these side effects.

Regional anesthesia by blocking the iliohypogastric and ilioinguinal nerves with local anesthetics (ropivacaine or bupivacaine), together with parenteral and oral analgesics, is a great measure for postoperative pain relief.[5]

Testicular Torsion

Acute onset of scrotal pain in the absence of trauma requires prompt investigation for testicular torsion. This is one of the few pediatric urological emergencies where surgery should be performed within 6 hours of onset of pain to save the testis.[8] General anesthesia with rapid sequence induction and endotracheal intubation is the usual technique in this situation. Surgical therapy usually relieves the pain; therefore, aggressive postoperative pain management is not normally required.

Urinary Bladder and Ureters

Bladder and Cloacal Exstrophy

Bladder exstrophy, a rare congenital anomaly with 2:1 male preponderance and a familial association, involves protrusion of the urinary bladder through a defect in the anterior abdominal wall. It is part of a spectrum of exstrophy–epispadius complex that may include cloacal exstrophy, spinal defects, and pelvic diastasis.[5]

A staged surgical repair is planned soon after birth, which involves closure of the bladder, abdominal wall, and possibly pelvic osteotomies. Epispadius repair is undertaken at 6 to 12 months of age, while bladder neck reconstruction is usually performed at 4 to 5 years, once bladder training has occurred.

Preoperative assessment should include evaluation of any cardiac anomalies, renal insufficiency, and electrolyte imbalance. General anesthesia for the initial repair is similar to that for most prolonged newborn surgeries; invasive hemodynamic monitoring, close attention to fluid and blood resuscitation and temperature maintenance, and postoperative intensive care constitute the usual management plan.[4] Caudal or epidural analgesia with a secured/tunneled catheter, using 0.2% ropivacaine, 0.1% lidocaine, or 0.125% bupivacaine with/without epinephrine, is usually initiated intraoperatively and continued up to 48 to 72 hours.[9] Local anesthetic toxicity should be kept in mind, especially with use of bupivacaine or if continued beyond 2 to 3 days.[10] Chloroprocaine is an attractive alternative in neonates and infants, especially in patients with liver impairment, or when higher infusion rates may be needed for large surgical incisions covering several dermatomes.[11]

Vesicoureteral Reflux

Vesicoureteral reflux (VUR) is a congenital defect, believed to be due to failure of ureteral development with abnormal insertion of the ureter into the bladder, resulting in retrograde flow into the ureters and kidneys during micturition. Secondary VUR usually results from urinary blockage following recurrent UTIs. Risk factors include female gender, age below 2 years, Caucasian race, and familial predilection. A voiding cystourethrogram can assist with assessment of the severity of reflux. Surgical intervention is usually required because if left untreated, VUR can lead to hydronephrosis, pyelonephritis, and progressive renal failure.

Ureteral reimplantation is a 3- to 4-hour open procedure under general endotracheal anesthesia with volatile anesthetics and muscle relaxants, paying close attention to normothermia and adequate urine flow. Effective postoperative analgesia can be achieved with caudal epidural block, or with transversus abdominis plane blocks (0.5 mL/kg 0.25% bupivacaine with 1:200,000 epinephrine). Postoperative bladder spasms can be treated with ketorolac and bethanechol.[12]

Laparoscopic techniques have been fairly successful but are associated with much longer surgical times.[13] Recently, endoscopic management of VUR under general anesthesia, with injection of tissue bulking substances at the vesicoureteral junction, has also been reported.[14]

While open ureteral reimplantation remains the gold standard for surgical correction of VUR, robotic-assisted laparoscopic ureteral reimplantation (RALUR) is increasingly being utilized. The latter provides the advantages of finer dissection and precise placement of intracorporeal sutures within a confined space, as well as lower postoperative analgesic requirements and decreased hospital stay.[15] However, RALUR is associated with longer operative times and increased costs; published outcomes are mixed and currently restricted to a few surgical facilities.[16]

Urolithiasis

Pediatric urolithiasis is much less common compared to adults; any metabolic (hypercalciuria, hyperoxaluria, cystinuria, etc.) patient should be investigated and treated preoperatively. Stones can be managed by extracorporeal shock-wave lithotripsy (ESWL), ureteroscopy, laser lithotripsy, percutaneous nephrolithotomy (PCNL) or via open approach. Deep sedation may be adequate for ESWL in older children; however, most cases will require general anesthesia with LMA or endotracheal tube, depending on the surgical procedure (muscle relaxation for ureteral stones). Postoperative management should include acetaminophen, ketorolac (IV 0.5 mg/kg), opioids, and prophylactic ondansetron for PONV.

Prune Belly Syndrome

Prune Belly syndrome is a male-dominated anomaly, consisting of a triad of anterior abdominal muscle deficiency with wrinkled overlying skin, urinary tract abnormalities, and undescended testes. This rare syndrome is often associated with orthopedic (congenital hip dislocation, scoliosis), gastrointestinal (malrotation, volvulus), and cardiac (tetralogy of Fallot, ventricular septal defect) abnormalities and with chromosomal defects (trisomy 18—primarily in girls—and trisomy 21).[17] Prognosis depends on the degree of renal impairment and pulmonary hypoplasia, with mortality approaching 50% by age 2 in severe cases.[18]

Children present to the surgical suite for correction of VUR, orchiopexy, or abdominal wall reconstruction. During management of general anesthesia in these cases, primary considerations should be directed to gastrointestinal, renal, and pulmonary issues. Postoperatively, vomiting and risk of aspiration after extubation are of concern, and respiratory tract infections are common. Continued postoperative ventilation may be the best approach for patients undergoing extensive abdominal procedures and when significant pulmonary disease is present.[5]

Kidneys and Renal Pelvis

Wilms Tumor

Also known as nephroblastoma, Wilms tumor is the commonest intra-abdominal tumor observed in children. It comprises about 5% of all cancers in children; approximately 500 to 600 new cases of Wilms tumor are diagnosed each year in the United States.[19] Most of these patients present with a painless abdominal mass between 3 and 4 years of age. About 10% of patients have a syndromic association, primarily Beckwith-Wiedemann syndrome (macrosomia, overgrowth syndrome) and Soto syndrome (overgrowth, distinctive facial features, learning disability). Almost 50% present with hypertension at diagnosis. Acquired von Willebrand disease may be seen in about 10% of patients.[4] Tailored multimodal therapy consists of radical nephrectomy, chemotherapy, and radiation. With progress in management of Wilms tumor over the past few decades, overall cure rates have exceeded 85%. Prognosis is primarily dependent on clinical staging and histological characteristics of the tumor.[20]

Most children presenting for radical nephrectomy should be evaluated preoperatively for concomitant syndromes, serum electrolytes, complete blood counts, coagulation profile, and renal function studies. Children with more extensive disease may undergo chemotherapy prior to surgery; cardiac assessment with echocardiography is recommended in these cases. Anesthetic considerations primarily pertain to the lengthy transabdominal retroperitoneal procedure (thermoregulation, positioning, fluid balance) and increased intra-abdominal pressure (intermittent inferior vena cava compression, ventilatory issues) in small children. Injury to major organs with potential for hemorrhage is also a concern during these procedures.[20] There is no particular drug choice for general endotracheal anesthesia (sedative, muscle relaxant) unless renal compromise has been documented (adjustment of renally excreted medications should be considered). Two large-bore peripheral IVs should be placed above the diaphragm; arterial monitoring is recommended for patients with large tumors or extensive disease. Postoperative analgesia is achieved with opioids or regional epidural analgesia (either caudal or thoracolumbar with threaded catheter to the level of the incision), provided the risk of coagulopathy is ruled out.

Ureteropelvic Junction Obstruction

Ureteropelvic junction (UPJ) obstruction usually occurs due to intrinsic or extrinsic compression of the ureter, resulting in hydronephrosis. The goal of surgery is to relieve UPJ obstruction at the renal pelvis. This is usually achieved with an open dismembered pyeloplasty, via an extraperitoneal flank incision.[12] Pediatric laparoscopic and robotic pyeloplasty are increasingly being used as an alternative to the open approach.[21]

Anesthetic considerations include proper patient positioning, adequate fluid resuscitation, and postoperative pain. Blood loss is usually not an issue. General endotracheal anesthesia with standard monitoring is the norm. For robotic surgery, additional concerns with positioning, immobilization, ventilation difficulties, etc., should be addressed.[22] Local infiltration with bupivacaine, and postoperative opioids with nonsteroidal anti-inflammatory drugs (NSAIDs) and ketorolac are reasonable measures for postoperative analgesia.

ANESTHETIC MANAGEMENT

Preoperative Evaluation

A comprehensive preoperative evaluation should include the patient's medical history and a physical examination (which can be difficult in an uncooperative child) with focus on comorbid conditions (cardiopulmonary, syndromic). Pertinent laboratory investigations should also be included based on clinical conditions and surgical procedure (electrolytes, creatinine levels, coagulation profile, hemoglobin, and platelet counts).

As with most pediatric cases, thorough preparation of the operating room (appropriate room temperature, warming blankets, padding appropriate for age and size, etc.) prior to entry of the patient is essential. In addition to spina bifida patients who are a known high-risk group for latex sensitization, other patients undergoing repeated urological interventions are also prone to latex sensitivity. Therefore, a latex-free environment should be utilized and discussed during time-out.[23]

Depending on the patient age, timely and adequate preoperative medication (midazolam, dexmedetomidine, ketamine through oral, intranasal, intramuscular, or intravenous route) will go a long way toward achieving a calm and comfortable patient, as well as allaying anxiety for the parents.

In-room setup for cases requires the usual attention to detail that is essential for these small-size patients.

Laryngoscope blades with correct (slim) handle, cuffed endotracheal tubes, oral airways, laryngeal mask airways (LMAs), etc. need to be age- or patient size–appropriate. Having a video laryngoscope (C-MAC*, GlideScope*) readily available is optimal when dealing with premature and syndromic children. Fluid delivery systems (buretrol and intravenous tubing, fluid warmers) should be free of air bubbles and ready to go before the patient enters the operating room. Pediatric suction tip and tubings need to be readily available, and appropriate ventilator settings should be programmed. Relevant anesthetic medications (sedatives, muscle relaxants, opioids), as well as resuscitative drugs, should be drawn up in appropriate-sized syringes, paying particular attention to appropriate dilutions as necessary.

Patients for genitourinary procedures may have impaired renal function and may be on chronic disease medications. All medications should be reviewed carefully, and specific instructions should be given regarding perioperative administration. Fluid administration and nil per os (NPO) guidelines should also be reviewed. A discussion with the pediatric nephrologist may be prudent to outline goals and expectations for perioperative management. If the patient has end-stage renal disease (ESRD) and on dialysis, the surgical procedure or diagnostic evaluation requiring anesthesia should be planned in between dialysis sessions (or at least 4 hours after dialysis) to allow for adequate volume and electrolyte equilibrium.

Secondary effects include abnormalities in the cardiovascular system; therefore, an electrocardiogram and/or a transthoracic echocardiogram may be beneficial to evaluate perioperative risk.

Systemic hypertension can be associated with renal insufficiency and subclinical cardiovascular disease.[24] In chronic hypertensive patients, wide fluctuations in blood pressure are expected intraoperatively especially if they are on medications such as angiotensin-converting enzyme inhibitors (ACEIs) or angiotensin II receptor blockers (ARBs). Patients with proteinuria or following renal transplantation may be on chronic steroid supplementation. As such, the daily oral dose should be continued and a stress dose of a glucocorticoid (1 mg/kg IV hydrocortisone) should be considered intraoperatively to prevent clinical manifestations of adrenal suppression such as refractory hypotension. Postoperative steroid administration should be discussed until resumption of usual medications orally.[4] Table 21-1 shows the relative equivalent doses and activities for IV steroids in comparison to oral prednisone.

Intraoperative Management

Anesthetic Technique

The type of anesthetic technique is dictated by the surgical procedure, level of patient cooperation, surgeon preference, and comfort level of the anesthesiologist. The overwhelming majority of cases are performed by general anesthesia—using face mask, LMA, endotracheal tube—as deemed appropriate. Regional anesthesia—using spinal, epidural, and peripheral nerve blocks—is usually performed in supplementation; it may be utilized as the sole anesthetic in isolated cases. Spinal anesthesia (0.5% preservative-free bupivacaine 1 mg/kg with/without epinephrine) has been described for infants undergoing urological procedures with an 89% success rate.[25] Caudal epidural blocks in sedated patients are a safe and effective means of providing postoperative analgesia for pediatric patients, including for neonates.[10]

Anesthetic Medications

Volatile inhalational agents are the mainstay of general anesthetic techniques, with sevoflurane with/without nitrous oxide being used for inhalation induction. Any intraoperative medications should be adjusted based on renal impairment if present with avoidance of nonsteroidal anti-inflammatory medications (unless explicitly discussed with surgical colleague). Fentanyl and other opioids (bolus/infusion/neuraxial) are administered in most patients. Dexmedetomidine is an excellent agent to alleviate anxiety (sedative agent) to prevent/treat emergence delirium in pediatric patients and to decrease perioperative opioid consumption. Antiemetics (ondansetron) and analgesics (acetaminophen) should also be strongly considered as adjuncts. Bupivacaine, lidocaine, and ropivacaine are primarily used for regional anesthesia and analgesia. Safe total amounts in mg/kg doses, when used with or without epinephrine, should be calculated prior to administration. Increased toxicity of bupivacaine, especially when used for caudal epidural analgesia in neonates, is a concern.

Table 21-1. Comparative Potency and Relative Equivalent Doses of Steroids

Steroid/Activity	Glucocorticoid Potency	Mineralocorticoid Potency	Equivalent Glucocorticoid Dose (mg)
Hydrocortisone	1	1	20
Methylprednisolone	5	0.5	4
Dexamethasone	30	0	0.75
Prednisone (po)	4	0.8	5

Monitoring

Standard noninvasive monitoring is adequate for the vast majority of cases (circumcision, orchiopexy, ureteral reimplantation). Invasive hemodynamic monitoring (arterial and central venous) is recommended for prolonged complex procedures, and for those with potential for major fluid shifts and significant blood loss. Measures to maintain optimal temperature (forced-air mattress, heated blanket) should be in place. Urine output should be monitored as an index of fluid status and perfusion.

Positioning

Laparoscopic and robotic surgeries are increasingly being utilized for pediatric urological procedures including pyeloplasty, nephrectomy, and antireflux surgery. Surgical advantages of minimally invasive surgery consist of better visualization of surgical field, mechanical improvements, stabilization of instruments, and improved ergonomics for the operating surgeon.[22] Anesthetic concerns for these procedures are related to specific positioning such as steep Trendelenburg and to inadequate patient access intraoperatively. Positioning may affect ventilation, intra-abdominal pressure, and in return cardiac output and systemic perfusion.

▶ Postoperative Care

Disposition after surgery to the outpatient recovery facility, post-anesthesia care unit (PACU), or intensive care unit (ICU) is dependent on (a) patient comorbidity, (b) type and outcome of surgery, and (c) intraoperative anesthetic course. Intraoperative management should include anticipation and prophylactic treatment for emergence delirium, PONV, and postoperative pain. Judicious administration of opioids and non-narcotic drugs (acetaminophen, ketorolac, etc.) should be complemented with intraoperative topical anesthetics and effective use of regional blocks whenever appropriate.

Ambulatory surgery patients should meet discharge criteria recommended for pediatric patients as age-appropriate. Premature children or patients with obstructive sleep apnea should be considered for an overnight stay.

For patients requiring inpatient stays, discharge from PACU should similarly meet age-appropriate criteria. Indwelling epidural or peripheral nerve catheters should be followed up religiously to ensure adequate pain relief, and to avert potential complications such as catheter migration, bleeding, or persistent neuropathy.

Patients requiring ICU postoperatively should be transferred to the respective unit with continued monitoring, oxygen supplementation (Ambu bag support when intubated), sedation, and analgesia. Resuscitative drugs and airway adjuncts should be carried with the patient during transport. Complete hand-off to the critical care team should be initiated outlining perioperative concerns and specific intraoperative management challenges, if any.

SUMMARY

Pediatric patients undergoing urological procedures are a diverse group of children. The acuity of the surgical intervention usually determines the perioperative anesthetic plan. Patient comorbidity is usually the greatest factor determining the rate of perioperative complications as well as the length of hospital stay. With growing experience and advanced training of pediatric urologists in laparoscopy and robotic surgery, it is incumbent upon pediatric anesthesiologists to gain familiarity and comfort in providing safe and effective perioperative care to pediatric patients undergoing minimally invasive genitourinary procedures.

REFERENCES

1. Policiano C, Djokovic D, Carvalho R, Monteiro C, Melo MA, Graça LM. Ultrasound antenatal detection of urinary tract anomalies in the last decade: outcome and prognosis. *J Matern Fetal Neonatal Med.* 2015;28(8):959-963.
2. Clayton DB, Brock JWIII. Prenatal ultrasound and urological anomalies. *Pediatr Clin North Am.* 2012;59(4):739-756.
3. Merten DF, Kirks DR. Diagnostic imaging of pediatric abdominal masses. *Pediatr Clin North Am.* 1985;32(6):1397-1425.
4. Hansen TG, Hennenberg SW, Lerman J. General abdominal and urologic surgery. In: Coté CJ, Lerman J, Anderson BJ, eds. *Coté and Lerman's A Practice of Anesthesia for Infants and Children.* 6th ed. Philadelphia, PA: Elsevier; 2019:669-689.
5. Williams RK, Lauro HV, Davis PJ. Anesthesia for general abdominal and urologic surgery. In: Davis PJ, Cladis FP, eds. *Smith's Anesthesia for Infants and Children.* 9th ed. Philadelphia, PA: Elsevier; 2017:789-816.
6. Bilgutay AN, Roth DR, Gonzales ETJr, et al. Posterior urethral valves: risk factors for progression to renal failure. *J Pediatr Urol.* 2016;12(3):179.e1-e7.
7. Houk CP, Hughes IA, Ahmed SF, Lee PA; Writing Committee for the International Intersex Consensus Conference Participants. Summary of consensus statement on intersex disorders and their management. International Intersex Consensus Conference. *Pediatrics.* 2006;118(2):753-757.
8. Bowlin PR, Gatti JM, Murphy JP. Pediatric testicular torsion. *Surg Clin North Am.* 2017;97(1):161-172.
9. Kost-Byerly S, Jackson EV, Yaster M, Kozlowski LJ, Mathews RI, Gearhart JP. Perioperative anesthetic and analgesic management of newborn bladder exstrophy repair. *J Pediatr Urol.* 2008;4(4):280-285.
10. Wiegele M, Marhofer P, Lönnqvist PA. Caudal epidural blocks in paediatric patients: a review and practical considerations. *Br J Anaesth.* 2019;122(4):509-517.
11. Veneziano G, Tobias JD. Chloroprocaine for epidural anesthesia in infants and children. Chloroprocaine for epidural anesthesia in infants and children. *Paediatr Anaesth.* 2017;27(6):581-590.
12. Litman RS. Urologic surgery. In: Litman RS, ed. *Basics of Pediatric Anesthesia.* Philadelphia, PA: Ron Litman; 2017:241-244.
13. Capozza N, Caione P. Vesicoureteral reflux: surgical and endoscopic treatment. *Pediatr Nephrol.* 2007;22(9):1261-1265. Epub 2007 February 3.
14. Rao KL, Menon P, Samujh R, et al. Endoscopic management of vesicoureteral reflux and long-term follow-up. *Indian Pediatr.* 2018;55(12):1046-1049.

15. Timberlake MD, Peters CA. Current status of robotic-assisted surgery for the treatment of vesicoureteral reflux in children. *Curr Opin Urol.* 2017;27(1):20-26.

16. Bowen DK, Faasse MA, Liu DB, Gong EM, Lindgren BW, Johnson EK. Use of pediatric open, laparoscopic and robot-assisted laparoscopic ureteral reimplantation in the United States: 2000 to 2012. *J Urol.* 2016;196(1):207-212.

17. Strand WR. Initial management of complex pediatric disorders: prunebelly syndrome, posterior urethral valves. *Urol Clin North Am.* 2004;31(3):399-415, vii.

18. Henderson AM, Vallis CJ, Sumner E. Anaesthesia in the prune-belly syndrome. A review of 36 cases. *Anaesthesia.* 1987;42(1):54-60.

19. Key statistics for Wilms tumors. Available at https://www.cancer.org/cancer/wilms-tumor/about/key-statistics.html. Accessed November 24, 2019.

20. Whyte SD, Mark Ansermino J. Anesthetic considerations in the management of Wilms' tumor. *Paediatr Anaesth.* 2006;16(5):504-513.

21. Muñoz CJ, Nguyen HT, Houck CS. Robotic surgery and anesthesia for pediatric urologic procedures. *Curr Opin Anaesthesiol.* 2016;29(3):337-344.

22. Spinelli G, Vargas M, Aprea G, Cortese G, Servillo G. Pediatric anesthesia for minimally invasive surgery in pediatric urology. *Transl Pediatr.* 2016;5(4):214-221.

23. Cremer R, Lorbacher M, Hering F, Engelskirchen R. Natural rubber latex sensitisation and allergy in patients with spina bifida, urogenital disorders and oesophageal atresia compared with a normal paediatric population. *Eur J Pediatr Surg.* 2007;17(3):194-198.

24. Vidi SR. Role of hypertension in progression of chronic kidney disease in children. *Curr Opin Pediatr.* 2018;30(2):247-251.

25. Whitaker EE, Wiemann BZ, DaJusta DG, et al. Spinal anesthesia for pediatric urological surgery: reducing the theoretic neurotoxic effects of general anesthesia. *J Pediatr Urol.* 2017;13(4):396-400.

Anesthesia for Orthopedic Procedures

Laura H. Leduc and Richard F. Knox

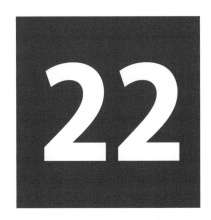

FOCUS POINTS

1. Somatosensory evoked potentials (SSEPs) indicate the integrity of the afferent pathways of the dorsal columns of the spinal cord.
2. Increased latency and decreased amplitude are indicators of potential injury to the spinal cord.
3. Motor evoked potentials (MEPs) are both more sensitive to anesthetic agents and spinal cord injury, but only function in the absence of neuromuscular paralysis.
4. Careful positioning is paramount to all procedures especially prone and those of long duration; it should be completed in collaboration with the surgeon, anesthesiologist, and nursing staff.
5. Postoperative visual loss (POVL) is a devastating complication of prone positioning and has been associated with hypotension, anemia, and direct external pressure.
6. Surgical wound infection prevention is the responsibility of all members of the health care team. It can be minimized by hand hygiene with feedback (monitoring of practitioners), frequent environmental cleaning, patient decolonization, improved line access methods, and infection surveillance.
7. Congenital and neuromuscular scoliosis patients tend to have significantly higher blood loss than patients with idiopathic scoliosis undergoing spinal fusion.
8. Maintaining a neutral cervical spine position and awareness of the potential for a difficult airway are the most important anesthetic considerations for patients with Klippel-Feil syndrome.
9. There are multiple forms of osteogenesis imperfecta ("brittle bone" disease), all of which require extreme care perioperatively to prevent fractures (padding, avoidance of frequent noninvasive blood pressures, etc.).
10. Patients with Marfan syndrome have skeletal, cardiovascular, and ocular abnormalities. The major cause of morbidity and mortality though is dilation of the aortic root leading to aortic dissection.
11. When an Ehlers-Danlos syndrome (EDS) child presents for surgery, particular attention should be given to bleeding tendencies with a low threshold to prepare blood products.
12. The most severe form of cerebral palsy is spastic quadriplegia with higher association of intellectual disability, seizures, and swallowing difficulties.
13. Cardiomyopathy is a major cause of death in patients with Duchenne muscular dystrophy (DMD) and all patients should undergo a cardiac evaluation with echocardiogram or cardiac MRI prior to an elective anesthetic.
14. Succinylcholine has been used without incident in spinal muscular atrophy (SMA) patients, but there is a potential for rhabdomyolysis and hyperkalemia and should be used with extreme caution.
15. Scoliosis repair requires careful planning that includes positioning, adequate access, invasive monitoring, and neuromonitoring (SSEP, MEP). The anesthetic plan should be tailored to the degree of surgical repair and the comorbidities of the patient.

16. The single most important risk factor for venous thromboembolism (VTE) in the pediatric population is the presence of a central venous catheter (CVC).

INTRODUCTION

Anesthesia for orthopedic surgery in children is determined as much by the patient's underlying health status and comorbidities as it is by the specific operation. The anesthetic plan varies depending on individual circumstances. In this chapter, we will outline many of the reasons patients present to the orthopedic operating room, both in elective and emergent circumstances. Conditions and syndromes most pertinent to orthopedic surgery will be described and particular anesthetic concerns will be highlighted.

Regional anesthesia is a critical component of pediatric orthopedic surgery. In pediatric anesthesia, regional procedures are often performed while the patient is under general anesthesia. Ideally, blocks are performed prior to surgery. Upper extremity surgeries are facilitated by blocks of the brachial plexus. Lower extremity surgeries are facilitated by blocks of the femoral and/or sciatic nerves. Epidural analgesia can be considered for any bilateral lower extremity procedure. Regional anesthesia is covered in more detail elsewhere in this text.

ANESTHETIC MANAGEMENT

Many aspects of anesthetic management for orthopedic procedures in children are similar to those for nonorthopedic procedures. This chapter highlights some of the issues most pertinent to the orthopedic operating rooms, including neuromonitoring, positioning, infection prevention, and tourniquet physiology.

▷ Neuromonitoring

Intraoperative neurophysiological monitoring is an integral component of surgery and anesthesia for major spine procedures. Monitoring of somatosensory evoked potentials (SSEPs) and motor evoked potentials (MEPs) has made identification of intraoperative ischemia to the spinal cord possible, which may enable the team to address the problem before irreversible damage occurs. Spinal cord perfusion is determined by the mean arterial pressure (MAP) minus the cerebrospinal fluid (CSF) pressure and is generally autoregulated within the range of 60 to 150 mm Hg. Spinal cord perfusion pressure is influenced by hypoxia, hypercarbia, and temperature. Inadequate spinal cord perfusion puts the patient at risk of neurological injury. Combined, SSEPs and MEPs provide a highly sensitive and specific measure of spinal cord function.

SSEPs indicate the integrity of the afferent pathways of the dorsal columns of the spinal cord. SSEP monitoring measures the average electrical response at the cortex to a peripheral stimulus. Most commonly, the posterior tibial or peroneal nerves are used for monitoring lower extremities and the ulnar nerve is used for monitoring upper extremities. Limitations of SSEPs include the delay associated with data collection, signal averaging, and the fact that the anterior spinal artery does not directly supply the dorsal columns.[1] Upon stimulation of a peripheral nerve, amplitude and latency of the cortical responses are monitored. Increased latency and decreased amplitude require evaluation as they are indicators of potential injury to the spinal cord.

MEPs provide a more sensitive measure of spinal cord function. The efferent motor pathways occur along the anterior portion of the spinal cord. MEPs are both more sensitive to anesthetic agents and spinal cord injury, but only function in the absence of neuromuscular paralysis. A stimulus is generated over the motor cortex of the scalp and the electrical response of the corresponding peripheral muscles is monitored. Most often, the tibialis anterior is used for this purpose. Upper extremity motor function is also monitored and can serve as a benchmark for anesthetic-induced decrease versus true neurological compromise.

Historically, a wake-up test was utilized to rule out the possibility of a motor deficit prior to closure after spine surgery. Currently this test is still performed although by fewer surgeons and sometimes only when there is concern for neurological injury based on neurophysiological monitoring. A wake-up test involves lightening the anesthetic until the patient can follow commands. The end point is to have the patient move their fingers and toes upon request. Anesthesia is deepened as soon as the wake-up test is complete. In the event that a patient can squeeze their fingers upon command, but no lower extremity movement is noted, a neurological injury is assumed.

Performing a safe and effective wake-up test requires skill and advance planning to occur efficiently. When possible, the patient can be prepared ahead of time for the test. Very few patients remember the wake-up test, especially when they have been prepared for it. The idea of the wake-up test is somewhat terrifying for patients, but most are reassured to know that even in the unlikely event that they have recall of the wake-up, they will not feel pain.

Communication with the surgeon to clarify timing of the test can be very helpful. All medications are discontinued in anticipation of the wake-up test. The patient should be placed on 100% oxygen. The surgeon packs the field with wet lap sponges and covers the wound. This is to prevent venous air embolism with deep inhalation and maintain sterility of the site. One person should be under the drapes to feel for movement of the toes. Two people should be at the head of the bed. One person can hold a hand and place a hand on the patient's head to prevent sudden movement and dislodging of the endotracheal tube. The other person can hold the other hand and be ready to manage the ventilator or administer medications when the test is complete.

The wake-up test has the potential for disaster if the patient self-extubates in the prone position or comes off the operating table completely. Therefore, a stretcher should be in the room and ready and all members of the team available to respond in case of an emergency. A wake-up test is only helpful in patients who can understand and respond to the command to "wiggle your toes." It can be performed in less than 5 minutes with planning, communication, and attention to the timing of any sedating medications that are long-acting.

Positioning

Careful positioning of pediatric patients is an important consideration in anesthesia care. It may be particularly challenging for patients with contractures for whom standardized operating room beds may not have adequate support. However, these same children may be specifically prone to positioning injury due to poor nutrition and chronic pressure points. Major orthopedic procedures may be associated with large volume blood loss and the resulting hypotension would place the patient at increased risk of pressure necrosis.

Peripheral nerve injury under anesthesia is thought to be related to stretching or compression of the nerve in addition to direct trauma caused by needle puncture or chemical toxicity. It is helpful to elicit a complete history of any underlying nerve damage during the preoperative interview, which can guide careful positioning. Additionally, during long procedures, pressure points, especially the face, can be periodically adjusted when the patient is positioned prone and the head when positioned supine. Fortunately, severe and permanent neurological dysfunction is rare from anesthesia and surgery.

Many orthopedic spine procedures are performed in the prone position. Confirmation of safe positioning prior to the start of the surgical procedure is the responsibility of the surgeon and circulating nurse in collaboration with the anesthesiologist. The face is usually in a foam headrest, which allows the ventilating circuit to exit without pressure or tension. The chest should be supported by chest-rolls placed carefully to avoid pressure on nipples. Shoulders should be abducted less than 90 degrees and the ulnar groove protected. Hips should be supported with particular attention to padding at the anterior superior iliac crests, knees should be clear of pressure, and feet should be supported on pillows, blankets, or pads. Male genitalia should be free of pressure as well. One benefit to SSEP monitoring is that there is potential for positioning injury to be identified prior to the occurrence of irreversible damage.

In addition to the importance of padding pressure points during prone positioning, there are some physiological changes pertinent to anesthesia in that position. Intraocular pressure is increased, which can cause decreased ocular perfusion pressure despite normal mean arterial pressures.[2] It is generally recommended that the bed be at a 15-degree reverse Trendelenburg position to protect the eyes. Postoperative visual loss (POVL) is a devastating complication during surgery and is poorly understood. Factors that may contribute include retinal ischemia, optic nerve ischemia, and optic vein engorgement in the setting of hypotension, anemia, and external pressure. However, POVL has occurred in the absence of any known risk factors.[3]

Prone positioning can compromise ventilation due to increased intra-abdominal pressure. Tables have been designed that allow the abdomen to hang free benefiting ventilation. Increased intra-abdominal pressure decreases venous return via compression of the inferior vena cava, thus resulting in decreased cardiac output and end-organ perfusion. Healthy patients may or may not demonstrate untoward effects from the physiological sequelae of prone positioning, but more fragile patients may develop hemodynamic and respiratory compromise.

Infection Prevention

Infections in orthopedic surgery patients can have far-reaching consequences due to the potential for hardware infection and infection deep in the tissues, joints, and bones, which can severely limit a patient's mobility and quality of life. The anesthesiologist plays an important role in the prevention of surgical site infections (SSIs) by using aseptic techniques and timely administering prophylactic antibiotics.

According to the Centers for Disease Control and Prevention (CDC), health care–associated infections (HAIs) are present in 1 in 25 in-hospital patients on any given day.[4] SSIs are a major component of HAIs and not only increase patient morbidity and mortality but also reflect poorly on a hospital system and will increasingly be tied to lower reimbursement rates. The financial burden of HAIs is estimated to be 30 billion dollars annually.[5]

Based on data collected in 2010 by the American College of Surgeons (ACS) National Surgical Quality Improvement Program-Pediatric (NSQIP-P), the overall rate of pediatric SSIs was 1.8% and the rate of neonatal SSIs was 3%.[6] Neonates are thought to be at higher risk of SSI due to their immature immune systems. This data does not demonstrate the difference that may be seen in SSI in sicker patients with chronic illnesses versus healthy patients presenting for straightforward outpatient operations.

According to a retrospective study of data collected over a 10-year period, children who did not receive antibiotic prophylaxis within the recommended 60-minute time frame were at a 1.7-fold increased risk of developing an SSI.

Identified modifiable risk factors for development of SSIs included incorrect dosing and time of administration of antibiotics.[7]

Another retrospective study from a 9-year period of data covering 16,031 patients indicated a rate of SSI of 0.99% (159 patients). Risk factors identified by this study included young age (neonates), African American race, postoperative ICU admission, urinary catheters, and implantable device placement. In this study, wound classification and antibiotic administration were not independent predictors of SSI.[8]

In addition to patient and surgical risk factors, and antibiotic administration, the anesthesia team can impact the development of HAIs. In particular, recurrent access of central lines may increase the risk of a HAI. The mantra now in practice is as follows: one syringe, one patient, one time, indicating that a syringe should only be used for administration of one dose to one patient and should not be refilled even with the same medication for the same patient.

Keeping the anesthesia work environment clean between cases is also essential in decreasing HAI and SSI. In addition to thorough cleaning between cases, hand hygiene among the anesthesia personnel is critical. Filters in the patient circuit can also help prevent bacterial transfer. Stopcock contamination is a significant problem for patients in the operating room. A comprehensive method to minimize bacterial transmission to patients in the anesthesia work area includes excellent hand hygiene with feedback (monitoring of practitioners), frequent environmental cleaning, patient decolonization, improved line access methods, and infection surveillance.[9]

Tourniquets

A tourniquet is a compression device often used during orthopedic surgery on an extremity to limit blood loss and maintain a clear operating field. It is usually placed on the patient prior to the surgical prep but not inflated until just prior to incision. The limb can be exsanguinated with an Esmarch bandage or by gravity and the tourniquet is then inflated to 50 to 100 mm Hg above the pressure required to occlude the arterial supply to the limb. To prevent injury the cuff should have a width that is greater than one-half the limb's diameter and should be inflated to the lowest pressure possible to satisfy the surgical requirements. Inflation time is monitored closely.[10]

While there is controversy over the maximum time a tourniquet can safely stay inflated, the general recommendation is not to exceed 2 hours. This is based on the fact that cellular changes appear to be reversible within 2 hours of ischemia.[10] When the safe ischemic time is exceeded, patients can have damage to muscle and nerves and develop neuropathy as a result. In patients who are prone to neuropathy for other reasons, the tourniquet time should be decreased.

Tourniquet pain is a phenomenon that can occur both in patients who are awake and in those who are under general anesthesia. It begins approximately 45 minutes into the tourniquet time. Patients who are anesthetized with a regional block but otherwise awake will note a dull ache that eventually becomes extremely painful. Patients under general anesthesia will often have increased blood pressure and heart rate when the tourniquet pain starts to set in. The pain does not respond well to narcotics and the hemodynamics, when necessary, can be treated with labetalol. The pain resolves when the tourniquet is deflated.

Tourniquet inflation increases blood pressure and central venous pressure. Likewise, with deflation the blood pressure and central venous pressure decrease.[10] For patients who are hemodynamically fragile, this may be relevant. Most children, however, do not have a dramatic hemodynamic response to inflation or deflation. The patient's core temperature will generally increase during tourniquet inflation and should be closely monitored to maintain euthermia.

With release of the tourniquet, there is an increase in carbon dioxide, which is most noticeable as increased end-tidal CO_2 in patients under general anesthesia. There is also a transient metabolic acidosis due to washout of the anaerobic metabolic byproducts such as lactate. These changes are generally self-limiting assuming the tourniquet time has been reasonable.

Blood Conservation

Some orthopedic operations and in particular spine surgeries are associated with significant blood loss. Congenital and neuromuscular scoliosis patients tend to have significantly higher blood loss than patients with idiopathic scoliosis undergoing spinal fusion. Neuromuscular patients have an almost seven times higher risk of losing greater than half of their blood volume during scoliosis surgery.[11] Optimal methods of mitigating blood loss transfusion are ongoing areas of interest. Some patients, such as the Jehovah's Witness population, will not accept blood products regardless of consequence, including death.

Blood loss is important because loss of oxygen-carrying red blood cells results in decreased delivery of oxygen to end-organs such as the kidneys, heart, and brain. Additionally, blood loss in excess of half the patient's blood volume and fluid replacement can result in dilutional coagulopathies, which lead to further hemorrhage and the risk of exsanguination. Predictors of blood loss for spine surgery include operative time, preoperative kyphosis, male sex, and mean arterial pressure.[12]

The determination of transfusion thresholds is an actively debated topic and ultimately is an individualized decision based on the risk/benefit ratio for each clinical situation. Healthy patients can tolerate significant anemia without known untoward effect, but patients with known cardiac impairment or other chronic illnesses may require a lower transfusion threshold for optimization of long-term outcomes.

In the past, deliberate hypotension was a common method of conserving blood loss. Despite the fact that it is effective for this purpose, it is no longer in common use for long spine surgeries. Prolonged hypotension can negatively affect perfusion to the spinal cord, kidneys, and eyes increasing the risk of potentially devastating consequences.

Hemodilution is another method of blood conservation but should be used with caution due to similar risk of anemia and loss of oxygen-carrying capacity. Cardiac indices and oxygen extraction increase during hemodilution and systemic vascular resistance, oxygen delivery, and mixed venous saturation decrease. When oxygen delivery becomes critical, lactic acidosis develops; therefore, close monitoring of hemoglobin is warranted. Complications of hemodilution include postoperative pulmonary edema, anasarca, and prolonged postoperative mechanical ventilation.[3]

Cell saver is often used for spine surgeries as a method of returning the patient's own blood to oneself. This is generally acceptable for Jehovah's Witness patients provided the blood is kept in a continuous circuit in connection with the patient. Contraindications to cell saver include tumor operations and allergy to the anticoagulant. Potential complications of the use of salvaged blood include air embolism and hemolytic and bleeding complications from centrifugation, cellular debris, or anticoagulant overdosage.[3]

Antifibrinolytic medications are increasingly used in long surgeries associated with high-volume blood loss. Both ε-aminocaproic acid (EACA) and tranexamic acid (TXA) can decrease blood loss in spine surgery for idiopathic and neuromuscular scoliosis surgery. TXA is a synthetic antifibrinolytic that acts by competitive blockade of the lysine-binding sites of plasminogen, plasmin, and tissue plasminogen activator resulting in a reversible blockade that slows fibrinolysis and degradation of clots. ε-aminocaproic acid acts via a similar mechanism but is 6 to 10 times less potent than TXA.

In one prospective randomized double-blind study by Sethna et al. in 2005, blood loss was reduced by 41% in the TXA group as compared with placebo. However, the amount of blood transfused was not different.[13] TXA was administered with a 100 mg/kg bolus followed by an infusion of 10 mg/kg/h until skin closure. This study indicated three variables predictive of blood loss including preoperative platelet count, American Society of Anesthesiologists (ASA) physical status, and treatment with TXA. No adverse events related to the TXA were present. A retrospective study by Yagi et al. in 2012 demonstrated significantly less intraoperative blood loss as well as significantly fewer blood products transfused in patients who received TXA.[14]

EACA has been shown to significantly decrease postoperative wound drainage in a prospective, randomized, double-blind study by Florentino-Pineda and colleagues in 2004.[15] A retrospective case control study by Thompson and colleagues in 2008 demonstrated that EACA was highly effective in decreasing perioperative blood loss and transfusion requirements in patients with neuromuscular scoliosis undergoing spine surgery.[16] EACA can be administered by bolus of 100 mg/kg, not to exceed 5 g, over 15 minutes followed by an infusion of 10 mg/kg/h until wound closure.[17]

Based on a prospective, randomized, double-blinded comparison of TXA and EACA by Halanski et al. in 2014, TXA use was associated with lower allogenic transfusion requirements, less alteration in postoperative clotting studies, and a trend toward lower blood loss in pediatric posterior spinal fusion patients.[18] However, due to flaws in the study such as an unequal distribution of patients undergoing Ponte osteotomies, their data is not sufficient to consider TXA to be more effective than EACA. Further investigation is warranted, especially considering the significantly increased cost associated with TXA over EACA.

Invasive arterial monitoring and frequent blood gas determinations are indicated for major orthopedic operations in order to keep close track of hemodynamics and blood loss. For any spine surgery, venous access in anticipation of large volume blood loss is essential. When peripheral access is inadequate, central access should be obtained prior to the start of the procedure since gaining access for line placement can be very difficult once the surgery has started. Significant bleeding can occur postoperatively, and patients should be monitored closely for the first few days after surgery.

SPECIFIC DISORDERS

While there are a multitude of genetic disorders, both inherited and sporadic, that have orthopedic and anesthetic implications, only a select few will be discussed in detail. Whenever one is faced with providing an anesthetic for a child with an unfamiliar disorder, at least a cursory literature review is indicated. Access to the basic components of syndromes and disorders is incredibly easy with access to the Internet. Some syndromes are known to have difficult airways, unstable cervical spines, or even predilection for malignant hyperthermia, and knowledge of the basics can be quite helpful. In many cases, parents have extensive knowledge of their child's rare condition and can be used as a resource where appropriate.

Arthrogryposis

Arthrogryposis is a term used to describe patients with joint contractures, which can result from multiple etiologies. The term derives from the Greek words "arthron" for "joint" and "gryposis" for "hooking." The joint contractures may be caused by muscular, neurological, or connective tissue anomalies. The "tes" are descriptive of patients who present with two or more congenital contractures of their joints. There are over 200 different disorders associated with arthrogryposis and approximately 1% of all births have associated joint contractures. The incidence of arthrogryposis is 1:5,000–10,000 live births and is equal between male and female infants.[19]

Arthrogryposis can be a result of intrauterine abnormalities such as fibroids or oligohydramnios and abnormalities of connective tissue development.[19] Neurological abnormalities are present in 70% to 80% of patients with arthrogryposis and are associated with patchy damage to the anterior horn cells of the spinal cord. Arthrogryposis is also associated with muscular dystrophies, intrauterine myositis, and mitochondrial diseases.

Classic arthrogryposis is called amyoplasia. It is a sporadic symmetric disorder where muscles are replaced by fibrous tissue. Multiple joints are involved including shoulders, elbows, hips, fingers, wrists, feet, and knees.[19] Distal arthrogryposis is a disorder of autosomal dominant inheritance primarily affecting the hands and feet. Typically, infants will have clenched fists with ulnar deviation of the fingers, medially overlapping fingers and club feet.[20]

Infants with arthrogryposis will generally have multiple joints involved and are best managed by a multidisciplinary team of therapists, surgeons, and primary physicians. Physical and occupational therapists can begin intervention early in the child's life with passive range of motion exercises and splinting and casting. Therapeutic goals include maximization of range of motion and function.[19]

Clubfoot deformities are common in patients with arthrogryposis. Treatment is initiated with serial casting followed by heel cord lengthening. Lifelong treatment is indicated to prevent recurrence of deformity. Treatment goals include maintenance of a stable, pain-free foot.[19]

Knee problems in arthrogryposis patients may be related to flexion, extension, subluxation, and stiffness. Occasionally, knee flexion can be associated with skin pterygiums and requires plastic Z lengthening procedures. Other flexion contractures may respond to hamstring lengthening with posterior knee capsular releases. The quadriceps muscle group is likely to be weak and easily fatigued. Quadriceps lengthening via release of the lateral and medial quadriceps and proximal detachment of the rectus femoris may need to be performed in the case of knee hyperextension.[19] Circular external fixation strategies or osteotomies and growth guidance may be used to manage knee flexion deformities. Hip dislocations are relatively common in patients with arthrogryposis. The hip joints are generally very stiff and require operative reduction about one year of age.[19]

Arthrogryposis of the upper extremities typically involves internally rotated arms, extended elbows, flexed wrists, and thumb in palm or clasp thumb deformities. Treatment begins early with splinting and occupational therapy. Surgery is generally performed between 1 and 12 months of age.[19] Maintaining elbow flexion is extremely important for independence with activities of daily living. Surgery may involve elbow release with reconstructive lengthening of the triceps and potentially muscle transfer to enable active elbow flexion. In cases where the wrist does not respond to hand therapy, partial corpectomies may be performed. Thumb adduction may be treated with an adductor release with an opponensplasty.[19]

Scoliosis is common in children with arthrogryposis and is associated with hip dislocations and compensatory lumbar lordosis.[19] If the curve continues to progress despite thoracolumbar spinal orthosis (TLSO) bracing, surgery may be indicated. Care of spinal deformity in particular is individualized as independent mobility may depend on spine flexibility.

Children with arthrogryposis will generally present for multiple orthopedic surgeries beginning during infancy. Particular care must be taken to provide a positive experience for children and their families so as not to contribute to a negative association with the hospital and surgery experience. Children who are traumatized early in life by a forceful hold of a mask during inhalation induction may carry anxiety into every hospitalization and surgery.

In addition to the orthopedic issues, infants may have associated conditions. Of particular relevance to anesthesia are micrognathia, trismus, short neck, limited mandibular excursion, and fusion of cervical vertebrae, which can cause difficult airway intubation.[20] There is also a potential for musculoskeletal deformities that can compromise respiratory function and lead to increased risk of restrictive lung disease, postoperative respiratory insufficiency, and aspiration. In general, patients with isolated distal arthrogryposis are less likely to have a difficult airway.[20]

Intravenous access in arthrogryposis patients can present unique challenges. In addition to a relative paucity of veins, limb contractures can make mechanical access to a vein difficult. Contractures and rotational changes can also result in veins appearing in relatively unexpected areas of the extremities. The common practice of inhalation induction and subsequent intravenous cannulation in healthy children carries an increased risk of potential difficulty in arthrogryposis. Careful preoperative evaluation of venous and airway anatomy may help prevent intraoperative anesthetic complications.

Meticulous attention to positioning is important in patients with arthrogryposis because they are at increased risk of fracture from joint contractures. If the patient has an associated muscular dystrophy, succinylcholine should be avoided due to the risk of hyperkalemia. Patients with arthrogryposis are not considered to be at increased risk of malignant hyperthermia but will sometimes exhibit a hypermetabolic state under anesthesia.[20]

▶ Juvenile Idiopathic Arthritis

Formerly known as juvenile rheumatoid arthritis, juvenile idiopathic arthritis (JIA) is the most common autoimmune disease of childhood. The worldwide incidence ranges from 0.8 to 22.6 per 100,000 children per year.

Approximately 100,000 children in the United States have JIA. The subtypes of JIA include oligoarthritis, polyarthritis, and systemic JIA. While the etiology of JIA is not clearly understood, there are likely both immunological and environmental factors. Associated immunological abnormalities cause an inflammatory synovitis, which can result in joint destruction if not treated.[21]

Diagnosis of JIA is clinical, and the differential diagnosis of joint pain is vast. Generally, patients with JIA present with arthritis defined as intra-articular swelling with two of the following: limitation in range of motion, tenderness or pain with movement, and warmth.[21] The joints are generally not erythematous, although they are swollen and painful. Patients with chronic temporomandibular joint disease can develop micrognathia. Patients may have cervical spine involvement with decreased neck extension and risk of atlantoaxial subluxation. Both jaw inflammation and spine involvement can lead to a difficult airway and tenuous neck stability.

Patients with JIA may present with laboratory abnormalities including increased white blood cell count and decreased red blood cell count. Patients with systemic JIA can develop macrophage activation syndrome (MAS), a potentially fatal complication. MAS is associated with a falling platelet count, extreme hyperferritinemia, evidence of macrophage hemophagocytosis in the bone marrow, increased liver enzymes, falling leukocyte count, persistent, continuous fever greater than or equal to 38°C, hypofibrinogenemia, and hypertriglyceridemia.[21]

Children with JIA have osteopenia, as well as increased levels of cytokines, which regulate bone metabolism and can result in abnormalities of skeletal growth. These children may present to the orthopedic operating rooms for surgery for limb length discrepancy, scoliosis, joint arthroplasties, and synovectomies. They might also present for limb and mandibular osteotomies, and trauma-related fractures frequent in children. They may be at increased risk of bleeding if platelets are low or if they are on chronic nonsteroidal anti-inflammatory medications. When the disease flares, they may be treated with oral steroids, and a careful history can help elicit whether stress-dosing is indicated perioperatively.

Klippel-Feil Syndrome

Klippel-Feil syndrome is a cervical spine disorder that results in a short neck due to fusion of cervical vertebrae. The traditional clinical triad is a short neck, low posterior hairline, and limited cervical mobility, but most patients do not exhibit all three signs. The incidence of Klippel-Feil syndrome is approximately 1:42,000 with a slight predilection for girls. Klippel-Feil may also be a phenotypic presentation associated with several other disorders including syndromes such as Goldenhar, Mohr, VACTERL (vertebral defects, anal atresia, cardiac defects, tracheo-esophageal fistula, renal anomalies, and limb abnormalities), and fetal alcohol.[22,23] The cervical spine in Klippel-Feil syndrome

may also have occipitocervical synostosis, odontoid abnormalities, and the proximal migration of the C2 vertebra known as basilar impression.[23]

In addition to the clinical triad, patients with Klippel-Feil syndrome may have sensorineural or conductive hearing loss, cleft lip, oligodontia, micrognathia, a webbed neck, and torticollis. They may have voice abnormalities due to malformed laryngeal cartilage. Congenital cardiac defects, including ventriculoseptal defect (VSD) and conduction delays, may be present (5% to 10% incidence). Many patients have winged scapula, vertebral anomalies including scoliosis, and renal abnormalities (double collecting systems, renal aplasia, and horseshoe kidney).[22-24]

Because the cervical spine becomes more immobile over time, the airway can become progressively more difficult to intubate. Therefore, a history of an uneventful anesthetic is not as reassuring as it would be in other patients with potentially difficult airways. Additionally, the cervical spine becomes hypermobile at levels above and below immobile joints causing increased risk of cervical spine injury with direct laryngoscopy. Seemingly minimal movement of the cervical spine under anesthesia can result in serious neurological sequelae and patients should be evaluated for neurological deficits and previously unidentified deficits should be investigated. For cooperative patients, the awake fiberoptic intubation has been the gold standard in airway management. However, most children are not able to tolerate the awake intubation and thus asleep fiberoptic intubation with spontaneous ventilation is appropriate. The widespread availability of the video laryngoscope in conjunction with in-line stabilization has enabled a view greater than that given by a traditional laryngoscope with minimal neck extension.

Postoperatively, patients with significant scoliosis have a higher risk of respiratory failure and may need to remain intubated in which case plans must be in place to maintain neutral neck position until the patient is fully awake. Patients with renal insufficiency may have a prolonged response to medications with renal clearance such as nondepolarizing neuromuscular blockers.

Skeletal Dysplasias

Achondroplasia and Dwarfism

Achondroplasia is the most common cause of short-limbed dwarfism.[25] It is an autosomal dominant disorder characterized by a disproportionately short stature. The incidence ranges between 1:15,000 and 1:40,000 births.[26] The clinical features result from abnormal cartilage formation especially at the epiphyseal growth plates. Patients with achondroplasia have a large head with a prominent forehead, depressed nasal bridge, prominent mandible, normal trunk, and short limbs. They can develop lordosis, thoracolumbar kyphosis, pelvic narrowing, and severe spinal stenosis. The spinal stenosis may present with cervical cord or thoracolumbar cord compression and cauda equina syndrome.[27]

Clinically, motor milestones are delayed in infants with achondroplasia due to hypotonia and the difficulty associated with balancing their disproportionately large heads. However, intelligence is normal in most achondroplastic dwarfs.

Patients with achondroplasia have comorbidities that include hydrocephalus, atlantoaxial instability, cleft palate, tracheomalacia, congenital heart disease, obstructive sleep apnea (OSA), pulmonary hypertension, and seizure disorders.[27] They may present to an orthopedic surgeon for repair of clubfoot, angular deformity, scoliosis, or spinal stenosis in addition to any of the common orthopedic complaints affecting children. Major preoperative issues include the potential for difficult airway management, cervical spine instability, abnormal respiratory mechanics, and OSA.

In patients with congenital heart disease, preoperative ECG, echocardiogram, and chest radiograph may be helpful. Patients with severe scoliosis are at risk for restrictive lung disease and pulmonary hypertension, further warranting a preoperative echocardiogram.

Intraoperatively, the anesthesiologist should take extreme care with positioning due to the potential for spinal cord injury and be cognizant of the potential for difficult airway and potential for subglottic stenosis, laryngomalacia, and tracheomalacia.

Postoperatively, patients are at risk for respiratory failure due to sleep apnea and the associated sensitivity to narcotic pain medications, as well as the altered pulmonary mechanics due to the lack of chest wall compliance. Nonopioid analgesics and regional anesthetics should be utilized whenever possible. Local anesthetic volume should be reduced in patients with achondroplasia undergoing neuraxial blocks due to their shorter height.

Osteogenesis Imperfecta

Also known as "brittle bone disease," osteogenesis imperfecta (OI) is a disorder of collagen formation. The defect in collagen may be qualitative or quantitative, either of which results in bones that are extremely fragile. The disease ranges in severity from mild to severe and incompatible with life. Children with the mild form of the disease have presented with multiple fractures during their childhood and their presentation can be mistakenly identified as resulting from child abuse.

Type I collagen is the basis of ligament, tendon, and bone formation. Defective structural collagen leads to compromised endochondral and intramembranous bone, poor ligament and tendon formation, and thin bone trabeculae.[27] Historically, OI was considered to be a triad of bone fragility, blue sclerae, and early deafness, but the complete triad does not hold true for most patients.[28]

OI type I is generally a mild form of the disease. In addition to recurrent fractures, blue sclerae, and early-onset hearing loss, children may exhibit hypermobile joints, easy bruising, thin skin, scoliosis, hernias, and mild short stature.[28] They may have dentinogenesis imperfecta, which is a disorder of tooth development resulting in discoloration and fragility of the dentition. Most patients with OI type I will have fractures in childhood but not as neonates. There is a decrease in fracture risk postpuberty but a resurgence in postmenopausal women.[29] Inheritance is autosomal dominant.

OI type II is generally a severe form of the disease and patients are either stillborn or die in the first year of life. Fractures may present in utero and the bones are extremely fragile. A small thorax contributes to respiratory insufficiency. There are abnormalities of the cerebral cortex including agyria, gliosis, and periventricular leukomalacia.[28] Inheritance may be either autosomal dominant or autosomal recessive.

Type III OI is the most severe, nonlethal form of the disease. Children will present at birth with fractures that occurred in utero. Postnatal fractures occur easily and heal poorly. There may be a "popcorn" appearance of the bones at the metaphyses.[28] Abnormalities of the thorax can result in respiratory insufficiency and patients can develop scoliosis and vertebral fractures. Patients will have an extreme short stature. They may have scleral changes, dentinogenesis imperfecta, hearing loss, and kyphoscoliosis.[28] Inheritance is either autosomal dominant or recessive.

Patients with type IV OI may also present with fractures in utero and bowing of the long bones. This type of OI is considered moderately severe and few patients will achieve independent ambulation.[28] Inheritance is autosomal dominant. OI types V to XI have been described and are beyond the scope of this text. They account for varying severity of bone fragility with and without the above-listed symptoms of blue sclerae, dentinogenesis imperfecta, ligamentous laxity, and rhizomelia.[28]

Osteogenesis Imperfecta	Disease Severity	Inheritance	Manifestations
Type I	Mild	Autosomal dominant	Blue sclerae, dentinogenesis imperfecta, childhood fractures
Type II	Severe	Autosomal dominant or recessive	Stillborn or death in first year of life
Type III	Severe	Autosomal dominant or recessive	Fractures in utero, "popcorn" calcifications
Type IV	Moderately severe	Autosomal dominant	Fractures in utero, bowing of long bones

Clinically, patients will present with multiple fractures, may develop scoliosis due to decreased strength of the ligaments, compression fractures, osteoporosis, and spondylolisthesis,[27] and have associated congenital heart disease [aortic root dilation, patent ductus arteriosus (PDA), atrial septal defect (ASD), VSD, and valvular defects].[27,29]

Patients with OI may present for elective, urgent, or emergent procedures. When possible, the preoperative evaluation should include investigation of associated cardiac anomalies with an echocardiogram. Patients who have severe kyphoscoliosis or other abnormalities of the thorax should be evaluated for restrictive lung disease. In patients with severe thoracic abnormalities there is a risk of cor pulmonale. The possibility of basilar impression, atlantoaxial instability, and cervical cord compression should not be overlooked.[27] Although not yet clearly characterized, there is a potential for platelet dysfunction.[29]

Intraoperatively, all pressure points must be padded, and great care must be taken to avoid fractures and injury to tendons and ligaments during positioning and throughout the surgery. Fractures from succinylcholine-induced fasciculations are possible and thus depolarizing neuromuscular blockade is relatively contraindicated. Fractures can also result from direct laryngoscopy and blood pressure cuffs. It may be appropriate to place an arterial catheter for longer operations and possibly avoid blood pressure cuff use for shorter operations given that the risk may outweigh the benefit. Patients with dentinogenesis imperfecta have a higher risk of dental damage.

Patients with OI are known to exhibit signs consistent with a hypermetabolic state such as hyperthermia but without the typical manifestations of malignant hyperthermia; to date there is no association with this potentially lethal disease.

Emergence of anesthesia should be as smooth as possible given the risk of fracture with agitation. This is of particular relevance in patients emerging from posterior spinal fusion due to the fact that they are at risk of dislodging hardware and injuring the spinal cord.

Osteopetrosis

Osteopetrosis is a bone disorder in which bones are sclerotic with increased density. It is also known as marble bone disease. It results from insufficient resorption of bone by osteoclasts. It can be inherited in an autosomal dominant or autosomal recessive manner.

The autosomal recessive form is severe and presents with an incidence of 1 in 250,000 births.[30] Generally, patients with this form will present in infancy with macrocephaly, hepatosplenomegaly, deafness, blindness, and severe anemia. There is bone sclerosis throughout and laboratory evaluation shows low calcium and phosphorus levels with elevated parathyroid hormone levels. Survival may extend into the second decade, but likely children will

have progressive cranial neuropathies, anemia, pathological fractures, and dental problems.[30]

The autosomal dominant form is mild and is much more frequent with an incidence of 1 in 20,000 births.[30] The body's failure to remodel growing bone results in narrowing of cranial nerve foramina and a decrease in functional bone marrow. Clinically, children with develop cranial nerve palsies, anemia, and compensatory extramedullary hematopoiesis in the liver and spleen.[30] They are also prone to pathological fractures and for this reason may present with some frequency to the orthopedic operating room.

Preoperatively, hematocrit and platelet count should be evaluated due to the potential for pancytopenia and hemorrhage. A calcium level may be indicated as well due to the risk of hypocalcemia-related seizures or tetany. Patients may have abnormal cells of immunity (white blood cells and macrophages) and are prone to infection. In more severe cases, infection may be the cause of demise in childhood. Patients may be on chronic steroids and stress doses of steroids should be considered.

Patients with osteopetrosis are at risk of difficult airway due to limitation of the mandibular movement, and restricted size of the oropharynx and nasal pharynx. Nasal intubation may be contraindicated due to the risk of bone growth limiting the size of the nasal cavity.[31] The risk of dental damage is also increased due to poor formation of teeth and higher likelihood of osteomyelitis of the mandible. Patients are at a greater risk of obstructive sleep apnea and considerations should be taken for increased sensitivity to narcotics and higher incidence of postoperative respiratory complications. Positioning with great care is of extreme importance due to the risk of pathological fractures intraoperatively.

Connective Tissue Disorders

Marfan Syndrome

Marfan syndrome is a connective tissue disease resulting from a defect in fibrillin, a major component of the connective tissue. Inheritance is autosomal dominant with high penetrance and incomplete expressivity, which results in a great degree of variability in presentation.[32] The incidence is 1 in 10,000 live births with approximately one-quarter of the cases sporadic.[33] Mutation in fibrillin-1 on chromosome 15 is present in 66% to 91% of cases; therefore, the inability to detect an abnormality on fibrillin-1 does not exclude the diagnosis.[34]

Patients with Marfan syndrome generally have skeletal, cardiovascular, and ocular pathology. They are tall with joint laxity and may have a wingspan greater than their height. They may have pectus excavatum or pectus carinatum. Their fingers are long and slender (arachnodactyly). Their heads are long and narrow (dolichocephaly) with enophthalmos, retrognathia or micrognathia, malar hypoplasia, a high arched palate, and downward slanting palpebral fissures.[33] They may have the "wrist sign," which is when the thumb overlaps the fifth finger when grasping the contralateral wrist, as well as the "thumb sign," which is when the thumb extends beyond the ulnar border of the hand when overlapped by the fingers. Other orthopedic considerations include scoliosis, kyphosis, chest asymmetry, hind foot deformity, severe flatfoot, acetabular protrusion, and reduced elbow extension.[34]

More than 50% of patients with Marfan syndrome develop scoliosis, but only 10% to 20% of those who develop it need treatment.[10] Generally, patients with Marfan syndrome have either atypical scoliosis or typical scoliosis with atypical features.[35] Atypical curve patterns include left thoracic curves, whereas right thoracic curves are more typical and thus more common. The natural history of scoliosis in patients with Marfan syndrome is more severe than in patients with adolescent idiopathic scoliosis (AIS).

The cardiovascular abnormalities associated with Marfan syndrome include mitral valve prolapse (MVP) with mitral insufficiency (MI), aortic insufficiency (AI), and a tendency toward aortic dissection and dilation of the ascending aorta. Cardiovascular symptoms may be present very early in life and any patient presenting for surgery should have a preoperative cardiac workup including a focused history, ECG, and echocardiography. Aortic dissection is the main cause of death in patients with undetected Marfan syndrome, and early diagnosis with treatment can prolong disease-free survival. Beta-blockers are an essential treatment because they have been shown to decrease the rate of aortic root dilation.[36]

From a pulmonary perspective, patients with Marfan syndrome are more prone to blebs and pneumothoraces. They have lower forced vital capacity due to the connective tissue abnormality and early airway closure. Chest deformities and scoliosis can impact vital capacity and total lung capacity and result in restrictive respiratory dysfunction. Pectus excavatum may result in cardiorespiratory dysfunction with dyspnea, decreased endurance, chest pain, and tachycardia.[37]

There is a high incidence of obstructive sleep apnea in patients with Marfan syndrome relative to the normal population. Untreated OSA may lead to an increased risk of aortic events, which may explain why patients with Marfan syndrome with OSA have a worse prognosis.[38] The etiology of the high incidence of OSA in these patients may be related to craniofacial abnormalities, tissue laxity, and high nasal airway resistance.[39] Multiple episodes of upper airway collapse followed by arousal cause additional stress on the aorta, which may lead to more rapid development of aortic dilation.[39]

Neurologically, patients are prone to dural ectasia, which is a widening of the dural sac. While the abnormality can occur anywhere along the spinal column, it is most likely to present in the lumbosacral region. There may be thinning of the cortex of the pedicles and laminae of the vertebrae and there may be an associated meningocele.[40]

Essentially, there is a disparity between the diameters of the dural sac and the vertebral body of the associated spine segment. The possibility of dural ectasia must be considered when planning neuraxial anesthesia. One population-based study demonstrated a prevalence of 90% for dural ectasia in patients with Marfan syndrome.[41]

The orthopedic operations for which patients with Marfan syndrome are most likely to present include scoliosis procedures and operations for foot deformity, angular deformity, and patella instability. In addition to a complete history and physical, cardiac workup may be indicated, and beta-blockers should be continued perioperatively. The patient's neck should be evaluated clinically and radiographically for atlantoaxial instability.

Intraoperatively, stable hemodynamics are essential. Maintaining low heart rate and avoiding hypertension can protect against acute aortic dissection intraoperatively and myocardial ischemia. Patients may have a higher requirement for neuraxial local anesthetics due to their height. Positioning must be done with great care due to joint laxity and potential for injury.

Ehlers-Danlos Syndrome

Ehlers-Danlos syndrome (EDS) is a diagnosis applied to a heterogenous group of connective tissue disorders characterized by joint hypermobility, skin laxity, and potential fragility of vascular structures. The incidence is estimated to be between 1:10,000 and 1:25,000 with an equal distribution between sexes and different ethnicities.

While as many as 10 subtypes of EDS have been described, the most commonly used nosology delineates 6 categories of disease pattern.[42] Most cases appear to be inherited in an autosomal dominant fashion and some are caused by mutations in genes encoding collagen type, or proteins that regulate collagen synthesis. Extreme variability in expression results in a broad range of clinical manifestations from insignificant to life-threatening. Table 22-1 provides an overview of the six categories and their characteristic profiles (modified from Weismann et al.).[43]

The classic and hypermobility types combinedly account for approximately 75% of EDS cases. These patients suffer frequent complications of joint hypermobility with recurrent dislocations as well as chronic joint and limb pain, which can result in the frequent need for pediatric orthopedic care. Vascular-type EDS children account for approximately 5% of cases. They commonly have club feet as well as tendon and muscle ruptures. The hallmark vascular and intestinal fragility can lead to catastrophic rupture. Children with kyphoscoliotic-type EDS frequently have congenital hypotonia and ocular fragility in addition to congenital and progressive scoliosis. Arthrochalasis-type EDS patients have an increased incidence of congenital bilateral hip dislocation and a propensity for recurrent subluxations. Dermatosparaxis-type patients have multiple skin-related features including redundancy,

Table 22-1. Ehlers-Danlos Syndrome Types

Type	Major Criteria	Minor Criteria
Classic	Joint hypermobility Skin hyperextensibility Atrophic scars	Smooth, velvety skin Easy bruising Muscle hypotonia Motor delay Positive family history
Hypermobility	Generalized joint hypermobility Skin hyperextensibility	Recurring joint dislocations Chronic joint/limb pain Positive family history
Vascular	Translucent thin skin Arterial/intestinal rupture Extensive bruising Characteristic facies	Acrogeria Hypermobility of small joints Tendon and muscle rupture Club feet Arteriovenous, carotid-cavernous sinus fistula Pneumothorax/hemothorax Positive family history, sudden death in close relative
Kyphoscoliotic	Congenital and progressive scoliosis Congenital hypotonia Scleral fragility and rupture of the ocular globe	Tissue fragility with easy bruising Arterial rupture Marfanoid habitus Microcornea Osteopenia/porosis Positive family history
Arthrochalasis	Congenital bilateral hip dislocations Generalized joint hypermobility with recurrent subluxations	Skin hyperextensibility Tissue fragility Easy bruising Hypotonia Kyphoscoliosis Osteopenia/porosis
Dermatosparaxis	Severe skin fragility Sagging, redundant skin	Doughy skin texture Easy bruising Large hernias

doughy texture, and hyperextensibility, but have fewer of the more severe traits seen in other EDS categories.

When an EDS child presents for surgery, particular attention should be given to bleeding tendencies, complications from past operations, and airway management issues. Further testing is dictated by the patient's history and the expected surgical risk. One should always have a low threshold for preparing blood products for EDS patients undergoing surgery. When formulating an anesthetic plan for an EDS patient, serious consideration of the risk/benefit ratio for every monitor and every type of access must be undertaken. Any procedure that requires a needle puncture carries with it a significantly increased risk of complication. Preemptive use of ultrasound for venous and arterial access is recommended as is utilizing the most experienced practitioner available. Even the interval time of automatic blood pressure devices and the tightness with which a pulse oximeter probe is applied can lead to excessive bruising or hemorrhage. Preoperative discussion with the surgical team should address the

need for tourniquets, foley catheters, gastric tubes, and any other invasive device. The preprocedure time out should also be used to ensure that everyone in the operating room is aware of the risks unique to EDS surgical patients. Additionally, extreme care must be taken with positioning and padding of all areas of the patient since joints can easily be dislocated or hyperextended, bruising can result from minimal pressure, and ocular and globe rupture can occur in prone positioning.

General anesthesia with volatile anesthetic or propofol is acceptable for EDS patients. Drugs that affect platelets should be either avoided or used with caution. Neuraxial blocks should be performed with caution or avoided due to the increased risk of hematoma formation. Regional blocks are an acceptable adjuvant therapy as long as ultrasound guidance is employed. Infiltration of incision sites with local anesthetics as well as locally injected anesthetics for dental procedures have been reported to have reduced efficacy in EDS patients.[44,45] Desmopressin (DDAVP) can be used prophylactically for procedures where large volume blood loss is a possibility. While the mechanism of effect is uncertain, studies of small groups of patients have demonstrated significant reductions in blood loss and related complications when desmopressin was given.[46]

During emergence, padding, and positioning must be meticulously maintained. Postoperatively, patients with casts, splints, and external fixation devices must be closely observed for signs of compartment syndrome. Postoperative nausea and vomiting (PONV) should be aggressively prevented as esophageal rupture has been reported during the recovery period.[47] When possible, EDS patients should be cared for in specialized facilities and monitored for at least 24 hours after surgery.

Neuromuscular Diseases

Cerebral Palsy

Cerebral palsy (CP) is a disorder of motor function that results from an irreversible insult to the developing brain. The brain damage causing CP may be due to a multitude of causes including infection, ischemia, and metabolic and genetic perturbations. Less than 10% of cases of CP are due to birth trauma, contrary to former beliefs.[48] In addition to a disorder of movement, patients may have difficulty with sensation, perception, cognition, communication, and behavior though many patients are of normal intelligence and function at a high level.[49]

The incidence of CP ranges from 1.5 to more than 4 per 1,000 live births worldwide. Approximately 1 in 323 children has CP. Most children with CP have spastic CP and 58.7% of children with CP can walk independently. Forty-one percent of children have concurrent epilepsy and nearly 7% have concurrent autism spectrum disorders.[48]

Risk factors for CP include low birth weight and premature birth as well as multiple birth pregnancies.[48] Preterm infants with intracerebral hemorrhage and periventricular leukomalacia are also at increased risk. Boys are at a higher risk than girls and are more likely to have a more severe degree of impairment.[49]

Symptoms of CP are highly variable between individuals and manifest in early childhood or infancy. CP is non-progressive, chronic, and not curable. Patients present for multiple orthopedic procedures due to spasticity, extremity contractures, scoliosis, and hip dislocation.

Different types of CP include spastic diplegia, spastic quadriplegia, spastic hemiplegia, and dyskinetic CP. The most severe form is spastic quadriplegia, which accounts for approximately 20% of cases.[49] There is a higher association of intellectual disability with this form as well as seizures and swallowing difficulties leading to recurrent aspiration pneumonias. Patients have increased tone and spasticity in all four extremities, decreased spontaneous movements, and brisk reflexes.

Spastic hemiplegia refers to patients with CP who have increased muscle tone and spasticity in the upper and lower extremities of either the left or right side of their bodies. Generally, the arm is more affected than the leg. Approximately one-third of patients with spastic hemiplegia have a seizure disorder and 25% have cognitive abnormalities.[49] Spastic hemiplegia may result from an intrauterine stroke or infection as well as other causes. Spastic diplegia is spasticity of both legs more so than the arms. It is associated with damage to the immature white matter in utero. Up to 70% of these children have periventricular leukomalacia.[49] The likelihood of seizure is far less than with spastic hemiplegia and these children are more likely to have normal intellect.

Dyskinetic CP, also known as athetoid, choreoathetoid, or extrapyramidal CP, accounts for approximately 20% of patients with CP. Infants are hypotonic with poor head control. Generally, the upper extremities are more affected than the lower extremities and patients will often have prominent tongue thrusting and drooling. Their movements may be athetoid (slow and writhing), choreoathetoid (jerky), or dystonic. These children are likely to have normal intellect but will experience difficulty with speech. Causes of dyskinetic CP include intrauterine or birth asphyxia, kernicterus, and metabolic disorders. There is cognitive impairment in approximately 50% of these children and 25% have a seizure disorder. In addition to chronic pain, they may develop hip displacement and contractures.[49]

Orthopedic procedures for which patients with CP will come to the operating room include injection of botulinum toxin (botox), release of the hip including adductor tenotomy or psoas transfer and release, hip reconstruction, rhizotomy, heel cord lengthening, scoliosis, and placement or change of intrathecal baclofen pumps.

There are no specific anesthesia contraindications for patients with CP. Succinylcholine is not more likely to cause hyperkalemia than in an otherwise healthy child and they are not at increased risk of developing malignant hyperthermia. Anesthesia will most often be dictated by the specific procedure, although many anesthesiologists have a low threshold for intubation in patients with copious oral secretions due to the increased risk of laryngospasm.

It is essential to remember that while many patients are limited in their ability to communicate with us, they are often not limited in their ability to understand. The caregiver is often a very helpful translator and can help identify anxiety and pain on behalf of the patient. Any anesthetic should be explained to the child in age-appropriate terms with reassuring tones. Many CP patients frequent the operating room and it is prudent to allow the patient and parent to have input into the anesthetic care, particularly with regard to intravenous placement prior to, or after, induction.

Short cases such as botox injections to spastic limbs often require only a mask anesthetic. In children who are otherwise healthy, this can safely be performed without the placement of an IV catheter. However, there are various reasons for placing an IV catheter in this situation, including signs of upper respiratory infection, excessive oral secretions, and concern for laryngospasm as well as access for medications such as ondansetron to help prevent PONV. Children with CP require a lower concentration of volatile anesthetic and have a longer emergence time than their healthy peers.[50]

Longer operations often require placing an endotracheal tube. Patients should be given their regular medications such as baclofen for spasticity and antiepileptics for seizure prevention preoperatively. Patients with CP have low pharyngeal tone and a high incidence of gastroesophageal reflux disease, and the endotracheal tube can help protect against aspiration. They have variable responses to neuromuscular relaxing drugs. Patients who take antiepileptic medications may be relatively insensitive to muscle relaxants due to induction of the cytochrome P-450 enzymes and other patients may have a prolonged recovery time. Extubation should be done with the patient completely reversed from neuromuscular blockade and as recovered from the anesthetic as possible.

Positioning for any procedure on a child with CP may be difficult due to multiple contractures. It is important to pad any bony surfaces to prevent pressure ulceration and nerve injury. The more painful orthopedic surgeries present difficulty with postoperative pain management. When indicated, regional anesthesia can be extremely helpful. Diazepam 0.1 mg/kg intravenously (or orally when tolerated postoperatively) treats muscle spasms and is an adjunct to pain management.

Duchenne Muscular Dystrophy

Muscular dystrophies are a heterogenous group of hereditary diseases of muscle, which present with progressive weakness. They are characterized by painless degeneration and atrophy of the skeletal muscles without denervation. Over time, muscle fibers are replaced with fibrous and fatty connective tissue. The defect is due to an absence of dystrophin, which results in failed integrity of the skeletal muscle membrane. This causes breakdown of the sarcolemma and an influx of extracellular calcium, activation of cellular proteases, inflammation, necrosis, and fibrotic infiltration.[51]

Duchenne muscular dystrophy (DMD) is the most common muscular dystrophy and has an incidence of approximately 1 in 3,500 births. It is an X-linked recessive disorder primarily affecting boys. There are documented cases in females with a range in severity of clinical course. Diagnosis is by proximal limb muscle biopsy with staining, which demonstrates an absence of dystrophin at the surface of the muscle fibers.[51]

Patients with DMD present with a waddling gait, frequent falls and difficulty climbing stairs, due to proximal muscle weakness. Calves hypertrophy, despite loss of functional muscle, is due to fatty infiltration. Combined with the proximal muscle weakness, pelvic girdle weakness causes "Gower's sign," which is when a child climbs up his legs to reach a standing position. Weakness in the shoulder girdle and thoracic muscles leads to thoracolumbar scoliosis for which these patients may require orthopedic surgery.

Generally, children will have normal development until 3 to 5 years of age at which point the muscle weakness becomes apparent and motor milestones may be lost. While the clinical course is variable, most children are unable to walk by 9 to 11 years of age.

Of importance in anesthesia is the development of dilated cardiomyopathy, which can occur at a very young age. Loss of dystrophin in the heart affects the L-type calcium channels resulting in increased intracellular calcium. This causes activation of proteases that degrade the contractile proteins leading to inflammation, myocardial cell death, and fibrosis. Cardiomyopathy is a major cause of death in patients with DMD and all patients should undergo a cardiac evaluation with echocardiogram or cardiac MRI prior to an elective anesthetic.[51] When patients present emergently, dilated cardiomyopathy with poor cardiac function should be presumed.

Patients with DMD are also at risk of postoperative respiratory failure. In severe cases, an intubation for an operation may even become a terminal intubation. All anesthetics should be performed at centers where pediatric intensive care is readily available. By the end of the first decade of life, pulmonary function tests (PFTs) will demonstrate decreases in inspiration, expiration, vital capacity, and total lung capacity, which may not be easily identified in the patient's history given poor exercise tolerance overall. There is benefit to extubating to Bi-Pap or CPAP. Preoperative preparation with noninvasive positive pressure ventilation and cough-assist devices can help facilitate transition back to independent respiratory effort.

The other major anesthetic consideration with DMD patients is the risk of life-threatening hyperkalemia in response to succinylcholine administration. Any paralytic agent should be given with caution given the underlying weakness in patients with DMD because they are more likely to have an increased response to nondepolarizing muscle relaxants in both peak effect and duration of action. Traditionally, volatile anesthetics were avoided in patients with DMD due to potential of triggering malignant hyperthermia. However, they are not contraindicated and can be used provided the patient's hemodynamics are maintained.

Spinal Muscular Atrophies

Spinal muscular atrophies (SMAs) are degenerative diseases of the anterior horn cells and lower brainstem nuclei that result in diffuse proximal muscle weakness. The degeneration begins in utero and continues to progress throughout infancy and childhood with varying degrees of severity. The incidence is approximately 1 in 6,000 to 1 in 10,000 people.[52]

SMA is characterized by hypotonia, hyporeflexia, and overall weakness especially in the lower extremities.

SMA22	Age of Onset	Disease Progression
Type 0	Neonatal period	Fatal during that period
Type 1: Werdnig-Hoffmann	Infantile	Respiratory failure, first year of life
Type 2	Late infantile	Most common (50% of SMA patients), slowly progressive
Type 3: Kugelberg-Welander	Juvenile	Chronic
Type 4	Adult	Slowly progressive

Most cases of SMA are autosomal recessive with a small minority of sporadic cases. They are caused by mutations or deletions of the survivor motor neuron 1 (*SMN-1*) gene on chromosome 5q. In some cases, survival motor neuron 2 (*SMN-2*) can take over function of the *SMN-1* gene, which may account for some of the variability in clinical severity of SMA.[22]

Treatment of SMA is mostly supportive involving chest physiotherapy, respiratory support, prevention of aspiration, and supplemental nutrition. Orthopedic intervention is often indicated for joint contractures including hip subluxations and dislocations as well as contractures and hypermobile joints of the upper extremities. Patients with SMA may present with spontaneous fractures due to osteopenia. Nearly all nonambulatory patients with SMA develop scoliosis with severe progression.[53]

Pulmonary compromise is present in children with SMA and patients are at increased risk of perioperative respiratory failure with decreased vital capacity and severe weakness of auxiliary respiratory muscles. Patients have difficulty clearing secretions and are prone to development of pulmonary infections, hypoventilation, and atelectasis. Some pulmonary function can be spared with early intervention for scoliosis.[53] Perioperatively, noninvasive positive pressure ventilation should be available and mechanical cough-assist devices may be helpful in preventing postoperative atelectasis and pneumonia.

Poor nutrition is a significant problem for patients with SMA and can increase perioperative complications. Some surgeons may opt to bolster nutritional status with gastric feedings or total parenteral nutrition (TPN) prior to major operations for scoliosis. Prolonged fasting should be avoided due to mitochondrial dysfunction with fatty acid oxidation.[53] Patients will also decondition very quickly over the course of a prolonged hospital stay, and physical therapists and occupational therapists are essential team members.

Anesthetics for patients with SMA should be considered at facilities with appropriate postoperative pediatric intensive care availability. Patients may require prolonged hospitalization especially after major scoliosis surgery. While there isn't a strong association between SMA and cardiomyopathy, preoperative echocardiogram may be indicated in patients with severe sleep apnea.

While most children do not present for surgery with advance directives in place, there is a potential for failed ventilatory wean after small operations for gastrostomy tube placement, which may result in a transition to comfort measures and hospice care.[54] Patients with SMA do not have an increased risk of cognitive disability and should be included in formulation of care plans, including the potential transition to comfort measures, as is age-appropriate. Avoiding hypoventilation and impairment of the respiratory drive is as critical as obtaining good pain control postoperatively.

In addition to narcotic and inhalation agent sensitivity, patients with SMA may have increased sensitivity to nondepolarizing neuromuscular blockers due to decreased choline acetyltransferase, which is a result of anterior horn cell degeneration.[22] This can result in a prolonged duration of action with otherwise short-acting muscle relaxants. Additionally, the nerve stimulator may not provide an accurate indication of recovery of neuromuscular function and thus muscle relaxants should be used with extreme caution. While succinylcholine has been used without incident in some patients with SMA, there is a potential for rhabdomyolysis and hyperkalemia due to the lower motor neuron denervation hypersensitivity and immobilization.[54]

The airway may be difficult to intubate in some patients with SMA due to atrophy of the masseter and other muscles of mastication. Regional anesthetics can be used, but paralysis of any muscles involved in respiration should be avoided. To decrease narcotic requirements postoperatively, surgeons should be asked to infiltrate the field with local anesthetic when appropriate.

The use of nusinersen (Spinraza, intrathecal administration), an SMN-2 antisense oligonucleotide, has provided an option to modify the disease course in patients with SMA with improvement in motor function and survival. Its current price tag in the United States makes it prohibitive for some patients.[55]

Neurofibromatosis

Neurofibromatosis type 1 (NF-1), the most prevalent type of neurofibromatosis, may have associated orthopedic considerations. It is an autosomal dominant condition affecting 1 in 3,000 live births.[56] The hallmark characteristic is multiple café au lait spots. Diagnosis is made via clinical features or genetic testing.

While neurofibromas generally involve the skin, they can form in many other places including peripheral nerves, blood vessels, viscera, and bone. Plexiform neurofibromas can result in deformity or overgrowth of a bone. Patients may develop sphenoid dysplasia, which is an osseous lesion or cortical thinning of long bones that may be associated with pseudoarthrosis. Congenital pseudoarthrosis is a spontaneous fracture that progresses to nonunion. It most often involves the tibia and the radius and severity can range from asymptomatic to severe requiring limb amputation.[57]

Children with NF-1 may have central nervous system abnormalities including learning disabilities and seizure disorders. Approximately 3% of patients will go on to develop malignant neoplasms and 10% of patients will develop scoliosis.[56] There is some association of NF-1 with pheochromocytoma, although this is rarely relevant to children. More likely, hypertension may develop in response to renal artery stenosis. Children can develop Moyamoya syndrome as a result of cerebral artery dysplasia, which can result in cerebral infarction and hemorrhage.

Patients may develop airway compromise from neurofibromas of the laryngeal, cervical, or mediastinal regions. Further respiratory compromise can result from severe kyphoscoliosis that remains untreated. In addition to airway considerations, anesthetic management for patients with neurofibromatosis depends on the underlying condition of presentation. Additionally, any signs or symptoms of increased intracranial pressure should be evaluated due to the possibility of intracranial lesions. Patients may have a variable response to both depolarizing and nondepolarizing neuromuscular relaxants.[57]

Neurofibromatosis-2 (NF-2) is a distinct entity from NF-1 and involves chromosome 22, as opposed to chromosome 17. Most patients will present in the second or third decade of life with acoustic schwannomas resulting in hearing loss, vestibular symptoms, or facial weakness.

Selected Lower Extremity Conditions

Blount Disease

Blount disease is a form of idiopathic tibia vara, more commonly known as "bowlegs." It is a result of abnormal endochondral ossification of the medial aspect of the proximal tibial physis leading to varus angulation and medial rotation of the tibia.[58] The infantile (age 1 to 3 years) type is most commonly seen in black females and the juvenile and adolescent types are more common in black males. Many patients are obese, although there has not been any causality described.

Young children with mild Blount disease are given a trial of orthotic management for up to one year. More severe disease and deformity that do not respond to noninvasive management are treated with surgery. The usual procedures are proximal tibial valgus osteotomies and fibular diaphyseal osteotomies. When the disease is severe, correction may also be indicated.

The anesthetic for patients with Blount disease may be complicated by the patient's underlying obesity, making airway, intravenous access, and positioning a challenge. The surgeon will usually inject local anesthetic and opioids with nonopioid adjuncts supporting postoperative pain management.

Slipped Capital Femoral Epiphysis

Slipped capital femoral epiphysis (SCFE) is a disorder of the hip in which the femoral head is displaced through the growth plate. It is most likely to present in patients during rapid growth in adolescence. Associated pain is in the groin, hip, or knee. The incidence of SCFE varies geographically with a much higher incidence in the northeastern United States (10 per 100,000) than in Japan (0.2 per 100,000). Obesity is a risk factor with approximately 60% of patients in the 90th percentile for weight.[59] Males are more likely than females to develop SCFE and there may be as many as 60% who have the disorder bilaterally, even when symptoms are only one-sided.[59]

SCFE may be acute, chronic, or acute-on-chronic. Acute SCFE occurs when a patient presents with 3 weeks or less of pain. It may be associated with a relatively minor injury. Patients with chronic SCFE present after a few months of pain, which may be vague in nature. Acute-on-chronic SCFE occurs in patients who have had greater than 3 weeks of prodromal symptoms and present with an acute exacerbation of the underlying pain. Radiographically, there is associated femoral neck remodeling with displacement of the capital epiphysis past the femoral neck.[59]

The most serious complications of SCFE are osteonecrosis and chondrolysis. Osteonecrosis is avascular necrosis and occurs due to injury to the blood supply of the femoral head. Chondrolysis is an acute loss of the articular cartilage in the hip. Patients who are unable to ambulate are considered to have unstable SCFE and are at greater risk of osteonecrosis of the hip. Those with stable SCFE ambulate and have a negligible risk of osteonecrosis.[59]

Treatment for SCFE involves pinning of the hip to prevent further progression of the slip and to stabilize the physis. The hip is not reduced due to the increased risk of osteonecrosis. Concerns of bilateral disease progression may lead to surgical intervention (prophylactically) on the contralateral side even with unilateral presentation.

Anesthesia for patients with SCFE may be urgent or emergent. Patients may have to be admitted to the hospital upon diagnosis and stabilized as soon as possible. Preoperative evaluation is dictated by whether or not the patient has any medical comorbidities. General anesthesia with an endotracheal tube is the preferred method of anesthesia to provide adequate muscle relaxation. Extubation at the end of the case, dictated by any additional comorbidities, is expected. Pain is usually managed with local anesthesia injected by the surgeon as well as intravenous pain medications both narcotic and adjuncts. Postoperative pain is generally not severe.

Clubfoot

Clubfoot, also known as congenital talipes equinovarus (CTEV), is a congenital deformity of the foot, which may be idiopathic or associated with many different conditions, including neuromuscular diseases and syndromes. The deformity involves forefoot adductus (medial deviation), midfoot cavus (high arch), hindfoot varus (back of the heel is rolled inward), and equinus (back of the heel is up). It is relatively common with an incidence of 1 in 1,000 births.[60]

Patients present for comprehensive release of clubfoot only after nonoperative treatment has failed. Most commonly, Ponseti casting is successful in correction of all but the equinus release, which can be performed via percutaneous tenotomy under local or general anesthesia.

When surgery is required, it is to provide a plantigrade, functional, and painless foot. Surgical release includes a comprehensive and systematic release of all the tight and contracted structures encountered. The term *posterior medial release* (PMR) describes the approach and may include lengthening of the Achilles tendon, toe flexors, plantar fascia, and abductor hallucis. Additionally, the joint capsules of the tibiotalar, calcaneal cuboid, and talar navicular will require releases as well. The subtalar will need to be addressed but with great care as medial and lateral releases can cause translation of this joint with significant pain and deformity. Throughout the entire procedure, the neurovascular structures are identified and protected. Pins and casting are often required for 6 to 8 weeks to hold the foot in a good position until healing has occurred.

Anesthesia for clubfoot surgeries in children is generally a combination of general with regional. General anesthesia can be either with an endotracheal tube or with a laryngeal mask airway depending on the patient's comorbidities and the length of the anticipated surgical procedure, as well as the preference of the surgeon and anesthesiologist. Some surgeons prefer prone positioning for the operation, which may impact the method of airway maintenance. While the anticipated surgical pain may be only moderate, young children may have a significant negative reaction to the full leg cast.

There are several options for regional anesthesia, including caudal, epidural, and peripheral nerve blocks. Generally, a caudal is performed after induction for young children, and popliteal and saphenous blocks are done in older children. Many children will need to return to the operating room for cast change under anesthesia approximately 2 weeks after the primary repair.

Developmental Dysplasia of the Hip

Developmental dysplasia of the hip (DDH) describes a phenomenon of joint laxity and instability that may result from multiple causes. There is a wide range in severity from mild dysplasia to dislocation. Some deformities are associated with underlying syndromes and others are isolated and idiopathic. Typical DDH describes the isolated deformity. Teratological DDH describes genetically influenced hip dysplasia.[61]

The incidence of DDH is highly variable and ethnically diverse. Caucasian newborns have approximately 1% incidence of DDH and 0.1% incidence of hip dislocation. The incidence is very high in Manitoba, Canada with 188.5 cases per 1000 babies. DDH is more common with a positive family history, breech presentation, or female sex, and in conditions such as oligohydramnios, large birth weight, and first pregnancy that may lead to intrauterine crowding.[61]

All neonates are screened for DDH because it is asymptomatic at birth and the joint will not develop appropriately if the hip is dislocated. As children get older, they may present with limited hip abduction and apparent asymmetry of the thigh and hip. Children who can walk may present with an awkward gait, a limp, or apparent leg-length discrepancy. Patients may develop an excessive secondary lordosis. Hip dysplasia, or failure to develop acetabular coverage, may be identified in teens. This scenario is more likely to occur when the dysphasia is bilateral since the newborn exam depends somewhat on asymmetry for diagnosis.

The goal in treatment of DDH is to maximize normal development of the hip joint, which requires that the femoral head be securely nestled within the acetabulum. Most children who are diagnosed with DDH as infants will respond to nonoperative interventions. Children who are older at diagnosis may come to the operating room for closed reduction. Once the hip is reduced, a spica cast is placed to maintain the reduction. If closed reduction fails or if the child is older than 2 years of age at diagnosis, the patient is likely to require an open reduction of the hip. Generally, a femoral shortening osteotomy is done at the same time due to the risk of osteonecrosis due to pressure on the proximal femur.[61]

Surgical complications include avascular necrosis of the femoral epiphysis, redislocation, residual subluxation, acetabular dysplasia, and wound infections.[61] Rare complications include bleeding or sciatic or peroneal nerve palsies.

Anesthesia for hip reduction, both open and closed, is usually general with or without epidural placement for postoperative pain management. Postoperative pain is moderate, and patients may be more distressed by the spica cast than by the incisions and hip reduction.

Leg-Length Discrepancy

While a difference in leg length of 1 cm is relatively common, people with a discrepancy of 2 cm or more are considered to have a pathological leg-length discrepancy. There are many congenital or acquired causes of a leg-length discrepancy. Patients will present with gait asymmetry. They may also develop secondary lumbar curvature.[62]

Treatment for leg-length discrepancy is variable depending on the amount of discrepancy, as well as the patient's comorbidities and preferences. For discrepancies of up to 2.5 cm, observation and use of shoe lift may be adequate. Operative procedures may involve limb-shortening or limb-lengthening techniques.

Epiphysiodesis is performed for patients with a discrepancy between 2 and 5 cm who are skeletally immature. It is a temporary or permanent growth cessation at the physis of the long leg. In percutaneous epiphysiodesis, the physis is permanently ablated with a drill and curette.[62] Alternatively, plates and screws can be inserted for temporary cessation of growth. Typically, the hardware would be removed when the legs have equalized.

Acute leg shortening may be necessary if the patient is already skeletally mature. This is usually performed at the femur as the risk of neurovascular compromise is increased when performed at the level of the lower leg.[62] Lengthening of the short leg is indicated when the leg-length discrepancy is greater than 5 cm.

The Ilizarov method is a common technique used for limb lengthening via distraction osteogenesis. The procedure involves placement of an external fixator. The bone is cut at the metaphyseal–diaphyseal junction and lengthening occurs gradually.[62] The major principles involve a low-energy osteotomy to preserve blood flow to the periosteum, a slow, incremental distraction to preserve soft-tissue blood supply, and continued full function of the extremity.[10]

The Ilizarov method can also be used in the treatment of acquired short limbs and defects from trauma, tumor excisions, fractures, and infections.[10] Surgical complications of leg-discrepancy procedures include pin-tract infections, wound infections, hypertension, joint subluxation, muscle contracture, premature consolidation, delayed union, implant-related problems, and fractures.[62]

Anesthesia for leg-length discrepancy surgery is guided foremost by the patient's comorbidities. Usually a combined approach is appropriate. After inducing general anesthesia, the preferred regional technique can be performed to provide postoperative pain control. Regional anesthesia should be discussed with the surgeon because a major surgical complication can be nerve damage and local-anesthetic-induced numbness might confuse postoperative evaluation. Additionally, patients are started in physical therapy as early as possible postoperatively and a continued dense block could interfere with safe mobility.

Postoperative pain can be moderate to severe, so regional anesthesia with intravenous narcotics and adjuvant analgesics such as acetaminophen and ketamine should be considered. Many surgeons will prefer to avoid nonsteroidal anti-inflammatory drugs (NSAIDs) due to the potential for impaired bone healing based on a retrospective review, which demonstrated a significant increase in the rate of nonunion after spinal fusion with the use of ketorolac.[63] An additional review article investigating the effect of NSAIDs on bone healing indicated that they do inhibit or delay fracture healing.[64]

Generally, there are no major hemodynamic shifts associated with leg-length discrepancy surgeries and invasive monitoring is not required. A single IV catheter that runs well is usually adequate.

Selected Upper Extremity Conditions

The upper limbs develop over weeks 4 to 8 of gestation. Limb anomalies are classified according to principles of limb development using a system called the OMT (Oberg, Manske, and Tonkin) scheme. Limb malformations are one of the most common types of anomalies.[65]

Amniotic Band Syndrome

Amniotic band syndrome (ABS) is a condition of circumferential bands around the limbs or digits resulting in significant loss of function and cosmesis. While the etiology of ABS may be either syndromic or not, treatment is similar for all patients. The hands are reconstructed by release of fused digits with skin grafting and release of bands where possible. These children present for surgery at a young age and may come back for recurrent surgeries as they grow, and scars need revision.

Anesthesia for patients with ABS is determined largely by any underlying conditions relating to the patient. The procedures are usually done under general anesthesia, but in many situations, upper extremity regional anesthesia can be very helpful for postoperative pain control, especially when limitation of narcotics is beneficial.

Syndactyly

Syndactyly is a webbing of the digits that results from a failure of apoptosis during limb development. Complete syndactyly involves the entire length of the digit, whereas incomplete syndactyly does not cover the length of the entire digit. Complex versus cutaneous syndactyly describes bony involvement. There may also be anomalies of the nerves, tendons, and muscles. Anesthesia considerations are like those listed for ABS earlier in this chapter.

Spine Deformity

Scoliosis

Scoliosis is an abnormal curvature of the spine in the coronal plane. The term *scoliosis* refers to a lateral curvature of the spine and derives from the Greek word "skolios," which means bent or curved. Scoliosis is a three-dimensional deformity with both curvature and rotation. The term *kyphosis* refers to anterior flexion of the spine, which can be a component of spinal deformity requiring surgery as well. Most scoliosis cases are idiopathic, but a significant number of children have neuromuscular, congenital, or syndromic scoliosis.

Idiopathic scoliosis may be infantile, juvenile, or adolescent with overall prevalence from 1% to 3% of skeletally immature patients.[66]

Scoliosis[66]	Age	Incidence (% of idiopathic cases)
Infantile	Birth to 3 years	0.5–4
Juvenile	3–10 years of age	8–16
Adolescent	≥11 years of age	70–80

Normal sagittal alignment includes cervical lordosis (concave curve), thoracic kyphosis (convex curve), and lumbar lordosis. Idiopathic scoliosis is a pathological exaggeration of the normal curvature of the spine, with additional rotation, and is a diagnosis of exclusion. Underlying intraspinal abnormalities such as tethered cord and syringomyelia must be ruled out. Evaluation of scoliosis begins clinically and is aided by radiographs. The curvature is defined by the Cobb angle (Figure 22-1). An angle of greater than 10 degrees is termed scoliosis.

Many patients with infantile idiopathic scoliosis will have spontaneous resolution of their spinal curvature. Those with developmental delay, presentation after 1 year of age, and larger curves are less likely to have this resolution. Far fewer patients with juvenile or AIS will have spontaneous resolution.

Congenital scoliosis refers to abnormality of the spine that is present from birth and usually results from abnormal development of the spine or ribs in utero. The clinical abnormality may not be immediately apparent at birth. Since the deformity results from an intrauterine insult, it is not surprising that many children will have other congenital abnormalities: 10% to 40% will have genitourinary abnormalities including unilateral renal agenesis, ureteral duplication, horseshoe kidney, and genital anomalies, 10% to 25% cardiac abnormalities, and 15% to 40% intraspinal anomalies such as tethered cord, teratomas, and closed spinal dysraphisms.[66]

Neuromuscular scoliosis is seen in children with underlying neuromuscular diseases and ones with spinal cord trauma. The scoliotic curve for these children results from muscular imbalance and sometimes spasticity. Neuromuscular scoliosis is positively associated with higher degrees of neurological impairment. It is present in more than 70% of patients with cerebral palsy and more than 90% of patients with Duchenne muscular dystrophy.[66] Virtually all patients who suffer a spinal cord injury prior to 10 years of age will develop scoliosis.

Many syndromes are strongly associated with scoliosis including Ehlers-Danlos, Marfan, Prader-Willi, neurofibromatosis, osteogenesis imperfecta, mucopolysaccharidosis, and rheumatoid arthritis.[10,66]

Specific treatment of scoliosis is based on the type of scoliosis, the rate of curve progression, the age of the patient, and the patient's goals. Otherwise healthy patients with scoliosis generally have a goal of maintaining the highest degree of function, with good cosmetic outcomes and as little risk as possible. Severely debilitated children may have a completely different end point such as prevention of curve progression and maintenance of alignment that best supports care of the child (ability to sit comfortably).

Preoperative evaluation for scoliosis surgery should be thorough given the potential for comorbidities and the fact that the operation is elective. In addition to a complete history and physical to elicit abnormalities and changes from baseline, radiographs, PFTs, electrocardiograms, echocardiograms, and coagulation studies are often helpful.

Chest radiographs are part of the surgical planning but are also relevant to the anesthesiologist. Thoracic curves can impact lung volumes and pulmonary compliance, even with a relatively small degree of curvature. Patients who have a curve of 65 degrees or more are likely to have restrictive lung disease based on PFTs and are at higher risk of postoperative respiratory complications. They may also have abnormalities in their central respiratory drive and upper airway function resulting in impaired clearance of secretions and recurrent infections putting them at risk of perioperative aspiration and need for postoperative mechanical ventilation.

Preoperative echocardiogram may be indicated even for patients with AIS. There is an increased incidence of mitral valve prolapse in patients with scoliosis and the study can provide valuable information on the degree of valve insufficiency. Patients with as little as 25 degrees of curvature can have increased pulmonary artery pressures, especially with exercise. Most patients will have pulmonary

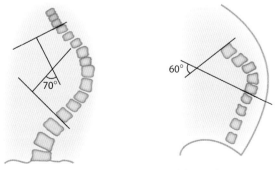

Posteroanterior   Lateral

▲ **Figure 22-1.** Cobb angle. (Reproduced with permission, from Freeman BS, Berger JS: *Anesthesiology Core Review: Part 2, Advanced Exam.* 2016. https://accessanesthesiology. mhmedical.com. Copyright © McGraw Hill LLC. All rights reserved.)

artery hypertension with exercise at a 70-degree curve and even at rest with a 110-degree curve.[3] Patients with pulmonary hypertension are at increased risk of perioperative right-sided heart failure and sudden death due to increased right ventricular (RV) afterload, hypoxemia, hypotension, and inadequate RV preload.[67] Tight hemodynamic parameters must be maintained for patients with pulmonary artery hypertension undergoing scoliosis surgery. Any child with a myopathy should have a preoperative electrocardiogram and echocardiogram due to the potential for associated cardiomyopathy.

Surgical goals in scoliosis surgery include stabilization of the spine and prevention of continued curve progression as well as improved cosmetic appearance and comfort. The approach may be anterior, posterior, or both. Anterior spinal surgery may be intended for complete treatment or for release of the spine to enhance the correction done posteriorly. Anterior spinal surgery is indicated for severe kyphosis. Thoracic curves are approached via thoracotomy or video-assisted thoracotomy on the convex side of the curve. Discectomies are performed in order to release the tension on the curvature. Thoracolumbar curves may be approached with a high subcostal incision and lumbar curves can be approached transabdominally or extraperitoneally.

Posterior spinal fusion is performed via bone grafting. The operation generally extends from one vertebra above the curve to the second vertebra below the curve. Raw bone is exposed via removal of the spinous processes. The bone graft is packed over the decorticated surface on the concave side. Instrumentation is performed to hold the spine stable during the healing of the bone resulting in spinal fusion.

Patients with neuromuscular scoliosis may require placement of growing rods at a young age. The hardware is placed and extended as the child grows. Newer rods have a magnetic extension system, which allows elongation of the rods without an operation. Anesthetic considerations for growing rod placement and removal are similar to those of posterior spinal fusion, although since the surgery is less involved, often an arterial line is not necessary, and the surgery may even be done as an outpatient procedure.

Spinal fusion for scoliosis is a major operation and requires general endotracheal anesthesia. The anesthesia team must be prepared for large volume blood loss and associated hemodynamic and electrolyte changes, complications of prone positioning, as well as rare complications such as pneumothorax, anaphylaxis, venous air embolism, and loss of motor or sensory evoked potentials.

Many patients presenting for scoliosis surgery will benefit from preoperative anxiolysis with midazolam intravenously or orally. Induction can be done via inhalation or intravenous routes. Standard of care for scoliosis surgery includes neuromonitoring and therefore the anesthetic plan will optimize this to the extent possible. An arterial line in addition to standard ASA monitors is indicated for

hemodynamic monitoring and frequent blood sampling. A central line may be necessary if there is inadequate peripheral access for the anticipated blood loss or if medications or CVP monitoring are indicated by the patient's comorbidities.

Once the patient is asleep, the neuromonitoring technician will place electrodes for SSEP and MEP monitoring. This can occur simultaneously with placement of additional lines and the foley catheter. The whole team should be present for prone positioning. The surgeon can direct positioning for the operation and the anesthesia team can ensure head and neck remain neutral and supported. Pressure points are particularly vulnerable during this operation because of duration and possible hypotension.

A small dose of rocuronium or vecuronium given with induction drugs is generally metabolized by the time the patient is ready for MEP monitoring. It is useful to look at the anesthetic depth at the time of MEP baselines because if there are MEP changes associated with the surgery, one can determine the relationship to anesthetic changes from baseline. Many institutions will run 0.5 MAC of isoflurane in conjunction with a propofol drip and a narcotic infusion to maintain an adequate anesthetic/analgesic depth.

Blood loss can be quite significant during spine surgery, especially for patients with neuromuscular scoliosis who may have a higher tendency toward bleeding, fragile tissues, and a smaller circulating blood volume relative to healthy patients presenting with AIS. Cell saver is utilized and can decrease the amount of allogeneic blood transfusion required. Transfusion triggers should be discussed as a team. They are variable and should account for anticipated ongoing blood loss. Exposed bony surfaces are a source of blood loss throughout the operation.

At the conclusion of a spine surgery, patients are usually emerged from anesthesia and extubated awake. The surgeon will often prefer a motor exam in the operating room when the patient has the mental capacity to follow commands. In cases where the patient is not suitable for extubation postoperatively, she or he can be transferred to a pediatric intensive care unit (PICU) for further management. This may be indicated for patients with severely compromised pulmonary function or poor baseline functioning as well as those who may have had major blood loss and resuscitation.

Scoliosis surgery is painful and there are a number of ways to manage the pain. For patients who can do so, a PCA is appropriate. Adjunctive pain medicines including acetaminophen and ketamine may be helpful. Many surgeons prefer to avoid ketorolac or ibuprofen due to the potential for inhibition of bone healing.

In addition to blood loss and positioning injuries, complications of scoliosis surgery can include coagulopathy, postoperative visual loss (POVL), infection, pneumothorax, neurological injury including paralysis, and cardiovascular collapse as a result of hemorrhage, anaphylaxis, or air embolism.

When there is an emergency during spine surgery, the surgeon focuses on controlling bleeding and covering the incision to maintain sterility in preparation for a quick "flip" to the supine position. A stretcher should always be available either inside or just outside the operating room for this purpose. The anesthesia team focuses on resuscitation and the differential diagnosis. Once the patient has been stabilized a decision needs to be collaboratively made whether to abort the surgery. Factors that must be considered include ongoing hemodynamic changes, bleeding and risk of bleeding, spine instability, and neurological injury as indicated by neurophysiological monitoring.

Acute Presentations

Fractures

Pediatric fractures differ from adult fractures in several ways. Pediatric bones have periosseous cartilage, physes, and a thicker, stronger, more osteogenic periosteum, which produces new bone more rapidly and in greater amounts. They are also lower in density and are more porous. These differences result in lower elasticity and bending strength.[68] Children are prone to remodeling and potential overgrowth at the site of the fracture. Injuries to the physes can cause progressive deformities and this type of fracture should be observed over the long term.

Fractures can alert the health care team to the potential for child abuse because they are the second most common manifestation of abuse, after skin changes such as bruising, burns, and abrasions.[68] Fractures that should raise suspicion of abuse include femur fractures in nonambulatory children, distal femoral metaphyseal corner fractures, posterior rib fractures, scapular spinous process fractures, and proximal humeral fractures.[68] These fractures are not definite indicators of abuse and there are situations in which underlying disease can mimic the fracture pattern of abuse such as osteogenesis imperfecta and osteomyelitis. Suspected nonaccidental trauma needs to be reported and managed by a specially trained team. However, the operating room may be an opportune time to examine the child and document injuries.

Fractures around the elbow in children require aggressive management to protect against malunion or nonunion.[68] The fractures may be transcondylar, supracondylar, and epiphyseal. Displaced supracondylar fractures may have associated neurovascular injury that may warrant immediate intervention. Operative treatment for distal humeral fractures is closed reduction and pinning when possible. Inadequate reductions can result in limitation of motion, cubitus varus or valgus, and nonunion or instability.[68]

Hip fractures in children are relatively uncommon but may present with surgical urgency. They result from high-impact trauma and are likely to have associated injuries. The rate of avascular necrosis is as high as 50% without urgent reduction, stable fixation, and spica casting.[68] In

the urgent setting, precautions against aspiration of gastric contents can be taken with a rapid sequence intubation. Regional anesthesia via a subarachnoid block or continuous epidural is less practical in this situation given the potential concurrent injuries and the risk of a full stomach or ileus.

Surgery for repair of fractures is indicated for displaced physeal fractures, displaced intra-articular fractures, unstable fractures, multiple injuries, open fractures, failure to achieve or maintain adequate reduction, and pathological fractures.[68] Surgical goals include restoration of alignment and stability. External fixation may be indicated for open fractures or fractures associated with other injuries as well as fractures associated with vascular or nerve injury.

Complications from fractures include growth arrest, or premature physeal closure, misalignment avascular necrosis, and compartment syndrome. Other risks include infection and neurovascular compromise postoperatively. There can be limb deformities from partial or complete closure of the physis. Complex regional pain syndrome is a rare but potentially debilitating complication.[68]

PERIOPERATIVE COMPLICATIONS

Venous Thromboembolism

Venous thromboembolism (VTE), including the clinical conditions of deep vein thrombosis (DVT) and pulmonary embolism (PE), is increasingly relevant to pediatric patients. The increased incidence is thought to be due to better surveillance and diagnosis and longer survival of children with chronic diseases.

The incidence of VTE in children increased by 70% from 2001 to 2007 (from 34 to 58 cases per 10,000 hospital admissions in tertiary care facilities).[69] Of patients admitted with a diagnosis of VTE in the same cohort, the incidence of PE was 11% and mortality was 8%.[69] The mortality of children who suffer from PE is 2.2%.[70,71] Infants younger than 1 year of age and adolescents are more likely than other children to develop VTE.

A high index of suspicion for VTE as well as a clear understanding of risk factors are essential in diagnosing and preventing the potentially catastrophic complication of massive PE. The single most important risk factor for VTE in the pediatric population is the presence of a central venous catheter (CVC).[70] More than 50% of DVTs in children and 80% of DVTs in newborns occur in patients with indwelling central lines.[71] Infection, including osteomyelitis, septic arthritis, septicemia, and local infection, was the second most common risk factor for VTE.[70] Other common risk factors for pediatric VTE include surgery, malignancy, trauma, heart disease, and nephrotic syndrome.

A venous thrombus can form when there is hemostasis and hypercoagulability or damage to the vessel endothelium which occur during trauma and surgery. Pulmonary embolism is the result of a dislodged thrombus from a deep vein. The thrombus can travel through the venous system until it reaches the right atrium and from there occlude the pulmonary arteries. An otherwise healthy child may remain asymptomatic with up to 50% of the pulmonary circulation occluded. With a massive PE, cardiopulmonary collapse can result from an acute increase in RV afterload, resulting in RV dilation and increased RV and PA pressures. Ultimately, cardiac output can be compromised, and death can result.

Awake adolescent patients are most likely to complain of pleuritic chest pain with a new onset PE. Younger patients may present with unexplained tachypnea. Intraoperative manifestations of a PE may include the sudden onset of hypoxemia, hypertension, and loss of end-tidal carbon dioxide (which indicates a loss of cardiac output). The diagnosis can be supported by intraoperative transesophageal echocardiogram (TEE) when available. When a PE is suspected intraoperatively, the surgery should be completed or aborted as quickly as possible. The diagnosis can be confirmed by CT or MRI once the patient is stabilized. Once diagnosis is made, initial therapy is likely a heparin infusion or low-molecular-weight heparin injection. A hematologist should be consulted for evaluation of underlying procoagulant states. A postsurgical patient may be best treated with unfractionated heparin due to the shorter half-life of the medication in the event of postoperative bleeding. Children who have less of a bleeding risk may benefit from low-molecular-weight heparin since it is dosed subcutaneously and does not need to have drug levels closely monitored.

Other complications include major hemorrhage as well as recurrent thrombus formation. Children are at risk of developing long-term disability from postthrombotic syndrome, which is a result of damage to the venous valves causing swelling and pain due to venous insufficiency. Other clinical manifestations of VTE may include cerebral sinovenous thrombosis, renal vein thrombosis, peripheral arterial thrombosis, and stroke as well as thrombotic storm, which is a rapidly progressive multifocal thrombosis that can result in multiorgan system dysfunction.[72]

Fat Embolism Syndrome

While fat embolism is nearly universal in patients with long bone fractures, fat embolism syndrome (FES) occurs with far less frequency. Fat emboli occur in as many as 90% of patients with long bone fractures, but symptomatic FES occurs in only 10% to 20% of patients with long bone or pelvic fractures. Symptomatic FES increases to 30% with multiple fractures.[10] The syndrome is characterized by a triad of hypoxemia, neurological changes, and a petechial rash. The onset of symptoms is approximately 48 to 72 hours after the injury and usually the first symptom is respiratory insufficiency. Most patients don't develop the complete triad of symptoms.

There are two theories of FES pathophysiology: mechanical and biochemical. The mechanical theory describes the direct damage caused by fat globules that are released into the pulmonary, neurological, and cutaneous systems. Essentially, fat globules are released at the site of injury and enter blood vessels. From the venous system, they can pass into the arterial system via the lungs or a patent foramen ovale (PFO). The biochemical theory describes the localized reaction of free fatty acids in the pulmonary microvasculature resulting in hemorrhage and inflammation. The resulting clinical syndrome is much like acute respiratory distress syndrome.[10]

Under anesthesia, the most likely presentation of FES is hypoxia without another explanation. The patient may exhibit a drop in the arterial oxygen concentration, hematocrit, platelet, and fibrinogen levels. Fulminant FES is most likely to occur 30 minutes after transfer to the operating room table. Clinically, the patient will exhibit progressive oxygen desaturation, hypotension, tachycardia, bradycardia, dysrhythmia, decreased lung compliance, pulmonary edema, and disseminated intravascular coagulation.[10] Treatment of FES is supportive. Patients may benefit from bronchoalveolar lavage to remove particles of fat and hemorrhage. This is also the most rapid and specific method of FES diagnosis. The mortality rate of FES in children is 33%.[10]

CONCLUSION

The variety of pediatric patients who present for orthopedic surgery is immense. Common themes which can improve care for patients intraoperatively include knowledge of the underlying disease process or pathophysiology, extreme care with positioning, attention to potential blood loss, and teamwork. Anesthesiologists can positively impact long-term outcomes by fostering a connection with each individual patient and family and leading the operative team through any crisis that may arise.

REFERENCES

1. Ferguson J, Hwang SW, Tataren Z, Samdani AF. Neuromonitoring changes in pediatric spinal deformity surgery: a single-institution experience. *J Neurosurg Pediatr*. 2014;13:247-254.
2. Cheng MA, Todorov A, Tempelhoff R, McHugh T, Crowder CM, Lauryssen C. The effect of prone positioning on intraocular pressure in anesthetized patients. *Anesthesiology*. 2001;95:1351-1355.
3. Zuckerberg AL, Yaster M. Anesthesia for pediatric orthopedic surgery. In: Davis PJ, Cladis FP, eds. *Smith's Anesthesia for Infants and Children*. 9th ed. Elsevier;2017:865-891.
4. CDC. HAI data. Available at https://www.cdc.gov/hai/surveillance/index.html. Accessed March 20, 2020.
5. National Nosocomial Infections Surveillance (NNIS) System Report, data summary from January 1992 through June 2004, issued October 2004. *Am J Infect Control*. 2004;32:470-485.
6. Bruny JL, Hall BL, Barnhart DC, et al. American College of Surgeons National Surgical Quality Improvement Program Pediatric: A beta phase report. *J Pediatr Surg*. 2013;48:74-80.

7. Shah GS, Christensen RE, Wagner DS, Pearce BK, Sweeney J, Tait AR. Retrospective evaluation of antimicrobial prophylaxis in prevention of surgical site infection in the pediatric population. *Pediatr Anesth*. 2014;24:994-998.

8. Bucher BT, Guth RM, Elward AM, et al. Risk factors and outcomes of surgical site infection in children. *J Am Coll Surg*. 2011;212(6):1033-1038.

9. Loftus RW, Koff MD, Birnbach DJ. The dynamics and implications of bacterial transmission events arising from the anesthesia work area. *Anesth Analg*. 2015;120(4):853-860.

10. Zuckerberg AL, Yaster M. Anesthesia for orthopedic surgery. In: Davis PJ, ed. *Smith's Anesthesia for Infants and Children*. 8th ed. Philadelphia, PA: Elsevier; 2011:842-869.

11. Edler A, Murray DJ, Forbes RB. Blood loss during posterior spinal fusion surgery in patients with neuromuscular disease: is there an increased risk? *Pediatr Anesth*. 2003;13:818-822.

12. Ialenti MN, Lonner BS, Verma K, Dean L, Valdevit A, Errico T. Predicting operative blood loss during spinal fusion for adolescent idiopathic scoliosis. *J Pediatr Orthoped*. 2013;33(4):372-376.

13. Sethna NF, Zurakowski D, Brustowicz RM, Bacsik J, Sullivan LJ, Shapiro F. Tranexamic acid reduces intraoperative blood loss in pediatric patients undergoing scoliosis surgery. *Anesthesiology*. 2005;102:727-732.

14. Yagi M, Hasegawa J, Nagoshi N, et al. Does the intraoperative tranexamic acid decrease operative blood loss during posterior spinal fusion for treatment of adolescent idiopathic scoliosis? *Spine (Phila Pa 1976)*. 2012;37(21):E1336-E1342.

15. Florentino-Pineda I, Thompson GH, Poe-Kochert C, Huang RP, Haber LL, Blakemore LC. The effect of Amicar on perioperative blood loss in idiopathic scoliosis: the results of a prospective, randomized double blind study. *Spine (Phila Pa 1976)*. 2004;29:233-238.

16. Thompson GH, Florentino-Pineda I, Poe-Kochert C, Armstrong DG, Son-Hing J. Role of amicar in surgery for neuromuscular scoliosis. *Spine*. 2008;33(24):2623-2629.

17. Florentino-Pineda I, Blakemore LC, Thompson GH, Poe-Kochert C, Adler P, Tripi P. The effect of epsilon-aminocaproic acid on perioperative blood loss in patients with idiopathic scoliosis undergoing posterior spinal fusion: a preliminary prospective study. *Spine (Phila Pa 1976)*. 2001;26(10):1147-1151.

18. Halanski MA, Cassidy JA, Hetzel S, Reischmann D, Hassan N. The efficacy of amicar versus tranexamic acid in pediatric spinal deformity surgery: a prospective, randomized, double-blinded pilot study. *Spine Deform*. 2014;2:191-197.

19. Horstmann HM, Conroy CM, Davidson RS. Chapter 682 arthrogryposis. In: Kliegman RM, Stanton BMD, Geme JS, Schor NF, eds. *Nelson Textbook of Pediatrics*. 20th ed. Philadelphia, PA: Elsevier; 2016:3310-3314.

20. Baum VC, O'Flaherty JE. Arthrogryposis. In: Baum VC, O'Flaherty JE, eds. *Anesthesia for Genetic, Metabolic, & Dysmorphic Syndromes of Childhood*. 3rd ed. Philadelphia, PA: Wolters Kluwer; 2015:42-43.

21. Wu EY, Bryan AR, Rabinovich CE. Juvenile idiopathic arthritis. In: Kliegman RM, Stanton BMD, Geme JS, Schor NF, eds. *Nelson Textbook of Pediatrics*. 20th ed. Philadelphia, PA: Elsevier; 2016:1160-1170.

22. Scott BK, Baranov D. Neurologic diseases. In: Fleisher LA, ed. *Anesthesia and Uncommon Diseases*. 6th ed. Philadelphia, PA: Elsevier; 2012:chap. 8:251-295. Print.

23. O'Toole P, Spiegel DA. The neck. In: Kliegman RM, Stanton BMD, Geme JS, Schor NF, eds. *Nelson Textbook of Pediatrics*. 20th ed. Philadelphia: Elsevier; 2016:chap. 680:3297-3301.

24. Baum VC, O'Flaherty JE. Klippel-Feil sequence. In: Baum VC, O'Flaherty JE, eds. *Anesthesia for Genetic, Metabolic, & Dysmorphic Syndromes of Childhood*. 3rd ed. Philadelphia, PA: Wolters Kluwer; 2015:231-232.

25. Boas SR. Skeletal diseases influencing pulmonary function. In: Kliegman RM, Stanton BMD, Geme JS, Schor NF, eds. *Nelson Textbook of Pediatrics*. 20th ed. Philadelphia, PA: Elsevier; 2016:chap. 417:2144-2146.

26. Horton WA, Hecht JT. Disorders involving transmembrane receptors. In: Kliegman RM, Stanton BMD, Geme JS, Schor NF, eds. *Nelson Textbook of Pediatrics*. 20th ed. Philadelphia, PA: Elsevier; 2016:chap. 696:3370-3372.

27. Tetzlaff JE, Benedetto PX. Skin and bone disorders. In: Fleisher LA, ed. *Anesthesia and Uncommon Diseases*. 6th ed. Philadelphia, PA: Elsevier; 2012:chap. 10:319-349.

28. Marini JC. Osteogenesis imperfecta. In: Kliegman RM, Stanton BMD, Geme JS, Schor NF, eds. *Nelson Textbook of Pediatrics*. 20th ed. Philadelphia, PA: Elsevier; 2016:chap. 701:3380-3384.

29. Baum VC, O'Flaherty JE. Osteogenesis imperfecta. In: Baum VC, O'Flaherty JE, eds. *Anesthesia for Genetic, Metabolic, & Dysmorphic Syndromes of Childhood*. 3rd ed. Philadelphia, PA: Wolters Kluwer; 2015:337-339.

30. Horton WA, Hecht JT. Disorders involving defective bone resorption. In: Kliegman RM, Stanton BMD, Geme JS, Schor NF, eds. *Nelson Textbook of Pediatrics*. 20th ed. Philadelphia, PA: Elsevier; 2016:chap. 699:3375-3376.

31. Baum VC, O'Flaherty JE. Osteopetrosis. In: Baum VC, O'Flaherty JE, eds. *Anesthesia for Genetic, Metabolic, & Dysmorphic Syndromes of Childhood*. 3rd ed. Philadelphia, PA: Wolters Kluwer; 2015:339-341.

32. Baum VC, O'Flaherty JE. Marfan syndrome. In: Baum VC, O'Flaherty JE, eds. *Anesthesia for Genetic, Metabolic, & Dysmorphic Syndromes of Childhood*. 3rd ed. Philadelphia, PA: Wolters Kluwer; 2015:267-269.

33. Doyle A, Doyle JJ, Dietz HC. Marfan syndrome. In: Kliegman RM, Stanton BMD, Geme JS, Schor NF. *Nelson Textbook of Pediatrics*. 20th ed. Philadelphia, PA: Elsevier; 2016:3384-3389.

34. De Maio F, Fichera A, De Luna V, Mancini F, Caterini R. Orthopaedic aspects of marfan syndrome: the experience of a referral center for diagnosis of rare diseases. *Adv Orthop*. 2016;2016:8275391.

35. Guard Y, Launay F, Edgard-Rosa G, Collignon P, Jouve J, Bollini G. Scoliotic curve patterns in patients with Marfan syndrome. *J Child Orthoped*. 2008;2:211-216.

36. Pepe G, Giusti B, Sticchi E, Abbate R, Genuine GF, Nistri S. Marfan syndrome: current perspectives. *Appl Clin Gene*. 2016;9:55-65. Available at http://dx.doi.org/10.2147/TACG.596233.

37. Baran S, Ignys A, Ingys I. Respiratory dysfunction in patients with Marfan syndrome. *J Physiol Pharmacol*. 2007;58(suppl 5):37-41.

38. Kohler M, Pitcher A, Blair E, et al. The impact of obstructive sleep apnea on aortic disease in Marfan's syndrome. *Respiration*. 2013;86:39-44.

39. Li M, Quanying H, Yinna W, Birong D, Jinhan H. High prevalence of obstructive sleep apnea in Marfan's syndrome. *Chinese Med J*. 2014;127 (17):3150-3155.

40. De Paepe A, Devereux RB, Dietz HC, et al. Revised diagnostic criteria for the Marfan syndrome. *Am J Med Genet*. 1996;62:417-26.

41. Veldhoen S, Stark V, Mueller GC, et al. Pediatric patients with Marfan syndrome: frequency of dural ectasia and its correlation with common cardiovascular manifestations. *Fortschr Röntgenstr*. 2014;186:61-66.

42. Beighton P, De Paepe A, Steinmann B, Tsipouras P, Wenstrup RJ. Ehrlers-Danlos syndromes: revised nosology, villefranche, 1997. Ehrlers-danlos National foundation (USA) and Ehrlers-danlos support group (UK). *Am J Med Genet.* 1998;77(1):31-37.

43. Weismann, Castori M, Malfait F, Wulf H. Recommendations for anesthesia and perioperative management in patients with Ehlers-Danlos syndrome(s). *Orph J Rare Dis.* 2014;9:109.

44. Arendt-Nielsen L, Kaalund S, Bjerring P, Hogsaa B. Insufficient effect of local analgesics in Ehlers Danlos type III patients (connective tissue disorder). *Acta Anaesthesiol Scand.* 1990;34:358-361.

45. Hakim AJ, Grahame R, Norris P, Hopper C. Local anaesthetic failure in joint hypermobility syndrome. *J Royal Soc Med.* 2005;98:84-85

46. Stine KC, Becton DL. DDAVP therapy controls bleeding in Ehlers-Danlos syndrome. *J Pediatr Hematol Oncol.* 1997;19:156-158.

47. Burcharth J, Rosenberg J. Gastrointestinal surgery and related complications in patients with Ehlers-Danlos syndrome: a systematic review. *Dig Surg.* 2012;29:349-357.

48. Data & statistics for cerebral palsy. Centers for Disease Control and Prevention, 02 May 2016. Available at https://www.cdc.gov/ncbddd/cp/data.html. Accessed January 25, 2017.

49. Johnston MV. Encephalopathies. In: Kliegman RM, Stanton BMD, Geme JS, Schor NF, eds. *Nelson Textbook of Pediatrics.* 20th ed. Philadelphia, PA: Elsevier; 2016:2896-2910.

50. Diu MW, Mancuso TJ. Pediatric diseases. In: Hines RL, Katherine E. Marschall KE, eds. *Stoelting's Anesthesia and Co-Existing Disease.* 6th ed. Philadelphia, PA: Elsevier; 2012:583-641.

51. Urban MK. Muscle diseases. In: Fleisher LA, ed. *Anesthesia and Uncommon Diseases.* 6th ed. Philadelphia, PA: Elsevier; 2012:296-318.

52. Spinal muscular atrophy. Available at https://ghr.nlm.nih.gov/condition/spinal-muscular-atrophy#statistics. Accessed April 12, 2017.

53. Haaker G, Fujak A. Proximal spinal muscular atrophy: current orthopedic perspective. *Applicat Clin Genet.* 2013;6:113-120.

54. Graham RJ, Athiraman U, Laubach AE, Sethna NF. Anesthesia and perioperative medical management of children with spinal muscular atrophy. *Pediatr Anesth.* 2009;19:1054-1063. Accessed April 12, 2017.

55. Finkel RS, Chiriboga CA, Vajsar J, et al. Treatment of infantile-onset spinal muscular atrophy with nusinersen: a phase 2, open-label, dose-escalation study. *Lancet.* 2016;388(10063):3017-3026.

56. Sahin M. Neurocutaneous syndromes. In: Kliegman RM, Stanton BMD, Geme JS, Schor NF. *Nelson Textbook of Pediatrics.* 20th ed. Philadelphia, PA: Elsevier; 2016:2874-2881.

57. Pasternak JJ, Lanier WL. Congenital anomalies of the brain. In: Hines RL, Marschall KE, eds. *Stoelting's Anesthesia and Co-Existing Disease.* 6th ed. Philadelphia, PA: Elsevier; 2012:218-254.

58. Baldwin KD, Wells L. Torsional and angular deformities. In: Kliegman RM, Stanton BMD, Geme JS, Schor NF, eds. *Nelson Textbook of Pediatrics.* 20th ed. Philadelphia, PA: Elsevier; 2016:3257-3263.

59. Sankar WN, Horn BD, Wells L, Dormans JP. The hip. In: Kliegman RM, Stanton BMD, Geme JS, Schor NF, eds. *Nelson Textbook of Pediatrics.* 20th ed. Philadelphia, PA: Elsevier; 2016:3274-3283.

60. Winell JJ, Davidson RS. The foot and toes. In: Kliegman RM, Stanton BMD, Geme JS, Schor NF, eds. *Nelson Textbook of Pediatrics.* 20th ed. Philadelphia, PA: Elsevier; 2016:3247-3257.

61. Wudbhav NS, Horn BD, Wells L, Dormans JP. The hip. In: Kliegman RM, Stanton BMD, Geme JS, Schor NF, eds. *Nelson Textbook of Pediatrics.* 20th ed. Philadelphia, PA: Elsevier; 2016:3274-3283.

62. Davidson RS. Leg-length discrepancy. In: Kliegman RM, Stanton BMD, Geme JS, Schor NF, eds. *Nelson Textbook of Pediatrics.* 20th ed. Philadelphia, PA: Elsevier; 2016:3264-3267.

63. Glassman SD, et al. The effect of postoperative nonsteroidal anti-inflammatory drug administration on spinal fusion. *Spine.* 1998;23(7):834-838.

64. Cottrell J, O'Connor JP. Effect of non-steroidal anti-inflammatory drugs on bone healing. *Pharmaceuticals.* 2010;3:1668-1693.

65. Wall LB, Goldfarb CA. Congenital upper limb deficiencies. In: Martus JE, ed. *Orthopaedic Knowledge Update Pediatrics 5.* Rosemont, IL: American Academy of Orthopaedic Surgeons; 2016:217-226.

66. Mistovich RJ, Spiegel DA. The Spine. In: Kliegman RM, Stanton BMD, Geme JS, Schor NF, eds. *Nelson Textbook of Pediatrics.* 20th ed. Philadelphia, PA: Elsevier; 2016:3283-3297.

67. Matei VA, Haddadin AS. Systemic and pulmonary arterial hypertension. In: Hines RL, Marschall KE, eds. *Stoelting's Anesthesia and Co-Existing Disease.* 6th ed. Philadelphia, PA: Elsevier; 2012:104-119.

68. Baldwin KD, Wells L, Dormans JP. Common fractures. In: Kliegman RM, Stanton BMD, Geme JS, Schor NF, eds. *Nelson Textbook of Pediatrics.* 20th ed. Philadelphia, PA: Elsevier; 2016:3314-3322.

69. Raffini L, Huang YS, Witmer C, Feudtner C. Dramatic increase in venous thromboembolism in children's hospitals in the United States from 2001 to 2007. *Pediatrics.* 2009;124(4):1001-1008. Accessed March 29, 2017.

70. Kim SJ, Sabharwal S. Risk factors for venous thromboembolism in hospitalized children and adolescents: a systemic review and pooled analysis. *J Pediatr Orthoped B.* 2014;23:389-393. Accessed March 29, 2017.

71. Nevin MA. Pulmonary embolism, infarction, and hemorrhage. In: Kliegman RM, Stanton BMD, Geme JS, Schor NF, eds. *Nelson Textbook of Pediatrics.* 20th ed. Philadelphia, PA: Elsevier; 2016:2123-2128.

72. Raffini LJ, Scott JP. Thrombotic disorders in children. In: Kliegman RM, Stanton BMD, Geme JS, Schor NF, eds. *Nelson Textbook of Pediatrics.* 20th ed. Philadelphia, PA: Elsevier; 2016:2394-2397.

Trauma and Special Emergencies

Cathie Tingey Jones

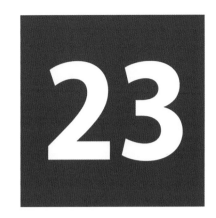

23

FOCUS POINTS

1. Trauma is the leading cause of pediatric mortality and these patients are best served at facilities equipped to treat children.
2. Injuries not in character with the play patterns of children should raise concerns for nonaccidental trauma.
3. The primary survey for pediatric patients is ABCDE: Airway, Breathing, Circulation, Disability, and Exposure.
4. It is important to prevent hypothermia in trauma patients to avoid the triad of acidosis, coagulopathy, and death.
5. Burn patients are in a hypermetabolic state and have altered pharmacodynamics of many drugs, including neuromuscular blockers. They can also become very tolerant to pain medications.
6. If inhalational injury is suspected in a burn patient, intubation should happen early.

Traumatic injuries are an important public health concern in pediatrics. Accidents are the leading cause of death in children over the age of 1. Unintentional injury was responsible for 17,603 deaths in the United States in patients ages 19 years and under in 2017.[1] Twenty-five children in the United States die from injuries every day.[2] Accidental injury also places a large cost burden on the health care system, exceeding $20 billion annually in costs.[3]

TYPES OF INJURY

Falls are the leading cause of nonfatal injuries in children from birth to age 14. Motor vehicle accidents are the leading cause of death for 5- to 19-year-olds. Drowning is the most common cause of death in children ages 1 to 4. Burns are also common causes of mortality from ages 1 to 9. Other types of unintentional injuries common in children are suffocation, poisoning, burns, and sports or recreation injuries.[2,4]

Non-Accidental Trauma

While many injuries are unintentional, child abuse, or non-accidental trauma, is a wide spread concern. Over 3 million reports of child abuse are filed annually in the United States. However, it is likely under-reported and under-detected. The majority of fatalities from child abuse in the United States are in children under 3 years of age, with the greatest percentage under 1 year of age.[5] For the protection of the child, it is important to consider early if the injury pattern is suggestive of intentional injury is suggestive of intentional injury.

Some injuries reflect normal childhood behavior and experiences. Toddlers learning to walk and climb are prone to falling. School-aged children are prone to playground accidents. Normal patterns of injury include shin bruises and forehead bumps for toddlers or forearm and elbow fractures from playground accidents. Patterns of injury that should raise concerns include bruising in areas that aren't usually bumped when walking or running (eg, thigh bruises), rib fractures, fracture of base or vault of skull, eye contusions, intracranial bleeding, multiple burns, and age younger than 1 year. Fractures of large bones, such as a femur, should also raise concern due to the amount of force needed for the fracture. Ribs are difficult to break due to the cartilaginous components of a child's chest. In accidental trauma, a child is more likely to have a pulmonary contusion without an overlying rib fracture.

Injury Prevention

Primary prevention in trauma aims to prevent the accident from ever happening. This includes improving traffic barriers or changing a dangerous intersection. Secondary prevention attempts to decrease the seriousness of the injury with aids such as car seats, seat belts, and air bags. Education to raise awareness about car seat safety, seat belt use, bicycle helmets, and household dangers is important to treat this problem. In the United States, the rate of death from unintentional injury has decreased due to implementation of injury prevention programs. Other injuries are unfortunately inflicted by family members or those caring for children. Parenting classes, childcare education, and stress reduction programs may be helpful in decreasing the incidence of these injuries as well.[2]

Tertiary prevention aims to minimize the problems and deterioration when the first two means fail. This includes appropriately identifying children with major trauma before hospital arrival. Many hospitals may not be equipped to deal with pediatric trauma. This allows referral to hospitals with the best resources to treat them and to activate transport teams if needed. Children have better outcomes when treated at centers equipped for pediatric trauma and should be preferentially triaged to pediatric trauma centers where available.[6]

PRESENTATION TO HOSPITAL

Before patients reach the emergency department, they usually have initial triage by Emergency Medical Systems (EMS). Appropriate triage is critical to identify seriously injured patients. The initial field triage considers Glasgow Coma Score, systolic blood pressure, and respiratory rate. This is the first point where a decision may be made to proceed to a designated trauma center. The second step looks at penetrating injuries, extremity, pelvic fractures, and chest wall instability. Steps 3 and 4 in field triage consider the mode of injury (fall from height >10 feet in children or high-risk auto crash) as well as if they are of extremes of age or have burns or other considerations.[7]

PRIMARY SURVEY

On presentation to the trauma center the primary survey, established from Advanced Trauma Life Support (ATLS), is key to establishing the patient's status in an organized manner. It has a simple mnemonic **ABCDE**: **A**irway, **B**reathing, **C**irculation, **D**isability, and **E**xposure. All of these assessments should be accomplished in the first 5 minutes after presentation.[8,9]

Some hospitals use aids to assist with the care of children. Luten and Broselow designed a system to help guide medical staff. Their system takes the length of the child, measured by the Broselow Tape, and approximates weight of the child. On the card, the appropriate equipment and dosing of common medications are listed. Some centers have carts stocked which correspond to the colors on the Broselow Tape and corresponding color-coded card.[10–12]

Many emergency departments are using ultrasound as part of their initial trauma assessment. A Focused Assessment with Sonography for Trauma (FAST) exam should be done immediately after the primary survey per ATLS guidelines. This can be done at the bedside in the emergency department. It looks at the four quadrants of the abdomen as well as assessing for the presence of hemothorax or pneumothorax checking pericardial fluid for signs tamponade. An extended FAST exam, E-FAST, adds the views to evaluate for pneumothorax.[13–16]

▶ Airway Maintenance with Cervical Spine Protection

The first step in the ATLS primary survey is ensuring a patent airway. Many EMS providers may not have experience or equipment for intubating a pediatric patient. The child may present to the emergency department with bag-valve-mask ventilation ensuing. Intubation is indicated if the patient has respiratory, circulatory, or neurological compromise.[8,9,17]

While cervical spine injuries are uncommon in children, it is important to maintain a neutral neck position during mask ventilation and intubation. In-line stabilization should be done before laryngoscopy to prevent the head from moving side to side and prevent flexion and extension.[16] Video laryngoscopy (VL) can be used but is not part of ATLS. VL has not been shown to improve mortality in trauma situations.[18]

▶ Breathing and Ventilation

Children presenting with breathing problems may have nasal flaring, grunting, or retractions. While assessing for adequacy of respirations, it is important to assess for intrathoracic pathology, such as a hemothorax or pneumothorax. This can be done with physical exam, portable x-ray, or bedside sonography. If a tension pneumothorax or hemothorax is found, a needle decompression or chest tube placement should occur in the trauma bay. A tension pneumothorax is more likely to cause hemodynamic instability in children and the institution of positive pressure ventilation may worsen vital signs.[9]

▶ Circulation with Hemorrhage Control

Adequacy of circulation should be determined at this step. Vascular access, if not already established in the field, should be obtained. Fluid resuscitation should be started or assessed (if underway) and laboratory studies obtained. External hemorrhage, if present, should be attempted to be controlled. If cardiac tamponade is present on FAST exam, a pericardiocentesis should be considered. If the cardiac arrest was witnessed after trauma, a thoracotomy should be considered. If there is no pulse, cardiac compressions should be started. The pelvis should also be examined for possible fracture or potential occult site of blood loss.[9]

Disability/Neurological Assessment

The patient's neurological status needs to be established. The Glasgow Coma Scale (GCS) is the most widely established way to communicate this, though it is modified slightly for young children (Table 23-1).

If the GCS is less than 8 or rapidly declining, intubation is indicated. The patient should be assessed for signs of potential herniation or spinal cord injury. If there is concern for herniation, moderate hyperventilation can be started, as well as osmotic agents if the patient is normotensive to temporize. The head of the patient's bed can also be elevated.

Exposure and Environmental Control

During the primary survey, the patient's clothing needs to be removed to fully evaluate the extent of his or her injury. If the patient is hypothermic, rewarming should be started.

SECONDARY SURVEY

After the primary survey, if the patient is stable, a secondary survey is done. It is a head to toe evaluation which includes a history and comprehensive physical and additional studies. If the patient is unstable and needs rapid operative care, it is important for this survey to be done after the patient is stabilized.

Injuries by System

Blunt trauma is the most common kind of traumatic injury in children. When a blunt force is applied to a child's body, multisystem trauma often occurs. Penetrating trauma typically comprises only 10% of injuries in children. While penetrating trauma is uncommon in pediatrics, it can lead to significant injury and disability. It is more likely to lead to operative intervention than blunt trauma.

Table 23-1. Modification of the Glasgow Coma Scale for Pediatric Patients

Type of Response	Score*	Age-Related Responses		
		>1 Year	<1 Year	
Eye-opening response	4	Spontaneous	Spontaneous	
	3	To verbal command	To shout	
	2	To pain	To pain	
	1	None	None	
		>1 Year	<1 Year	
Motor response	6	Obeys commands	Spontaneous	
	5	Localizes pain	Localizes pain	
	4	Withdraws to pain	Withdraws to pain	
	3	Abnormal flexion to pain (decorticate)	Abnormal flexion to pain (decorticate)	
	2	Abnormal extension to pain (decorticate)	Abnormal extension to pain (decorticate)	
	1	None	None	
		>5 Years	2–5 Years	0–2 Years
Verbal response	5	Oriented and converses	Appropriate words, phrases	Babbles, coos appropriately
Verbal response	5	Oriented and converses	Appropriate words, phrases	Babbles, coos appropriately
	4	Confused conversation	Inappropriate words	Cries but is consolable
	3	Inappropriate words	Persistent crying or screaming to pain	Persistent crying or screaming to pain
	2	Incomprehensive sounds	Grunts or moans to pain	Grunts or moans to pain
	1	None	None	None

*Scoring: severe, <9; moderate, 9–12; mild, 13–15.

Source: Modified with permission, from James HE, Anas NG, Perkin RM, eds. *Brain Insults in Infants and Children: Pathophysiology and Management.* 1985. Copyright © Grune and Stratton Inc. All rights reserved.

A surgeon should be consulted early in presentation if there are gunshot or stab wounds to the head, neck, chest, or abdomen. Gunshot wounds (GSWs) are classified by the velocity of the weapon: low, medium, and high. Low-velocity GSWs take an erratic path through soft tissue as they follow tissue planes and rarely penetrate bone. Medium- and high-velocity weapons make a more direct path through the body and cause injury when they enter and exit the body.

Head

Traumatic brain injury (TBI) is a significant public health concern. It is the most common cause of death and long-term disability from injury regardless of age. Most pediatric head trauma is minor and does not need operative intervention or hospitalization. Observation is still important, as signs of TBI may arise after discharge. In children with head injury, systemic blood pressure needs to be maintained in order to maintain cerebral perfusion pressure. While most children present with a systolic blood pressure (SBP) greater than 90 mm Hg, children who present with SBP less than 90 mm Hg had three times greater mortality than those who present with a SBP greater than 90 mm Hg.[19,20]

Neck

Children are less likely to have cervical spine fractures than adults. Their spines are more cartilaginous and the vertebrae are not completely ossified. When injury occurs from a substantial force, such as from a motor vehicle accident or fall, a C-spine injury is more likely. Cervical spine injury in children is typically in a more cephalad location: C3 or above. If a C-spine injury is suspected, or if patient's mental status is decreased or altered, the C-spine should be immobilized until further studies can be done. Fear, pain, age, and stranger anxiety can be confounding factors when examining for cervical spine injury. In nonverbal children, the examiner has to rely on facial expression, guarding & other less reliable inputs.[21,22]

It can be difficult to rule out cervical spine injury in children based on x-rays alone. There is a phenomenon called **S**pinal **C**ord **I**njury **W**ith**O**ut **R**adiographic **A**bnormality (SCIWORA). This may occur in 25% to 50% of children with spinal cord injuries. According to ATLS guidelines, a CT scan of the neck, to evaluate for fracture, may replace x-rays. While this has increased the number of fractures found, ligamentous injuries cannot be found on x-ray or CT. If there is concern for a ligamentous injury or SCIWORA, an MRI should be obtained when the patient is stable.[23,24]

Pseudosubluxation of the cervical spine is also a common finding in children. It appears as an anterior displacement of C2 on C3. The person examining the child needs to elucidate if it is a true subluxation or benign pseudo-subluxation. The appearance of pseudosubluxation on x-ray can be reduced by placing the child's head in sniffing position when the film is taken. This should only be done after consultation with the surgeon due to the risk of spinal cord injury. Older children who can cooperate can have an open mouth film taken. This allows evaluation of the more cephalad vertebrae and helps rule out a fracture and accounts for the potential pseudosubluxation.

Some children with genetic syndromes have predispositions to cervical spine injury, such as Down and Klippel–Feil syndromes. If there are findings, either clinical or radiographic, suggestive of injury, consultation with a specialist is recommended.[21-24]

Chest

Thoracic trauma is the second leading cause of traumatic death in children. Patients with abnormal vital signs, significant bony tenderness, or abnormal breath or heart sounds may have intrathoracic injury, and warrant additional evaluation. Due to a more cartilaginous thorax, internal injuries may be masked due to the lack of fractures. If a child has a rib fracture, without an underlying pulmonary contusion, it should raise the clinical suspicions for non-accidental trauma. Patients with rib fractures may require aggressive pain treatment to breathe adequately.

Abdominal

Children are more prone to abdominal trauma than adults. With a more compact torso, there is a smaller area to disperse the force. The organs are often larger, relative to the patient's size, and may project below the costal margin. They also have less abdominal fat to cushion them from the trauma. Approximately 5% to 10% of pediatric blunt trauma have intraabdominal injury.[25] Mortality after blunt trauma is generally low but increases as injury to organs and vessels are injured.

Children that have intraabdominal injuries and are hemodynamically unstable, despite fluid resuscitation, warrant operative intervention. Signs of hemorrhagic shock include tachycardia, narrow pulse pressures, prolonged capillary refill time, pallor, altered mental status, and decreased urine output. Other external signs to look for are ecchymoses, abrasions, tire marks, seat belt signs, abdominal tenderness or distension, and absent bowel sounds.[26]

Extremities

Some injuries to extremities may require immediate operative intervention. These include situations when there is neurovascular compromise to the extremity. The extremities should be examined for swelling, contusions, deformities, tenderness, and presence of pulses. If the patient is able to participate in the exam, sensation in extremities should be checked.

Anesthetic Care and Planning

When the patient is stable and time allows, a full preoperative evaluation should be conducted. Along with the traumatic presentation, this includes past medical and surgical history, family history of problems with anesthesia, review of systems, and time of last meal. If surgery needs to proceed rapidly, the preop assessment can be truncated to include many salient points.

NPO

When planning for the trauma anesthetic, if nil per os (NPO) status is unknown, it should be assumed that the patient has a full stomach. Gastric residual volume is greater in children undergoing emergency surgery versus elective surgery. Precautions should be taken to reduce the chance of aspiration. These may be pharmacological or mechanical, such as elevating the head of the bed during induction. A rapid sequence induction may be considered.[27]

Vascular Access

Adequate intravascular access is essential to post-trauma resuscitation. In pediatrics, the patient may have been uncooperative with intravenous (IV) catheter placement by EMS. Placing an IV catheter in a moving vehicle presents an extra level of difficulty, and decreased intravascular volume may increase the challenge. If the child arrives at the hospital without a peripheral intravenous (PIV) line, and a PIV line is not easily obtainable, an intraosseous (IO) line should be considered. Urgent life-saving care should not be delayed for placement of a central venous line without attempting an IO line. An IO line can be placed quickly with minimal discomfort for the patient. It is traditionally placed below the tibial tuberosity in children. The humerus and sternum have also been used.

Local anesthesia is typically not used for IO placement as the patient is often in extremis. After sterile preparation of the skin, the needle is inserted at 90 degrees to the skin and tibia. The needle is advanced using constant pressure and a rotating motion until a "give" is felt. This suggests that the needle has gone through the outer cortex of the bone and into the marrow. The stylet is removed from the needle and a syringe attached. Using the syringe, marrow or blood should be aspirated and can be sent for lab tests if needed. If no marrow is obtained, fluid should freely flow to gravity through the needle. The surrounding area can be palpated for extravasation of fluid. Fluid may flow slowly, so medication should be followed by a saline flush. An ultrasound can confirm placement of the IO needle. It is important not to insert the needle too far in small children as it can come out the backside of the bone. IO needles should be replaced as soon as more definitive access can be obtained.[28,29]

Central venous access can be obtained via the Seldinger technique. The femoral vein can be easily accessed in an awake child. Placing the patient in a cervical collar, if there is concern for head and neck injury, can also impede central venous access. If an internal jugular or subclavian location is preferred the patient may require some sedation. Ultrasound guidance can be used to facilitate visualization of the vessel and placement of the central line. Nonpediatric centers may be limited in what catheters they have for central access in pediatric patients.

Airway

If the patient has not had his or her airway secured prior to arrival in the operating room, adequate equipment should be available. Personnel should also be available to maintain in-line stabilization to protect the cervical spine if it has not been cleared. Additional equipment and personnel should be ready and available if there are concerns that the airway will be difficult to manage.

Blood and Fluid Resuscitation

Massive hemorrhage is uncommon in the pediatric population. When it occurs, it is typically the result of injury to solid viscera or major vascular structures. Traumatic injury severe enough to cause exsanguination typically results in death at the scene of the accident. In both adults and children, approximately 25% of trauma patients receive blood transfusions.

Children typically maintain their blood pressure for a longer period than adults following blood loss. The first sign of blood loss in a child may be tachycardia, which may appear when 10% to 20% of the patient's blood volume is lost. Hypotension typically does not present until 25% or more of the patient's blood volume has been lost. The presence of hypotension due to hypovolemia is a concerning sign and may signal impending cardiovascular collapse.

The primary goal of resuscitation is to maintain the patient's intravascular volume. Massive transfusion and fluid resuscitation after injury may result in a coagulopathy. Massive transfusion in children is defined as replacement of 1 blood volume in 24 hours or 50% of the blood volume in 3 hours.[30] The coagulopathy is usually from the dilution of clotting factors and thrombocytopenia. Hypothermia may also contribute to clotting problems, and should be actively treated. Fibrinolysis or disseminated intravascular coagulation (DIC) may also occur after a traumatic injury, but like hypothermia, they are not the most likely cause of coagulopathy. The "triad of death" consists of coagulopathy, hypothermia, and acidosis.[30–32]

It is important to know your institution's ability to handle a massive transfusion. Whenever possible, pediatric patients with anticipated need for transfusion should be triaged to a center with this capability. The blood bank should be notified as soon as it is anticipated that large volumes of blood may be needed to allow time for preparation. Additional personnel such as additional anesthesia providers, nurses, or other operating room staff may be

Massive Hemorrhage

Defined: Hemodynamic instability with blood loss > ~ 40 mL/kg or expecting needing to replace patient's total blood volume over 24 hours or less

- Contact Blood Bank to activate pediatric massive transfusion protocol (MTP)
- Send blood sample for type & cross
- If typed blood is not available, use uncrossmatched O negative PRBCs and AB+ plasma until type specific blood is available
- Recommend transfusing at ratio of 1 PRBC: 1FFP: 1 platelet unit
- Treat for Hemoglobin (hgb) <7, Platelet <50,000, INR>1.5, Fibrinogen <100 mg/dL
  - PRBC 10-20 mL/kg (4 mL/kg increases Hgb by 1)
  - FFP 10-15 mL/kg
  - Platelets 2-3 mL/kg or 1unit/10 kg
  - Cryoprecipitate 5 mL/kg or 1U/5 kg
- Maintain normothermia
- Check labs frequently to monitor CBC, Electrolytes, ABG, PT/PTT/INR, Fibrinogen & lactate
- Monitor for hyperkalemia, give calcium gluconate 50-100 mg/kg or calcium chloride 20 mg/kg if needed
- Watch for signs of citrate toxicity: hypocalcemia and hypomagnesemia
  - Calcium: CaGluconate 30-50 mg/kg or CaChloride10-20 mg/kg
  - Magnesium: if Mg<1.5 mg/dL, Mg Sulfate 50 mg/kg
- When bleeding is under control, contact blood bank to stop MTP

▲ **Figure 23-1.** Massive hemorrhage critical events checklist. (Data from Society for Pediatric Anesthesia. *Critical Events Checklist*. 2018. https://www.pedsanesthesia.org/critical-events-checklist/. Copyright © Society for Pediatric Anesthesia. All rights reserved.)

needed to check blood products as well as get the blood components from the blood bank.[7]

There is not a fixed formula for when to transfuse packed red blood cells (PRBCs), platelets, or clotting factors in pediatric trauma. Most of the studies have been carried out in adults and extrapolated to pediatrics. Transfusion exclusively of PRBCs is known to dilute clotting factors and platelets. The adult trauma literature suggests that transfusing plasma and platelets early in trauma care can prevent some of the acute coagulopathy.[34,35] Many adult centers use a 6:6:1 transfusion strategy (6 units PRBCs:6 units FFP:1 unit of pooled platelets) for trauma patients expected to receive a large volume of blood. There is one pediatric study in combat trauma patients that showed higher mortality in patients receiving balanced component transfusion.[36] However, other pediatric studies support the balanced approach.[37,38] There is also some evidence to support the use of antifibrinolytics such as tranexamic acid in trauma patients, including pediatric trauma. It has been shown to be associated with decreased mortality in combat patients; however, this may not extrapolate to blunt trauma patients.[39–42]

Other problems with massive transfusion are hypothermia and hyperkalemia. Warming the blood products prior to transfusing prevents the blood products from contributing to hypothermia. Hyperkalemia is more common when older blood products are transfused, due to the higher amount of lysed RBCs in the unit. This potassium load can be diminished by transfusing the freshest blood possible. Another option to lower the potassium is washing the blood cells prior to transfusion. As the RBCs need time to be washed, this is typically not something that can be done in the setting of rapid or massive transfusion.

Temperature Regulation

Operating room temperature is the most important factor influencing heat loss in surgical patients. The average surgical patient will maintain his or her core temperature if the room temperature is 23°C for adults or 26 °C for infants. Maintaining normothermia is important to help with peripheral perfusion, as well as preventing worsening coagulation from hypothermia.

Depending on the nature and extent of injuries, not all patients can have all of their definitive treatment on their initial trip to the operating room. The concept of "damage control surgery" has evolved in adults and pediatrics. The initial, life- and limb-threatening issues are treated surgically in the operating room. Then, if needed, the abdomen or other injured parts of the body are packed or a wound-vacuum system is used, and the patient is taken to the intensive care unit for further management of critical medical issues. This may require diuresis, stabilization of acid-base status, or completion of the secondary survey before the patient is ready to return to operating room to finish his or her surgical care.[43,44]

SPECIAL EMERGENCIES

▷ Burns

Burns are the fifth leading cause of death in children in the United States.[2] While mortality has declined due to advances in burn care and prevention, burn injury requires intensive treatment and has long-term disability. It is important to identify and treat injuries early, resuscitate appropriately, and refer to a burn center early in care in children with major burns.

Scald burns represent 65% of burns in children under age of five in the United States. Family education should occur whenever a child presents with scald burns. Turning down the temperature of the water heater to less than 120°F and turning in pan handles on the stove are simple measures that can decrease the incidence of these burns.[2] Scald injuries, although common, can be representative of non-accidental trauma to the child. Signs suggestive of non-accidental scald burns are injury inconsistent with the story, clear edges of the burn (as if the patient were submerged in the hot water), and lack of splash marks.[44-46]

Older children are more likely to be injured from actual fire and flames. Fireworks can cause severe burns to the hands, face, and eyes of older children. Electrical burns cause direct thermal damage. Chemical burns vary based on the substance and the duration of contact.[47]

Burns can be superficial, superficial partial-thickness, deep partial-thickness, or full-thickness. *Superficial* burns involve the epidermis. They are painful but heal quickly and without scarring. *Superficial partial-thickness* burns involve the epidermis and portions of the dermis. They typically form blisters. *Deep partial-thickness* burns extend into the deeper dermis. They damage hair follicles and glandular tissue; they can be difficult to distinguish from full-thickness burns. *Full-thickness* burns destroy the dermis and extend into the subcutaneous tissue. They are often white or black on the surface. As nerves are damaged in full-thickness burns, they are less painful than partial-thickness burns.[45]

Rule of 9s

The amount of body surface burned is typically estimated by the "Rule of 9s." A reference chart (see Figure 23-2) can be used to help estimate the portion of the body surface area burned. Palm size represents approximately 1% of a patient's total body surface area. Small children do not have the same rule of 9s as adults. Their head is larger relative to the rest of their body and represents a larger percent of total body surface area (TBSA) (see Figure 23-2), though the overall process of estimation is the same.

Severity of the burn is impacted by depth, TBSA, location of the injury, and the presence or absence of inhalation injury.[46]

Fluid Resuscitation

The Parkland formula represents the approximate crystalloid fluid needs over the initial 24 hours in a burn patient. It is meant as a guide for adequate fluid resuscitation so patients are not under-resuscitated. The formula is as follows: 4 mL × weight in kg × TBSA (%) burned plus normal maintenance fluid requirements. Half of the fluid should be given in the first 8 hours, with the remaining half given over the subsequent 16 hours. Urine output (UO) needs to be maintained at 1 mL/kg/h as it acts as a marker of organ perfusion. If the UO falls, additional fluids should be given. Children under 30 kg need to maintain UO of 1 to 2 mL/kg/h, while children 30 kg and greater need to maintain 0.5 to 1 mL/kg/h.

While the Parkland formula is most commonly used, it is not the only formula for burn victim's fluid resuscitation. Another formula, the Brooke formula, uses less fluid overall. Originally, the Brooke formula employed the use of colloids. The modified Brooke formula uses 2 mL × weight in kg × TBSA (%) burned. Additionally, it also titrates fluids to urine output. The Parkland formula is more commonly used in children as they have relatively higher daily fluid requirements than adults. Both formulas provide an estimate, and volume status should be monitored carefully.[44]

The use of colloids is controversial in burn patients. Some centers employ their use after 24 hours of resuscitation, others use them only when a patient's albumin levels decrease. As significant capillary leakage occurs in burned tissue, some experts feel colloids do not carry a significant benefit. There is currently no consensus on colloid use.[47-49]

The first 48 hours of a burn injury are considered the acute phase. During the acute phase the patient typically loses a large amount of protein and is hypovolemic. In the subsequent phase, after 48 hours, the patient enters a hypermetabolic phase. Early burn excision and grafting decreases the metabolic demands of the burn patient. As the patient's metabolic demands are highest in the first few days following a burn, early excision and grafting will help with healing and improve the patient's physiology.

Inhalational Injury and Intubation

Inhalational injury from smoke to the tracheobronchial tree is a concern whenever burn patients present. This is especially true with fires in enclosed spaces, such as house fires. Combustion of materials in a closed space can consume significant amounts of oxygen, leaving the patient in a hypoxic environment. Though the number of patients with true inhalational injury is small, when it does occur there is a high risk of morbidity and mortality. Patients with a high likelihood of inhalational injury should be intubated early.

Thermal damage, asphyxiation, and pulmonary irritation are the main mechanisms that lead to smoke inhalation injury. Thermal damage is typically limited to the oropharynx as heat typically dissipates by the time the air reaches the trachea. External signs of inhalational injury include facial burns, blistering/edema of the oropharynx, mucosal lesions, scorched nasal hairs, carbonaceous sputum, sooty secretions, singed eyebrows, hoarseness, and stridor.

The incidence of inhalational injury increases as the TBSA percentage increases. Intubation should be strongly

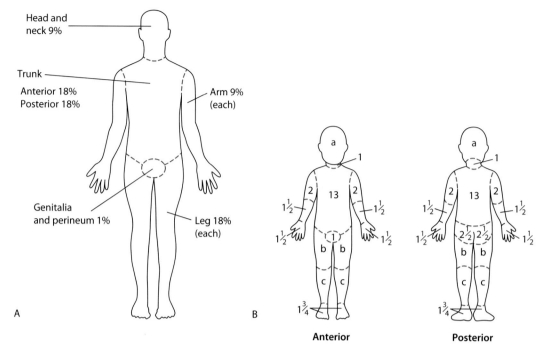

Relative percentage of body surface area (% BSA) affected by growth

Body part	Age				
	0 yr	1 yr	5 yr	10 yr	15 yr
a = 1/2 of head	9 1/2	8 1/2	6 1/2	5 1/2	4 1/2
b = 1/2 of 1 thigh	2 3/4	3 1/4	4	4 1/4	4 1/2
c = 1/2 of 1 lower leg	2 1/2	2 1/2	2 3/4	3	3 1/4

▲ **Figure 23-2.** Rule of Nines for calculating Body Surface Area (BSA) percentage burned. (A) Shows the BSA percentages for an adult using the Rule of Nines. (B) The table and associated drawing show how the Rule of Nines changes with age as a child's head is a large portion of their BSA when they are an infant but as they age their legs become a larger portion of their BSA. (Redrawn with permission, from Artz CP, JA Moncrief: *The Treatment of Burns.* 2nd ed. 1969. Copyright © WB Saunders Company. All rights reserved.)

considered when the TBSA is 30% or greater. In burns that exceed 30% of the TBSA, if bronchopulmonary injury is present, mortality increases to 70%. Along with swelling that may come from fluid resuscitation, patients which a large TBSA often develop progressive upper airway edema in the first 48 hours, even if there was no inhalational component. This can make delayed intubation difficult and even impossible. If a patient needs to be transferred to a higher eschelon of care, consideration should be given to securing his or her airway prior to transport.[50–54]

Carbon Monoxide

Carbon monoxide (CO) is an odorless, colorless gas and is a major component of smoke in fires. Burns from enclosed spaces place the patient at risk for CO poisoning. CO binds hemoglobin with a greater affinity than oxygen. It also causes a left shift of the oxyhemoglobin dissociation curve. This reduces the ability of the red blood cells to off-load oxygen and can lead to hypoxia in the tissues. CO can also bind to heme molecules in myoglobin and decrease oxygen diffusion into muscle, including in the heart.[55,56]

CO and oxyhemoglobin absorb the same wavelength (660 nM) of light. This will falsely elevate standard pulse oximetry as carboxyhemoglobin is misread as oxyhemoglobin. The amount of CO in the blood is likely best detected by co-oximetry. Co-oximeters measure absorption at several wavelengths of light and can distinguish carboxyhemoglobin from oxyhemoglobin. Affected patients who may be able to be treated with 100% oxygen should improve with time. If they are severely affected and have

CO encephalopathy, they may require hyperbaric oxygen treatment.[44,55,56]

Cyanide (CN) poisoning can also occur after a fire due to incomplete combustion of nitrogen-containing materials. CN is a colorless gas with a bitter almond odor. It is produced by the combustion of plastic, polyurethane, wool, silk, nitriles, rubber, and paper products. CN stimulates the chemoreceptors in the carotid and aortic bodies, which can lead to hyperpnea. It interferes with metabolism on the cellular level by inhibiting cytochrome *c* oxidase and affecting the mitochondria. This converts the cell to anaerobic metabolism and lactic acidosis ensues. One of the ways it can be diagnosed is with a high mixed venous oxygen saturation. CN toxicity can be treated by sodium thiosulfate or hydroxocobalamin.[44,57]

Eschars

Eschars, which are from the dead and denatured dermis, often form over burned tissue and may form rapidly. They can form at any location in the body. Eschars that form over circumferential burns over the abdomen or thorax may impede the patient's ability to breathe. As edema increases in the first 24 hours, eschars may become tourniquet-like. They may act like restrictive lung disease if there is thoracic wall involvement or lead to abdominal compartment syndrome, with decreased cardiac output, venous return, and urinary output.[58]

Extremities should also be monitored for signs of ischemia from circumferential eschars as well. Warnings signs showing an escharotomy is needed are as follows: (5 Ps)— pain, pallor, paresthesia, paralysis, and pulselessness. If these signs are ignored and an emergent escharotomy is not undertaken it can lead to limb loss.[44]

Thermoregulation

When patients are burned, burns disrupt their integumentary system. The patient's ability to regulate and maintain his or her temperature is decreased due to large raw surfaces. Core temperatures are higher in burn patients (38 to 39°C). Heat loss is proportional to the TBSA burned. Denervated areas can no longer vasoconstrict in response to cold, further complicating the issue. Maintaining normothermia is especially important as heat production adds to already high metabolic demands. Ultimately skin grafting helps prevent the fluid and heat loss at the burned sites.

Anesthesia leads to thermoregulatory vasodilation, which causes a redistribution of body heat from the core to the patient's periphery. Burn patients maintain temperature best with an ambient temperature of 30 to 31°C. This minimizes radiant heat loss. Convective warming, while very effective in most patients, is often difficult to use in burn patients. It can be challenging to use a convective warmer on a patient who needs large areas of skin exposed to debride the wound, harvest skin, and place the skin grafts. Warming IV fluids can prevent further heat loss but is not an effective way to warm patients. For each 1 L of fluid warmed, it prevents the body temperature from losing 0.25°C. The inability to warm fluids significantly above the patient's body temperature is a barrier to this technology.[44]

Nutrition

Burn injury patients require good nutrition to promote healing. Burn injuries create a hypermetabolic state; the larger the area burned, the higher the metabolic rate. Enteral feeding is important to introduce calories, maintain gastrointestinal motility, and protect the mucosa. Without enteral feeds, the risk of infection and sepsis increases. While parenteral feeds can be used, they do not help maintain the integrity of the mucosal barrier in the gut. The mucosal barrier helps prevent bacterial translocation. Feeding can also help decrease the incidence of stress ulcers following a burn. Gastroduodenal ulcers are a common problem, unless the patient is getting enteral feeds or is treated with preventative measures such as proton pump inhibitor (PPI), histamine-2 receptor antagonists, or neutralizing agents.[59–61]

If the patient is unable to take food by mouth, a feeding tube should be placed early to help with caloric intake as well as the other benefits of enteral feeding. A post-pyloric feeding tube is helpful in maintaining round-the-clock feeding in patients with large burns. There is no consensus if post-pyloric feeds should be stopped before anesthesia or sedation. If the patient is not hemodynamically stable and on vasoactive agents, enteral feeding may be held until the patient is more stable. Some sources advocate enteral feeding via a feeding tube in patients with a 30% to 40% TBSA burn as it will be difficult to meet their caloric requirements by oral feeding. For children the estimated protein requirements are 3 g/kg/day after a burn.[44]

Other Changes

Acute Phase

The acute phase is immediately after the burn. As there are systemic release of vasoactive substances and cytokines, the cardiac output is transiently low. The myocardial function is depressed, the blood is viscous, systemic vascular resistance (SVR) is high, and intravascular volume is low. There can be airway obstruction and edema (presenting as bronchospasm and laryngospasm), along with potential carbon monoxide poisoning. The kidneys usually have a low glomerular filtration rate (GFR). In patients with either electrical burns or crush injuries, they may develop myoglobinuria. The liver is often poorly perfused at this point manifested with increasing liver enzymes. There may be hemoconcentration as fluids leave the intravascular space. There may be mucosal damage in the gastrointestinal tract, release of endotoxins, and neurological changes secondary to cerebral edema and increased intracranial pressure.[44,46,62]

Late Phase

After the acute phase passes, the patient enters into hypermetabolic phase and things again change throughout the body. The cardiac output increases and SVR decreases. Patients may be persistently tachycardic and hypertensive. They may develop tracheal stenosis, pneumonia, or tracheobronchitis. There can also be significant sloughing of the mucosa in the airway. The kidneys will see an increase in GFR, tubular dysfunction, as well as breakdown of glucose, lipids, and muscle. The patients may develop anemia, and have stress ulcers and ileus. Their neurological changes may include a personality change, delirium, seizures, or even coma.[44,46]

▶ Neuromuscular Blocking Drugs (NMBDs)

Burn injury can lead to the upregulation of fetal and mature acetylcholine receptors. This usually leads to a resistance to nondepolarizing muscle relaxants (NMBDs) and an increased sensitivity to depolarizing muscle relaxants such as succinylcholine. This is noted to occur between 24 and 72 after injury. This also occurs after stroke, spinal cord injury, prolonged immobility, prolonged exposure to neuromuscular blockers, multiple sclerosis, and Guillain-Barré syndrome. While burn injury upregulates the receptors, they are downregulated in myasthenia gravis, anticholinesterase poisoning, and organophosphate poisoning.[63–66]

Resistance to nondepolarizing NMBDs is typically seen in patients with at least 25% burns. It may take months to years for the receptors to return to normal. Potassium has been noted to markedly increase in burn patients following succinylcholine (SCh) use. SCh has been safely administered in the first 24 hours of a burn injury. After this period, the muscle receptors are likely already altered and SCh should be avoided. Over time, as normal skin regrows, normal acetylcholine receptors return. While it is not known exactly how long to avoid SCh, a conservative estimate avoids the use from 24 to 48 hours after injury and for the next 1 to 2 years.[67,68]

PAIN MANAGEMENT AFTER BURNS

Proper pain treatment minimizes the burn patient's metabolic demands, which aids healing. It is important to manage the patient's analgesic and anti-anxiety medications well. The patient undergoes multiple procedures: burn dressing changes, debridement, skin grafting, physical therapy, and scar tissue resections or releases. Pain tends to be the most intense from the freshly harvested donor sites as they have the greatest number of nerve endings. A tumescent solution can be used by the surgeons intraoperatively to help decrease the pain.[68–70]

Burn patients often need rapid escalations of their doses of analgesics. Some of this is likely from tolerance; however, the opiate receptors likely undergo thermal-injury changes which cause the doses to rapidly escalate. The nerve endings may also change from burn and grafting procedures. Once the skin wound is closed, the need for opiates rapidly decreases. Opiates and anxiolytics should be slowly titrated down to minimize withdrawal symptoms. Alpha-2 agonists have also been used to prevent withdrawal.[46,71]

Many analgesics can be used to treat the pain from burns. Fentanyl, morphine, and hydromorphone are options. Methadone and ketamine, with their N-methyl-D-aspartate (NMDA) antagonist activity, may decrease the hyperalgesia and minimize opioid tolerance. Dexmedetomidine is also being used for anxiolysis and pain treatment in burn patients. Nonsteroidal anti-inflammatory drugs (NSAIDs) and acetaminophen can also be considered but the patients need to closely be watched for renal or hepatic problems. Remifentanil may also contribute to hyperalgesia and should likely be avoided due to that reason.[72–75]

Pain is better treated in burn patients on a regular standing schedule, rather than as needed (PRN). Boluses of pain medications should be given prior to therapies and dressing changes; however, they should not be limited to those times. Stool softeners should be started to prevent side effects from the opiates. Diphenhydramine should be considered in patients, especially children, who have healing burns. Shear forces from itching or scratching at the graft site can cause graft failure. Pruritus may result from medication effects or from granulation tissue growth.[44]

CONCLUSION

Trauma and burns are both significant public health concerns to children today. They both are prime examples of areas where education as well as team-based care can have great opportunities for positive impacts on the health of children. Knowing about the physiological concerns, as well as the concerns for different health care systems, can improve the care delivered to this group of patients.

REFERENCES

1. Center for Disease Control and Prevention. 10 Leading causes of death by age group, United States—2017. Available at https://www.cdc.gov/injury/images/lc-charts/leading_causes_of_death_by_age_group_2017_1100w850h.jpg.
2. Center for Disease Control and Prevention. National Action Plan for Child Injury Prevention. Available at https://www.cdc.gov/safechild/pdf/cdc-childhoodinjury.pdf. Updated 2012.
3. Center for Disease Control and Prevention. *Data & Statistics (WISQARS): Cost of Injury Reports*. Available at

https://wisqars.cdc.gov:8443/costT. Updated 2015. Available at http://www.cdc.gov/injury/wisqars/index.html.

4. Centers for Disease Control and Prevention (CDC) MMWR. Vital signs: unintentional injury deaths among persons aged 0–19 years—United States, 2000–2009. *Morb Mortal Wkly Rep.* 2012;61:270.

5. U.S. Department of Health and Human Services, Administration for Children and Families, Administration on Children, Youth, and Families, Children's Bureau. Child maltreatment 2014. Available at https://www.acf.hhs.gov/cb/resource/child-maltreatment-2014. Accessed January 9, 2017.

6. American Academy of Pediatics. Management of pediatric trauma. *Pediatrics.* 2008;121:849-854.

7. *Guidelines for Field Triage of Injured Patients: Recommendations of the National Expert Panel on Field Triage* (2011). Available at https://www.cdc.gov/mmwr/pdf/rr/rr6101.pdf. Accessed October 10, 2016.

8. Kortbeek JB, Al Turki SA, Ali J, et al. Advanced trauma life support, 8th edition: the evidence for change. *J Trauma.* 2008;64:1638-1650.

9. American College of Surgeons, Committee on Trauma: Advanced trauma life support (ATLS). 8th ed 2008 American College of Surgeons Chicago.

10. Luten R. Error and time delay in pediatric trauma resuscitation: addressing the problem with color-coded resuscitation aids. *Surg Clin North Am.* 2002;82:303-314.

11. Agarwal S, Swanson S, Murphy A, et al. Comparing the utility of a standard pediatric resuscitation cart with a pediatric resuscitation cart based on the Broselow tape: a randomized, controlled, crossover trial involving simulated resuscitation scenarios. *Pediatrics.* 2005;116:e326-e333.

12. Rosenberg M, Greenberger S, Rawal A, et al. Comparison of Broselow tape measurements versus physician estimations of pediatric weights. *Am J Emerg Med.* 2011;29:482-488.

13. Schonfeld D, Lee LK. Blunt abdominal trauma in children. *Curr Opin Pediatr.* 2012;24(3):314-318.

14. Blackbourne LH, Soffer D, McKenney M, et al. Secondary ultrasound examination increases the sensitivity of the FAST exam in blunt trauma. *J Trauma.* 2004;57(5):934-938.

15. Heller K, Reardon R, Joing S. Ultrasound use in trauma: the FAST exam. *Acad Emerg Med.* 2007 Jun;14(6):525.

16. Warner KJ, Carlbom D, Cooke CR. Paramedic training for proficient prehospital endotracheal intubation. *Prehosp Emerg Care.* 2010;14:103-108.

17. Vanderhave KL, Chiravuri S, Caird MS, et al. Cervical spine trauma in children and adults: perioperative considerations. *J Am Acad Orthop Surg.* 2011;19:319-327.

18. Yeatts DJ, Dutton RP, Hu PF et al. Effect of video laryngoscopy on trauma patient survival: a randomized controlled trial. *J Trauma Acute Care Surg.* 2013;75(2):212-219.

19. Koepsell TD, Rivara FP, Vavilala MS, et al. Incidence and descriptive epidemiologic features of traumatic brain injury in King County, Washington. *Pediatrics.* 2011;128: 946-954.

20. Savitsky E, Eastridge B. *Combat Casualty Care: Lessons Learned from OEF and OIF.* Fort Detrick, MD: Borden Institute; 2012:565-576.

21. Parent S, Mac-Thiong JM, Roy-Beaudry M, et al. Spinal cord injury in the pediatric population: a systematic review of the literature. *J Neurotrauma.* 2011;28:1515-1524.

22. Easter JS, Barkin R, Rosen CL, et al. Cervical spine injuries in children, part II: management and special considerations. *J Emerg Med.* 2011;41:252-256.

23. Pang D. Spinal cord injury without radiographic abnormality in children, 2 decades later. *Neurosurgery.* 2004;55:1325-1342.

24. Yucesoy K, Yuksel KZ. SCIWORA in MRI era. *Clin Neurol Neurosurg.* 2008;110:429-433.

25. Holmes, Lillis K, Monroe D, et al. Identifying children at very low risk of clinically important blunt abdominal injuries. *Ann Emerg Med.* 2013;62(2):107.

26. Marwan A, Harmon CM, Georgeson KE, et al. Use of laparoscopy in the management of pediatric abdominal trauma. *J Trauma.* 2010;69:761-764.

27. Sagarin MJ, Chiang V, Sakles JC, et al. Rapid sequence intubation for pediatric emergency airway management. *Pediatr Emerg Care.* 2002;18:417-423.

28. Tobias JD, Ross AK. Intraosseous infusions: a review for the anesthesiologist with a focus on pediatric use. *Anesth Analg.* 2010;110(2):391-401.

29. Guy J, Haley K, Zuspan SJ. Use of intraosseous infusion in the pediatric trauma patient. *J Pediatr Surg.* 1993;28(2):158-161.

30. Maw G, Furyk C. Pediatric massive transfusion: a systematic review. *Pediatr Emerg Care.* 2018;34(8):594-598.

31. Holcomb JB, et al. Damage control resuscitation: directly addressing the early coagulopathy of trauma. *J Trauma.* 2007;62:307-310.

32. Dehmer JJ, Adamson WT. Massive transfusion and blood product use in the pediatric trauma patient. *Semin Pediatr Surg.* 2010;19:286-291.

33. Massive hemorrhage. In: Pedi Crisis: Critical Events Checklists. Available at https://www.pedsanesthesia.org/wp-content/uploads/2018/08/SPAPediCrisisChecklistsJuly2018.pdf. Accessed March 29.

34. Holcomb JB, Tilley BC, Baraniuk S, et al. Transfusion of plasma, platelets, and red blood cells in a 1:1:1 vs a 1:1:2 ratio and mortality in patients with severe trauma: the PROPPR randomized clinical trial. *JAMA.* 2015; 313:471-482.

35. Fraga GP, Bansal V, Coimbra R. Transfusion of blood products in trauma: an update. *J Emerg Med.* 2010;39:253-260.

36. Edwards ME, Lustik MB, Clark ME, et al. The effects of balanced blood component resuscitation and crystalloid administration in pediatric trauma patients requiring transfusion in Afghanistan and Iraq 2002 to 2012. *J Trauma Acute Care Surg.* 2015;78:330-335.

37. Hwu RS, Spinella PC, Keller MS, et al. The effect of massive transfusion protocol implementation on pediatric trauma care. *Transfusion.* 2016;56:2712-2719.

38. Chidster SJ, Williams N, Wang W, et al. A pediatric massive transfusion protocol. *J Trauma Acute Care Surg.* 2012;73:1273-1277.

39. Eckert MJ, Wertin TM, Tyner SD, et al. Tranexamic acid administration to the pediatric trauma patients in a combat setting: the pediatric trauma and tranexamic acid study (PED-TRAX). *J Trauma Acut Care Surg.* 2014;77:852-858.

40. The CRASH-2 Collaborators. The importance of early treatment with tranexamic acid in bleeding trauma patients: an exploratory analysis of the CRASH-2 randomised controlled trial. *Lancet.* 2011;377(9771):1096-1101.

41. The CRASH-2 Collaborators. Effects of tranexamic acid on death, vascular occlusive events, and blood transfusion in trauma patients with significant haemorrhage (CRASH-2): a randomised, placebo-controlled trial. *Lancet.* 2010;376(9734):23-32.

42. Leeper CM, Neal MD, McKenna CJ, et al. Trending fibrinolytic dysregulation: fibrinolysis shutdown in the days after injury is associated with poor outcome in severely injured children. *Ann Surg.* 2017;266:508-515.

43. Fabian TC. Damage control in trauma: laparotomy wound management acute to chronic. *Surg Clin North Am.* 2007;87(1):73-93, vi.

44. Savitsky E, Eastridge B. *Combat Casualty Care: Lessons Learned from OEF and OIF*. Fort Detrick, MD: Borden Institute; 2012:596-631.

45. Souza AL, Nelson NG, McKenzie LB. Pediatric burn injuries treated in US emergency departments between 1990 and 2006. *Pediatrics.* 2009;124:1424-1430.

46. Fuzaylov G, Fidkowski CW. Anesthetic considerations for major burn injury in pediatric patients. *Paediatr Anaesth.* 2009;19:202-211.

47. Lawrence A, Faraklas I, Watkins H, et al. Colloid administration normalizes resuscitation ratio and ameliorates "fluid creep." *J Burn Care Res.* 2010;31:40-47.

48. Faraklas I, Lam U, Cochran A, Stoddard G, Saffle J. Colloid normalizes resuscitation ratio in pediatric burns. *J Burn Care Res.* 2011;32:91-97.

49. Lawrence A, Faraklas I, Watkins H, et al. Colloid administration normalizes resuscitation ratio and ameliorates "fluid creep." *J Burn Care Res.* 2010;31:40-47.

50. Tredget EE, Shankowsky HA, Taerum TV, Moysa GL, Alton JD. The role of inhalation injury in burn trauma: a Canadian experience. *Ann Surg.* 1990;212:720-727.

51. Fein A, Leff A, Hopewell PC. Pathophysiology and management of the complications resulting from fire and the inhaled products of combustion: review of the literature. *Crit Care Med.* 1980;8:94-98.

52. Barillo DJ, Goode R, Esch V. Cyanide poisoning in victims of fire: analysis of 364 cases and review of the literature. *J Burn Care Rehabil.* 1994;15:46-57.

53. McCall JE, Cahill TJ. Respiratory care of the burn patient. *J Burn Care Rehabil.* 2005;26:200-206.

54. Palmieri TL, Warner P, Mlcak RP, et al. Inhalation injury in children: a 10 year experience at Shriners Hospitals for Children. *J Burn Care Res.* 2009;30:206-208.

55. Walker AR. Emergency department management of house fire burns and carbon monoxide poisoning in children. *Curr Opin Pediatr.* 1996;8:239-242.

56. Barker SJ, Tremper KK. The effect of carbon monoxide inhalation on pulse oximetry and transcutaneous PO2. *Anesthesiology.* 1987;66:677-679.

57. Barker SJ, Tremper KK, Hyatt J. Effects of methemoglobinemia on pulse oximetry and mixed venous oximetry. *Anesthesiology.* 1989;70:112-117.

58. Quinby WCJr. Restrictive effects of thoracic burns in children. *J Trauma.* 1972;12:646-655.

59. Deitch EA, Rutan R, Waymack JP. Trauma, shock, and gut translocation. *New Horiz.* 1996;4:289-299.

60. Khorasani EN, Mansouri F. Effect of early enteral nutrition on morbidity and mortality in children with burns. *Burns.* 2010;36:1067-1071.

61. Andel D, Kamolz LP, Donner A, et al. Impact of intraoperative duodenal feeding on the oxygen balance of the splanchnic region in severely burned patients. *Burns.* 2005;31:302-305.

62. Gupta KL, Kumar R, Sekhar MS, Sakhuja V, Chugh KS. Myoglobinuric acute renal failure following electrical injury. *Ren Fail.* 1991;13:23-25.

63. Martyn JA, Fukushima Y, Chon JY, Yang HS. Muscle relaxants in burns, trauma, and critical illness. *Int Anesthesiol Clin.* 2006;44:123-143.

64. Martyn J, Goldhill DR, Goudsouzian NG. Clinical pharmacology of muscle relaxants in patients with burns. *J Clin Pharmacol.* 1986;26:680-685.

65. Han T, Kim H, Bae J, Kim K, Martyn JA. Neuromuscular pharmacodynamics of rocuronium in patients with major burns. *Anesth Analg.* 2004;99:386-392.

66. Gronert GA, Theye RA. Pathophysiology of hyperkalemia induced by succinylcholine. *Anesthesiology.* 1975;43:89-99.

67. Martyn JA, Richtsfeld M. Succinylcholine-induced hyperkalemia in acquired pathologic states: etiologic factors and molecular mechanisms. *Anesthesiology.* 2006;104:158-169.

68. Stoddard FJ, Ronfeldt H, Kagan J, et al. Young burned children: the course of acute stress and physiological and behavioral responses. *Am J Psychiatry.* 2006;163:1084-1090.

69. Stoddard FJ, Saxe G, Ronfeldt H, et al. Acute stress symptoms in young children with burns. *J Am Acad Child Adolesc Psychiatry.* 2006;45:87-93.

70. Kavanagh C. Psychological intervention with the severely burned child: report of an experimental comparison of two approaches and their effects on psychological sequelae. *J Am Acad Child Psychiatry.* 1983;22:145-156.

71. Angst MS, Clark JD. Opioid-induced hyperalgesia: a qualitative systematic review. *Anesthesiology.* 2006;104:570-587.

72. Owens VF, Palmieri TL, Comroe CM, et al. Ketamine: a safe and effective agent for painful procedures in the pediatric burn patient. *J Burn Care Res.* 2006;27:211-216.

73. Walker J, Maccallum M, Fischer C, et al. Sedation using dexmedetomidine in pediatric burn patients. *J Burn Care Res.* 2006;27:206-210.

74. Potts AL, Anderson BJ, Warman GR, et al. Dexmedetomidine pharmacokinetics in pediatric intensive care: a pooled analysis. *Paediatr Anaesth.* 2009;19:1119-1129.

75. Potts AL, Warman GR, Anderson BJ. Dexmedetomidine disposition in children: a population analysis. *Paediatr Anaesth.* 2008;18:722-730.

76. Kirkpatrick AW1, Simons RK, Brown R, et al. The hand-held FAST: experience with hand-held trauma sonography in a level-I urban trauma center. *Injury.* 2002;33(4):303-308.

Anesthesia for Renal Transplantation

Barbara Meinecke

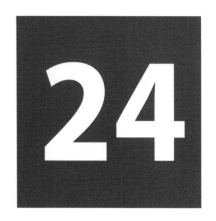

INTRODUCTION

End-stage renal disease (ESRD) is a complex and difficult problem in pediatric medicine. It causes significant metabolic and physiological derangements as the disease progresses leading to growth retardation, chronic anemia, electrolyte abnormalities, and systemic hypertension. Dialysis can be a life-prolonging treatment; however, renal transplant is considered to be the therapy of choice for patients with ESRD. Transplantation has the advantages of better quality of life, increased survival, and decreased health cost over time. Younger patients who undergo transplantation tend to have greater benefit and survival.[1,2]

EPIDEMIOLOGY

The Organ Procurement and Transplant Network (OPTN) manages the national transplant registry of the United States. The 2017 OPTN data shows 1,022 patients ages 17 and under on the active waiting list. This represents 1.05% of the 96,628 patients on the active waiting list.[3,4] The North American Pediatric Renal Trials and Collaborative Studies (NAPRTCS) group has been following a similar small cohort of patients since 1987 in order to better characterize the epidemiology and outcomes of this unique population. They have obtained voluntary participation from all U.S. and Canadian centers performing a minimum of four pediatric renal transplants per year.[5] As of the 2014 Annual Report, 12,189 transplants have been reported for 11,186 patients (Table 24-1). Congenital and structural abnormalities account for a majority of cases of pediatric renal failure. In contrast, the leading causes of adult renal failure are diabetes mellitus, hypertensive nephrosclerosis, and glomerular disease.

Table 24-1. Index Transplants: Recipient and Transplant Characteristics

Recipient and Transplant Characteristics	N	%
Total	11186	100.0
Sex		
Male	6606	59.1
Female	4580	40.9
Race		
White	6605	59.0
Black	1911	17.1
Hispanic	1910	17.1
Other	760	6.8
Primary Diagnosis		
Kidney Aplasia/Hypoplasia/Dysplasia	1769	15.8
Obstructive uropathy	1713	15.3
Focal segmental glomerulosclerosis	1308	11.7
Reflux nephropathy	576	5.1
Chronic glomerulonephritis	344	3.1
Polycystic disease	339	3.0
Medullary cystic disease	305	2.7
Congenital nephrotic syndrome	289	2.6
Hemolytic uremic syndrome	288	2.6
Prune belly	279	2.5
Familial nephritis	247	2.2
Cystinosis	225	2.0
Idiopathic crescentic glomerulonephritis	195	1.7
Membranoproliferative glomerulonephritis type 1	191	1.7
Pyelonephritis/interstitial nephritis	189	1.7
SLE nephritis	172	1.5
Renal infarct	144	1.3
Berger's (IgA) nephritis	135	1.2
Henoch–Schonlein nephritis	115	1.0
Membranoproliferative glomerulonephritis type 2	87	0.8
Wegener's granulomatosis	71	0.6
Wilms tumor	59	0.5
Oxalosis	58	0.5
Drash syndrome	57	0.5
Membranous nephropathy	51	0.5
Other systemic immunological disease	34	0.3
Sickle cell nephropathy	16	0.1
Diabetic glomerulonephritis	11	0.1
Other	1223	10.9
Unknown	692	6.2

Source: Reproduced with permission, from North American Pediatric Renal Trials and Collaborative Studies. *NAPRTCS 2014 Annual Transplant Report.* Copyright © The Emmes Company, LLC. All rights reserved.

PATHOPHYSIOLOGY

The kidneys perform a number of functions, including filtration of metabolic waste products, volume regulation, and hormone production. Dysfunction in any of these roles leads to wide-spread systemic problems. Metabolic derangements are the most common. As the glomerular filtration rate falls, the kidney's ability to remove acids, urea, and potassium decreases. Hyponatremia and volume overload occur due to decreased ability to excrete free water. Initiation of dialysis can help correct electrolyte and fluid levels but can cause significant hypotension from aggressive fluid removal.

Hyperphosphatemia results from the kidney's inability to adequately excrete phosphate. The excess phosphate then binds serum calcium and magnesium, causing levels of both to decrease. Hypocalcemia induces increased production of parathyroid hormone, stimulating osteoclast activity, causing further bone destruction in an attempt to raise serum calcium levels. This ongoing problem leaves the patient prone to fractures.

Damage to the cardiovascular system can occur through multiple routes in patients with chronic renal failure.[6] Hyperkalemia is particularly problematic due to its effects on the cardiac conduction system, leading to potentially lethal arrhythmias if high enough (ECG changes can be seen with potassium levels as low as 6 mmol/L) levels are reached. Systemic hypertension develops due to chronic fluid overload, and increased activity of the renin-angiotensin-aldosterone system in response to diminished renal perfusion. Erythropoietin production is decreased leading to chronic anemia. This decrease in oxygen-carrying capacity further stresses the cardiovascular system with a need for increased output to meet oxygen demand. Young patients with early-onset renal disease often have premature coronary artery calcification.[7] Hyperhomocysteinemia associated with cardiovascular disease in adults is often found in young patients with renal disease, and can be a biomarker for disease progression.[8] Uremic cardiomyopathy as a result of uremia is a cluster of symptoms including left ventricular (LV) hypertrophy, LV dilation, and LV systolic and diastolic dysfunctions.[9]

Besides its effects on the cardiovascular system, uremia also has detrimental effects on the neurological, hematologic, and gastrointestinal systems. Acute uremia can often cause seizures and coma, as well as peripheral neuropathy and encephalopathy in patients with chronic disease.[10] Platelet dysfunction is a multifactorial problem in uremic patients as a result of the underlying disturbance of the α-granules (containing platelet factor 4, transforming growth factor β1, platelet-derived growth factor, fibronectin, serotonin, and factors V and XIII). There is also derangement of the arachidonic acid and prostaglandin metabolism, leading to impaired synthesis and release of thromboxane A_2 which in turn reduces adhesion and aggregation of platelets.[11]

Uremic enteropathy is another serious complication of chronic renal disease. Urea is an irritant to the gastrointestinal mucosal surface causing changes in the microbiome, as well as changes to the gut barrier integrity.[12] This alters nutrient and drug absorption and excretion. Evidence also suggests that mechanical dysfunction (eg, delayed gastric emptying) is part of this syndrome. Anorexia is frequently seen in uremic patients, thus putting the child at significant risk for growth retardation. The need for protein and calories must be carefully balanced against excessive protein intake, which can worsen metabolic acidosis. Recombinant growth hormone has been used as a treatment in children with renal disease to help prevent height deficits without acceleration for the disease process.[13]

SURGICAL TECHNIQUE

Historically, renal transplantation in smaller children (<20 kg) differed in approach from adult renal transplant. A midline incision was made, and the kidney was placed intraabdominally, with vascular connections to the vena cava and aorta. Since the late 1990s, this approach has largely been abandoned in favor of the adult approach which involves a curvilinear right lower quadrant incision and retroperitoneal placement of donor kidney. The right side is favored because of easier access to the vena cava for anastomosis. This approach has been successful in small children and infants. The decision to whether anastomoses are performed to either aorta and vena cava or iliac vessels depends on the size of the patient and the length of the donor vessels present. After revascularization of the kidney, a ureterocystostomy is performed, followed by abdominal closure and completion of the procedure.[14]

PREOPERATIVE EVALUATION

There are two routes for renal transplantation: living donor and cadaveric donor. In the case of a living donor, the operation is an elective surgery with adequate time to optimize any fluid deficits or excess, metabolic derangements, and nil per os (NPO) status. With a cadaveric renal donor, there may not be time to completely optimize the patient for surgery. In either case, a CBC and an electrolyte panel should be drawn the day of surgery to evaluate the degree of anemia and electrolyte derangement prior to proceeding to the operating room. A physical exam should be conducted such as in any other surgery and should include vital signs and weight and assessment of the airway and cardiopulmonary status of the patient. Once obtained, anthropometric parameters and blood pressure should be compared against others in patient's recent past to determine true baselines. Evaluation of fluid status is particularly important. Dialysis history should be reviewed to help determine if the child is volume overloaded, or potentially intravascularly depleted if dialysis has recently occurred. If an arteriovenous fistula is present, this should be noted and protected during all parts of surgery (eg, no arterial or venous lines, or blood pressure cuff on that extremity).

Most chronic medications should be continued up to the time of surgery. Antihypertensive medications in particular, if taken up to the morning of the procedure, may prevent rebound hypertension intraoperatively, though cautious use of angiotensin-converting enzyme (ACE) inhibitors and angiotensin II receptor blockers (ARBs) is recommended since they may cause persistent refractory hypotension.

INTRAOPERATIVE MANAGEMENT

Vascular Access and Monitoring

Vascular access can be a challenge even in healthy children. Children with renal failure have been subjected to countless lab draws and peripheral IV placements, causing stenosis and scarring of peripheral veins. Central-line placement may also be difficult if the child has had several dialysis lines placed. If access is estimated to be particularly difficult, arrangements should be made for preoperative assistance from interventional radiology.

Standard, noninvasive monitors should be placed prior to induction of anesthesia to monitor for hemodynamic changes. Invasive monitors (arterial line, central venous catheter) should be placed after induction. A central venous line is important for several reasons. It allows for monitoring of central venous pressure (CVP), infusion of vasoactive medications, and infusion of certain types of immunosuppressive medications. An arterial line should be considered on a case-by-case basis. Smaller children and infants do not tolerate the third-spacing and fluid shifts caused by pre-reperfusion volume loading making an arterial line essential for optimal intra- and postoperative management. Larger children and teenagers tolerate this better, and typically do not require an arterial line. Avoiding an arterial line if possible is also beneficial in that it better preserves a possible future dialysis fistula site. Near-infrared spectroscopy (NIRS) is another measure of tissue perfusion that can help guide intraoperative fluid and inotrope management. It has been proven to correlate with ultrasound data and can be used to monitor the graft postoperatively in real time.[15,16]

Induction

Premedication with oral or intravenous midazolam is often used to decrease preoperative anxiety. The decision between an inhaled induction and intravenous induction depends on the patient's NPO status and overall cardiovascular stability. An inhalational induction with sevoflurane with or without nitrous oxide is an appropriate plan for an NPO-appropriate patient with clinically normal gastric function. In patients with severe systemic hypertension, or suspected volume-depletion from recent dialysis, a carefully titrated intravenous induction with hypnotic and narcotic medications will likely have more hemodynamic stability. A rapid-sequence induction may be needed if a patient is not NPO appropriate or has known gastroparesis.

Several medications depend on the kidney for metabolism or clearance of metabolites. Not only can immediate graft function after transplant not be assumed, but protein-binding and volume status will not be immediately normalized as well. Medications should be planned with this in mind. Drugs with organ-independent elimination, those that do not depend on the kidney for metabolism or elimination of metabolites, and those with inactive metabolites, are excellent choices for patients in renal failure. Succinylcholine can be used in patients with normal serum potassium levels. Sugammadex has been proven to be safe and effective in patients with renal failure; however, the recovery was slower than that of patients with normal renal function. Sugammadex and sugammadex-rocuronium complexes are cleared by hemodialysis.[17–19]

Intraoperative Management

Maintenance of anesthesia can be accomplished with either a general, or general and regional anesthesia approach. Children who had epidural analgesia for renal transplantation did receive larger volumes of fluid intraoperatively, but also demonstrated a tendency toward better hemodynamic stability.[20] There is some evidence that a continuous transversus abdominus plane (TAP) block can be used to effectively reduce the need for narcotic pain medications postoperatively, but that has not been studied in the pediatric population.[21] As with all abdominal cases, nitrous oxide should be avoided to prevent abdominal distention.

Immunosuppressive therapy is typically started in the operating room. An immuno-induction agent is selected by the transplant team prior to commencement of the operation. Induction agents include polyclonal antibodies—antithymocyte globulin (thymoglobulin), and monoclonal antibodies—basiliximab (Simulect, *Novartis*) and daclizumab (Zenapax, *Biogen*). Thymoglobulin is a rabbit polyclonal antibody against human lymphocytes used to cause lymphocyte depletion. This allows for administration of calcineurin inhibitors (maintenance agent), which can be nephrotoxic to the new graft, to be delayed. Thymoglobulin should be given over 4 hours via a central venous catheter to prevent chemical thrombophlebitis of smaller peripheral veins. Premedication with diphenhydramine and hydrocortisone can reduce cytokine-release reactions associated with it. Basiliximab and daclizumab are monoclonal antibodies against the IL-2 receptor, targeting the proliferative T-cell response of the immune system. These agents have the advantage of not causing a cytokine-release reaction and are thus better tolerated by the patient. Alemtuzumab (Lemtrada, *Boyer*) is a newer monoclonal antibody that targets the CD-52 surface protein. Maintenance immunosuppressive agents are administered later in the postoperative period.[22,23]

Providing optimal hemodynamics for graft reperfusion is extremely important. Patients require volume-loading to augment their mean arterial pressure to combat the decrease in blood pressure due to diversion of volume into the new organ. This can be particularly problematic in small children and infants where this represents a much larger fraction of their total blood volume. Recommendations for CVP range from 8 to 12 mm Hg to 16 to 20 mm Hg, with most centers targeting the middle of these ranges (12 to 15 mm Hg). Mean arterial pressure should be raised to greater than 65 mm Hg. Crystalloid, colloid, blood products, and potentially inotropic infusions may be required to achieve this. After aortic unclamping, sodium bicarbonate may be needed if acidosis is severe. Mannitol and/or furosemide may be given to promote diuresis.

Immediate Postoperative Management

At the end of the operation anesthetic agents should be discontinued, neuromuscular blockade reversed, and the patient assessed for extubation. Extubation may be delayed in smaller patients with ongoing need for volume or pressor infusion to maintain organ perfusion pressure or in patients who have had significant volume loading and resulting pulmonary edema. This is generally less of an issue in larger children with more size-matched kidneys. Intravenous and enteral fluid supplementation may be required long into the postoperative period to adequately maintain perfusion pressure. Decreased perfusion pressure carries higher risk of acute tubular necrosis (ATN) and graft loss.

POSTOPERATIVE COMPLICATIONS, LONG-TERM ISSUES, AND OUTCOMES

Graft Loss

Causes of graft loss in the immediate postoperative period include primary nonfunction of the new organ and thrombosis of vessels, though these can also occur at any time. Patients are often monitored in an intensive care setting to closely follow hemodynamics, track urine output, and periodically check the vessels by ultrasound. Acute rejection can occur at any time but can often be reversed with prompt and aggressive treatment. The overall frequency of acute rejection reactions has been decreasing over time as improvements in immunosuppressive regimens have been made (Table 24-2). The frequency of chronic graft dysfunction is a more insidious and long-term issue. Incidence of each of these increases over time (Figure 24-1).[24]

Malignancy

Malignancy is a potential complication after transplant surgery. Many of these malignancies are due to opportunistic viral infection, or reactivation of latent virus from

Table 24-2. Frequency of Acute Rejections Over Time and Comparing Source of Graft

	Frequency of Acute Rejections					
	1987–2013					
	Total*		Living Donor		Deceased Donor	
	N	%	N	%	N	%
All transplants	12116	100.0	6100	100.0	6016	100.0
Transplants with at least 1 rejection	5399	44.6	2449	40.2	2950	49.0
Number of acute rejections						
0	6717	55.4	3651	59.9	3066	51.0
1	2801	23.1	1329	21.8	1472	24.5
2	1285	10.6	606	9.9	679	11.3
3	665	5.5	270	4.4	395	6.6
≥4	648	5.4	244	4.0	404	6.7
Transplants with at least 1 rejection by transplant era						
1987–1991	1874/2692	69.6	780/1210	64.5	1094/1482	73.8
1992–1996	1754/3169	55.4	807/1603	50.3	947/1566	60.5
1997–2001	1000/2720	36.8	537/1599	33.6	463/1121	41.3
2002–2006	548/2151	25.5	249/1133	22.0	299/1018	29.4
2007–2013	223/1384	16.1	76/555	13.7	147/829	17.7

*Total with known donor source.

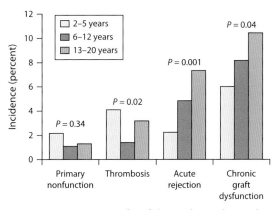

▲ **Figure 24-1.** Causes of graft loss, relationship with recipient age. (Reproduced with permission, from Hwang AH, Cho YW, Cicciarelli J, et al. Risk Factors for Short- and Long-Term Survival of Primary cadaveric renal allografts in Pediatric Recipients: a UNOS Analysis. *Transplantation.* 2005; 80: 466-70.)

immunosuppressive therapy. Post-transplant lymphoproliferative disease (PTLD) is the most common type. This develops from latent Epstein–Barr virus (EBV), from prior infection, that is allowed to go unchecked with immunosuppressive therapy. Latent EBV can be present in the patient prior to transplant, but a seronegative recipient can be exposed by a graft received from a seropositive donor. The risk of developing PTLD increases over time. Comparing across multiple years, the overall incidence of PTLD increased, and seemed to coincide with more powerful immunosuppressive medications coming into use[25] (Figure 24-2E). Human papilloma virus (HPV)–related malignancies (anal, perineal, cervical) and human herpes virus 8–related malignancies (Kaposi sarcoma) can also occur with immunosuppression.[26,27]

Outcomes

Overall, both graft and patient survival rates have improved since the 1980s when pediatric renal transplant became a more common operation (Figure 24-2A–C). Improvements in surgical technique, immunosuppressive therapy, and donor selection have contributed to this success.

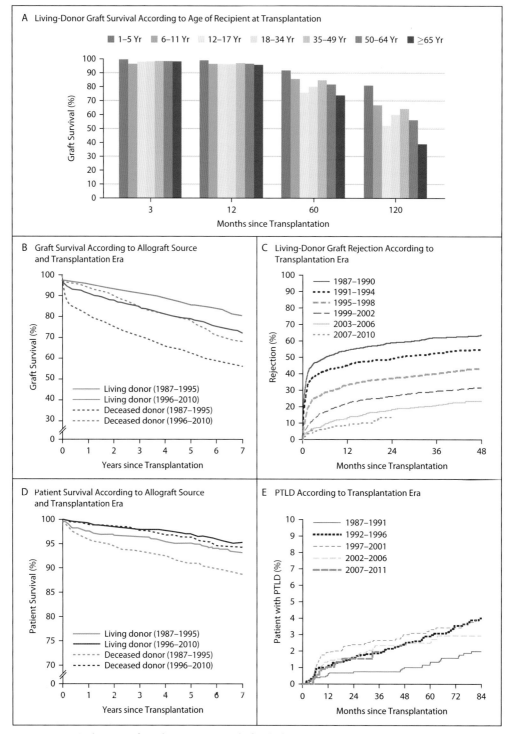

▲ **Figure 24-2 A–E.** Pediatric graft and patient survival after kidney transplant. (Reproduced with permission, from Dharnidharka VR, Fiorina P, Harmon WE. Kidney transplantation in children. *N Engl J Med.* 2014; 371(6):550–558.)

Living-donor recipients tend to fare better over time compared to cadaveric-donor recipients (Figure 24-2D).[28]

Unfortunately, despite these advances, adolescents have the worst outcomes based on graft survival and represent higher risk for retransplant. A likely reason for this is medication noncompliance. More research needs to be done into methods of education and tracking to help improve the outcomes in this group.[29]

REFERENCES

1. McDonald SP, Craig JC. Long-term survival of children with end-stage renal disease. *N Engl J Med.* 2004;350:2654-2662.
2. Dharnidharka VR, Fiorina P, Harmon WE. kidney transplantation in children. *N Engl J Med.* 2014;371:549-558.
3. OPTN: latest data reports. Accessed September 11, 2017. Available at http://optn.transplant.hrsa.gov/data/view-data-reports/national-data/#.
4. UNOS database. Accessed September 5, 2017. Available at https://optn.transplant.hrsa/data/view-data-reports/national-data/#.
5. NAPRTCS 2014 Annual Transplantation Report. Accessed September 5, 2017. Available at https://web.emmes.com/study/ped/annlrept/annualrept2014.pdf.
6. Gansevoort RT, Correa-Rotter R, Hemmelgarn BR, et al. Chronic kidney disease and cardiovascular risk: epidemiology, mechanisms, and prevention. *Lancet.* 2013;382:339-352.
7. Goodman WG, Goldin J, Kuizon BD, et al. Coronary-artery calcification in young adults with end-stage renal disease who are undergoing dialysis. *N Engl J Med.* 2000;342:1478-1483.
8. Amin HK, El-Sayed MK, Leheta OF. Homocysteine as a predictive biomarker in early diagnosis of renal failure susceptibility and prognostic diagnosis for end stage renal disease. *Renal Failure.* 2016;38(8):1267-1275.
9. Alhaj E, Alhaj N, Rahman I, et al. Uremic cardiomyopathy: an underdiagnosed disease. *Congest Heart Fail.* 2013;19(4):E40-E45.
10. Baluarte JH. Neurological complications of renal disease. *Semin Pediatr Neurol.* 2017;24(1):25-32.
11. Lutz J, Menke J, Sollinger D, et al. Haemostasis in chronic kidney disease. *Nephrol Dial Transplant.* 2014;29(1):29-40.
12. Grant CJ, Harrison LE, Hoad CL, et al. Patients with chronic kidney disease have abnormal upper gastro-intestinal tract digestive function: a study of uremic enteropathy. *J Gastroenterol Hepatol.* 2017;32:372-377.
13. Mehls O, Lindberg A, Haffner D, et al. Long-term growth hormone treatment in short children with CKD does not accelerate decline of renal function: results from the KIGS Registry and ESCAPE trial. *Pediatr Nephrol.* 2015;30(12):2145-2151.
14. Magee JC. Renal transplantation. In: Coran AG, Adzick NS, eds. *Pediatric Surgery.* 7th ed. Philadelphia, PA: Elsevier Mosby; 2012:617-629:chap. 46.
15. Vidal E, Amigoni A, Brugnolaro V, et al. Near-infrared spectroscopy as continuous real-time monitoring for kidney graft perfusion. *Pediatr Nephrol.* 2014;29(5):909-914.
16. Malakasioti G, Marks SD, Watson T, et al. Continuous monitoring of kidney transplant perfusion with near-infrared spectroscopy. *Nephrol Dialysis Transplant.* 2018;33(10):1863-1869.
17. Cammu G, Van Vlem M, van den Heuvel L, et al. Dialysability of sugammadex and its complex with rocuronium in intensive care patients with severe renal impairment. *Brit J Anaesth.* 2012;109(3):382-390.
18. Staals LM, Snoeck MMJ, Driessen JJ, Flockton EA, Heeringa M, Hunter JM. Multicentre, parallel-group, comparative trial evaluating the efficacy and safety of sugammadex in patents with end-stage renal failure or normal renal function. *Brit J Anesth.* 2008;101(4):492-497.
19. De Souza CM, Tardelli MA, Tedesco H, et al. Efficacy and safety of sugammadex in the reversal of deep neuromuscular blockade induced by rocuronium in patients with end-stage renal disease. *Eur J Anaesthesiol.* 2015;32:681-686.
20. Coupe N, O'Brien M, Gibson P, de Lima J. Anesthesia for pediatric renal transplantation with and without epidural analgesia—a review of 7 years of experience. *Pedatr Anesth.* 2005;15(3):220-228.
21. Faraq E, Guirguis MN, Helou M, et al. Continuous transversus abdominis plane block catheter analgesia for postoperative pain control in renal transplant. *J Anesth.* 2015;29(1):4-8.
22. Blondet NM, Healey PJ, Hsu E. Immunosuppression in the pediatric transplant recipient. *Semin Pediatr Surg.* 2017;26:193-198.
23. Smith JM, Nemeth TL, McDonald RA. Current immunosuppressive agents: efficacy, side effects, and utilization. *Pediatr Clin N Am.* 2003;50:1283-1300.
24. Hwang AH, Cho YW, Cicciarelli J, et al. Risk factors for short- and long-term survival of primary cadaveric renal allografts in pediatric recipients: a UNOS analysis. *Transplantation.* 2005;80:466-470.
25. Patel HS, Silver ARJ, Northover JMA. Anal cancer in renal transplant patients. *Int J Colorect Dis.* 2007;22(1):1-5.
26. Chin-Hong P. Human papillomavirus in kidney transplant recipients. *Semin Nephrol.* 2016;36(5):397-404.
27. Lebbe C, Legendre C, Frances C. Karposi sarcoma in transplantation. *Transplant Rev.* 2008;22(4):252-261.
28. Cladis, FP., Blasiole, B., Anixter, MB., Cain, JG., Davis, PJ. Organ transplantation. In: Coté C, Lerman J, Anderson B, eds. *A Practice of Anesthesia for Infants and Children.* 5th ed. Philadelphia, PA Elsevier; 2013:607-611:chap. 29.
29. Dobbles F, Ruppar T, De Geest S, et al. Adherence to the immunosuppressive regimen in pediatric kidney transplant recipients: a systematic review. *Pediatr Transplant.* 2010;14:603-613.

Anesthesia for Liver Transplantation

John (Jake) P. Scott and George M. Hoffman

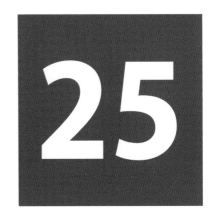

FOCUS POINTS

1. Most common etiology of end-stage liver disease (ESLD) in children is cirrhosis secondary to biliary atresia.
2. ESLD involves nearly every organ system.
3. The primary pulmonary manifestation of ESLD is arterial hypoxemia.
4. The most common cause of fulminant hepatic failure (FHF) is acute viral hepatitis.
5. Indications for the highest priority status (1A) for liver transplantation include FHF and hepatic arterial thrombosis or primary graft nonfunction post-transplant.
6. There are three surgical phases in liver transplantation: preanhepatic, anhepatic, and neohepatic.
7. Postreperfusion syndrome (PRS) during the neohepatic phase is associated with increased perioperative morbidity and mortality.
8. Postoperative complications following liver transplantation include bleeding, vascular occlusion events, rejection, and primary nonfunction.

CASE

A 9-year-old boy with history of biliary atresia post Kasai procedure presents with hyperbilirubinemia, transaminitis, and altered mental status. Acute hepatic failure with hepatic encephalopathy is diagnosed and he is placed on the highest priority status (1A) for liver transplantation.

HISTORY

Dr. Thomas Starzl performed the first pediatric liver transplant (LT) in a 3-year-old girl with biliary atresia in 1963. The recipient expired in the operating room secondary to intraoperative bleeding. In 1967, the first successful pediatric LT was performed.[1] Prior to the introduction of cyclosporine, 2-year survival following LT was less than 30% with rudimentary immunosuppression regimens consisting of corticosteroids and aza-thioprine.[2-4] Following the introduction of cyclosporine in 1979 survival rates increased. Current 1-year survival rates exceed 80%.[5] Initially few centers performed pediatric LTs, but this has increased significantly over the past three decades. Currently, there are more than 100 centers approved to perform pediatric LT in the United States; however, only 16 centers perform more than 10 pediatric LT annually.[6]

Less than 10% of all LTs are performed in children. According to the United States Organ Procurement and Transplantation Network (OPTN) more than 145,000 LTs were performed in the United States between 1998 and 2016, and approximately 1600 were performed in children.[5] Current survival rates for deceased donor LT (DDLT) are greater than 90% in some centers (Figure 25-1A), with higher survival rates for live donor LT.[5] Inadequate cadaveric organ supply has resulted in unacceptably high pretransplant waitlist mortality (Figure 25-1B). Innovative techniques to optimize hepatic graft supply for pediatric LT include reduced liver, split liver, and live donor LT (Figure 25-1C). However, split and reduced LTs have lower graft survival compared to whole organ cadaveric and live donor transplants.[7]

Pediatric anesthesiologists are key members of the multidisciplinary teams needed to ensure optimal pediatric LT outcomes. Pediatric anesthesiologists must participate in

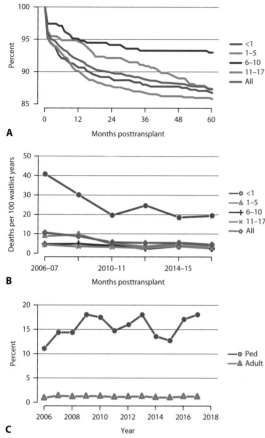

Figure 25-1. A. Patient survival among pediatric liver transplant recipients: deceased donor. **B.** Pretransplant mortality rates among pediatric patients waitlisted for a liver transplant, by age. **C.** Percentage of split liver transplants compared to total transplants performed among pediatric and liver transplant recipients. (Reproduced with permission, from Kasiske BL, Israni AK, Snyder JJ, et al. OPTN/SRTR 2017 Annual Data Report: Liver: *Am J Trans.* 2019; 19(S2): 184-283.)

all phases of perioperative care including patient selection, preoperative optimization, intraoperative management, and postoperative care. This essentiality is highlighted by a United Network for Organ Sharing (UNOS) mandate requiring all LT centers (including pediatric centers) to designate a Director of Liver Transplant Anesthesia (UNOS Bylaws, Appendix B, Attachment I, Section XIII). This chapter will focus on the perioperative management of pediatric LT.

INDICATIONS

Indications for pediatric LT include end-stage liver disease (ESLD), metabolic disorders, hepatic malignancy,

and fulminant hepatic failure. The most common form of pediatric ESLD is cirrhosis secondary to biliary atresia. This disease is caused by obstruction or agenesis of the extrahepatic biliary tree resulting in cholestasis and progressive cirrhosis. Prior to introduction of the Kasai hepatoportoenterostomy 2-year survival for children born with biliary atresia was less than 10%.[8] The Kasai procedure increased survival rates, but most patients will still develop hepatic failure requiring LT by age 10.[8,9] Other indications for pediatric LT include metabolic disorders (22%), fulminant hepatic failure (11%), hepatic neoplasms (9%), autoimmune diseases (4%), and other miscellaneous conditions (13%).[5]

PATHOPHYSIOLOGY OF END-STAGE LIVER DISEASE

End-stage liver disease is defined as irreversible hepatic fibrosis and cirrhosis resulting in portal hypertension and the loss of synthetic function and toxin clearance. Complications of ESLD involve nearly every organ system.

Patients with ESLD typically exhibit hyperdynamic circulatory physiology with high cardiac output and low systemic vascular resistance. Cardiac output is increased secondary to both stroke volume and heart rate. Systemic vascular resistance is reduced as a consequence of vasodilatory splanchnic peptide release and systemic arterial shunt (intrapulmonary, portopulmonary, etc.) development. Patients with ESLD typically have maldistributed systemic bloodflow and abnormal oxygen utilization with elevated systemic venous oxygen saturation.[10] Low-resistance splanchnic bloodflow is increased, stealing bloodflow from vital organs. Compensatory increases in sympathetic nervous and renin-angiotensin-aldosterone tone decrease responsiveness to exogenous and endogenous vasoactive agents. In rare instances, children with ESLD develop cirrhotic cardiomyopathy with reduced ejection fraction and diastolic dysfunction.[11] Congenital heart malformations associated with progressive hepatic failure are common with biliary atresia or Alagille syndrome.[12]

The primary pulmonary manifestation of ESLD is arterial hypoxemia. Cyanosis in liver failure is multifactorial due to intrapulmonary shunt, restrictive lung disease, and abnormal hypoxic pulmonary vasoconstriction. Severe pulmonary complications of ESLD include hepatopulmonary syndrome (HPS) and portopulmonary hypertension (PPH). Hepatopulmonary syndrome is defined as liver dysfunction and arterial hypoxemia in the presence of intrapulmonary arteriovenous malformations.[13] The diagnosis is established by ruling intracardiac shunt and demonstrating intrapulmonary arteriovenous shunt on bubble echocardiogram or ventilation perfusion scan.[14] The development of HPS has been linked to increased mortality.[15,16] There are no specific treatments for HPS, but LT is curative. Increased portal and pulmonary vascular resistance (PVR) are diagnostic of PPH. This entity may be complicated by acute right ventricular ischemia and sudden cardiac death. For severe PPH, pretransplant pulmonary vasodilator therapy (inhaled nitric oxide, prostacyclin, and sildenafil) may be indicated and has been linked to reduced pulmonary artery pressures allowing for successful LT.[17,18]

Coexistent renal dysfunction (prerenal azotemia, acute tubular necrosis, or hepatorenal syndrome) is common with ESLD. Intravascular volume depletion due to ascites, hypoalbuminemia, and diuretic therapy frequently results in prerenal azotemia. Treatment involves fluid administration and decreased diuretic administration. Acute tubular necrosis (ATN) may occur due to acute alterations in renal blood flow (RBF) and renal ischemia, especially with increased intraabdominal pressure from ascites. Management of ATN includes optimization of RBF and in severe instances renal replacement therapy (RRT). Hepatorenal syndrome (HRS) is the rapid development of acute kidney injury (AKI) that may progress to acute renal failure requiring RRT.[19–21] Oliguria with arterial hypertension and low urinary sodium is diagnostic of hepatorenal syndrome. The etiology of HRS is not completely understood but is thought to be secondary to renal arteriolar vasoconstriction and maldistribution of renal blood flow. An inciting stressor (infection, bleeding, etc.) generally precedes HRS. Liver transplantation has been shown to reverse HRS; however, patients may require intraoperative dialysis during LT.

Gastrointestinal complications of ESLD included portal hypertension, gastrointestinal bleeding, dysmotility, malabsorption, malnutrition, and growth failure. Portal hypertension is associated with the development of varices, prone to acute bleeding, and may require transfusion and sclerotherapy. Abnormal gastrointestinal motility and delayed gastric emptying increase the risk of aspiration during anesthesia. Ascites development is a source of protein loss with loss of plasma proteins and increased risk of peritonitis.

The neurological sequelae of liver disease are life-threatening. Hepatic encephalopathy (HE) is common in acute and chronic liver failure. Symptoms range from altered sensorium to obtundation with decorticate and decerebrate posturing, cerebral edema, intracranial hypertension, and uncal herniation (Table 25-1).[22–24] The etiology of HE is likely multifactorial. Neurotoxins (ammonia, false neurotransmitters) exerting GABA-like effects are thought to play a role.[25] Similar to HRS, precipitating events (sepsis, bleeding) frequently precede the development of HE. Treatment includes supportive therapies (ICP monitoring, temperature regulation) and gastrointestinal decontamination (lactulose, rifaximine).[26]

Table 25-1. Grades of Hepatic Encephalopathy and Associated Clinical Findings

Grade	Clinical Signs	Asterixis	EEG Findings
I	Altered sleep-wake cycle	Minimal	Minimal
II	Drowsy, irritable, altered mood	Obvious	Generalized Slowing
III	Unresponsive to verbal stimuli, hyperreflexia, positive Babinski	Reduced	More pronounced slowing
IV	Obtunded, decerebrate or decorticate posturing to painful stimuli	Absent	Generalized slowing with reduced amplitude to flat EEG

Hematological changes in ESLD include thrombocytopenia due to hypersplenism, and reduced synthesis of coagulation factors. Hepatically derived procoagulant and anticoagulant factors are decreased in ESLD affecting both the intrinsic and extrinsic coagulation pathways. Children with ESLD have increased risk of both bleeding and thrombosis.

FULMINANT HEPATIC FAILURE

The United Network for Organ Sharing (UNOS) defines FHF as the onset of HE within 8 weeks of the first symptoms of liver disease in the absence of preexisting liver disease. The most common cause of FHF is acute viral hepatitis (hepatitis A, B, C, D, E; EBV; CMV; enterovirus; etc.). Other causes include toxin exposure (acetaminophen), metabolic disease (neonatal hemochromatosis, Wilson disease), and idiopathic forms. Encephalopathy may be absent, late, or difficult to recognize. Patients with FHF with coagulopathy (INR > 2.0) and/or the presence of encephalopathy secondary to liver failure (grade II or greater) require higher level monitoring in the PICU.[24] FHF is a disease associated with significant mortality and is an indication for emergent Status 1A listing.. Benzodiazepines should be avoided in FHF as they increase false neurotransmitters and may precipitate encephalopathy. Infection is a common cause of pre-transplant mortality. Children with FHF are at high risk of infection secondary to the impaired cellular and humoral immunity and empiric antimicrobial (bacterial and fungal) therapy is indicated.[27] Organisms responsible for life threatening infections in FHF include: S. Aureus, other Gram-Positive bacteria, E. coli, and Candida.[27]

PRETRANSPLANT EVALUATION

The pretransplant evaluation process is an essential component of pediatric liver transplantation. In 2014, the American Association for the study of Liver Diseases, the American Society of Transplantation and The North American society for Pediatric Gastroenterology set forth "Guidelines for the Pediatric Patient Undergoing Evaluation for Liver Transplantation".[12] These guidelines recommend that pediatric transplant centers develop multidisciplinary patient selection committees for the purpose of evaluating candidates for liver transplantation prior to listing. These teams will typically include transplant surgeons, hepatologists, anesthesiologists, intensivists, psychologists, social workers, nurses, dieticians, and pharmacists. The first task of these transplant evaluation teams is to identify the timing of initiation of the pretransplant workup, which may range from emergent to elective. Patients with fulminant or acute hepatic failure may be critically ill and at risk for death and permanent neurological injury. These patients will typically be listed in an emergent or urgent fashion.

These committees also serve to identify, evaluate, and manage comorbidities of ESLD. A comprehensive multiorgan system assessment is critical to the pretransplant evaluation process. Patients with malnutrition may require enteral or parenteral supplementation. Management of ascites includes diuretic therapy. Porto systemic shunt procedures may be recommended in the setting of respiratory compromise secondary to ascites.[12] Assessment of cardiorespiratory status should include evaluation of HPS and PPH with room air pulse oximetry and trans thoracic echocardiogram. If concern for HPS is identified with pulse oximetry then agitated saline bubble test should be performed with TTE to evaluate for right to left shunt. If TTE shows evidence of right ventricular hypertension then PPHN evaluation with cardiac catheterization should be performed with direct pulmonary artery pressure measurements.

Following completion of the evaluation candidates will be listed and stratified according to severity of illness. Patients who are most critically ill with acute liver failure receive the highest priority status (Status 1A). Indications for status 1A listing include FHF, or hepatic artery thrombosis or primary graft nonfunction following liver transplantation. Status 1B is reserved for chronically ill children with life threatening comorbidities who receive special exceptions. All other patients with chronic liver disease awaiting cadaveric livers have been stratified according to the Pediatric End-Stage Liver Disease (PELD) score and Model for End-Stage Liver Disease (MELD) scoring systems. The PELD score is applied to children age less than 12 years and incorporates age, weight, height, bilirubin level, albumin level, and international normalized ratio (INR). The MELD score is for children older than 12 years and incorporates serum bilirubin, creatinine, and INR, as well as the need for renal replacement therapy. The MELD and PELD scores were designed to reduce pretransplant mortality without increase in posttransplant outcomes.[28] These scoring systems, implemented in 2002, predict pretransplant waitlist mortality and assist with organ allocation better than the previously used Child-Turcotte-Pugh Score, which incorporated subjective measures.[29,30] The observation of elevated waitlist mortality in hyponatremic adults with ESLD candidates has led to the recent application of the MELD Na score.[31]

INTRAOPERATIVE MANAGEMENT

▶ Operating Room Set Up

The operating room configuration for LT should resemble other major blood loss procedures (cardiopulmonary bypass or trauma). Dual fluid warmers with Y type blood administration sets and multiple invasive pressure lines set up should be available. Rapid infusion devices should be available for infants greater than 20 kg. A balanced salt solution containing dextrose carrier should be attached to a manifold such that vasoactive and inotropic medications may be administered at a constant rate. Multiple syringe pumps must also be available for drips on a pump tree. Available vasoactive infusions should be able to support cardiac output (epinephrine) and vasomotor tone (norepinephrine and vasopressin). Bolus resuscitative drugs should include epinephrine and phenylephrine in 10 mcg/mL and 100 mcg/mL dilutions in 10-mL syringes as well as atropine, calcium chloride, and sodium bicarbonate. Additional medications should include antibiotics (ie, ampicillin-sulbactam), immunosuppressants (ie, methylprednisolone, basiliximab), and heparin (1000 U/mL).

The blood bank must be notified of the potential LT when the organ is accepted to ensure that blood products are available. The quantity required varies based on patient weight and on additional risk factors for bleeding (previous abdominal surgery, decreased synthetic function with coagulopathy, hypersplenism with thrombocytopenia). The minimum available products should be 2 adult packed red blood cell (PRBC) units/10 kg, 2 adult fresh frozen plasma (FFP) units/10 kg, and 1 single-donor platelet (SDP) unit/10 kg. Blood products should be pre-checked and placed in the room-specific refrigerator or cooler within the operating room. Platelets must not be refrigerated but placed on a rocker.

Patients undergoing LT have multiple risk factors for perioperative hypothermia including intraabdominal surgery, massive fluid shifts, and hypothermic graft implantation. The patients will lose heat rapidly after abdominal incision. Hypothermia increases the risk of coagulopathy, infection, and dysrhythmias. The operating room should be warmed prior to patient arrival. Additional warming methods should be employed such as forced air heating devices, circulating water heating blanket, heated, humidified circuits, heating lamps, and fluid warmers.

Anesthetic Induction

Preservation of cardiorespiratory homeostasis is essential during induction of anesthesia for LT. Premedication with midazolam is generally acceptable but should be avoided in patients with HE. Intravenous induction is preferred. Patients with ESLD are at risk for aspiration due to delayed gastric emptying as well as increased intraabdominal pressure from hepatomegaly and ascites. Rapid sequence induction with cricoid pressure is routinely performed to mitigate risk of aspiration. Placement of an appropriately sized cuffed endotracheal tube is recommended as dynamic changes in ventilatory mechanics are routine during dissection of the diseased liver. There may also be significant size discordance between the donor graft and the recipient abdomen, further contributing to reduced compliance postoperatively.

Standard monitors include electrocardiogram, two pulse oximeters (one upper extremity, one lower extremity in case of cross-clamping of the aorta), capnography, and core body temperature. Advanced invasive and non-invasive monitoring should include arterial and central venous pressures (CVPs) as well as two-site (cerebral and somatic) near-infrared spectroscopy (NIRS), although NIRS may only be useful as a trend monitor with hyperbilirubinemia. Two large-bore IV catheters should ideally be placed in upper extremities in case of cross-clamping. If venovenous bypass (VVB) is to be potentially used, a discussion with the surgeon should take place regarding the extremity to be used or avoided for IV placement. Generally, the left side is preferred for VVB. Arterial access should be obtained in an upper extremity in anticipation of abdominal aorta cross-clamp during anastomosis of the hepatic artery with placement of the noninvasive blood pressure cuff on a lower extremity. Central venous access is generally placed in the internal jugular vein with ultrasound guidance. When long-term durable central venous access is required, the surgeon will place a tunneled Hickman or Broviac catheter. Care must be taken when placing an orogastric tube as these patients may have esophageal varices and are generally coagulopathic. Nasogastric tubes should be avoided in coagulopathic patients.

MAINTENANCE OF ANESTHESIA

Maintenance of anesthesia typically involves a balanced anesthetic technique consisting of a volatile agent (sevoflurane or isoflurane) along with an opioid (fentanyl or sufentanil). Cisatricurium is a neuromuscular blocking agent metabolized by Hoffman elimination and not dependent on hepatic metabolism, which may be useful in the setting of ESLD, particularly when early postoperative extubation is planned.

Coagulation Monitoring

The American Society of Anesthesiologists (ASA) recommends advanced viscoelastic coagulation monitoring during cases where major blood loss is expected.[32] Preoperative coagulation assessment via routine hemostatic assays (PT, aPTT, INR platelet count) is not predictive of perioperative bleeding during liver transplantation.[33–36] Goal-directed transfusion algorithms based on viscoelastic assays (thromboelastography, rotational thromboelastometry) have been shown to reduce blood product exposure. In addition to help diagnose the specific elements of clot formation that contribute to coagulopathy, these assays may also be useful for identification of hypercoagulable states and fibrinolysis that are known to occur in the setting of hepatic failure.[32,37]

Surgery

There are three surgical phases: preanhepatic, anhepatic, and neohepatic.

Preanhepatic Phase

The preanhepatic phase involves abdominal dissection with ultimate removal of the diseased liver. Significant alterations in preload occur during this period secondary to bleeding and reduced systemic venous return with manipulation of the mesentery and liver prior to explantation. Bleeding is increased with adhesions from previous abdominal surgery (ie, Kasai procedure, liver transplant). Anesthetic goals during the preanhepatic phase include maintenance of a relatively low CVP without limiting cardiac output and perfusion.[38] Blood losses should be replaced, and coagulopathy corrected. Vasopressin may be used to redistribute splanchnic bloodflow to the central circulation and reduce portal venous pressure and bleeding.

Anhepatic Phase

The anhepatic phase begins with clamping of the infrahepatic and suprahepatic vena cavae. Thereafter the hepatic artery and portal vein are cross-clamped, and the liver is removed. Caval clamping decreases venous return such that cardiac output may be reduced by up to 30%; however, children with portal hypertension may have collaterals mitigating preload limitation. This is not the case in the setting of acute fulminant hepatic failure. Required interventions include volume resuscitation and vasoactive and inotropic medication administration. When cardiac output remains critically limited despite corrective measures, VVB (typically femoral—axillary) is indicated. Direct feedback to the surgeon from the anesthesiologist during test clamping is essential in this decision-making process.

Maintenance of cardiorespiratory, hematological, and metabolic homeostasis is essential during the anhepatic phase.[39] Labs should be checked regularly (every 30 minutes) and prior to reperfusion so that electrolyte and acid-base status may be optimized. Hypokalemia is generally not corrected prior to reperfusion, as potassium levels will increase with reperfusion. Transfusion of packed red blood cells (PRBCs) (hematocrit 60% to 70%) in isolation without reconstitution in FFP may lead to a higher-than-desired recipient hematocrit and associated hyperviscosity. We routinely reconstitute packed PRBCs and FFP for all intraoperative transfusions after initiation of the anhepatic phase to maintain hemodilution (goal Hct 30 or less) and coagulation factor levels. Prior to reperfusion of the neohepatic graft, acid-base, electrolyte (calcium and potassium), and intravascular volume status should be optimized.

Neohepatic Phase

Reperfusion marks the end of anhepatic phase and the start of the neohepatic phase. Reperfusion of the liver occurs with release of the portal venous, infrahepatic, and suprahepatic vena caval clamps. Preservation fluid is typically flushed out of the graft prior to reperfusion; however, there is frequently residual cold, acidotic, hyperkalemic solution within the graft which may cause circulatory depression.[39] Cardiovascular instability may ensue with bradycardia, hypotension, elevated PVR and right heart failure, malignant ventricular arrhythmias, and circulatory collapse. Postreperfusion syndrome (PRS) is defined as a 30% reduction in baseline blood pressure for more than 1 minute within 5 minutes of reperfusion. PRS is associated with increased perioperative morbidity (transfusion, renal failure, hospital length of stay) and mortality.[40] Increased PVR with PRS may require pulmonary vasodilator therapy (inhaled nitric oxide). Metabolic abnormalities should be corrected immediately after reperfusion. Thereafter most metabolic derangements will self-correct if the liver is functioning properly.

Following reperfusion, the hepatic artery anastomosis is performed. Biliary drainage is constructed as either direct end-to-end anastomosis or Roux-en-Y hepaticojejunostomy. Depending on patient physiological status, the biliary reconstruction may be delayed in the setting of a staged abdominal closure. Abdominal closure will increase intraabdominal pressure, especially with large donor organs. Graft perfusion may be compromised in this setting. Ventilatory mechanics and renal somatic NIRS trends should be followed closely during closure. Loss of the lower extremity pulse oximeter tracing is a late finding of high intraabdominal pressures. Bladder pressure monitoring may be useful to detect abdominal compartment syndrome.

POSTOPERATIVE MANAGEMENT

Hemodynamics

Hemodynamic support of the newly transplanted liver following reperfusion includes preservation of cardiac output and oxygen delivery through maintenance of adequate end-organ perfusion and avoidance of systemic venous hypertension. Maintenance of neohepatic perfusion without venous congestion is critical in the early postoperative period following LT. Hepatic perfusion pressure (HPP) is calculated by subtracting the CVP from the mean arterial blood pressure (HPP = MAP − CVP). The HPP should be maintained to at least 40 mm Hg. It is also critical to keep the systemic venous pressure within normal limits (less than 10 mm Hg) as systemic venous hypertension is associated with hepatic venous congestion and potential compromise of hepatic artery and portal venous blood flow, increasing the risk of thrombosis.

Anticoagulation

Pediatric LT is associated with an increased incidence of neohepatic thrombotic complications. Due to the high morbidity associated with neohepatic hepatic artery thrombosis (HAT) and portal vein thrombosis (PVT), hepatic artery thrombosis anticoagulation is initiated early after hemostasis is achieved. Heparin infusions are started once adequate hemostasis has been established before exiting the operating room. The goal is therapeutic anticoagulation within the first 24 hours. Post-LT aPTT and anti-Xa levels are used to guide heparin management. Early initiation of antiplatelet therapy with aspirin is employed to reduce the incidence of HAT.

POSTOPERATIVE COMPLICATIONS

Postoperative complications following liver transplantation include bleeding, vascular occlusion events, rejection, and primary nonfunction. The overall incidence of post-LT complications approaches 10%. Surgical reexploration may be indicated for graft threatening lesions or for postoperative hepatic failure of unclear etiology. Bleeding and hemodynamic lability may be significant during these procedures requiring anticipatory planning by the anesthesiology team.

Postoperative vascular complications are more common following pediatric LT than in adults. Hepatic artery thrombosis (HAT) occurs in 1% to 2% of pediatric LTs and is associated with significant morbidity and mortality.[41] The celiac trunk is the only arterial source of neohepatic arterial bloodflow. Risk factors for HAT include long donor-organ cold ischemic time, hypotension, mesenteric vasoconstriction, and hepatic venous congestion. Hepatic arterial flow limitation from thrombosis may range from stenosis to occlusion. Persistent transaminitis [aspartate aminotransferase (AST), alanine aminotransferase (ALT)], elevated lactate dehydrogenase (LDH), or coagulopathy (INR) post-LT should prompt immediate imaging with Doppler ultrasonography. Early diagnosis and treatment are critical to graft and patient survival. Surgical reexploration is generally indicated for suspected postoperative hepatic artery stenosis.

Fulminant hepatic failure following HAT requires urgent retransplantation.[41]

Portal vein thrombosis (PVT) is more frequent in children transplanted for biliary atresia due to portal vein hypoplasia.[41] The overall incidence of PVT is 5% to 10%.[41] Concern for post-LT PVT requires Doppler ultrasonography. Treatment for early PVT may involve surgical reexploration, anastomotic revision, and thrombectomy. Recrudescence of portal hypertension (GI bleeding, thrombocytopenia) is suggestive of late PVT. Catheter-based balloon dilation may be helpful for portal vein stenosis.[41]

Acute rejection is common following pediatric LT. There may be no symptoms, but a clinical presentation can consist of fever, right upper quadrant and back pain, irritability, and malaise. Transaminitis with leukocytosis and eosinophilia suggest rejection. Liver biopsy is the gold standard for diagnosis; however, donor-derived cell-free DNA offers the promise of noninvasive diagnosis of rejection. Treatment of rejection involves increasing immunosuppression. Antibody-mediated rejection may be treated with immunoglobulin, plasmapheresis, and CD-20 antibody (ie, rituximab).

Primary nonfunction (PNF) is suggested by signs of hepatic failure without evidence of vascular compromise or rejection. Persistent transaminitis, lactic acidosis, coagulopathy, and bleeding are common with PNF. Hyperammonemia with encephalopathy is life-threatening complications of PNF. Treatment is supportive initially, but urgent retransplantation is indicated in fulminant graft nonfunction.

CONCLUSION

The perioperative care of children undergoing LT requires a thorough understanding of physiology of ESLD and the unique challenges associated with each perioperative phase of care. Pediatric anesthesiologists possess the skills and training necessary to assume vital leadership roles on multidisciplinary pediatric LT teams allowing continued improvement in outcomes for this vulnerable patient population.

REFERENCES

1. Starzl TE, Groth CG, Brettschneider L, et al. Orthotopic homotransplantation of the human liver. *Ann Surg.* 1968;168(3):392-415.
2. Gordon RD, Bismuth H. Liver transplant registry report. *Transplant Proc.* 1991;23(1 pt 1):58-60.
3. Gordon RD, Todo S, Tzakis AG, et al. Liver transplantation under cyclosporine: a decade of experience. *Transplant Proc.* 1991;23(1 pt 2):1393-1396.
4. Otte JB. History of pediatric liver transplantation. Where are we coming from? Where do we stand? *Pediatr Transplant.* 2002;6(5):378-387.
5. (OPTN) OPaTN. National Data 2017. Available at https://optn.transplant.hrsa.gov/data/view-data-reports/national-data/. Accessed March 19, 2019.
6. Rana A, Pallister Z, Halazun K, et al. Pediatric liver transplant center volume and the likelihood of transplantation. *Pediatrics.* 2015;136(1):e99-e107.
7. Diamond IR, Fecteau A, Millis JM, et al. Impact of graft type on outcome in pediatric liver transplantation: a report from studies of pediatric liver transplantation (SPLIT). *Ann Surg.* 2007;246(2):301-310.
8. Laurent J, Gauthier F, Bernard O, et al. Long-term outcome after surgery for biliary atresia. Study of 40 patients surviving for more than 10 years. *Gastroenterology.* 1990;99(6):1793-1797.
9. Kasai M, Mochizuki I, Ohkohchi N, et al. Surgical limitation for biliary atresia: indication for liver transplantation. *J Pediatr Surg.* 1989;24(9):851-854.
10. Jugan E, Albaladejo P, Jayais P, et al. Continuous monitoring of mixed venous oxygen saturation during orthotopic liver transplantation. *J Cardiothorac Vasc Anesth.* 1992;6(3):283-286.
11. Myers RP, Lee SS. Cirrhotic cardiomyopathy and liver transplantation. *Liver Transpl.* 2000;6(4 suppl 1):S44-S52.
12. Squires RH, Ng V, Romero R, et al. Evaluation of the pediatric patient for liver transplantation: 2014 practice guideline by the American Association for the Study of Liver Diseases, American Society of Transplantation and the North American Society for Pediatric Gastroenterology, Hepatology and Nutrition. *Hepatology.* 2014;60(1):362-398.
13. Krowka MJ. Hepatopulmonary syndromes. *Gut.* 2000;46(1):1-4.
14. Mazzeo AT, Lucanto T, Santamaria LB. Hepatopulmonary syndrome: a concern for the anesthetist? Pre-operative evaluation of hypoxemic patients with liver disease. *Acta Anaesthesiol Scand.* 2004;48(2):178-186.
15. Krowka MJ, Mandell MS, Ramsay MA, et al. Hepatopulmonary syndrome and portopulmonary hypertension: a report of the multicenter liver transplant database. *Liver Transpl.* 2004;10(2):174-182.
16. Krowka MJ, Porayko MK, Plevak DJ, et al. Hepatopulmonary syndrome with progressive hypoxemia as an indication for liver transplantation: case reports and literature review. *Mayo Clin Proc.* 1997;72(1):44-53.
17. Ghofrani HA, Wiedemann R, Rose F, et al. Combination therapy with oral sildenafil and inhaled iloprost for severe pulmonary hypertension. *Ann Intern Med.* 2002;136(7):515-522.
18. Makisalo H, Koivusalo A, Vakkuri A, et al. Sildenafil for portopulmonary hypertension in a patient undergoing liver transplantation. *Liver Transpl.* 2004;10(7):945-950.
19. Iwatsuki S, Popovtzer MM, Corman JL, et al. Recovery from "hepatorenal syndrome" after orthotopic liver transplantation. *N Engl J Med.* 1973;289(22):1155-1159.
20. Gonwa TA, Poplawski S, Paulsen W, et al. Hepatorenal syndrome and orthotopic liver transplantation. *Transplant Proc.* 1989;21(1 pt 2):2419-2420.
21. Gonwa TA, Poplawski S, Paulsen W, et al. Pathogenesis and outcome of hepatorenal syndrome in patients undergoing orthotopic liver transplant. *Transplantation.* 1989;47(2):395-397.
22. Ardizzone G, Arrigo A, Schellino MM, et al. Neurological complications of liver cirrhosis and orthotopic liver transplant. *Transplant Proc.* 2006;38(3):789-792.
23. Raghavan M, Marik PE. Therapy of intracranial hypertension in patients with fulminant hepatic failure. *Neurocrit Care.* 2006;4(2):179-189.
24. Wendon J, Lee W. Encephalopathy and cerebral edema in the setting of acute liver failure: pathogenesis and management. *Neurocrit Care.* 2008;9(1):97-102.

25. Basile AS, Jones EA. Ammonia and GABA-ergic neurotransmission: interrelated factors in the pathogenesis of hepatic encephalopathy. *Hepatology*. 1997;25(6):1303-1305.

26. Larsen FS, Wendon J. Prevention and management of brain edema in patients with acute liver failure. *Liver Transpl*. 2008;14(suppl 2):S90-S96.

27. Kelly DA. *Diseases of the Liver and Biliary System in Children*. 3rd ed. Oxford, UK: Blackwell; 2009.

28. Bourdeaux C, Tri TT, Gras J, et al. PELD score and post-transplant outcome in pediatric liver transplantation: a retrospective study of 100 recipients. *Transplantation*. 2005;79(9):1273-1276.

29. Barshes NR, Lee TC, Udell IW, et al. The pediatric end-stage liver disease (PELD) model as a predictor of survival benefit and posttransplant survival in pediatric liver transplant recipients. *Liver Transpl*. 2006;12(3):475-480.

30. Edwards EB, Harper AM. The impact of MELD on OPTN liver allocation: preliminary results. *Clin Transpl*. 2002;21-28.

31. Sharma P, Schaubel DE, Goodrich NP, et al. Serum sodium and survival benefit of liver transplantation. *Liver Transpl*. 2015;21(3):308-313.

32. American Society of Anesthesiologists Task Force on Perioperative Blood M. Practice guidelines for perioperative blood management: an updated report by the American Society of Anesthesiologists Task Force on Perioperative Blood Management. *Anesthesiology*. 2015;122(2):241-275.

33. Reyle-Hahn M, Rossaint R. Coagulation techniques are not important in directing blood product transfusion during liver transplantation. *Liver Transpl Surg*. 1997;3(6):659-663; discussion 63-65.

34. Steib A, Freys G, Lehmann C, et al. Intraoperative blood losses and transfusion requirements during adult liver transplantation remain difficult to predict. *Can J Anaesth*. 2001;48(11):1075-1079.

35. Massicotte L, Beaulieu D, Thibeault L, et al. Coagulation defects do not predict blood product requirements during liver transplantation. *Transplantation*. 2008;85(7):956-962.

36. Carlier M, Van Obbergh LJ, Veyckemans F, et al. Hemostasis in children undergoing liver transplantation. *Semin Thromb Hemost*. 1993;19(3):218-222.

37. Kang Y. Thromboelastography in liver transplantation. *Semin Thromb Hemost*. 1995;21(suppl 4):34-44.

38. Massicotte L, Lenis S, Thibeault L, et al. Effect of low central venous pressure and phlebotomy on blood product transfusion requirements during liver transplantations. *Liver Transpl*. 2006;12(1):117-123.

39. Yudkowitz FS, Chietero M. Anesthetic issues in pediatric liver transplantation. *Pediatr Transplant*. 2005;9(5):666-672.

40. Siniscalchi A, Gamberini L, Laici C, et al. Post reperfusion syndrome during liver transplantation: From pathophysiology to therapy and preventive strategies. *World J Gastroenterol*. 2016;22(4):1551-1569.

41. Tiao GM, Alonso MH, Ryckman FC. Pediatric liver transplantation. *Semin Pediatr Surg*. 2006;15(3):218-227.

Anesthesia for Fetal Surgery

Elaina E. Lin and Kha M. Tran

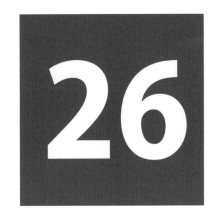

26

FOCUS POINTS

1. What are the indications for fetal surgery?
2. What are the maternal and fetal physiological considerations?
3. What are the surgical considerations and how can the anesthetic plan best facilitate surgical conditions?

INTRODUCTION

Fetal surgery is a rapidly evolving field in which the developing fetus receives therapy with the goal of decreasing mortality and/or morbidity. It provides unique challenges and requires the integration of both obstetric and pediatric anesthesia practice. Fetal therapies range from minimally invasive techniques to open mid-gestation procedures to near-term procedures performed with the fetus partially delivered while on placental circulation. In this chapter, we describe the indications for fetal surgery, review the principles for providing anesthesia for these cases, and outline the anesthetic approach to minimally invasive, open mid-gestation, and ex utero intrapartum treatment (EXIT) procedures.

A BRIEF HISTORY OF FETAL SURGERY

The first successful fetal therapy in humans began in the 1960s when hydrops fetalis caused by Rh sensitization was treated with in utero transfusion. However, successful exposure of the fetus would have to wait until the 1980s when better prenatal imaging techniques such as sonography and MRI, surgical techniques, and safer anesthetic agents were available. Select milestones in fetal surgery include the first congenital cystic adenomatous malformation (CCAM) resection in 1984, congenital diaphragmatic hernia (CDH) repair in 1989, aortic valvuloplasty in 1991, sacrococcygeal tumor (SCT) resection in 1992, laser ablation of placental vessels in 1995, EXIT procedure in 1995, fetoscopic surgery in 1996, myelomeningocele (MMC) open repair in 1997, hypoplastic left heart balloon septoplasty and valve dilation in 2004, and hypoplastic left heart laser atrial septotomy in 2005.[1] Many of these therapies have since become standard of care and the field of fetal surgery continues to evolve rapidly.

INDICATIONS FOR FETAL SURGERY

While many fetal anomalies can be detected prenatally with sonography and MRI, only select cases have compelling physiological rational for intrauterine therapy. Untreated, the risk of death or severe disability to the fetus must be high. The risk of surgery to the mother should be relatively low. In twin-twin transfusion syndrome, blood passes unequally between twins that share a placenta. The smaller donor twin pumps blood to the larger recipient twin. Twin reversed arterial perfusion (TRAP) sequence is a severe form of twin-twin transfusion syndrome in which one twin is developmentally normal and the other has a serious condition such as a missing heart or missing head that prevents it from surviving on its own. The goal of therapy in twin syndromes is to interrupt the blood flow between the twins. This can be accomplished under visualization with a fetoscope and laser coagulation of the shared vessels. In the case of TRAP syndrome, radiofrequency ablation or ligation of the cord of the abnormal twin can be used to stop the blood flow to the abnormal twin (Figure 26-1). These surgeries are usually performed at 18 to 25 weeks' gestation.[2]

Thoracic diseases such as CCAM, pulmonary sequestration, and other intrathoracic masses can cause severe

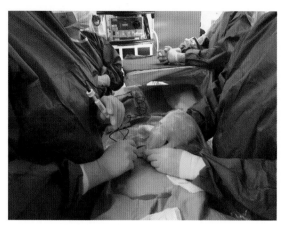

▲ **Figure 26-1.** Minimally invasive radiofrequency ablation (RFA) for twin reversed arterial perfusion (TRAP) sequence. Procedure is performed under ultrasound guidance. (Used with permission, from Dr. Lin and Dr. Tran. The Children's Hospital of Philadelphia.)

pulmonary hypoplasia and heart failure. Depending on the size, location, and composition of the lesion, treatments can range from minimally invasive ultrasound-guided cyst drainage to full laparotomy, hysterotomy, and surgical resection of the lesion. Minimally invasive cyst drainage is generally performed at 18 to 25 weeks' gestation.[3] Open mid-gestation resection is an option if the pulmonary lesion is preventing sufficient lung development to be incompatible with ex-uterine life or such severe heart failure that the fetus is not expected to survive. The goal of open mid-gestation resection or debulking is to remove enough of the mass to allow the lungs and heart to remodel and develop during the rest of gestation. After surgery, the fetus is returned to the uterus and pregnancy continued to as close to term as possible.[4] EXIT procedure is an option that allows for the controlled resection of large fetal lung lesions at delivery. Performing the surgery while on placental bypass avoids acute respiratory decompensation related to mediastinal shift, air trapping, and compression of the normal lung during surgery.[5]

Congenital cardiac malformations can be treated with minimally invasive techniques. Severe aortic stenosis is treated with fetal aortic valvuloplasty[6] and hypoplastic left heart syndrome (HLHS) with an intact atrial septum is treated with atrial septostomy.[7] Pericardial teratomas that are large enough to cause hydrops can be resected or debulked with an open mid-gestation procedure (Figure 26-2A–H).[8]

Myelomeningocele repair is performed at 22 to 26 weeks gestation. The mother undergoes laparotomy and hysterotomy and the defect is exposed. It is then closed primarily or with a patch (Figure 26-3A–B) and the fetus is returned to the uterus with the goal of continuing

pregnancy until 37 weeks' gestation, at which time the fetus is delivered via C-section. Maternal complications after open fetal myelomeningocele repair include membrane separation, preterm premature rupture of membranes, preterm labor, and need for blood transfusion.[9] Sacrococcygeal teratomas are resected in utero generally around 20 to 25 weeks' gestation if the highly vascular tumors are causing life-threatening high-output cardiac failure and fetal hydrops.[10]

Fetal neck masses such as cervical teratomas and lymphangiomas are masses that can grow so large as to block the fetal airway and esophagus. These airway malformations usually do not present a problem for the fetus while they are on placental circulation. However, these lesions are not compatible with ex utero life as the airway obstruction prevents the neonate from breathing normally. These lesions are managed by EXIT procedure, in which the airway is secured while the fetus is still on placental circulation, and the placenta is acting as the organ of respiration. This involves maternal laparotomy and hysterectomy. The securing of the airway is accomplished by intubation, tracheostomy, and/or partial or full mass resection (Figure 26-4). After the airway is secured, the umbilical cord is cut and the fetus is delivered immediately after the procedure. These procedures are usually performed as close to term as possible to minimize the problems associated with prematurity.[11] Congenital high airway obstruction syndrome (CHAOS) is a syndrome in which there is blockage of the upper airway of the fetus from laryngeal cysts, webs, or atresia. CHAOS can prevent the fluid, which is normally produced by the lungs, from draining into the amniotic space; the lungs may become massively distended, causing cardiac compression, heart failure, and fetal demise. If the CHAOS is causing life-threatening hydrops, the fetus may be treated with a mid-gestation percutaneous laser decompression to relieve the tracheal obstruction. The fetus may then subsequently be delivered via EXIT procedure or cesarean section depending on the anticipated residual obstruction (Table 26-1).[12]

Fetal surgery for other conditions such as repair of posterior urethral valves causing bladder outlet obstruction,[13] aqueductal stenosis of the fourth ventricle causing hydrocephalus, and diaphragmatic hernia with liver in the chest causing severe pulmonary hypoplasia have been attempted in the past but with poor results. However, new techniques are under development for these conditions.

CONTRAINDICATIONS

Contraindications to fetal surgery include maternal medical disease such as morbid obesity, cardiac disease, maternal hypertension that would increase the risk of preeclampsia or preterm delivery, or psychosocial factors that would put the mother at high risk for morbidity or mortality, and other concomitant fatal or severely disabling abnormalities in the fetus.

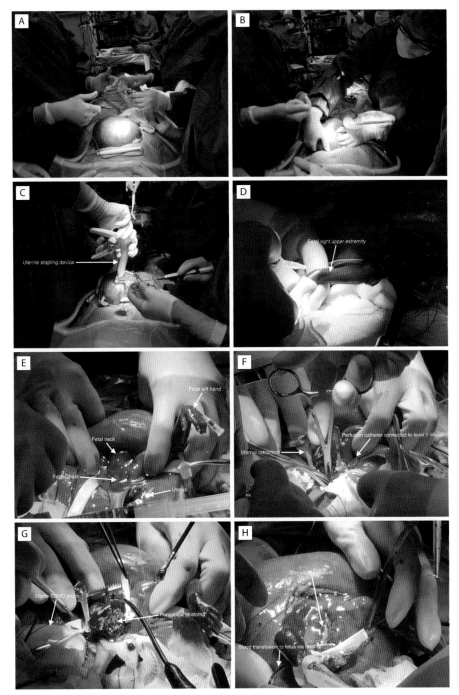

▲ **Figure 26-2.** **A**. With an anterior placenta, the uterus is externalized to expose the posterior aspect for incision. **B**. Fetus undergoes version with ultrasound guidance to place it in correct position for surgical exposure. **C**. Uterine stapler is used to incise uterus while maintaining hemostasis. **D**. Peripheral IV catheter is placed in right upper extremity of fetus. **E**. Bilateral upper extremities and fetal chest are exposed through hysterotomy site. **F**. Fetal sternotomy is performed. Perfusion catheter infuses body temperature lactated ringers into uterine cavity to replace lost amniotic fluid. **G**. Fetal pericardial teratoma is exposed for resection. Continuous echocardiography is used to monitor fetal heart rate, heart function, valvular dysfunction, and volume status. **H**. Fetal chest after sternal closure prior to return of fetus to uterus. (Used with permission, from Dr. Lin and Dr. Tran. The Children's Hospital of Philadelphia.)

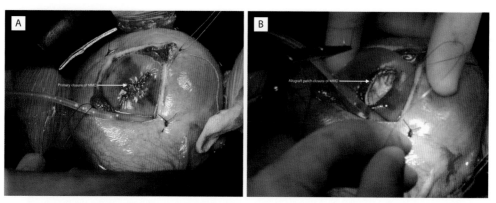

▲ **Figure 26-3.** **A.** Fetal myelomeningocele with primary closure. **B.** Fetal myelomeningocele with allograft patch closure. (Used with permission, from Dr. Lin and Dr. Tran. The Children's Hospital of Philadelphia.)

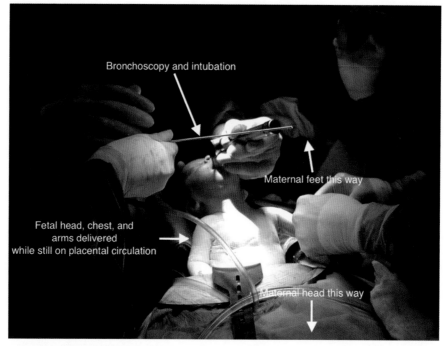

▲ **Figure 26-4.** Fetus with cervical lymphangioma delivered via EXIT procedure for bronchoscopy and intubation. (Used with permission, from Dr. Lin and Dr. Tran. The Children's Hospital of Philadelphia.)

PRINCIPLES IN PROVIDING ANESTHESIA FOR FETAL SURGERY

▷ Maternal Factors

Maternal Physiology

The mother undergoes significant physiological changes during pregnancy. She is at increased risk of aspiration due to the following factors: enlargement of the uterus pushing up on the gastroesophageal junction and causing sphincter incompetence, slower gastric emptying rate, and increased gastrin production increasing acidic content of stomach. Therefore, as of mid to late second trimester, the pregnant patient should be treated as a full stomach with measures to minimize risk of aspiration.

Maternal respiration also undergoes significant changes during pregnancy. Functional residual capacity decreases due to the gravid uterus. Minute ventilation increases by

Table 26-1. Fetal Surgery Treatment Options

Fetal Anomaly	Surgical Management
Twin syndromes • TTTS • TRAP	• Amnioreduction • Fetoscopic laser photocoagulation • Fetoscopic radiofrequency ablation
Lung lesions • CCAM • BPS	• Minimally invasive thoracoamniotic shunt placement • Mid-gestation surgical resection • EXIT procedure surgical resection
Heart lesions • Aortic stenosis • HLHS with intact atrial septum • Pericardial teratoma	• Percutaneous balloon aortic valvuloplasty • Percutaneous balloon atrial septostomy • Mid-gestation surgical resection
Neurological lesions • MMC	• Primary closure or patch closure of MMC
Airway lesions • Large cervical mass • CHAOS	• EXIT procedure intubation, tracheostomy, partial or complete resection of lesion • Mid-gestation laser decompression
Abdominal lesions • CDH	• Fetoscopic temporary tracheal occlusion

[(uterine arterial – uterine venous pressure)/uterine vascular resistance]. Many factors, including medications, surgical manipulation of the uterus, maternal hemodynamics, and maternal respiration, can affect uterine blood flow. Hypotension, caval compression, uterine contraction, valsalva, and hypocapnia decrease uterine blood flow. However, some anesthetic interventions such as use of vasopressors, regional anesthesia, volatile anesthetic agents, vasodilators, and magnesium can have variable effect on uterine blood flow.

The location of the placenta (anterior vs. posterior) will affect the surgical approach so that incision is not made through the placenta. Uterine relaxation in mid-gestation procedures during and after the procedure to prevent preterm labor is vital. Volatile anesthetics are powerful tocolytics and are currently used to provide uterine relaxation during surgery. Intravenous nitroglycerin is a powerful tocolytic with fast onset of action and limited duration. However, the tocolytic effects of these drugs must be balanced with the maternal hypotension, decrease in uteroplacental perfusion, and decrease in fetal cardiovascular function also caused by use of high doses of volatile anesthetics.[18] To maintain placental blood flow, maternal blood pressure must be maintained, often with the assistance of vasopressors. There is also the danger of placental abruption if uterine tone is too high or amniotic fluid is lost too rapidly after hysterotomy. Compression or kinking of the umbilical cord must also be avoided. Some medications cross the placenta from mother to fetus.[19] Drugs that are lipid soluble, not ionized, and of low molecular weight cross the placenta more easily.

Fetal Factors

Fetal physiology is unique from that of children or adults. The fetal circulation is a parallel system. The combined cardiac output (sum of left and right ventricular output) is 425 to 550 mL/kg/min, with the right ventricle contributing 60% to 70% of the combined cardiac output. The fetal myocardium is stiffer than that of adults and therefore cardiac output is more heart-rate dependent than preload dependent.[20] The fetal blood volume is approximately 120 to 162 cc/kg estimated fetal weight at 16 to 22 weeks, and 93 cc/kg estimated fetal weight by 31 weeks. However, two-thirds of the blood volume is on the placental side. Fetuses are hypocoagulable as compared to infants, with coagulation factors increasing with gestational age. The anesthetic requirements of fetuses are lower than that of their pregnant mothers.[21] While there is substantial evidence of fetal autonomic and endocrine response to noxious stimuli,[22,23] it is unclear as to whether fetuses have conscious perception of pain. Pharmacological interventions can be delivered to the fetus via placental blood transmission from the mother, or via umbilical artery, fetal intravenous, and fetal intramuscular administration. One should consider providing pharmacological intervention

50% and increases oxygen consumption, increasing the risk for hypoxia. The airway may also become edematous and along with increased breast size may make intubation more challenging.[14]

Compression of the inferior vena cava and aorta by the gravid uterus can cause decrease in systemic venous return and uterine perfusion, hypotension, and hypoxia. The mother should be put in left uterine displacement to minimize the compression. The pregnant patient requires less anesthetic as compared to the same patient in the nonpregnant state. Minimal alveolar concentration (MAC) is thought to be reduced by 30%[15,16] due to increased progesterone and endorphins. Epidural anesthetics also have increased effect due to decreased protein levels, pH changes in the cerebrospinal fluid, increased nerve sensitivity, and hormonal changes.[17]

Uteroplacental Physiology

Adequate uterine blood flow is necessary for placental and fetal perfusion. Uterine blood flow depends on the pressure gradient between the uterine artery and uterine vein and is inversely proportional to uterine vascular resistance to blunt the fetal stress response to surgical stimuli via one or more of these routes.

Preoperative Evaluation and Preparation

Fetal anomalies are usually first diagnosed by ultrasound. After initial suspicion of anomaly, further imaging via detailed fetal ultrasound, MRI, echocardiography, and chromosomal analysis may be warranted to better understand the anomaly and any other associated disorders. A comprehensive prenatal team of maternal fetal medicine specialists, surgeons, neonatologists, geneticists, psychologists, and social workers must work together to diagnose and counsel patients with their treatment options. Prior to any fetal intervention, the mother must also have a complete workup, including a thorough history and physical, electrocardiogram, blood work, and other diagnostic tests that may be warranted in order to devise a safe anesthetic plan.

Anesthesia for Minimally Invasive Fetal Surgery

Minimally invasive surgery involves using a percutaneous approach with a fiberscope and/or visualization by transabdominal ultrasound. The anesthetic approach to these cases can be quite variable, depending on the procedure and surgical and maternal factors. Surgical factors to consider include position of the placenta, umbilical cord, location of the lesion, duration of the procedure, and experience of the surgeons. Maternal factors to consider include any comorbidities and preoperative level of maternal discomfort and anxiety. Local anesthesia, sedation, general anesthesia, and regional anesthesia are all potential approaches to these cases. Local anesthesia or sedation may be appropriate for the procedure that is not anticipated to have a long duration with a mother that is able to cooperate. General anesthesia or regional anesthesia may be more appropriate for longer procedures or where maternal anxiety or discomfort makes cooperation more difficult. In general, the risk of blood loss is low in these cases and one peripheral IV catheter should suffice. Postoperative pain is usually minimal due to the small incision size. Postoperative tocolysis is usually achieved with oral nifedipine, with the addition of intravenous magnesium if needed.[24] There is the potential for fetal distress during minimally invasive surgery. Depending on the gestational age at the time of procedure, the fetus may or may not be viable outside the womb. In the event that the fetus is viable, staff should be prepared to perform emergency cesarean section and fetal resuscitation, if required.

Anesthesia for Open Mid-Gestation Fetal Surgery

Open fetal surgery requires that both the mother and fetus be anesthetized and the uterus be relaxed during the procedure to prevent uteroplacental compromise. This is generally achieved with general endotracheal tube anesthesia with high doses of volatile anesthetic (>2 MAC volatile agent). However, some centers prefer to use moderate doses of volatile anesthetic supplemented with intravenous anesthesia with the thought that this may decrease fetal cardiac dysfunction.[25] Prior to induction of anesthesia, a type and cross should be completed for the mother with type-specific red blood cells available for the mother in case of hemorrhage. O-negative red blood cells should be prepared for the fetus and cross-checked against the mother's sample, with the addition of AB-negative fresh frozen plasma and platelets if needed. Resuscitation medications for the fetus (atropine and epinephrine) as well as analgesia (fentanyl) and muscle relaxant (vecuronium) should be prepared in unit dosing based on the estimated fetal weight from the most recent ultrasound.

On the day of surgery, the mother should be appropriately NPO. An intravenous line is placed in the preoperative area. A preoperative low thoracic/high lumbar epidural is placed in the preoperative area for postoperative pain control. A good postoperative analgesia for the mother is associated with less uterine irritability.[26] An epidural test dose is administered to ensure it is not intravascular, but a bolus dose is not recommended as this may exacerbate the anticipated hypotension from high doses of volatile anesthetic. On arrival to the operating suite, the mother is placed in left uterine displacement. After preoxygenation, the mother is then induced with a rapid sequence induction and an endotracheal tube is placed. A second intravenous line is placed as well as an arterial line for careful monitoring of hemodynamics. A Foley catheter is placed. Volatile anesthetic is increased to >2 MAC and uterine tone is assessed by the surgeon prior to hysterotomy. Uterine relaxation may be augmented with the use of intravenous nitroglycerin. The maternal blood pressure will almost certainly require support with vasopressors, generally achieved with a phenylephrine infusion and ephedrine boluses as needed. Maternal fluid administration is limited to decrease the incidence of pulmonary edema.[27,28] At the authors' institution, fetal cardiac function is monitored with intraoperative fetal echocardiography. If the fetal cardiac function appears to be depressed, the volatile anesthetic is decreased and the umbilical cord is checked to make sure that there is no compression or kinks. If cardiac dysfunction persists, fetal resuscitation medications can be given through the umbilical vein, intramuscular, or through a fetal intravenous line if one is placed. Fetal intravenous lines are generally placed in open mid-gestation procedures such as resection of lung lesions or sacrococcygeal tumors where at least one fetal limb is externalized from the uterus. In cases of severe cardiac dysfunction, intraoperative fetal chest compressions may be necessary.

Toward the end of the procedure, intravenous magnesium sulfate is initiated for tocolysis. The epidural is dosed for postoperative pain control. Serious postoperative complications include preterm labor, pulmonary edema, amniotic fluid leak, chorioamniotic membrane separation, and fetal demise.[15]

Anesthesia for EXIT Procedure

The preoperative preparation, anesthetic induction, and preincision preparation for an EXIT procedure are similar to that of an open mid-gestation procedure. For an obstructive airway lesion, the EXIT procedure may involve intubation of the fetus, tracheostomy, bronchoscopy, and/or partial or complete resection of the obstructive airway lesion prior to clamping the cord. In the case of large CCAM, the lesion is resected while on placental circulation. In either situation, it is important that no ventilation of the fetal lungs take place until the cord is ready to be clamped. Otherwise, the fetus will transition from fetal to neonatal physiology prematurely, with loss of placental support. The difference in the EXIT procedure compared to the open mid-gestation procedure is that the fetus is delivered immediately after the procedure. Therefore, magnesium sulfate is not needed for tocolysis, and oxytocin is administered after the cord is clamped to prevent uterine atony and hemorrhage. Given the fact that high levels of volatile agent were used to promote uterine relaxation during the procedure, additional medications such as methylergonovine and prostaglandin F2 alpha are occasionally required. Crystalloid administration may be more liberal during these cases as there is less risk of pulmonary edema. In the event that the surgical procedure cannot be completed on placental circulation (due to events such as premature placental separation, maternal complications, fetal intolerance) and the fetus must emergently be separated from the mother, a second operating room should already be setup and a second operating room team should be immediately available to resuscitate and manage the neonate (Table 26-2).[24,29]

Intraoperative Fetal Monitoring and Resuscitation

Fetal monitoring during fetal procedures depends on the procedure being performed, risk of fetal compromise, and availability of certain monitoring techniques at the local institution. Fetal monitoring may range from preoperative and postoperative monitoring of fetal heart rate to continuous fetal echocardiography. In the case of open procedures, fetal heart rate and oxygen saturation may be monitored with pulse oximeter attached to an externalized fetal limb. Depending on the gestational age, normal fetal heart rate is expected to be 120 to 160 beats per minute. Normal fetal oxygen saturation is expected to be 40% to 60%.[30] Blood samples drawn from the umbilical artery may also be sent for laboratory analysis. When available, continuous intraoperative fetal echocardiography may be helpful in monitoring fetal well-being during the procedure and helping to guide anesthetic management and fetal resuscitation if needed.[31]

Table 26-2. Anesthetic Techniques for Fetal Surgery

	Minimally Invasive Surgery	Open Fetal Surgery	EXIT Procedure
Maternal anesthesia	• Generally well tolerated with IV sedation • Regional anesthesia or general anesthesia can also be used, especially if there is a concern that fetus may have to be delivered by emergent c-section	• General anesthesia with epidural for postoperative pain control • Regional anesthesia with nitroglycerin for uterine relaxation	• General anesthesia with or without epidural for postoperative pain control
Fetal anesthesia	• Transplacental drug delivery from mother	• Transplacental drug delivery from mother • IM or IV narcotics, muscle relaxant, or resuscitation medications • Umbilical vein resuscitation medications	• Transplacental drug delivery from mother • IM or IV narcotics, muscle relaxant, or resuscitation medications • Umbilical vein resuscitation medications
Intraoperative tocolysis	• No—tocolysis contraindicated	• Yes—with high dose volatile agent, IV nitroglycerin, IV magnesium sulfate	• Yes—with high dose volatile agent, IV nitroglycerin
Risk of preterm labor	• Minimally increased	• Significantly increased	• Not applicable—fetus delivered at end of procedure

In instances of fetal distress, resuscitation medications may be administered to the fetus through the umbilical vein, an intramuscular injection, or an intravenous line if available. Maternal factors such as hypotension, impaired venous return, and insufficient amniotic fluid should be considered and treated if relevant. Uteroplacental factors such as a compressed or kinked umbilical cord or uterine contractility should be evaluated and ameliorated.

Future Directions

Fetal surgery is a field that continues to grow. New techniques, such as minimally invasive endoscopic myelomeningocele repair,[32,33] continue to be developed. Providing anesthesia for these procedures requires detailed understanding of both maternal and fetal physiology and the anesthetic plan must balance the physiology of two patients at the same time. Further research is needed to refine anesthetic technique as the field continues to evolve.

Practical High-Yield Concepts and Tips for the Practitioner

- First do no harm; maternal safety is paramount.
- The anesthetic plan must incorporate maternal and fetal physiology as well as an understanding of the surgical needs of the case.
- Preoperative, intraoperative, and postoperative communication and coordination of care among multiple teams (surgery, maternal fetal medicine, neonatology, anesthesia, and nursing) are imperative.
- Anesthesia for minimally invasive cases can range from light sedation to general anesthesia.
- Anesthesia for open mid-gestation cases must facilitate intraoperative uterine relaxation and postoperative tocolysis.
- Anesthesia for EXIT procedures must facilitate intraoperative uterine relaxation but normal postpartum uterine contractility. Post-EXIT care of a potentially critical neonate requires the coordination of a neonatology team and secondary operating room team for the neonate.

REFERENCES

1. Jancelewicz T, Harrison MR. A history of fetal surgery. *Clin Perinatol*. 2009;36(2):227-236, vii.
2. Moldenhauer JS, Johnson MP. Diagnosis and management of complicated monochorionic twins. *Clin Obstet Gynecol*. 2015;58(3):632-642.
3. Peranteau WH, Adzick NS, Boelig MM, et al. Thoracoamniotic shunts for the management of fetal lung lesions and pleural effusions: a single-institution review and predictors of survival in 75 cases. *J Pediatr Surg*. 2015;50(2):301-305.
4. Cass DL, Olutoye OO, Ayres NA, et al. Defining hydrops and indications for open fetal surgery for fetuses with lung masses and vascular tumors. *J Pediatr Surg*. 2012;47(1):40-45.
5. Hedrick HL, Flake AW, Crombleholme TM, et al. The ex utero intrapartum therapy procedure for high-risk fetal lung lesions. *J Pediatr Surg*. 2005;40(6):1038-1043; discussion 1044.
6. Marshall AC, Tworetzky W, Bergersen L, et al. Aortic valvuloplasty in the fetus: technical characteristics of successful balloon dilation. *J Pediatr*. 2005;147(4):535-539.
7. Marshall AC, Levine J, Morash D, et al. Results of in utero atrial septoplasty in fetuses with hypoplastic left heart syndrome. *Prenat Diagn*. 2008;28(11):1023-1028.
8. Rychik J, Khalek N, Gaynor JW, et al. Fetal intrapericardial teratoma: natural history and management including successful in utero surgery. *Am J Obstet Gynecol*. 2016;215(6):780.e1-780.e7.
9. Moldenhauer JS, Soni S, Rintoul NE, et al. Fetal myelomeningocele repair: the post-MOMS experience at the Children's Hospital of Philadelphia. *Fetal Diagn Ther*. 2015;37(3):235-240.
10. Hedrick HL, Flake AW, Crombleholme TM, et al. Sacrococcygeal teratoma: prenatal assessment, fetal intervention, and outcome. *J Pediatr Surg*. 2004;39(3):430-438.
11. Laje P, Howell LJ, Johnson MP, Hedrick HL, Flake AW, Adzick NS. Perinatal management of congenital oropharyngeal tumors: the ex utero intrapartum treatment (EXIT) approach. *J Pediatr Surg*. 2013;48(10):2005-2010.
12. Kohl T, Van de Vondel P, Stressig R, et al. Percutaneous fetoscopic laser decompression of congenital high airway obstruction syndrome (CHAOS) from laryngeal atresia via a single trocar—current technical constraints and potential solutions for future interventions. *Fetal Diagn Ther*. 2009;25(1):67-71.
13. Nassr AA, Shazly SAM, Abdelmagied AM, et al. Effectiveness of vesico-amniotic shunt in fetuses with congenital lower urinary tract obstruction: an updated systematic review and meta-analysis. *Ultrasound Obstet Gynecol*. 2017;49(6):696-703.
14. Mushambi MC, Jaladi S. Airway management and training in obstetric anaesthesia. *Curr Opin Anaesthesiol*. 2016;29(3):261-267.
15. Tran KM. Anesthesia for fetal surgery. *Semin Fetal Neonatal Med*. 2010;15(1):40-45.
16. Chan MT, Mainland P, Gin T. Minimum alveolar concentration of halothane and enflurane are decreased in early pregnancy. *Anesthesiology*. 1996;85(4):782-786.
17. Kanto J. Obstetric analgesia. Clinical pharmacokinetic considerations. *Clin Pharmacokinet*. 1986;11(4):283-298.
18. Rychik J, Tian Z, Cohen MS, et al. Acute cardiovascular effects of fetal surgery in the human. *Circulation*. 2004;110(12):1549-1556.
19. Tran KM, Maxwell LG, Cohen DE, et al. Quantification of serum fentanyl concentrations from umbilical cord blood during ex utero intrapartum therapy. *Anesth Analg*. 2012;114(6):1265-1267.
20. Rychik J. Fetal cardiovascular physiology. *Pediatr Cardiol*. 2004;25(3):201-209.
21. Gregory GA, Wade JG, Beihl DR, Ong BY, Sitar DS. Fetal anesthetic requirement (MAC) for halothane. *Anesth Analg*. 1983;62(1):9-14.
22. Lee SJ, Ralston HJ, Drey EA, Partridge JC, Rosen MA. Fetal pain: a systematic multidisciplinary review of the evidence. *JAMA*. 2005;294(8):947-954.
23. Smith RP, Gitau R, Glover V, Fisk NM. Pain and stress in the human fetus. *Eur J Obstet Gynecol Reprod Biol*. 2000;92(1):161-165.
24. Van de Velde M, De Buck F. Fetal and maternal analgesia/anesthesia for fetal procedures. *Fetal Diagn Ther*. 2012;31(4):201-209.

25. Ngamprasertwong P, Michelfelder EC, Arbabi S, et al. Anesthetic techniques for fetal surgery: effects of maternal anesthesia on intraoperative fetal outcomes in a sheep model. *Anesthesiology*. 2013;118(4):796-808.

26. Tame JD, Abrams LM, Ding XY, Yen A, Giussani DA, Nathanielsz PW. Level of postoperative analgesia is a critical factor in regulation of myometrial contractility after laparotomy in the pregnant baboon: implications for human fetal surgery. *Am J Obstet Gynecol*. 1999;180(5):1196-1201.

27. DiFederico EM, Burlingame JM, Kilpatrick SJ, Harrison M, Matthay MA. Pulmonary edema in obstetric patients is rapidly resolved except in the presence of infection or of nitroglycerin tocolysis after open fetal surgery. *Am J Obstet Gynecol*. 1998;179(4):925-933.

28. Duron VD, Watson-Smith D, Benzuly SE, et al. Maternal and fetal safety of fluid-restrictive general anesthesia for endoscopic fetal surgery in monochorionic twin gestations. *J Clin Anesth*. 2014;26(3):184-190.

29. Lin EE, Moldenhauer JS, Tran KM, Cohen DE, Adzick NS. anesthetic management of 65 cases of ex utero intrapartum therapy: a 13-year single-center experience. *Anesth Analg*. 2016;123(2):411-417.

30. Nikolov A, Dimitrov A, Vakrilova L, Iarukova N, Tsankova M, Krusteva K. [Reference values range of the fetal oxygen saturation and its dispersal during labor without cardiotocographic evidence for fetal distress]. *Akush Ginekol (Sofiia)*. 2005;44(1):24-31.

31. Rychik J, Cohen D, Tran KM, et al. The role of echocardiography in the intraoperative management of the fetus undergoing myelomeningocele repair. *Fetal Diagn Ther*. 2015;37(3):172-178.

32. Verbeek RJ, Heep A, Maurits NM, et al. Fetal endoscopic myelomeningocele closure preserves segmental neurological function. *Dev Med Child Neurol*. 2012;54(1):15-22.

33. Pedreira DAL, Zanon N, Nishikuni K, et al. Endoscopic surgery for the antenatal treatment of myelomeningocele: the CECAM trial. *Am J Obstet Gynecol*. 2016;214(1):111.e1-111.e11.

Procedures in Pediatric Anesthesia

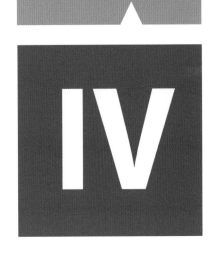

Advanced Airway Techniques

Patrick N. Olomu, Edgar E. Kiss, and Asif Khan

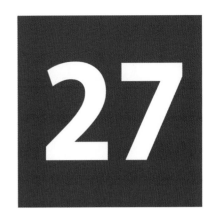

1. Knowledge of proper supraglottic airway insertion techniques, tests for position and performance, and maneuvers to correct malpositions are critical to successful use and the prevention of complications.

2. Video laryngoscopy provides better views of the glottis compared to direct laryngoscopy, although intubation times may be prolonged. Skill acquisition in elective cases before use in complex difficult airway situations is recommended. Corrective maneuvers in the "Can see, can't intubate" situation must be learned.

3. Difficult airway management in pediatric patients is associated with a high incidence of severe complications. Risk factors for complications are: greater than two laryngoscopy attempts, direct laryngoscopy persistence (direct laryngoscopy for first three attempts), and weight under 10 kg.

4. Supplemental oxygenation during pediatric difficult airway management is an important intervention that may reduce the incidence of severe complications.

5. Fiberoptic intubation in the small infant is challenging and requires great attention to every detail. Practicing this technique in elective normal airways is likely to result in greater rate of successful intubation when faced with a difficult airway.

6. Adequate preparation and planning decreases the need for surgical airway access. Use of a small angiocatheter technique is the preferred initial approach for front of neck access in children 1 to 8 years of age.

7. Simple airway maneuvers such as two-handed mask ventilation and adjunctive airway devices are critical in management of the difficult pediatric airway.

SUPRAGLOTTIC AIRWAY DEVICES

Supraglottic airway devices (SGAs) are devices with a ventilation opening(s) located above the glottis. Other terms that have been used include extraglottic airway devices (EADs) and periglottic airway devices (PADs). Supraglottic airway devices have also been abbreviated as SADs, but this usage is less common than SGAs. In general, SGAs may be considered a hybrid device between a face mask and an endotracheal tube (ETT). Over 30 devices are currently on the market but only a few of these are clinically useful in pediatric patients.

CLASSIFICATION OF SGAs

SGAs may be classified by brand type or by degree of sophistication.[1] The Laryngeal Mask Airway™ is the first brand and remains the most commonly used brand. Since its development in the late1980s, several brands have been developed and are increasingly being used in anesthetic practice (Figure 27-1). Other brands are classified as the non-LMA™ family of devices.

First-generation devices are basic airway tubes, consisting essentially of a mask bowl, an airway tube, and an inflation line. Second-generation devices have a separate channel for gastric access (Figure 27-2). This channel allows decompression of the stomach and may offer more safety.[2–6]

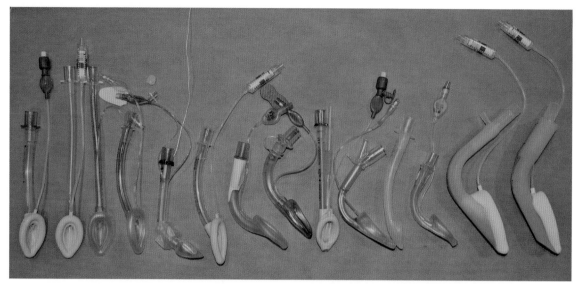

▲ **Figure 27-1.** Supraglottic airway devices. Left to right: LMA Classic, LMA Flexible with Cuff pilot valve, LMA Flexible PVC, LMA Unique, Cobra Perilaryngeal Airway, LMA Unique Silicone Cuff, Ambu Aura-i laryngeal mask, Air-Q ILA, LMA ProSeal, LMA Supreme, i-gel, Ambu AuraGain, LMA Protector, LMA Gastro. (Used with permission, from Dr. Patrick N. Olomu, University of Texas Southwestern Medical Center/Children's Health System of Texas - Dallas.)

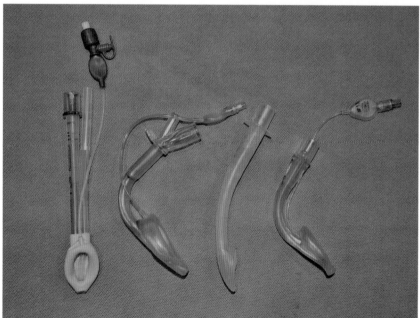

▲ **Figure 27-2.** Second-generation SGAs. Left to right: LMA ProSeal, LMA Supreme, i-gel, Ambu AuraGain. (Used with permission, from Dr. Patrick N. Olomu, University of Texas Southwestern Medical Center/Children's Health System of Texas - Dallas.)

More recently, third-generation devices have been developed (Figure 27-4). These are highly sophisticated devices that are designed for advanced surgical procedures or endoscope insertion.

▶ The Laryngeal Mask Airway™

The Laryngeal Mask Airway™ (LMA™, LMA Company, Henley, England, the United Kingdom) was invented by Dr. Archie Brain, a British anesthetist, in 1988.[7] It gained

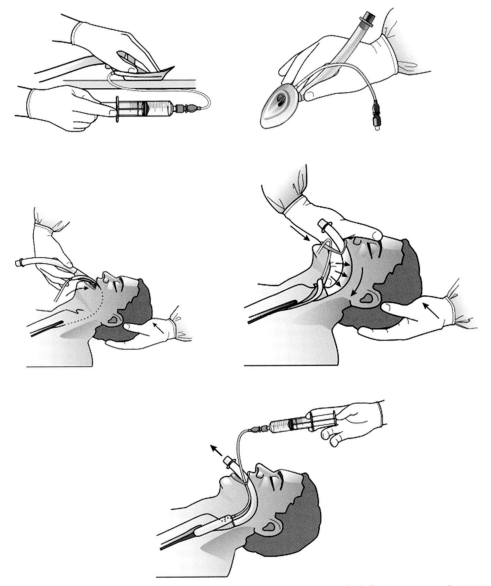

▲ **Figure 27-3.** First-generation LMA™ insertion technique. (Image courtesy of Teleflex Incorporated. © 2020 Teleflex Incorporated. All rights reserved.)

the Food and Drug Administration (FDA) approval in 1991. Over 200 million uses have been reported.

The LMA Classic™

The LMA Classic is the original SGA. It is made of medical grade silicone. When correctly placed, it creates a low-pressure seal with the supraglottic tissues and pharynx. The manufacturer guarantees each device for up to 40 uses. It is a general purpose LMA and is used for minor peripheral surgical procedures and radiological imaging such as

magnetic resonance imaging. The maximum allowable cuff pressure is 60 cm H_2O.[8]

LMA Unique™

The LMA Unique™ (Teleflex® Inc., Morrisville, NC, the United States) is the same device as the LMA Classic except that it is made of medical grade polyvinyl chloride (PVC). It is designed for single use and the prevention of disease transmission. The indications for use are the same as the LMA Classic. In the United States, the LMA Unique has largely replaced the LMA Classic.

LMA Unique Silicone Cuff

The LMA Unique Silicone Cuff incorporates an integral intracuff pressure monitor. This obviates the need for a separate manometer. Cuff pressure monitor is rarely used despite mounting evidence of significant iatrogenic complications from cuff overinflation.[9] Routine cuff manometry has been recommended by several authors and may become a standard requirement in the near future.[10–13]

LMA Flexible

The LMA Flexible™ is a special purpose LMA designed for head and neck procedures. It is made of steel reinforced silicone or PVC airway tube to reduce the risk of kinking. The silicone version is extremely floppy and may be difficult to insert by novice users. The longer, narrower, and extremely flexible airway tube allows for fixation in any position. It is used extensively for pediatric ophthalmologic procedures, especially eye muscle surgeries. It is also used for adenotonsillectomy by expert users, especially in certain European and Commonwealth countries. It is estimated that 15% to 60% of anesthesiologists in the United Kingdom and Australia use the Flexible LMA for adenotonsillectomy.[14] Such widespread use is uncommon in the United States. The insertion technique is similar to the LMA Classic, but may be difficult for inexperienced users. Stabilization of the posterior aspect of the mask bowl on the hard palate usually facilitates insertion.

► Classic Insertion Technique for First-Generation LMA™ Devices

Following inhalational induction with sevoflurane and intravenous access, propofol (1 to 2 mg/kg) may be administered to facilitate insertion. If intravenous access proves difficult, the LMA can usually be inserted under deep vapor anesthesia in most children. Generous lubrication of the posterior aspect of the mask is important for smooth insertion and reduced risk of traumatic placement (Figure 27-3). Spontaneous ventilation is commonly utilized but low-pressure mechanical ventilation (<15 cm H_2O peak pressures) may be used. The lower esophageal sphincter (LES) pressure is lower in pediatric patients; therefore high inflation pressures may cause gastric insufflation.

LMA ProSeal

The LMA ProSeal™ is the original second-generation LMA device.[15] Adult sizes were introduced in 2000 and pediatric sizes followed 3 years later. Half sizes were introduced in 2004. It is made of medical grade silicone and is reusable up to 40 times. A drain tube for gastric access runs alongside the airway tube and exits at the tip of the mask. Larger sizes (sizes 3 and higher) have an additional dorsal cuff for improved seal. The wedge-shaped mask provides better plugging of the hypopharynx and an enhanced seal.[16–19] Leak pressures are 5 to 15 cm H_2O higher than the same size LMA Unique.[2] The airway tube is steel reinforced and has an integral bite block proximally and an insertion strap distally. Three insertion techniques have been described: (1) digital (index finger in insertion strap), (2) use of an introducer tool in insertion strap, and (3) bougie-assisted. The manufacturer recommends inserting the device fully deflated and well lubricated. Separation of the alimentary and airway tracts occurs when the device is correctly placed. Diagnostic tests have been described[20–22] but are rarely performed. The ProSeal LMA may be used for invasive mechanical ventilation and for advanced surgical procedures.[23] Reported complications with its use are glottic insertion, mask fold over, epiglottic downfolding, and upper airway obstruction.

LMA Supreme

The LMA Supreme™, like the LMA ProSeal, is a second-generation SGA that is designed for advanced surgical procedures.[24] It is made of medical grade PVC and is designed for single use. Unlike the ProSeal, it lacks a posterior cuff. The airway tube is pre-curved and elliptical in shape and is bisected into two separate channels by the drain tube, which facilitates gastric access. The mask bowl is cone-shaped and provides a better plug of the hypopharynx and the glottis, thus providing a better overall seal. Leak pressures are similar to the ProSeal LMA.[25,26] In a study comparing the LMA Supreme to the LMA Unique, Jagannathan and coworkers observed no added benefit of increasing intracuff pressure from 40 to 60 cm H_2O as leak pressures were essentially unchanged.[27] Gastric insufflation rates were lower with the LMA Supreme, an advantage when invasive mechanical ventilation is used. The manufacturer recommends insertion with the mask fully deflated and with the head in the neutral or sniffing position. The manufacturer also recommends applying a piece of tape from cheek to cheek over the fixation tab prior to cuff inflation. This reduces the likelihood of outward migration during cuff inflation and may improve the seal with the airway and hypopharynx. When correctly placed, separation of the airway tract and the alimentary tract is achieved. The LMA Supreme may therefore be suitable for more invasive surgical procedures. Diagnostic tests for the LMA Supreme and ProSeal have been described but these are rarely performed.[28] The device is available in all sizes and half sizes and may be used as a conduit for intubation.

Newer Devices (Third-Generation Devices)

In recent years, new special purpose advanced LMAs have been developed. These include the LMA Protector and the LMA Gastro (Figure 27-4). There is no evidence that these devices are in wide use in pediatric patients. The size 3 is the smallest size and may be suitable for teenage patients.

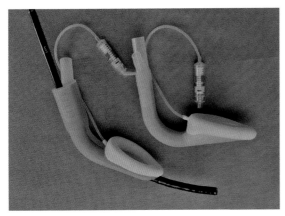

▲ **Figure 27-4.** Third-generation LMA devices. LMA Gastro with endoscope and LMA Protector. (Used with permission, from Dr. Patrick N. Olomu, University of Texas Southwestern Medical Center/Children's Health System of Texas - Dallas.)

Complications of LMA use are airway activation, oxygen desaturation, airway trauma, sore throat, hoarseness, and nerve injury. Many of these complications are the result of cuff overinflation and use of nonstandard insertion techniques.

Non-LMA™ Supraglottic Airway Devices (See Figures 27-1 & 27-2)

Air-Q Intubating Laryngeal Airway

The Air-Q® Intubating Laryngeal Airway (Cookgas, St. Louis, MO, the United States) is a non-LMA™ SGA used for routine anesthesia and as a conduit for intubation. It is manufactured of medical grade silicone. The design features appear to have advantages over earlier SGAs as a conduit for intubation in small children.[29,30] The wider, shorter, and curved airway tube as well as the detachable 15-mm connector allow for easier placement of the ETT and removal of the air-Q after intubation. It is available in three pediatric sizes: 1, 1.5, and 2. The weight recommendation and insertion technique are the same for the first-generation LMA™ devices. The manufacturer also recommends a gentle jaw lift to move the epiglottis more anteriorly and off the path of the advancing device. The larger sizes may be used for older children. Because of the wider airway tube, a larger ETT may be inserted through a relatively small air-Q. A fiberoptic bronchoscope (FOB) is recommended for intubation through the air-Q. A removal stylet is available to facilitate removal of the air-Q following endotracheal intubation.

Ambu Devices

The Ambu AuraOnce (Ambu USA, Columbia, MD, the United States) is a single-use SGA with a preformed curve. The Ambu Aura-i laryngeal mask is a modification of the original AuraOnce that is designed to facilitate intubation. Pediatric size recommendations are similar to the LMA™ with some consideration for the patient's height. The airway tube of the Aura-i is shorter, wider, and stiffer than the same-size AuraOnce. An integral bite block is present in the proximal portion. All pediatric sizes are available for clinical use. Insertion technique is similar to other first-generation devices. The Aura-i performed similarly to the air-Q as a conduit for tracheal intubation in children.[31]

Ambu-AuraGain

This second-generation SGA incorporates a drain tube in addition to the other features of the AuraOnce and Aura-i. It therefore can be used for routine anesthesia, as a conduit for intubation, and for more invasive procedures. It is available in all pediatric sizes. Markings on the device indicate its size, maximum ETT size, and maximum gastric tube size.

i-gel

The i-gel™ (Intersurgical Ltd., Wokingham, Berkshire, the United Kingdom) is a single-use second-generation SGA developed by Dr. Muhammed Nasir, a British anesthetist. Pediatric sizes were introduced in 2009. It is made of a thermoplastic elastomer gel and lacks a cuff. Its larger size may offer more stability and less risk of axial rotation. The airway tube has an integral bite block. The mask has an epiglottic rest for prevention of epiglottic downfolding. It is available in five full sizes and two pediatric half sizes (1.5 and 2.5). An integral drain tube is available in sizes 1.5 and higher. Despite the absence of a cuff, the i-gel appears to provide high seal pressures comparable to other second-generation SGAs.[32–35] It may also be used as a conduit for intubation.

DIRECT LARYNGOSCOPY

Direct laryngoscopy (DL) is used to visualize the glottis by aligning the oral, pharyngeal, and laryngeal axes. It is also called "line of sight" intubation, as a straight line is created between the eye and the glottis. An ETT can then be easily placed through the glottis and into the trachea. Endotracheal intubation is indicated for many elective and emergency procedures, especially when controlled mechanical ventilation is required. Prior to performance of DL, a thorough history and physical examination must be performed. Any contraindications or indicators of difficulty must be identified and documented.

Equipment, supplies, suction, and medications must be carefully prepared and assistance must be immediately available. Several formulae for the appropriate ETT size in pediatric patients have been described. The most widely used is $(Age + 16)/4$ for an uncuffed ETT.[36] This formula is for children 2 years or older. Another commonly used method is to use the tube that approximates the size of the child's small finger. Despite a lack of scientific validation, this method has proven clinically useful.[37] Two uncuffed tubes with an internal diameter of 0.5 mm smaller and larger should be immediately available should they be required. The leak pressure (the airway pressure at which an audible leak is heard) should be between 15 and 25 cm H_2O. This range allows for effective positive pressure ventilation without excessive mucosal pressure. If no audible leak is heard above 25 cm H_2O, a decision should be made whether to downsize the tube. The ease of initial tube placement and surgical duration are important considerations. A dose of dexamethasone (0.5 mg/kg) should be administered, if no contraindications exists, for airway swelling and postoperative nausea and vomiting prophylaxis. If a cuffed ETT is chosen, a half-size reduction is recommended. A full-size reduction may be required in certain patients at higher risk for airway swelling. When a cuffed tube is used, the gas leak can be easily controlled by inflating the cuff.

The initial depth of the ETT (cm) is as follows:

Oral: 3 × [ETT internal diameter (mm)]

Nasal: 3 × [ETT internal diameter (mm)] + 2 cm

An alternate formula is as follows:

Oral: (Age/2) + 12 cm

Nasal: (Age/2) + 15 cm

Historically, straight Miller-type blades are used for intubation in infants and small children under 8 years. They are believed to offer a better mechanical advantage when lifting the floppy epiglottis. Curved Macintosh blades may be used in older children over 8 years. Most experienced laryngoscopists can use both blade types interchangeably in infants and small children.

Standard practice for oral intubation begins with first extending the head and slightly flexing the neck.[38,39] Next, the blade (held in the left hand) is introduced from the right side of the mouth and the tongue is simultaneously "swept" to the left and displaced into the submental space. Gentle advancement of the blade will expose the tip of the epiglottis. The tip of a straight blade "lifts" the epiglottis from behind, exposing the glottic aperture. A curved blade is advanced in front of the epiglottis and into the vallecula. A gentle lifting action indirectly displaces the epiglottis and exposes the glottis. All "lifting" actions must be in the upward and forward direction. The teeth or gum line should never be used as a pivot point to lift the laryngeal structures as this can result in airway trauma. External laryngeal manipulation may facilitate visualization of the glottis.

NASOTRACHEAL INTUBATION

Nasotracheal intubation (NTI) was first described by Kuhn in 1902,[40] and then popularized in the 1920s by Magill.[41] This technique is commonly used for dental procedures, intraoral surgeries, or circumstances where orotracheal intubation is not an option (eg, intraoral mass or trismus). The nasal route is also an important path for fiberoptic intubation (FOI) as it provides a more direct route when compared to the oral route. The medial wall of the nasal cavity is formed by the nasal septum. The lateral wall is formed by the medial wall of the orbit and characterized by three nasal conchae (turbinates). With the inferior turbinate being the most prominent, it has the highest risk of being sheered with passage of an ETT, which would lead to massive epistaxis. Superiorly, the nasal cavity narrows toward the cribriform plate of the ethmoid bone, which separates it from the anterior cranial fossa. The nasotracheal route is contraindicated in patients with suspected basilar fractures since damage to the cribriform plate can lead to intracranial placement of the ETT. The sphenopalatine artery provides a majority of the blood supply to the nasal cavity. It forms anastomoses with other arteries in the anterior portion of the nasal septum called Kieselbach's plexus, also known as Little's area. This location is the most common source of epistaxis with placement of a nasal ETT. This technique is contraindicated in patients with a significant coagulopathy given the risk of bleeding. Assessment of the patient prior to this technique should include an evaluation for nasal polyps or septum deviation. Preparation for the procedure includes topicalization of the nasal airway with vasoconstrictors such as oxymetazoline or cocaine to minimize epistaxis, and the use of serial dilation with incrementally sized nasopharyngeal airways (NPAs) lubricated with a local anesthetic such as lidocaine. The right naris is traditionally preferred over the left since it makes subsequent laryngoscopy easier and facilitates use of the Magill forceps (Figure 27-5). With insertion of the ETT into the naris, the bevel should be facing the lateral wall, thereby orienting the tip of the tube toward the medial wall and away from the turbinates located on the lateral wall. The ETT should be passed posteriorly and parallel to the hard palate. Any resistance should not be forced forward, but rather withdrawn, rotated, and advanced again. A loss of resistance indicates passage into the oropharynx, at which point direct or video laryngoscopy should be performed to visualize the ETT. Using a Magill forceps, the tip of the ETT should be aligned with the glottic opening and then advanced (Figure 27-6). In situations where direct or video laryngoscopy is not possible, fiberoptic remains the gold standard. Abrons and coworkers recently described a NPA guided, bougie assisted (Seldinger technique), NTI.[42] The authors observed similar intubation success rates, decreased incidence and severity of nasopharyngeal trauma, and decreased requirement for transoral manipulation with a Magill's forceps.

ENDOTRACHEAL TUBES

▶ Microcuff

Microcuff tubes (Microcuff Pediatric Tracheal Tube, Microcuff GmbH, Weinheim, Germany; Microcuff PET, Kimberly Clark, Health Care, Atlanta, GA, the United States)

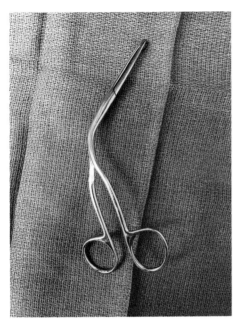

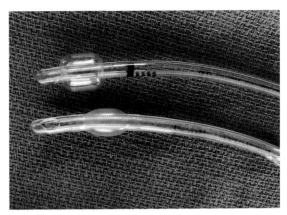

▲ **Figure 27-7.** The cuff of a Microcuff® endotracheal tube (top) next to a traditional endotracheal tube cuff (bottom), note the more distal, uniform, and cylindrical cuff of the Microcuff tube. (Used with permission, from Dr. Patrick N. Olomu, University of Texas Southwestern Medical Center/Children's Health System of Texas - Dallas.)

▲ **Figure 27-5.** Magill forceps. (Used with permission, from Dr. Patrick N. Olomu, University of Texas Southwestern Medical Center/Children's Health System of Texas - Dallas.)

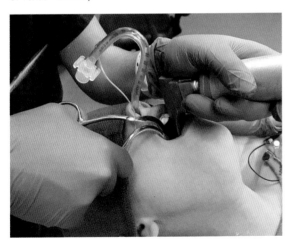

▲ **Figure 27-6.** Demonstrating advancement of a nasotracheal tube with a Magill forceps under visualization with direct laryngoscopy. (Used with permission, from Dr. Patrick N. Olomu, University of Texas Southwestern Medical Center/Children's Health System of Texas - Dallas.)

are unique high-volume/low-pressure cuffed ETTs. The hallmark of the microcuff is its ultra-thin (10 μm) polyurethane cuff, which replaces the thicker (50 to 70 μm) PVC cuff of traditional ETTs (Figure 27-7). With removal of the Murphy eye, the cuff is placed more distally on the shaft of the tube to ensure cuff placement below the subglottis. The cylindrical shape of the cuff makes uniform and complete contact with the tracheal wall without the formation of folds or channels. This allows for an airway seal at cuff pressures of approximately 10 cm H_2O, significantly lower than the 20 cm H_2O routinely required of traditional cuffed ETTs. Microcuff tubes have the potential to reduce tracheal mucosal edema, post-extubation stridor, and minimize the tube exchanges seen with sizing uncuffed ETT.[43] As with all ETTs, microcuff tubes require routine cuff pressure evaluation during their use. With ultra-thin polyurethane being highly permeable to nitrous oxide, these tubes are exceptionally vulnerable to hyperinflation with nitrous oxide use. When adopting the use of microcuff tubes, it is important to consider a cost–benefit analysis, since the cost of microcuff tubes can be several times that of traditional ETT.

Parker Flex-Tip

This ETT is designed to facilitate atraumatic intubation past the vocal cords, large nasal turbinates, or other possible areas at risk for trauma. The flexible, curved, and tapered tip of the tube allows for smooth passage while limiting the risk of it getting hung up (Figure 27-8). Other unique features of the tube include a downward facing bevel, and a murphy eye on each side of the tip. This tube is available in various designs, such as nasal, reinforced, uncuffed, and oral.

Reinforced

Armored or reinforced tubes are defined by the flexible spiral wire that fortifies the wall of the ETT (Figure 27-9). The flexibility of the wire allows the tube to hold any

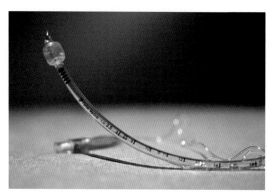

▲ **Figure 27-8.** Parker Flex Thin-Cuff endotracheal tube. (Used with permission, from Dr. Patrick N. Olomu, University of Texas Southwestern Medical Center/Children's Health System of Texas - Dallas.)

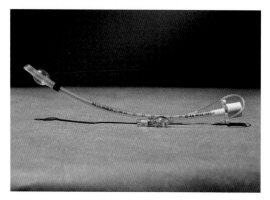

▲ **Figure 27-9.** Reinforced endotracheal tube. (Used with permission, from Dr. Patrick N. Olomu, University of Texas Southwestern Medical Center/Children's Health System of Texas - Dallas.)

formed shape and makes it kink-resistant. These features make the tube ideal for situations where there might be a risk for obstruction or kinking by surgical equipment, airways with unique angles, or prone positioning. While these tubes are kink-resistant relative to standard ETTs, they can be kinked by significant force. Once kinked, the spiral wire will not re-expand; therefore, it is important to safeguard against any significant force that might permanently kink and obstruct the tube. It is always prudent to use a bite block whenever possible when using a reinforced tube.

VIDEO LARYNGOSCOPY

Video laryngoscopes are devices that provide an indirect view of the larynx by using miniaturized video cameras and a light source. The image is transmitted to a display screen. Video laryngoscopes provide a wide angle and magnified view of the glottis and pharynx. In general, video laryngoscopes provide a one to two grade improvement in the Cormack and Lehane grade when compared to DL. Intubation times are, however, prolonged when compared to DL.[44–47] Their ability to see around the corner offers advantages in certain difficult intubation situations. Several devices have been introduced over the past 15 years and some of these are shown in Figure 27-10.

▶ Classification of Video Laryngoscope Blades

Video laryngoscopes are classified into three groups: standard geometry blades (nonangulated video laryngoscope blades), hyperangulated blades (angulated video laryngoscope blades), and channeled devices. Normal geometry blade types are similar to the commonly used Macintosh and Miller DL blades and include the C-MAC, Storz DCI, Truview, and GlideScope® Direct. The hyper-angulated

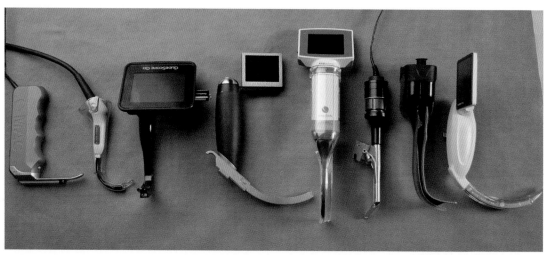

▲ **Figure 27-10.** Video laryngoscopes. Left to right: C-MAC, GlideScope Cobalt baton and Stat blade, GlideScope Go portable monitor, McGrath MAC Series 5, King Vision, Truview PCD, Airtraq, McGrath MAC. (Used with permission, from Dr. Patrick N. Olomu, University of Texas Southwestern Medical Center/Children's Health System of Texas - Dallas.)

Table 27-1. Overview of Commonly Used Video Laryngoscopes

Brand	Manufacturer	Blade Type	Pediatric Blades	Anti-Fogging Mechanism	Oxygen Insufflation	Use for Direct Laryngoscopy	Recording Capability	Blade Use	Field of View (Degrees)
GlideScope	Verathon Inc.	Hyperangulated	Yes	Yes	No	No	Yes	Single and reusable	45–53
C-MAC	Storz	Standard geometry and hyperangulated D-blade	Yes	Yes	Yes (separate attachment on blade)	Yes	Yes	Reusable and single	80–90
TruView PCD	Truphatek	Standard geometry	Yes	Yes (by oxygen flow)	Yes	No	Yes	Reusable	42
King Vision	Ambu Medical	Hyperangulated and channeled	Yes	Yes	No	No	Yes	Single	54
McGrath MAC	Aircraft Medical and Medtronic	Standard geometry	Yes	No	No	Yes	No	Single	N/I
PAWS	Pentax and Ambu Medical	Channeled	Yes	No	No	No	Yes	Single	N/I
Airtraq	Prodol Meditech and Teleflex	Channeled	Yes	Yes	No	No	Yes	Single	60

N/I, no information.
Source: Dr. Patrick N. Olomu, University of Texas Southwestern Medical Center/Children's Health System of Texas - Dallas, Dr. Edgar E. Kiss, University of Texas Southwestern Medical Center/Children's Health System of Texas - Dallas, Dr. Asif Khan, Boston Children's Hospital/Harvard Medical School.

blades are the GlidesScope, King Vision, McGrath series 5, McGrath MAC, and the Storz D-Blade. Video laryngoscopes with a guiding channel are as follows: the Airtraq, King Vision, and Pentax Airway Scope. An overview of video laryngoscopes is presented in Table 27-1.

Standard Geometry Blades (Nonangulated Video Laryngoscope Blades)

C-MAC Video Laryngoscope (Karl Storz, Tuttlingen, Germany)—This is the latest iteration of the Storz DCI system (Figure 27-11). It is a normal geometry blade, similar to the Macintosh and Miller blades. The complex optical system consists of a high-definition miniaturized camera, very bright LED, and a wide-angle lens. The image is transmitted by cable to a 7-inch monitor. A portable pocket monitor is also available. Miller #0, #1, and MAC #0 blades are available for infants and young toddlers. Disposable Miller 0 and 1 blades have recently been introduced and are used with the pediatric C-MAC imager (Figure 27-12).

Truview Picture Capture Device (PCD) Video Laryngoscope (Truphatek International Limited, Netanya, Israel)—The Truview PCD has reusable steel blades for use in infants and adults (Figure 27-13). The optical tube has a lens and a prism. A 46-degree inferior refraction provides an improved view of the larynx. A side port for deep oxygen insufflation is also available. The oxygen flow also defogs the lens and clears secretions. Use of the Truview PCD has been shown to delay oxygen desaturation during laryngoscopy in children.[48]

Hyperangulated Blades

GlideScope® Video Laryngoscope (Verathon Medical, Bothell, WA, USA)—The GlideScope® video laryngoscope is the first modern video laryngoscope and was introduced in 2001.[49] The Cobalt system is the most commonly used in children (Figure 27-14). It consists of the video baton, which is enshrouded by a disposable blade. Sizes 0, 1, 2, and 2.5 are available for pediatric patients. Olomu and co-workers found a high first-attempt success rate and improved glottic views in infants and children weighing less than 10 kg.[50] Sizes 3 and 4 are used in older children and have a larger video baton. Recently, the GlideScope® Spectrum system (Figure 27-15) was introduced into pediatric practice. The camera and LED are integrated into the blade, removing the need for a separate baton. The black single-use blades are more ergonomic, have a lower profile, and allow for improved maneuverability. Images are transferred to the monitor via a "smart connector" cable that attaches to a High-Definition Multimedia Interface (HDMI) output on the blade. Furthermore, the brighter LED light and reduced ambient light distortion provide a much higher image resolution. Sizes 1 and 2 blades are available for pediatric use and are

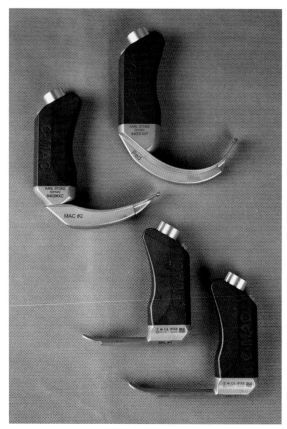

▲ **Figure 27-11.** C-MAC. New C-MAC standard pediatric blades and D blade (top right). (Used with permission, from Dr. Patrick N. Olomu, University of Texas Southwestern Medical Center/Children's Health System of Texas - Dallas.)

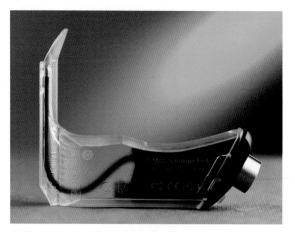

▲ **Figure 27-12.** C-MAC S Pediatric Imager with single use Miller #0 blade. (Used with permission, from Dr. Patrick N. Olomu, University of Texas Southwestern Medical Center/Children's Health System of Texas - Dallas.)

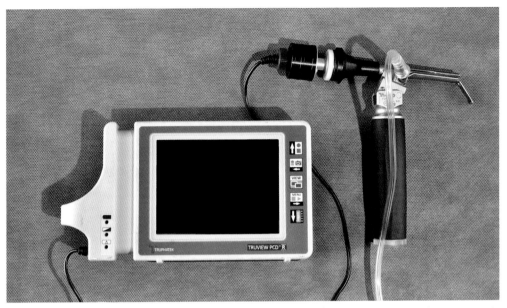

▲ **Figure 27-13.** Truview PCD video laryngoscope. (Used with permission, from Dr. Patrick N. Olomu, University of Texas Southwestern Medical Center/Children's Health System of Texas - Dallas.)

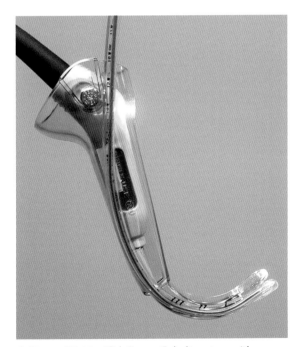

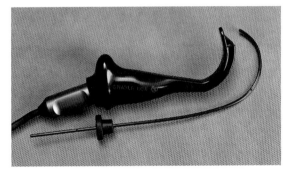

▲ **Figure 27-15.** GlideScope Spectrum with pediatric Glidrite® stylet. (Used with permission, from Dr. Patrick N. Olomu, University of Texas Southwestern Medical Center/Children's Health System of Texas - Dallas.)

▲ **Figure 27-14.** GlideScope Cobalt system with appropriately styletted endotracheal tube. (Used with permission, from Dr. Patrick N. Olomu, University of Texas Southwestern Medical Center/Children's Health System of Texas - Dallas.)

accompanied by an appropriately curved stylet (Gliderite®). Both blades were found to be highly effective for intubation in normal infant, difficult infant, and child manikin models.[51]

Steps for proper use of the GlideScope® video laryngoscope are as follows: prepare and check equipment, select patient-appropriate baton/blade, select appropriate ETT, insert stylet into ETT and shape to approximate the curve of the blade, slowly insert the blade midline into the mouth and visualize oropharyngeal structures looking for any abnormalities, center the uvula in the middle at the bottom of the screen, advance the blade slowly until the tip of the epiglottis is visualized, continue advancing the blade until the best view of the glottis is obtained, center the image as close as possible to the imaginary center of the monitor, and insert the tube directly behind the blade or from the right side. Look in the mouth to follow the tube until the tip of the tube appears on the monitor, advance the ETT to the glottic opening, and slowly remove the stylet.

In "can see, can't intubate" situations, the following steps may be beneficial: ensure image is centered on the display screen, gently back up the stylet and advance ETT slowly while rotating the ETT clockwise or counter-clockwise, and aligning the glottic aperture with the ETT by intentionally decreasing the airway grade (by decreasing the traction on the tongue). Reverse loading of the ETT on the stylet may also be attempted. This is done by placing the

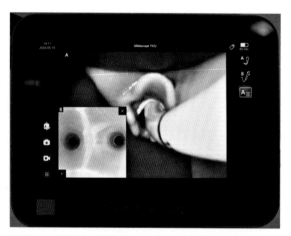

▲ **Figure 27-16.** GlideScope Core touchscreen monitor. (Used with permission, from Dr. Patrick N. Olomu, University of Texas Southwestern Medical Center/Children's Health System of Texas - Dallas.)

Murphy eye of the ETT anteriorly. Stylet withdrawal returns ETT to its original form in a rotational movement facilitating intubation. A FOB may also be used as a maneuverable stylet to advance the ETT into the trachea. Most recently, Verathon has released a new monitor for comprehensive airway visualization. The GlideScope® Core™ (Figure 27-16) offers a high-resolution 10-inch touchscreen monitor with simultaneous (picture-in-picture) display. This allows simultaneous displays of both the video laryngoscope and flexible digital scope (BFlex™) images. Each of these modalities may be used alone or in combination (see the section "Hybrid (Combined) Techniques"). The monitor also has an integral pulse oximeter for line-of-sight monitoring of oxygenation during difficult airway management.

C-MAC Video Laryngoscope (Karl Storz, Tuttlingen, Germany)—The pediatric D (Dörges) blade is a hyperangulated blade designed for extremely difficult airways (Figure 27-11). It allows the use to "see around the corner." This blade may be unsuitable for small infants. An adult-size blade is also available and may be used in older children. Single-use adult D blades for use with an adult imager have recently been introduced.

King Vision Video Laryngoscope—The King Vision® Video Laryngoscope (Ambu USA, Columbia, MD, the United States) is a portable hyperangulated blade for indirect laryngoscopy. The video baton has an integrated camera, an LED light source, and a portable monitor (Figure 27-17). The disposable blade enshrouds the baton and the image is projected on a 2.4-inch monitor. Sizes 1, 2, and 2C (Channeled) blades are available for pediatric use (Figure 27-18). Even though no recording capability is available on the portable monitor, an output port allows projection to compatible monitors in the operating room. Λ 10-mm mouth opening is required for the standard blade, while the channeled blade requires a 13-mm mouth opening. A recent study comparing the King Vision Video laryngoscope to a standard Miller

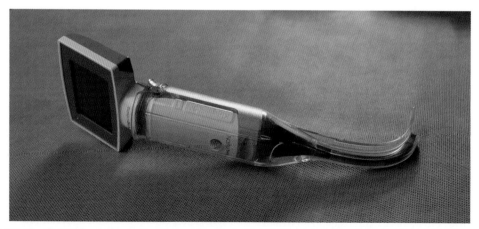

▲ **Figure 27-17.** King Vision video laryngoscope (regular). (Used with permission, from Dr. Patrick N. Olomu, University of Texas Southwestern Medical Center/Children's Health System of Texas - Dallas.)

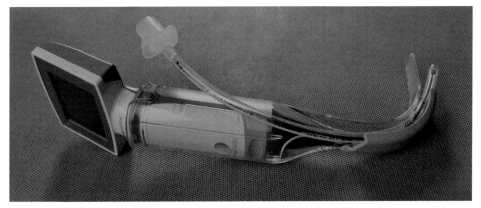

▲ **Figure 27-18.** King Vision blade with guiding channel. (Used with permission, from Dr. Patrick N. Olomu, University of Texas Southwestern Medical Center/Children's Health System of Texas - Dallas.)

direct laryngoscope found the King Vision to be equally effective for tracheal intubation in children 2 years or younger.[52]

McGrath Series 5—The McGrath® Series 5 (Aircraft Medical, Edinburgh, UK) is the original portable video laryngoscope (Figure 27-10). The adjustable steel blade may be fastened from the equivalent of a size 3 to 5 MAC blade sizes. The blade may also be disarticulated from the handle and inserted into the mouth before rearticulation. Only one disposable blade size is available.

McGrath MAC—The McGrath® MAC (Aircraft Medical, Medtronic Medical, Dublin, Ireland) is the improved version of the McGrath Series 5. The ergonomic handle houses a lithium battery and a larger monitor (Figure 27-10) Unlike series 5, the steel blade is not adjustable. The device comes with a standard size 3 blade and two smaller pediatric blades (sizes 1 and 2). Four standard blade sizes (1-4) are available for clinical use. Recently, a hyperangulated size 3 X-blade was introduced for the very difficult airways. A new third generation device has also recently been introduced, with higher image resolution, brighter LED light, and auto shut-off to conserve battery drainage.

Channeled Devices

Airtraq Optical Laryngoscope

The Airtraq® (Prodol Meditec, Vizcaya, Spain) is the prototype channeled device (Figure 27-19). The optical tube consists of a series of prisms and lenses that transfer the image to an eyepiece. A camera head or an adapter can then transfer the image to an external monitor, a clip-on monitor, or a smartphone screen. The specialized Airtraq camera can also project the image wirelessly to a larger monitor such as an iPad. Color-coded devices are available in several sizes from infants to adults. The gray and purple colors are for infant and young toddlers, respectively (Figure 27-20). The device is inserted in the midline

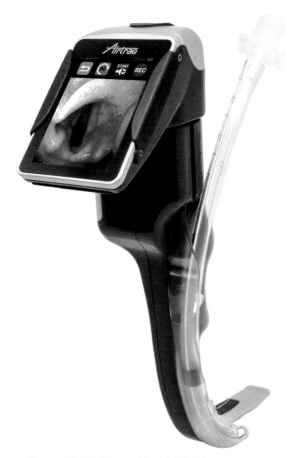

▲ **Figure 27-19.** Airtraq SP with Wi-Fi Camera and endotracheal tube. (Image courtesy of Teleflex Incorporated. © 2020 Teleflex Incorporated. All rights reserved.)

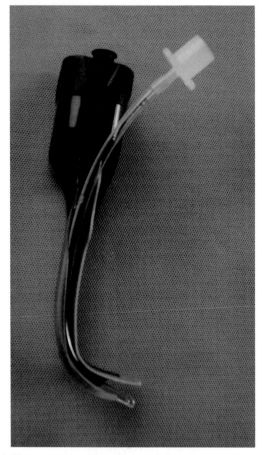

▲ **Figure 27-20.** Infant Airtraq with endotracheal tube. (Used with permission, from Dr. Edgar E. Kiss, University of Texas Southwestern Medical Center/Children's Health System of Texas - Dallas.)

and advanced slowly until the epiglottis is visualized. Further advancement to the vallecula or gently lifting of the epiglottis provides a clear and magnified view of the glottis. Centering the image on the monitor appears to facilitate insertion. The ETT is slowly advanced through the glottis and into the trachea. The proximal part of the ETT is then "peeled away" from the guiding channel. The Airtraq may be used with a FOB as part of a combined technique should ETT advancement proves difficult. The Airtraq provides a better view of the larynx compared with DL, but time to intubation is longer.[53]

FIBEROPTIC BRONCHOSCOPES

The history of bronchoscopy began in the late 1870s when Gustav Killian used a rigid bronchoscope to successfully extract a foreign body from a farmer's respiratory tract.[54,55] However, it was not until 1968 that Machida Endoscope and Olympus produced the FOB initially proposed by Shigeto

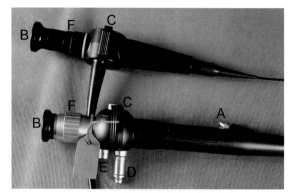

▲ **FIGURE 27-21.** Parts of the fiber-optic bronchoscope. Top: neonate fiber-optic bronchoscope (FOB). Bottom: child/adult-sized FOB. The handle consists of the working channel (A), lens (B), distal flexible tip control lever (C), light source adaptor port (D), suction valve port (E), and focus ring (F). (Used with permission, from Dr. Edgar E. Kiss, University of Texas Southwestern Medical Center/Children's Health System of Texas - Dallas.)

Ikeda in 1966. The FOB was quickly recognized for its unique characteristics and became an instrument of choice for difficult intubation management and other diagnostic purposes. Olympus, Pentax, Vision Sciences, Ambu, and Karl Storz are current major manufacturers of various bronchoscopes.[56-61]

▶ Design

The handle, insertion tube, and flexible tip are the three main parts of the fiberscope. A light source that is either battery powered or connected to an external light source is attached to the handle. The visual section of the handle located proximally is composed of an eyepiece and lens, a video output adaptor, or a video screen with an integrated camera. The focus is adjusted by a focus ring near the handle (Figures 27-21 and 27-22). The insertion tube is the part of the FOB that goes into the patient and ranges from 50 to 65 cm in length, depending on the manufacturer. Its outer diameter (OD) determines the minimum internal diameter (ID) of the ETT in which the FOB can pass. The neonate and infant FOB made by Pentax and Olympus have the smallest external diameter of 2.4 and 2.2 mm, respectively, and will accommodate an ETT as small as 2.5 mm (ID). The flexible tip can bend as much as 350 degrees using the controller on the back of the handle. However, the glass fibers are sensitive to excessive bending and pressure especially if the tip of the FOB is still in the ETT, which can damage the scope (Figure 27-23). The working channel runs the length of the FOB to the tip of the scope. This channel allows for administration of medication and adding suction. Connecting oxygen to the working channel should be avoided in infants and some children as this may cause overinflation of the lungs resulting in barotrauma.[62–64] "Single-use" FOB either with a disposable sheath-like protective barrier (Vision Sciences) or completely disposable digital bronchoscopes (Ambu® aScope™, Storz Five S, and Verathon BFlex™) have recently been developed to help avoid cross-contamination and protect immunocompromised patients (Figures 27-24 through 27-26). These "non-fiber-optic" scopes use a CMOS (complementary metal oxide semiconductor) sensor, thereby eliminating fiberoptic wires that are prone to breakage.[65–67]

Indications and Contraindications for Use of Fiberoptic Intubation in Pediatrics

Fiberoptic intubation (FOI) has become the "gold standard" for patients where traditional DL may be difficult or even impossible. It can be used to intubate in various patient positions, through the nasopharynx or orally, troubleshoot ventilation problems, and confirm ETT position during conventional ventilation or single lung ventilation. In patients with concern for an unstable cervical spine, FOI has been shown to result in minimal cervical spine motion.[68] Due to the wide range of syndromes with the possibility of associated congenital abnormalities in infants and children, the FOB is an important tool for managing the pediatric difficult airway.[69,70] The contraindications for FOI are few but include lack of skill and training with the FOB, near complete total airway obstruction, and significant amounts of blood in the airway that may obscure the distal lens.[62] Passing the ETT blindly over the FOB may cause trauma to airway structures, especially the vocal cords. A combined technique with video laryngoscopy (Figure 27-27) or direct laryngoscopy can allow for better visualization of the ETT passage past the cords.

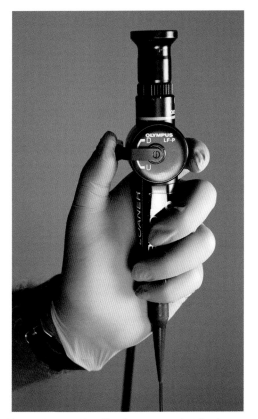

▲ **Figure 27-22.** Handle of a neonate intubating bronchoscope. The thumb is positioned to maneuver the flexible tip up or down while the other opposite hand guides the distal end of the insertion tube. (Used with permission, from Dr. Edgar E. Kiss, University of Texas Southwestern Medical Center/Children's Health System of Texas - Dallas.)

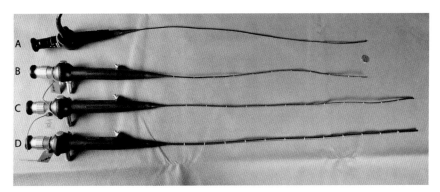

▲ **Figure 27-23.** Various sizes of intubating fiber-optic bronchoscopes. (A) Olympus neonate bronchoscope with external diameter of 2.2 mm, lacking a working channel; (B), (C), (D) Karl Storz FOBs sizes 2.8-, 3.7-, 5.2-mm external diameter include a working channel. Penny included for scale. (Used with permission, from Dr. Edgar E. Kiss, University of Texas Southwestern Medical Center/Children's Health System of Texas - Dallas.)

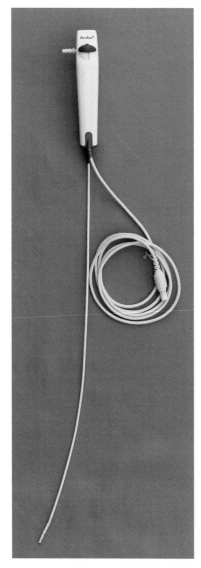

▲ **Figure 27-24.** Ambu aScope single-use digital scope. (Used with permission, from Dr. Patrick N. Olomu, University of Texas Southwestern Medical Center/Children's Health System of Texas - Dallas.)

▶ Planning and Techniques

The anesthetic management of the pediatric patient with a difficult airway starts with a thorough review of the medical record including all prior anesthetics and a detailed history and physical examination. Usually, the ability to mask ventilate or not is a critically important factor and greatly influences the airway management plan. If the FOB is chosen to be deployed or as a backup, all components should be checked for functionality and visually inspected for damage. Once the appropriate FOB size is selected for the

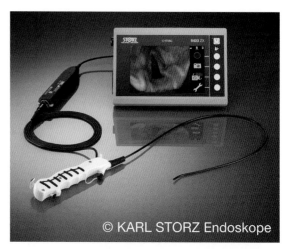

▲ **Figure 27-25.** Storz Five S single-use digital scope (pediatric). (Image courtesy of KARL STORZ. ©2020KARL STORZ Endoscopy-America, Inc. All rights reserved.)

patient, the ETT is loaded onto the lightly lubricated insertion tube and held in place proximally by a piece of tape. Some newer digital scopes have a tube-holding mechanism. All other routine and backup airway management devices should be inspected prior to induction of anesthesia.

Adolescents and young adults will have the greatest success rates of awake FOB intubation with mild sedation and local anesthetic topicalization of the airway. However, a vast majority of patients with difficult airways also have coexisting developmental delays that will make an awake attempt nearly impossible.[71] For this reason, FOB intubation in infants and children are mostly performed under general anesthesia (GA) or moderate to deep sedation depending on the situation. Patient preparation without intravenous access includes premedication with an oral anxiolytic (midazolam 0.5 to 0.7 mg/kg). If the patient has intravenous (IV) access, midazolam intravenously (0.1 mg/kg up to 2 mg) usually provides enough anxiolysis for separation from the parents. Intramuscular ketamine combined with midazolam and glycopyrrolate as well as intranasal dexmedetomidine or midazolam with lidocaine administration are also options in uncooperative patients. In patients who still do not tolerate peripheral intravenous access after premedication, inhalation induction with a nonpungent inhalational agent (sevoflurane) is acceptable. The vasodilatory effect of inhalation anesthetics aids in obtaining an IV access shortly after induction. The recent advent of vein-viewer technology and improved ultrasound-guided PIV techniques increase the likelihood of success.

After the patient is brought to the operating suite and standard anesthesia monitors are placed, anesthesia is induced either via the inhalational or intravenous routes. Maintenance of spontaneous ventilation is desirable while performing FOI until a definitive airway is established. Spontaneous ventilation can be achieved with titration of

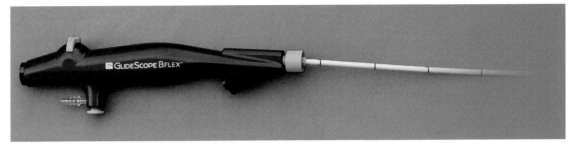

▲ **Figure 27-26.** Verathon Bflex single-use digital scope. (Used with permission, from Dr. Patrick N. Olomu, University of Texas Southwestern Medical Center/Children's Health System of Texas - Dallas.)

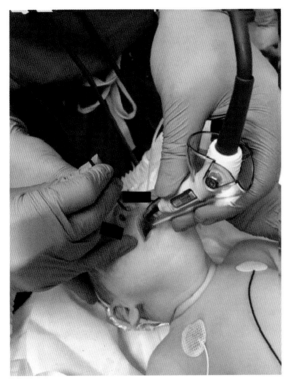

▲ **Figure 27-27.** Combined technique. Video laryngoscopy used to aid in visualization of nasal endotracheal tube passage through the cords over the fiber-optic scope. (Used with permission, from Dr. Patrick N. Olomu, University of Texas Southwestern Medical Center/Children's Health System of Texas - Dallas.)

propofol and minimizing any narcotics. Due to its narrow therapeutic margin, propofol may cause apnea and must therefore be administered very slowly in this situation. Ketamine has a lower incidence of apnea and may be titrated to desired effect. Dexmedetomidine is devoid of airway depressive effects but may cause intraoperative hypotension and prolonged sedation during recovery.

Supplemental oxygen should be provided during FOI attempts through either nasal cannula, high-flow nasal cannula, or oral RAE tube taped to side of mouth.[72] A modified NPA with a 15-mm ETT connector may also be used with an anesthesia breathing system (Figure 27-34). Glycopyrrolate at the antisialogogue dose of 5 mcg/kg should be administered prior to FOI attempts, especially if ketamine is used.

Nasotracheal intubation offers the most direct route for passage of the FOB into the trachea. The bed is lowered and the patient is positioned with the head in a neutral position. An ETT tube half-size smaller than for the oral route should be used for NTI. Oxymetazoline 0.05% or phenylephrine 0.5% intranasal sprays increase the nasal airway lumen size and decrease the risk of bleeding. Lidocaine 2% to 4% spray/gel/paste may also be applied intranasally but may not be necessary if the patient is under GA. The FOB is inserted into one of the nares and advanced under direct visualization. A lubricated breakaway NPA may be used in older children to aid in passage of the FOB.[73] Care must be taken not to damage the adenoid tissue. The "spray as you go" of local anesthetic consisting of lidocaine 2% or 4% helps avoid hemodynamic changes during attempts making sure to avoid LA toxicity.[74] A jaw thrust and/or tongue pull will help open the posterior oropharynx for better exposure of airway structures. Gauze is used to pull the tongue forward but a stitch at the tip of the tongue may also help in extreme circumstances. The tip of the FOB usually requires some degree of forward flexion to advance through the vocal cords but quickly needs to be relaxed or retroflexed to continue down the trachea. The ETT is then advanced over the FOB into the trachea being mindful of any resistance met along the way. Forcing the ETT when resistance is met may cause trauma, vocal cord injury, or damage to the FOB.

For oral FOIs, the FOB is inserted through the mouth, down the midline avoiding any blind advancement and follows the same steps outlined above. Care must be taken when progressing below the level of the vocal cords, keeping in mind that the funnel-shaped infant larynx is narrowest at the level of the cricoid cartilage.[75]

Failure of FOB-Assisted Intubation

The lack of experience with the FOB has been heralded as the most common cause of failure of FOIs. A support system of experienced personnel who are ready to assist and quickly troubleshoot will likely increase the success rates and minimize the risks. Other reasons for difficulties include the FOB tip exiting through the Murphy's eye of the ETT, hanging up at the arytenoids, and mistaking the esophagus for the trachea due to indentation-like rings in the esophageal anatomy. Since fogging, blood, and secretions can make identifying structures difficult, some have advocated concurrent use of the video laryngoscopy to visualize the passage of the FOB and ETT through the vocal cords.[62,76]

PRINCIPLES OF DIFFICULT AIRWAY MANAGEMENT

The American Society of Anesthesiologists (ASA) defines a difficult airway (DA) as: "The clinical situation in which a conventionally trained anesthesiologist experiences difficulty with face mask ventilation of the upper airway, difficulty with tracheal intubation, or both." The overall incidence of difficult laryngoscopy (Cormack and Lehane grade III/IV) in pediatric patients is 1.35% with a higher incidence in infants (4.7% vs. 0.7%) compared to older children.[77] Fiadjoe et al. found an incidence of 2 to 5 difficult intubations per 1000 intubations based on findings from the Multicenter Pediatric Difficult Intubation Registry (PeDIR).[78] Predictors of DA include micrognathia (small jaw), midface hypoplasia, obstructive sleep apnea, microtia (especially when bilateral), and neck immobility. The six most common syndromes associated with difficult intubation are Pierre Robin sequence, hemifacial microsomia, Klippel–Feil sequence, Treacher Collins syndrome, epidermolysis bullosa, and Hurler syndrome (unpublished report from the Multicenter PeDIR database). The majority of DA patients have a known syndrome whereas a small fraction have an unknown syndrome or no syndrome at all. Management of the difficult airway begins with a detailed history and physical examination. A history of any coexisting medical problems, especially congenital heart disease, should be sought. Records of prior anesthetic management should be carefully reviewed.

Physical examination should focus on mouth size and opening, jaw size, tongue size and neck mobility. Imaging of the airway and associated structures may be required in a small subset of patients with severe disease. Such imaging may include plain radiographs, computerized tomography, magnetic resonance imaging, and ultrasonography. A comprehensive plan for airway management should include the following: experience of the staff/team, sedation/induction technique, availability of ancillary devices/techniques, method of intubation, method of oxygenation during and between attempts, and a logical order of technique/device selection. The common adage is that plans A, B, and C must be clearly defined and communicated to all team members. A plan for rescue and extubation must also be made. Team members should always debrief following DA management. Most institutions will have a difficult airway cart in the operating room and at other locations, such as the pediatric intensive care unit and the emergency department. Their contents will depend on local needs and preferences. In general, it should include a wide array of basic and advanced airway devices and a device for a surgical airway.

COMPLICATIONS OF DIFFICULT AIRWAY MANAGEMENT

Complications of difficult airway management are classified as severe and nonsevere.[78] Severe complications include severe hypoxemia, pneumothorax, severe airway trauma, aspiration, esophageal intubation with delayed recognition, emergent surgical airway, and cardiac arrest. Non-severe complications are minor airway trauma, pharyngeal bleeding and epistaxis, arrhythmias without hemodynamic consequences, bronchospasm, laryngospasm, esophageal intubation with immediate recognition, and short-lived hypoxemia (10% below preintubation saturation and lasting <45 seconds). Risk factors for severe complications are weight under 10 kg, greater than two intubation attempts, and persistence with direct laryngoscopy (DL for first three attempts).[78] Administration of supplemental oxygen during difficult airway management can prevent severe hypoxemia and other severe complications. For use of nasal cannula, modified oral RAE tube to the side of the mouth, and use of a modified NPA see the section "Ancillary Airway Techniques."

EXTUBATION OF THE DIFFICULT AIRWAY

Post-extubation respiratory complications occur very frequently.[79] Extubation planning is therefore a critical part of difficult airway management. Consideration must be given to location of the planned extubation, staffing, and techniques to maintain an airway. Most importantly, equipment for reintubation must be immediately available. If airway trauma occurred during difficult airway management, steroids should be given and delayed extubation may be indicated. An airway exchange catheter or guidewire may be used for airway access following extubation. In general, awake extubation is recommended following difficult airway management. Extubation planning should be documented and clearly communicated to all staff caring for the patient. Special attention must be given to location, timing, and position of extubation. Complications of a poorly conducted extubation are airway activation, excessive coughing, hypoxemia, upper airway obstruction, and airway trauma.

Airway Exchange Catheters

The indications for ETT exchange are varied and include change in ETT size or type, change in ETT route (ie, nasal to oral or vice versa), ruptured or leaking cuff, or ETT obstruction. Exchange of an ETT can be easily facilitated using an airway exchange catheter (AEC). An AEC is a semi-rigid thin catheter with a hollow lumen and a blunt tip. The long length of the AEC allows for it to be threaded into an ETT to maintain access to the airway when the ETT is removed. A replacement ETT can be simply "railroaded" over the AEC left in place, thereby easily facilitating tube exchange. When advancing the replacement ETT over the AEC, direct or video laryngoscopy can be used to displace the tongue and any soft tissue obstructing the path of the ETT. Replacement of the ETT under visualization can also prevent the ETT from getting caught in the piriform fossa or blocked by the arytenoid cartilages. Most exchange catheters allow for ventilation, in an emergency situation, through their hollow lumen and distal holes. For the Cook airway exchange catheters (Cook Critical Care, Bloomington, IN), a Luer-Lock jet adapter and a 15-mm connector allow for jet ventilation and connection to the anesthesia circuit, respectively (Figure 27-28). An AEC may also be placed prior to extubation of a suspected difficult airway or critically ill patient who might fail extubation and require reintubation. If placed before removal of the ETT and left in place post-extubation, the AEC can act as a quick and easy conduit for reintubation.

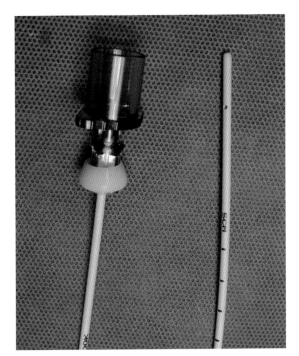

▲ **Figure 27-28.** Cook Airway Exchange Catheter (8.0F) showing Rapi-Fit™ 15-mm adapter. (Used with permission, from Dr. Patrick N. Olomu, University of Texas Southwestern Medical Center/Children's Health System of Texas - Dallas.)

FRONT OF NECK ACCESS (FONA) IN PEDIATRIC PATIENTS

FONA refers to all invasive airway access techniques performed in the anterior neck, from the cricothyroid membrane (CTM) to the anterior tracheal wall. The incidence of emergency front of neck access (FONA) in pediatric patients is extremely low.[80] When they occur, they are associated with a high mortality rate.[80] Many anesthesiologists have never and will likely never perform one in their careers. From birth to adolescence, trachea length doubles, tracheal diameter triples, and tracheal cross-sectional area increases sixfold.[81] The neonatal CTM measures 2.6 mm × 3.0 mm compared to 10.4 mm × 8.2 mm wide in the adult. The mean newborn tracheal length is about 4 cm.

FONA is indicated in "can't intubate, can't oxygenate" situations. FONA in pediatric patients can be achieved by one of four methods: small cannula (angiocatheter) cricothyroidotomy, large cannula cricothyroidotomy (Seldinger), large cannula cricothyroidotomy (non-Seldinger or scalpel), and emergency tracheostomy by a surgeon. Anesthesiologists are generally more familiar and comfortable with the angiocatheter and Seldinger techniques. In the small cannula technique, a 14–18G angiocatheter is introduced into the inferior aspect of the of the CTM. Aspiration of air confirms intratracheal placement. The catheter is advanced

and the needle removed. The catheter may be connected to a jet ventilator or other similar devices. Care must be taken to ensure upper airway patency to avoid the risk of barotrauma. Injury to surrounding structures must be avoided. Various brands are available for large cannula technique in children and adults. The Melker Emergency Cricothyrotomy Catheter set (Seldinger, Cook Medical, Inc., Bloomington, IN, USA) is available in a 3.5 mm and 4.2 mm internal diameter sizes (Figure 27-29). A cut down (scalpel) set is also available in a 5.0 mm internal diameter size. A Universal Set, consisting of both types, is also available but only in the 5.0 mm internal diameter size (Figure 27-30). In the Seldinger technique, a needle is inserted through a small skin incision over the cricothyroid membrane. Tracheal entry is confirmed by aspiration of air. A guidewire is placed and the needle or catheter is removed. A tapered dilator and catheter are inserted as a unit over the wire and into the trachea. The guidewire and dilator are then removed as a unit leaving the catheter in place. A guidewire may also be used with an existing small cannula (angiocatheter). In the surgical approach, a vertical midline incision is made over the cricothyroid membrane and carried down to the laryngeal structures. A horizontal incision is made near the inferior edge of the cricothyroid membrane. Tracheal hooks

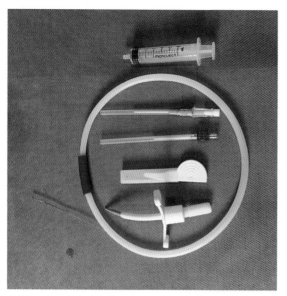

▲ **Figure 27-29.** Melker Emergency Cricothyrotomy Set (Seldinger). (Used with permission, from Dr. Patrick N. Olomu, University of Texas Southwestern Medical Center/Children's Health System of Texas - Dallas.)

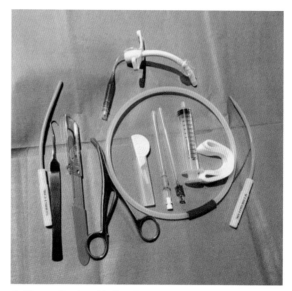

▲ **Figure 27-30.** Melker Emergency Universal Cricothyrotomy Set (Seldinger and Scalpel). (Used with permission, from Dr. Patrick N. Olomu, University of Texas Southwestern Medical Center/Children's Health System of Texas - Dallas.)

are used to retract the inferior margin of the thyroid cartilage superiorly. The CTM incision is then dilated using a Trousseau dilator or simply widened by gently turning the blade. The catheter-dilator assembly is inserted into the trachea as a unit and the dilator removed. Alternatively, an appropriately sized ETT may be placed. There is increasing evidence that the small cannula (angiocatheter) technique should be the first FONA technique in children 1 to 8 years of age.[82] Complications of FONA are bleeding, creation of a false passage, and damage to surrounding structures. Anesthesiologists should familiarize themselves with these techniques using manikin or animal models, especially at review courses and conferences.

HYBRID (COMBINED) TECHNIQUES

The recognition that no individual technique guarantees success has led to the utilization of hybrid (combined) techniques. Hybrid techniques utilize two or more modalities for management of the difficult airway. The most commonly used hybrid techniques are as follows: FOB intubation through a supraglottic airway (Figures 27-31 and 27-32), video laryngoscopy–assisted FOI, and retrograde-assisted FOI.[33,76,83–90] When a fiberoptic or digital bronchoscope is used in combination with a video laryngoscope, simultaneous upper and lower airway visualization is achieved. This typically requires two separate monitors depending on local availability. The new GlideScope Core™ (Figure 27-16) picture-in-picture modality allows both views

to be displayed simultaneously on a touchscreen monitor (see the section "GlideScope"). Practitioners must gain experience in the performance of these techniques to minimize the risk of serious complications.

▶ Ancillary Airway Techniques

Two-Handed Mask Ventilation

There will be situations with mask ventilation when the ability to obtain an adequate seal or maintain a patent airway for ventilation can be difficult to accomplish with one hand. If an oral or nasal airway does not result in improved ventilation, two-handed mask ventilation should be considered. With this technique, one person uses both hands to mask seal the patient, while a second person compresses the reservoir bag to ventilate. When mask sealing with both hands, the left and right hands are both applying a jaw thrust while the thumbs and index fingers are maintaining a seal (Figure 27-33). This maximizes the ability to lift the mandible, thereby elevating the hyoid bone and tongue off the posterior pharyngeal wall and alleviating any soft tissue obstruction. The second person has the ability to feel the effectiveness of ventilation via the reservoir bag, while also applying CPAP to the airway if necessary. This technique can also be accomplished by a solo anesthesia provider, where the provider performs a two-handed mask seal while the anesthesia machine is activated to ventilate the patient.

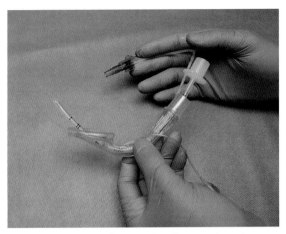

▲ **Figure 27-31.** Ambu AuraGain laryngeal mask with ETT and gastric suction catheter. (Used with permission, from Dr. Patrick N. Olomu, University of Texas Southwestern Medical Center/Children's Health System of Texas - Dallas.)

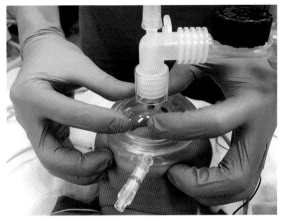

▲ **Figure 27-33.** Two-handed mask ventilation. Note the placement of the third and fourth fingers on the mandible, and not the soft tissue. (Used with permission, from Dr. Patrick N. Olomu, University of Texas Southwestern Medical Center/Children's Health System of Texas - Dallas.)

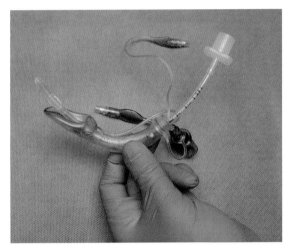

▲ **Figure 27-32.** Air-Q ILMA with ETT. Note the detachable 15-mm connector. (Used with permission, from Dr. Patrick N. Olomu, University of Texas Southwestern Medical Center/Children's Health System of Texas - Dallas.)

Nasopharyngeal Airways

The NPA is a plastic or rubber cylinder of various sizes that is placed in the naris to alleviate airway obstruction between the tongue and the posterior pharyngeal wall. The appropriate size NPA for each patient is based upon the visual width of the naris, which is typically similar to the width of the patient's fifth finger. The ideal position of the NPA is approximately 10 mm above the epiglottis and should ideally clear the tongue base.[91] The distance from the naris to the angle of the mandible is the approximate length the

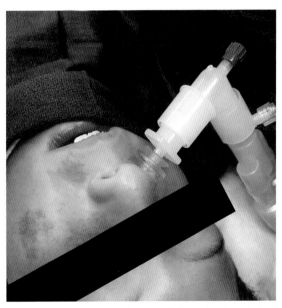

▲ **Figure 27-34.** A nasopharyngeal airway in place that has been connected to the anesthesia circuit via a 15-mm adapter from an endotracheal tube. (Used with permission, from Dr. Patrick N. Olomu, University of Texas Southwestern Medical Center/Children's Health System of Texas - Dallas.)

NPA needs to achieve this ideal position. Prior to insertion, the NPA should be lubricated with a water-based lubricant to facilitate passage. Use of lidocaine gel may improve patient tolerance. In addition to this, the nasal passage should be inspected for patency, nasal polyps, or any septal deviation that might complicate placement of an NPA. The naris can be topicalized with vasoconstrictor sprays or

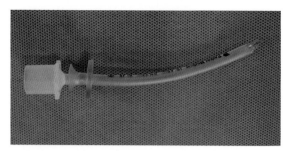

▲ **Figure 27-35.** Nasopharyngeal airway with a Flex-Tip®, slidable depth ring, and a 15-mm connector. (Used with permission, from Dr. Patrick N. Olomu, University of Texas Southwestern Medical Center/Children's Health System of Texas - Dallas.)

drops to minimize the risk of epistaxis. Upon insertion, the NPA should be advanced gently with the concave side parallel to the hard palate. This will result in the NPA advancing downward toward the posterior nasopharynx, rather than upwards toward the cribriform plate of the ethmoid bone which can lead to intracranial placement of the NPA. Difficulty with passage of an NPA can be overcome with a 90 degrees counterclockwise rotation of the NPA, use of a smaller size, or switching to the other naris. In the awake or semiconscious patient, where a gag reflex remains intact, an NPA is an alternative airway device to an oropharyngeal airway (OPA). It also has advantages over an OPA in situations of oral trauma and limited mouth opening. Furthermore, as a less stimulating airway device, it can be used in situations of increased intracranial pressure. Upon emergence, the NPA can be an excellent device if there is any concern of residual airway obstruction, as commonly seen in pediatric patients undergoing adenotonsillectomy for severe obstructive sleep apnea. Contraindications to use of an NPA are bleeding disorders, anticoagulation, or suspected basilar skull fractures. An NPA can be connected to the anesthesia circuit with the 15-mm connector from an ETT (Figure 27-34). Newer designs with a Flex-Tip®, a slidable depth ring, and a 15-mm connector (Figure 27-35) are now available (Parker Medical and Mercury Medical, Clearwater, FL, the United States). The correct NPA French size is the ETT internal diameter multiplied by 4. Ventilating through an NPA can be a beneficial technique when managing a difficult airway or performing FOI.

VIDEOS

Video 27-1. Insertion technique for LMA Unique. Note fully deflated mask.

Video 27-2. Insertion technique for LMA Supreme. Note tape application prior to mask inflation to prevent outward migration and loss of seal.

Video 27-3. Insertion technique for the Air-Q Intubating Laryngeal Airway.

Video 27-4. Insertion of the Ambu AuraGain laryngeal mask.

Video 27-5. Video intubation with GlideScope Cobalt blade and generic stylet.

Video 27-6. Video intubation with portable GlideScope (Glidescope® Go™), pediatric Spectrum blade, and pediatric Gliderite stylet.

Video 27-7. Video intubation using King Vision channeled blade.

Video 27-8. Combined Air-Q ILA and fiberoptic intubation.

Video 27-9. Combined GlideScope and fiberoptic intubation (Ambu aScope digital scope) showing both views.

Video 27-10. Combined C-MAC video laryngoscope and fiber-optic intubation (internal C-MAC view only).

Videos can be accessed at https://accessanesthesiology.mhmedical.com/.

REFERENCES

1. Brimacombe J. A proposed classification system for extraglottic airway devices. *Anesthesiology.* 2004;101(2):559.
2. Brimacombe J. Laryngeal mask. In: *Anesthesia: Principles and Practice.* 2nd ed. Philadelphia, PA: Saunders (Elsevier); 2005:505-537.
3. Mark DA. Protection from aspiration with the LMA-ProSeal after vomiting: a case report. *Can J Anaesth.* 2003;50(1):78–80.
4. Keller C, Brimacombe J, von Goedecke A, Lirk P. Airway protection with the ProSeal laryngeal mask airway in a child. *Paediatr Anaesth.* 2004 Dec;14(12):1021-1022.
5. Goldmann K, Jakob C. Prevention of aspiration under general anesthesia by use of the size 2$^{1/2}$ ProSeal laryngeal mask airway in a 6-year old boy: a case report. *Paediatr Anaesth.* 2005;15(10):886-889.
6. Keller C, Brimacombe J, Kleinsasser A, Löckinger A. Does the ProSeal laryngeal mask airway prevent aspiration of regurgitated fluids? *Anesth Analg.* 2000;91:1017-1020.
7. Brain AIJ. The laryngeal mask: a new concept in airway management. *Br. J. Anaesth.* 1983;55:801-805.
8. LMA. *LMA™ Instruction Manual.* San Diego, CA: LMA North America; 2003.
9. Wong D, Tam A, Mehta V, Raveendran R, Riad W, Chung FF. New supraglottic airway with built-in pressure indicator decreases postoperative pharyngolaryngeal symptoms: a randomized controlled trial. *Canad J Anesth.* 2013;60:1197-2003.
10. Bick E, Bailes I, Patel A, Brain AI. Fewer sore throats and a better seal: why routine manometry for laryngeal mask airways must become the standard of care. *Anaesthesia (editorial).* 2014;69(12):1304-1308.
11. Van Zundert T, Brimacombe J. Comparison of cuff pressure changes in silicone and PVC laryngeal masks during nitrous oxide anaesthesia in spontaneously breathing children. *Anaesthesiol Intens Ther.* 2012;44:63-70.

12. Seet E, Yousaf F, Gupta S, Subramanyam R, Wong DT, Chung F. Use of manometry for laryngeal mask airway reduces post-operative pharyngolaryngeal adverse events. *Anaesthesiology.* 2010;112:652-657.

13. Von Ungern-Sternberg BS. Cuff Pressure monitoring in paediatric laryngeal mask airways – is it worth the pain? *Australas Anaesth.* 2009:55-57.

14. Brimacombe J. *Laryngeal Mask Anesthesia: Principles and Practice.* 2nd ed. Philadelphia, PA: Saunders (Elsevier); 2005:445-467.

15. Brain AIJ, Verghese C, Strube PJ. The LMA ProSeal: a laryngeal mask with an oesophageal vent. *Br. J. Anaesth.* 2000;84:650-654.

16. Brimacombe J, Keller C. The ProSeal laryngeal mask airway—a randomized crossover study with the standard laryngeal mask in paralyzed anesthetized patients. *Anesthesiology.* 2000;93:104-109.

17. Goldmann K, Jakob C. Size 2 ProSeal™ laryngeal mask airway: a randomized, crossover investigation with the standard laryngeal mask in paediatric patients. *Br J Anaesth.* 2005;94:385-389.

18. Goldmann K, Roettger C, et al. The size 1.5 ProSeal™ laryngeal mask airway in infants: a randomized, crossover, investigation with the Classic™ laryngeal mask airway. *Anesth Analg.* 2006;102:205-416.

19. Lopez-Gil M, Brimacombe J. The ProSeal™ laryngeal mask airway in children. *Pediatric Anesthesia.* 2005;15:229-234.

20. O'Connor CJ Jr, Borromeo CJ, et al. Assessing ProSeal laryngeal mask positioning: the suprasternal notch test. *Anesth Analg.* 2002;94:1374-1375.

21. Stix MS, O'Connor CJ Jr. Depth of insertion of the ProSeal™ laryngeal mask airway. *Br J Anaesth.* 2003;90:235-237.

22. Sanders JC, Olomu PN, et al. Detection, frequency, and prediction of problems in the use of the ProSeal laryngeal mask airway in children. *Pediatr Anesth.* 2008;18:1183-1189.

23. Sinha A, Sharma B, et al. Proseal™ as an alternative to endotracheal intubation in pediatric laparoscopy. *Pediatr Anesth.* 2007;17:327-332.

24. Verghese C, Ramaswamy B. LMA-Supreme™: a new single-use LMA™ with gastric access: a report on its clinical efficacy. *Br. J. Anaesth.* 2008;101:405-410.

25. Jagannathan N, Sohn LE, et al. A randomized comparison of the LMA Supreme™ and LMA ProSeal™ in Children. *Anaesthesia.* 2012;67(6):632-639.

26. Hosten T, Gurkan Y, et al. A new supraglottic airway device: LMA-Supreme, comparison with LMA-ProSeal. *Acta Anaesthesiol Scand.* 2009;53(7):852-857.

27. Jagannathan N, Sohn L, et al. A randomized comparison of the laryngeal mask airway supreme™ and laryngeal mask Unique™ in infants and children: does cuff pressure influence leak pressure? *Pediatr Anesth.* 2013;(23):927-933.

28. Nobuyuki-Hai T, Olomu PN, et al. Laryngeal mask airway supreme in children: a retrospective audit. *J. Anesth Perioper Med.* 2016;3:241-246.

29. Jagannathan N, Sohn LE, et al. A randomized crossover comparison between the Laryngeal Mask Airway-Unique and the Air-Q Intubating Laryngeal Airway in children. *Pediatr Anesth.* 2012;22(2):161-167.

30. Jagannathan N, Kho MF, et al. Retrospective audit of the Air-Q Intubating Laryngeal Mask Airway as a conduit for tracheal intubation in pediatric patients with a difficult airway. *Pediatric Anesthesia.* 2011;(21):422-427.

31. Jagannathan N, Sohn LE, et al. A randomized trial comparing the Ambu® Aura-i™ with the air-Q™ intubating laryngeal airway as conduits for tracheal intubation in children. *Pediatr Anesth.* 2012;22(12):1197-1204.

32. Hughes C, Place K, et al. A clinical evaluation of the i-gel supraglottic airway device in children. *Pediatr Anesth.* 2012;22(8):765-771.

33. Gasteiger L, Brimacombe J, et al. *Acta Anaesthesiol Scand.* 2012;56(10):1321-1324.

34. Goyal R, Shukla RN, et al. Comparison of size 2 i-gel supraglottic airway with LMA-ProSeal LMA in spontaneously breathing children undergoing elective surgery. *Pediatr Anesth.* 2012;22(4):355-359.

35. Mitra S, Das B, et al. Comparison of size 2.5 i-gel with ProSeal LMA in anaesthetized paralyzed children undergoing elective surgery. *N Am J Medical Sci.* 2012;4(10):453-457.

36. Morgan GAR, Steward DJ. A preformed paediatric orotracheal tube design based on anatomical measurements. *Can Anaesth Soc J.* 1982;29:9-11.

37. Motoyoma EK, Davis PJ. *Smith's Anesthesia for Infants and Children.* 7th ed. Philadelphia, PA: Mosby (Elsevier); 2006:336.

38. Motoyoma EK, Davis PJ. *Smith's Anesthesia for Infants and Children.* 7th ed. Philadelphia, PA: Mosby (Elsevier); 2006:338-341.

39. Aitkenhead AR, Smith G. *Textbook of Anesthesia.* 3rd ed. Edinburgh, UK: Churchill Livingstone; 1996:326-329.

40. Kuhn F. Die pernasale tube. *München Med Wochenschr.* 1992;49:1456.

41. Magill IW. Endotracheal anesthesia. *Am J Surg.* 1936;34:450.

42. Abrons RO, Zimmerman MB, El-Hattab YMS. Nasotracheal intubation over a bougie vs. non-bougie intubation: a prospective randomized, controlled trial in older children and adults using videolaryngoscopy. *Anaesthesia.* 2017;72(12):1491-1500.

43. Weiss M, Dullenkopf A, Fischer JE, Keller C, Gerber AC; European Paediatric Endotracheal Intubation Study Group. Prospective randomized controlled multi-centre trial of cuffed or uncuffed endotracheal tubes in small children. *Br J Anaesth.* 2009;103(6):867-873.

44. Sun Y, Lu Y, et al. Pediatric video laryngoscope versus direct laryngoscope: a meta-analysis of randomized controlled trials. *Paediatr Anaesth.* 2014;24:1056-1065.

45. Redel A, Karademir F, et al. Validation of the GlideScope video laryngoscope in pediatric patients. *Paediatr Anaesth.* 2009;19:667-671.

46. Kim JT, Na HS, et al. GlideScope video laryngoscope: a randomized clinical trial in 203 paediatric patients. *Br. J. Anaesth.* 2008;101:531-534.

47. Fiadjoe JE, Gurnaney H, et al. A prospective randomized equivalence trial of the GlideScope Cobalt video laryngoscope to traditional direct laryngoscopy in neonates and infants. *Anesthesiology.* 2012;116:622-628.

48. Steiner JW, Sessler DI, et al. Use of deep laryngeal oxygen insufflation during laryngoscopy in children: a randomized clinical trial. *Br J Anaesth.* 2016;117(3):350-357.

49. Cooper RM, Pacey JA, et al. Early clinical experience with a new videolaryngoscope (GlideScope) in 728 patients. *Can J Anaesth.* 2005;52(2):191-198.

50. Olomu PN, Khan A, et al. Glidescope Cobalt AVL video baton for intubation in infants weighing less than 10 kilograms. *J Anesth Perioper Med.* 2016;3:236-240.

51. Olomu PN, Khan A. Assessment of the GlideScope spectrum single-use video laryngoscope blades and stylet for use in pediatrics: a manikin study. *Anesthesiology.* 2016; Abstract (A3191).

52. Jagannathan N, Hajduk J, Sohn L, et al. Randomized equivalence trial of the King Vision aBlade videolaryngoscope with the Miller direct laryngoscope for routine tracheal intubation in children <2 years of age. *Br J Anaesth.* 2017;118(6):932-937.

53. White MC, Marsh CJ, et al. A randomized, controlled trial comparing the AirTraq™ optical laryngoscope with conventional laryngoscopy in infants and children. *Anaesthesia.* 2012;67:226-231.

54. Kollofrath O. Entfernung eines Knochenstücks aus dem rechten Bronchus auf natürlichem Wege und unter Anwendung der directen Laryngoscopie. *MMW.* 1897;38:1038-1039.

55. Becker HD, Marsh BR. History of the rigid bronchoscope. In: Bollinger CT, Mathur PN, editors. *Interventional bronchoscopy,* vol 30. Basel, Switzerland: Karger, Prog Respir Res; 2000: 2-15.

56. Burkle C, Zepeda Z, et al. A historical perspective on use of the laryngoscope as a tool in anesthesiology. *Anesthesiology.* 2004;100:1003-1006.

57. Ikeda S, Yanai N, et al. Flexible bronchoscope. *Keio J Med.* 1968;17:1-16.

58. Taylor PA, Towey RM. The bronchoscope as an aid to endotracheal intubation. *Br J Anaesth.* 1972;44:611-612.

59. Davis NJ. A new fiberoptic laryngoscope for nasal intubation. *Anesth Analg.* 1973;52:807.

60. Raj PP, Forestner J, et al. Techniques for fiberoptic laryngoscopy in anesthesia. *Anesth Analg.* 1974;53:708-714.

61. Wang JF, Reves JG, et al. Use of the fiberscope for difficult endotracheal intubation. *Ala J Med Sci.* 1976;13:247-251.

62. Gil KSL, Diemunsch PA. Fiberoptic and flexible endoscopic-aided techniques. In: Hagberg C. *Benumof and Hagberg's Airway Management.* 3rd ed. Philadelphia, PA: Elsevier; 2013:365-411.

63. Iannoli ED, Litman RS. Tension pneumothorax during flexible fiberoptic bronchoscopy in a newborn. *Anesth Analg.* 2002;94:512-513.

64. Mayordomo-Colunga J, Rey C, et al. Iatrogenic tension pneumothorax in children: Two case reports. *J Med Case Rep.* 2009;3:7390.

65. Colt H, Beamis J, et al. Novel flexible bronchoscope and single-use disposable-sheath endoscope system: a preliminary technology evaluation. *Chest.* 2000;118:183-187.

66. Pujol E, López AM, et al. Use of the Ambu® aScope™ in 10 patients with predicted difficult intubation. *Anaesthesia.* 2000;65:1037-1040.

67. Piepho T, Werner C, et al. Evaluation of the novel, single-use, flexible aScope for endotracheal intubation in the simulated difficult airway and first clinical experiences. *Anaesthesia.* 2010;65:820-825.

68. Wong DM, Prabhu A, et al. Cervical spine motion during flexible bronchoscopy compared with the Lo-Pro GlideScope. *Br J Anaesth.* 2009;102:424-430.

69. Frova G, Sorbello M. Algorithms for difficult airway management: a review. *Minerva Anestesiol.* 2009;75:201-209.

70. Holm-Knudsen R, Eriksen K, Rasmussen LS. Using a nasopharyngeal airway during fiberoptic intubation in small children with a difficult airway. *Paediatr Anaesth.* 2005;15:839-845.

71. Altman K, Wetmore R, et al. Congenital airway abnormalities in patients requiring hospitalization. *Arch Otolaryngol Head Neck Surg.* 1999;125:525-528.

72. Fiadjoe JE, Litman RS. Oxygen supplementation during prolonged tracheal intubation should be the standard of care. *Br J Anaesth.* 2016 Oct;117(4):417-418.

73. Beattie C. The modified nasal trumpet maneuver. *Anesth Analg.* 2002;94:467-469.

74. Webb AR, Fernando S, et al. Local anesthesia for fiberoptic bronchoscopy: transcricoid injection or the "spray as you go" technique? *Thorax.* 1990;45:474-477.

75. Holzki J, Brown KA, et al. The anatomy of the pediatric airway: Has our knowledge changed in 120 years? A review of historical and recent investigations of the anatomy of the pediatric larynx. *Paediatr Anaesth.* 2018;28:13-22.

76. Doyle DJ. GlideScope-assisted fiberoptic intubation: a new airway teaching method. *Anesthesiology.* 2004;101:1252.

77. Heinrich S, Birkholz T, et al. Incidence and predictors of difficult laryngoscopy in 11,219 pediatric anesthesia procedures. *Paediatr Anaesth.* 2012;22(8):929-936.

78. Fiadjoe EM, Nishisaki A, et al. Airway management complications in children with difficult tracheal intubation from the Pediatric Difficult Intubation (PeDI) registry: a prospective cohort analysis. *Lancet Resp Med.* 2016;4(1):37-48.

79. Karmarka S, Varshney S. Tracheal extubation. *Contin Edu Anaesth Crit Care Pain.* 2008;8(6):214-220.

80. Sabato SC, Long E. An institutional approach to the management of the 'Can't Intubate, Can't Oxygenate' emergency in children. *Paediatr Anaesth.* 2016;26(8):784-793.

81. Monnier P. Applied surgical anatomy of the larynx and trachea. In: Monnier P, ed. *Pediatric Airway Surgery.* Berlin, Heidelberg: Springer; 2011:7-29.

82. Black AE, Flynn PER, et al. Development of a guideline for the management of the unanticipated difficult airway in pediatric practice. *Paediatr Anaesth.* 25(2015):346-362.

83. Burjek NE, Nishisaki A, et al. Videolaryngoscopy versus fiberoptic intubation through a supraglottic airway in children with a difficult airway: an analysis from the Multicenter Pediatric Difficult Intubation Registry. *Anesthesiology.* 2017;127(3):432-440.

84. Jagannathan N, Kho MF, et al. Retrospective audit of the Air-Q Intubating Laryngeal Airway as a conduit for tracheal intubation in pediatric patients with a difficult airway. *Paediatr Anaesth.* 2011 Apr;21(4):433-437.

85. Lenhardt R, Burkhart MT, et al. Is video laryngoscope-assisted flexible tracheoscope intubation feasible for patients with predicted difficult airway? a prospective, randomized clinical trial. *Anesth Analg.* 2014;118:1259-1265.

86. Blasius K, Gooden C. A pediatric difficult airway managed with a glidescope-assisted fiberoptic intubation. *Pediatr Anesthesiol.* 2011(Abstract), CSF 141.

87. Barr B, Olomu P, et al. Feasibility of combined videolaryngoscopy and fiberoptic intubation for the pediatric difficult airway: a multicenter analysis from the Pediatric Airway Registry (PeDIR). *Pediatr Anesthesiol (winter).* 2015 (Abstract), 305-A-18.

88. Moore MS, Wong AB. Glidescope intubation assisted by fiberoptic scope. *Anesthesiology.* 2007;106:885.

89. Sukernik MR, Bezinover D, et al. Combination of glidescope with fiberoptic bronchoscope for optimization of difficult endotracheal intubation. A case series of three patients. Available at http://www.priory.com/medicine/Glidescope_bronchoscope.htm. Accessed November 1, 2017.

90. Audenaert SM, Montgomery CL, et al. Retrograde-assisted fiberoptic tracheal intubation in children with difficult airways. *Anesth Analg.* 1991;73:660-664.

91. Stoneham MD. The nasopharyngeal airway. Assessment of position by fiberoptic laryngoscopy. *Anaesthesia.* 1993;48(7):575-580.

Intravenous Access

Jennifer Hernandez, Sana Ullah, and Luis M. Zabala

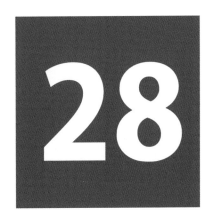

FOCUS POINTS

1. Establishing and maintaining adequate and reliable vascular access is one of the most critical aspects of pediatric anesthesiology.
2. Internal jugular, subclavian, and femoral central venous access sites are commonly used in pediatrics. Considerations for site selection include indications for placement, anticipated duration, patient-specific factors, and operator experience.
3. Infectious complications can be markedly reduced with universal precautions and good aseptic technique. Strict sterile barrier precautions should be employed including a mask, cap, sterile gown, and gloves. Chlorhexidine solutions are preferred to the use of povidone-iodine solutions for skin preparation.
4. Ultrasound guidance is recommended for central venous cannulation in children. It is also commonly used during placement of peripherally inserted central catheters and difficult peripheral venous line placement.

CENTRAL VENOUS ACCESS

Indications

Although there are no absolute indications for intraoperative central venous pressure (CVP) monitoring in pediatrics, the insertion of a central venous catheter (CVC) is warranted if it contributes to the management of a safe anesthetic. CVP monitoring can provide an estimate of right ventricular filling pressures and intravascular volume status. This information can be used to guide fluid resuscitation during procedures associated with significant blood loss, large fluid shifts, and hemodynamic instability. CVCs also serve as reliable access for the central administration of vasoactive medications, delivery of blood products, blood sampling, and central venous oxygen tension analysis. A multi-orifice CVC positioned at the superior vena cava (SVC) and right atrial (RA) junction allows for aspiration of entrained air in patients at risk for venous air emboli. Finally, insertion of a CVC may be the only option in cases where establishment of peripheral intravenous access is unsuccessful.

In children with chronic diseases, several therapeutic interventions that extend beyond the operating room are made possible with the use of specialized CVCs. In larger cardiac patients, these catheters can serve as conduits for the insertion of transvenous electrodes for cardiac pacing and the placement of pulmonary artery catheters for more comprehensive hemodynamic monitoring. In critically ill patients, these catheters can also be used for temporary hemodialysis, continuous venovenous hemofiltration, and plasmapheresis. Administration of chemotherapy, long-term antibiotics, parenteral nutrition, and the delivery of other chronic continuous intravenous medications such as epoprostenol and milrinone are also common indications for CVCs in pediatric patients. This long-term access requirement usually involves the surgical placement of tunneled catheters that provide better long-term stability and reduced infection risk such as a subcutaneous port, Broviac, or Hickman catheter.

Contraindications

As in adults, there are no absolute contraindications to the placement of CVCs in children. Relative contraindications include coagulopathy/thrombocytopenia, localized infection over the insertion site, target vessel stenosis/thrombosis, anatomical abnormalities/tumor presence, and parental/patient refusal. The use of antimicrobial/antiseptic impregnated CVCs has increased in recent years in pediatric patients in whom catheter is expected to remain in place for greater than 5 days. It is important to note that use of minocycline/rifampin or chlorhexidine/silver sulfadiazine impregnated catheters is contraindicated in patients with allergies to these coatings.

Insertion Site

Various sites can be used for central cannulation in children. Commonly used CVC placement sites for intraoperative use in pediatrics include internal jugular, subclavian, and femoral veins. Considerations prior to site selection should include clinical setting and indication, risks, anticipated duration of use, and operator skill/experience. Intraoperative accessibility makes the internal jugular and subclavian veins favorable for anesthesiologists. Their location at the head of the operating room table allow for direct visualization of the insertion site, permitting routine insertion site assessment, intravascular confirmation with the application of negative pressure/aspiration, and troubleshooting ease when necessary. The more distal location of the femoral veins may be preferable in trauma settings allowing for neck immobilization, as well as simultaneous airway management and resuscitation efforts.

While all insertion sites share common complications such as potential for vessel injury, inadvertent arterial puncture, hematoma formation, embolic events, risk of thrombosis, and infection, each site confers its own unique safety profile that should be considered in the context of patient-specific factors. Practice guidelines issued in 2012 by the American Society of Anesthesiologists Task Force on Central Venous Access state that insertion site selection should be based on clinical necessity, should not be contaminated, or at risk for future contamination.[1] A working group comprised of members from various professional organizations and disciplines, which was led by the Society of Critical Care Medicine, published guidelines for the prevention of intravascular catheter-related infections in 2011. The group's recommendation for the avoidance of femoral venous access was based on category 1A evidence. To reduce infection risk, the subclavian site was recommended over the internal jugular and femoral sites in adults (category 1B).[2] Unfortunately, there is an absence of compelling data in the pediatric literature with respect to this issue.[3]

INTERNAL JUGULAR VEIN

Anatomy

The right internal jugular vein (RIJV) is commonly a preferred site for central venous cannulation because of its anatomical location, distinct surface landmarks, and straight trajectory to the SVC and RA. The vessel initially runs deep to the sternocleidomastoid muscle (SCM), but courses closer to the skin surface within the triangle formed by the sternal and clavicular heads of the SCM and the clavicle. Although the IJV is located anterolateral to the common carotid artery (CCA) in most cases, a wide range of anatomical variations exist.[4,5] An early study that used ultrasound to examine the venous anatomy in children under the age of 6 found that up to 18% had variability of vessel positioning that could result in inadvertent arterial puncture, failed cannulation, or injury.[6] For this reason, real-time direct ultrasound (US) guidance is now commonly used to reduce complications with IJV cannulation.[7,8]

Technique

Intraoperative cannulation of the IJV is typically performed following induction of general anesthesia and endotracheal intubation. When placed in other settings, measures should be taken to make the patient comfortable to both facilitate placement and reduce complications associated with patient movement. Supplemental oxygen should be administered and pulse oximetry, blood pressure, and the electrocardiogram (ECG) should be monitored. As with all invasive procedures, a procedural time out is recommended prior to patient positioning. The patient is positioned on a shoulder roll to provide adequate neck extension and the head is rotated approximately 45° to the contralateral side. Care must be taken to avoid excessive head rotation as this can alter the anatomy and cause the IJV to directly overlie the CA.[9] After identification of surface landmarks, Trendelenburg positioning (15° to 20°) is often utilized to both decrease the risk of air embolus and improve cannulation success by increasing the cross-sectional diameter of the vessel.

Universal precautions and good aseptic technique are required during catheter insertion. Hand hygiene with either antiseptic soaps or alcohol-based products has repeatedly been shown to reduce central line–associated bloodstream infection (CLABSI) rates.[10] Strict sterile barrier precautions should be employed including a mask, cap, sterile gown, and gloves. The anterolateral neck is prepped widely from just below the earlobe and along the clavicle toward the sternoclavicular joint. Chlorhexidine solutions have been shown to reduce the risk of catheter colonization and are preferred to the use of povidone-iodine solutions.[10-12] A large sterile drape is then applied over the patient with care to maintain sterility.

Three percutaneous approaches have been described: central, anterior, and posterior. In the central approach, the carotid pulse is palpated with the nondominant hand. A needle mounted on a slip tip syringe (3 to 5 mL) is then inserted at the apex of the triangle formed by the two heads of the SCM, just lateral to the carotid pulse.

The needle should be angled 20° to 45° above the skin surface. With gentle aspiration, the needle is then advanced in the direction of the ipsilateral nipple. The IJV is accessed at a needle depth of 1.0 to 1.5 cm beneath the skin surface in most patients. The landmark for the anterior approach is the midpoint of the anterior edge of sternal head of the SCM, halfway between the angle of the mandible and the sternum. The carotid pulse is palpated along the medial border of the sternal head. The needle is then inserted just lateral to the palpated pulse, along the anterior margin of the SCM and is directed toward the ipsilateral nipple. In the posterior approach, a useful landmark is the point at which the external jugular vein crosses the lateral edge of the SCM, cephalad to its bifurcation into the sternal and clavicular heads. The needle is inserted approximately 1 cm superior to this point and is advanced along the underbelly of the SCM in the direction of the sternal notch.

Although cannulation of the IJV using the landmark technique is considered a safe approach for experienced providers, several publications have demonstrated a reduction in complications when ultrasonography is used to facilitate the placement of CVCs in pediatric patients. Studies have examined the use of both static US (preprocedural identification of an optimal entry site with the determination of vessel anatomy and course) and real-time US during IJV cannulation. In randomized studies of infants undergoing elective congenital heart disease surgery, the use of US has been associated with a higher success rates, lower rates of arterial puncture, decreased number of total attempts, and shorter procedural/cannulation time.[4,13] The use of ultrasonography during CVC placement is increasingly becoming the standard of care, as several medical organizations and professional groups have issued recommendations and guidelines supporting its use.[14-16]

Irrespective of the approach, most CVCs are placed using the Seldinger technique. Upon venipuncture with a small-bore needle and the establishment of dark, non-pulsatile free venous flow, the needle is stabilized and the syringe is removed. Care must be taken to prevent air entrainment. A long, thin guidewire with either a J-tip or a soft, pliable tip is then inserted through the needle. The guidewire should be advanced into the vessel lumen with little or no resistance. It is important to monitor the ECG during this step to detect the occurrence of arrhythmias that can be elicited with wire advancement into the heart. If arrhythmias occur, the wire should gently be withdrawn until they cease. The needle is then removed while stabilizing the wire. When using landmark methods, it is recommended that venous cannulation is confirmed prior to dilator or CVC placement in the event of unintentional arterial puncture. This can be accomplished by a fluid-column test, where sterile intravenous tubing is attached to the needle or angiocatheter hub and allowed to fill retrograde with blood. The open distal end of the tubing is then raised and held upright at a distance above the patient's approximate venous pressure. The height of the fluid column should correspond to the CVP and demonstrate respiratory variation. A fall in the column of blood should be observed with vertical elevation of the tubing. In the event of inadvertent arterial cannulation, pulsatile blood will quickly fill the entire tubing and will likely escape at the distal end. Alternatively, a sterile transducer can be attached to determine the vessel's waveform and directly measure the pressure. Once venous cannulation is confirmed, the guidewire is reinserted. If US guidance is used, intravenous wire placement should be verified prior to dilator insertion. The insertion site is often enlarged with a No. 11 scalpel tip, and a rigid, tapered-tip vessel dilator is commonly used to dilate the underlying tissue tract prior to catheter insertion. While maintaining control of the guidewire, the dilator is advanced 1 to 2 cm with gentle rotation close to the tip. Once the dilator is removed, the CVC can then be advanced over the guidewire. Adequate control of the external end of the guidewire usually requires that the wire be retracted out of the patient until the distal end extends beyond the catheter hub. This helps prevent wire embolization during catheter advancement through the skin. The CVC should be advanced to an approximate depth that positions the catheter tip at the cavoatrial junction. The guidewire is subsequently withdrawn and blood return should be confirmed in all ports. The catheter is then secured in place with sutures and the skin around the insertion site is cleaned and dried with sterile gauze. A sterile occlusive dressing is then applied and the lumens are connected to monitoring or infusion tubing via Luer-lock connectors.

Although the left IJV (LIJV) can be cannulated with any of the approaches described above, anatomic asymmetries make this vessel a less favorable choice. Whereas the RIJV follows a direct inferior course to the SVC, the nonlinear course of the LIJV complicates vascular access and increases injury risk. Both the guidewire and the catheter must navigate an angulation at the junction of the LIJV and the left subclavian vein (LSCV), where the vessels merge to form the innominate vein. This is also the location where the thoracic duct enters the venous system, which increases the potential for pleural effusion and chylothorax. The innominate vein then courses to the right as it continues its inferior course, where it enters the SVC almost perpendicularly. At any point along this path, the distal tip of either the guidewire or the catheter may impinge on the vessel wall thereby increasing the potential for injury. Additional factors complicating left-sided cannulation include an increased potential for pneumothorax (pleural apex higher on left) and less practitioner familiarity with the left-sided technique.

SUBCLAVIAN VEIN

Anatomy

The subclavian vein (SCV) is a continuation of the axillary vein as it passes over the first rib and courses medially under the medial third of the clavicle where it joins the IJV behind the sternoclavicular joint to form the brachiocephalic trunk. The subclavian artery lies just posterior to the SCV as it passes over the first rib, and in most patients its pulsation can be readily felt in the supraclavicular fossa. This is a useful landmark, as the SCV lies just anterior and medial to the artery. Using the anatomical landmarks technique, the SCV can be accessed by directing the needle under the clavicle just anterior and medial to the palpable subclavian artery.

Technique

SCV cannulation is not used as frequently for central venous access due to the higher risk of pneumothorax and arterial injury, as compared with internal jugular or femoral venous sites. It can be used when access to the head and neck is limited, or when movement of the neck is not possible due to trauma or airway manipulations. It is the most popular route for long-term venous access due to its easier fixation, making it more comfortable for patients as mobility is not restricted.

Disadvantages include the significant risk of pneumothorax (higher on the left due to the apex of the left lung being higher); injury to the subclavian artery which, if it occurs, is not very amenable to digital pressure and may be problematic in coagulopathic patients; misplacement of the line into the ipsilateral internal jugular vein (right > left side); vessel perforation, especially from a left sided line, due to the catheter tip rubbing against the SVC; and vessel stenosis from large bore catheters used for dialysis—this may cause future problems with hemodialysis access. A subclavian central line placed by the infraclavicular approach is not recommended for cardiac surgery as it may become compressed between the clavicle and first rib when the sternal retractor is placed. Approximately 0.5% of normal patients and approximately 5% to 15% of patients with congenital heart disease have a persistent left SVC, which usually drains into the coronary sinus, but may empty into the left atrium. This may increase the risk of systemic particulate and air embolism via the central line.

There are two common approaches to SCV cannulation—infraclavicular (most common) and supraclavicular.[17,18] The supraclavicular approach avoids the "pinching off" of the catheter between the clavicle and first rib, and may be preferable during cases involving sternotomy. Cannulation may be done using anatomical landmarks or with the use of real-time US imaging. US-guided vascular access is rapidly becoming the standard of care in many institutions due to the higher success rate and fewer complications.[19]

Technical considerations to improve the success rate of SCV cannulation include placing the patient in Trendelenburg position, keeping the head in neutral position, orientating the needle bevel caudally, inserting the J-tip of the wire so it exits the needle inferiorly, and turning the head to the ipsilateral side during wire placement to decrease misplacement into the IJV. A rolled towel placed longitudinally between the scapulae is not necessary as it may drop the shoulder posteriorly and reduce the size of the vein by compressing it between the clavicle and first rib. The use of real-time US is highly recommended to visualize the anatomy.

FEMORAL VEIN

Anatomy

The FV is accessed 1 cm below the inguinal ligament, just medial to the femoral artery. The mnemonic NAVEL can be used to remember the anatomical structures—proceeding lateral to medial —Nerve, Artery, Vein, "Empty" space, and Lymphatics. Although traditional landmark techniques have been used, the use of US increases the success rate and reduces arterial puncture. An US study has shown that there is partial or complete overlap of the FV with the femoral artery in up to 12% of pediatric patients.[20] Although either side can be used for access, for patients with cardiac disease, the left side is preferable, leaving the right side available for cardiac catheterization procedures. In addition, there is less overlap of the two vessels on the left side, which may reduce the risk of arterial puncture.[21]

Technique

The femoral vein is used frequently for central venous access in children. It is readily accessible, particularly in resuscitation situations where access to the upper body is limited, relatively superficial, avoids the risk of pneumothorax, and manual pressure can be readily applied in case of arterial puncture. It is especially useful in functional single-ventricle patients in whom upper body central venous cannulation may cause thrombosis, which can have catastrophic consequences. Complications include arterial puncture, thrombosis (particularly after multiple attempts), femoral nerve injury, and rarely, retroperitoneal hematoma.

Procedural aspects for successful FV catheterization include (1) placing a small rolled towel under the pelvis to "open" up the groin, (2) reversing Trendelenburg and moderate abduction of the leg to increase venous pooling and increase vessel diameter, (3) digital pressure above the FV or abdominal compression to increase the size, and (4) using real-time US imaging.[22]

PERIPHERAL VENOUS ACCESS

Peripheral intravenous (PIV) catheter placement is one of the most common invasive procedures performed in hospitals today. The ability to obtain and secure PIV access is an essential skill for pediatric anesthesiologists. In most circumstances, this is a relatively simple procedure based on visualization and palpation of the vein. This traditional method of PIV cannulation requires knowledge of vascular anatomy, and experience allows for anticipation of anatomic variables. PIV cannulation in the pediatric population emphasizes the utilization of upper extremity veins, via the basilic, cephalic, or dorsal veins of the hands. Another common site of traditional cannulation technique based on consistent anatomic location is the greater saphenous vein. Three characteristics make the saphenous vein ideal for cannulation based on anatomical landmarks: (1) its consistency (one can depend upon its presence just anterior to the medial malleolus); (2) being the only structure of importance in that location (no arteries or tendons that could get damaged); and (3) the vein lying on the periosteum (providing a tough and solid base for cannulation). Universal precautions are applicable for all PIV placements. Gloves must be worn while starting all IV placements and alcohol swab/chlorhexidine must be used prior to venipuncture.

In the pediatric population, venous access is generally performed following inhalation induction of anesthesia. Exceptions to this rule are critically ill children, full stomach precautions, and comorbid conditions in which inhalation induction of anesthesia represents a prohibitive hemodynamic risk. In these special circumstances, PIV must be secured prior to anesthesia induction, regardless of age or difficulty. Administration of 50% nitrous oxide in selected patients prior to induction of anesthesia may represent a viable and safe alternative for securing IV access, specifically in those patients in which movement may put at risk the only target for a successful IV access.[23]

The extent of the surgical procedure guides the need for fluid therapy and therefore access. The fluid infusion rate is proportional to the radius to the power of four, and inversely proportional to length; therefore, longer and smaller diameter PIV catheters are associated with slower infusion rates. Catheter size is a limitation for rapid rate of infusion in neonates and small infants, due to the size of their peripheral veins. Recommended sizes are 24 ga 1″ to 22 ga 1″ catheters for newborns through 6 months of age, and 22 ga 1″ to 20 ga 1.25″ catheters from 6 months to 3 years.

Obtaining vascular access is difficult in 35% of the patients who present to the emergency department.[24] Other studies have reported first rate success as low as 53% in the pediatric population.[25] With multiple failed attempts at cannulation, patients experience pain, parental anxiety, and delays in their care. The difficult IV access (DIVA) score is a clinical prediction rule (CPR) developed to determine success rates for IV placement in children. Initially described by Yen et al. there are four variables, each weighted score including (a) age (3 points if less than 1 year, 1 point if 1 to 2 years, and 0 points if older than

PERIPHERAL INTRAVENOUS CANNULATION TECHNIQUE

Apply a tourniquet above the site chosen for access. Clean the site with antiseptic solution. With the non-dominant hand stabilize the vein and apply counter tension to the skin. This can also be achieved by padding the extremity with towels and anchoring the distal skin with tape to a rigid surface (OR table) (Figure. 28-1). Follow this by using the dominant hand to insert the stylet through the skin and reduce the angle as you advance through the vein. Once a flashback of blood is seen in the back chamber of the stylet, advance the catheter in the vein while keeping tension on the skin. Then remove the needle and secure the IV tubing. The great saphenous vein (Figure. 28-1) is a large and anatomically reliable vein in patients of all ages. It may be hard to visualize and palpate, but it is easily accessible on the medial aspect of the foot where it ascends between the medial malleolus and the medial edge of the tibia.

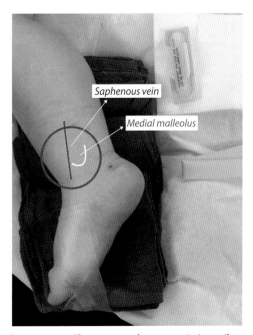

▲ **Figure 28-1.** The great saphenous vein is easily accessible on the medial aspect of the foot where it ascends between the medial malleolus and the medial edge of the tibia. (Used with permission, from Dr. Luis M. Zabala, Medical Director of Pediatric Cardiac Anesthesia. University of Texas Southwestern Medical Center/Children's Health System of Texas - Dallas.)

2 years); (b) vein visibility (2 points if not visible and 0 points if visible); (c) vein palpability (2 points if nonpalpable and 0 points if palpable); and (d) gestational age (3 points for prematurity <38 weeks of gestation and 0 points if term).[26] Patients with score of 4 or more were 50% more likely than the mean success rate to have failed IV placement on the first attempt. This rule is useful in determining which children would benefit from interventions that may improve successful intravenous placement. The alternative to traditional landmark-driven, palpation, or blind technique is the utilization of any of the available technologies to aid peripheral venous cannulation.

Of the available technologies, the most used in clinical practice are transilluminators, near-infrared light technology, and US. Transillumination technology is based on the transmission of light through tissue. It was first described in 1975 by Kuhns et al., who used it to cannulate peripheral veins of obese children undergoing radiologic studies.[27] Many different devices fall into the category of transilluminators, including light emitted by otoscopes, fiber-optic cables attached to cold light sources and more recently light-emitting diodes (LEDs).[28,29] One serious concern with this technology is the amount of heat generated by the light source and the possibility of burns. Transilluminator-assisted PIV cannulation is used widely in the neonatal population. A meta-analysis of three pediatric randomized control trials (RCTs) found a trend toward a lower risk of first-attempt failure compared to the traditional landmark (visualization and palpation) technique, though it was not statistically significant. One RCT found that the use of transillumination in a subgroup of patients younger than 2 years was associated with a significantly decreased risk of first attempt cannulation failure, suggesting that perhaps the technology is better suited for patients younger than 2 years of age.[30] Near-infrared (NIR) technology aids vessel visualization by emitting NIR light toward the patient's skin which is then differentially absorbed by blood and tissue based on wavelengths. The light that reflects back from the veins is processed by the device. Many devices using NIR technology are coupled with advanced technologies to display an image of superficial vasculature (from 0 to 8 mm below the skin surface) directly onto the patient's skin or to an alternate display. The most commonly used device is the Vein Viewer (Luminetx Technologies Corporation, Memphis, TN). Others include the AccuVein® and the VeinLuminator™. The literature reports conflicting results from the use of this technology. Three RCTs comparing PIV cannulation using an NIR light device with the traditional method found that the use of the device had no impact on PIV cannulation first-attempt failure.[30] Despite disappointing evidence of its utility and efficacy based on multiple studies, NIR technology offers many benefits: allows for rapid assessment of viable targets, easily identifies the valve of a vein, and allows assessment of the catheter/vein ratio (optimal ratio to avoid thrombosis = 3:1).[31–33]

Bedside ultrasonography has been shown to facilitate central venous access in pediatric patients and real-time 2D US needle visualization throughout the cannulation process is today considered the gold standard technique.[34,35] US technology involves the transmission of high-frequency waves aimed at a body part. These waves interact with tissues and can be absorbed, transmitted, or reflected. The reflected waves (bounced waves or "Echoes") are used by the receiver to create 2D image on a screen. The role of US for peripheral venous access has expanded, particularly with difficult access.[36,37] A recent meta-analysis found that US guidance increases the likelihood of successful cannulation in difficult access patients.[38] According to the international evidence-based recommendations on US-guided vascular access, US guidance should be considered when difficult intravenous access is required, and blind deep antecubital fossa puncture should not be attempted.[39]

US-guided peripheral access demands complete understanding of peripheral venous anatomy and comfort with the equipment. Other basic concepts include selection of an appropriate vein, image optimization, and US orientation. Maximizing the image heavily relies on adjusting the gain to differentiate fluid-filled structures such as veins from those reflecting US waves or echoes (muscle or subcutaneous tissue). Depth should also be adjusted so that the view of target structures is maximized allowing for

PERIPHERAL VENOUS US-GUIDED TECHNIQUE

Station setup is critically important for successful peripheral venous access (Figure. 28-2). **Preliminary scan of basilic, cephalic, antecubital, and greater saphenous veins is performed to establish preferred site of puncture.** *The ideal vein is large, superficial, and clearly differentiated from arterial structure (compression test). After having the appropriate equipment, and the selected vein for cannulation, the patient's arm should be propped up with towels and the distal skin secured with tape to a rigid structure (OR table) attempting to stabilize the vein and facilitate entry of the need through the skin. A tourniquet is placed proximal to the site selected and sterile antiseptic solution applied. Out-of-plane (short axis) allows visualization of the vessel in its short-axis view. The needle tip is seen from its skin point of entry and follows its progression through the subcutaneous tissue to the target below. Short axis illustrates whether the needle is aimed directly over the target. The in-plane technique (long axis) displays correct angle of entry and conformation of the catheter after needle withdrawal within the vein lumen. This technique demands exact alignment of the needle shaft with the ultrasound beam.*

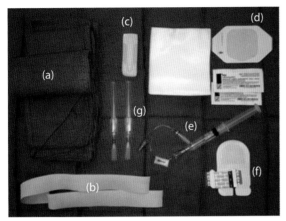

▲ **Figure 28-2.** Station setup for successful peripheral venous access: (a) roll of towels used to place beneath the upper or lower extremity limb used for access to create stability, (b) tourniquet, (c) chlorhexidine pad, (d) conductive gel and transparent adhesive to cover the ultrasound probe, (e) saline connector, (f) adhesive securing mechanism, and (g) appropriately sized intravenous catheters. All elements for peripheral ultrasound cannulation should be available prior to initiation of the procedure. (Used with permission, from Dr. Luis M. Zabala, Medical Director of Pediatric Cardiac Anesthesia. University of Texas Southwestern Medical Center/Children's Health System of Texas - Dallas.)

posterior structures to also be seen. Orientation of the US probe in relation to the screen is crucial to successful cannulation. Each transducer has an indicator that correlates with the active indicator on the screen of the monitor. A common practice is to match the marker of the transducer at the left of the patient with the marker on the upper left hand of the screen.

PERIPHERALLY INSERTED CENTRAL CATHETER (PICC) LINES

A peripherally inserted central catheter, or PICC, is defined as a catheter inserted percutaneously via a peripheral vein with the tip residing in a central vein. These lines are intended for medium- to long-term venous access in patients who require parenteral therapy or frequent phlebotomy. PICCs are used widely in the pediatric inpatient and outpatient population. Indications include intravenous therapy for greater than 14 days, stable patient requiring intravenous therapy with peripherally incompatible solutions, infusions of vesicants, parenteral nutrition, chemically irritating, frequent phlebotomy, patients in palliative care or hospice, among others. Small vessel, infection at the site of puncture, previous thrombosis of proximal vessel, phlebitis, burn or sclerosis, and emergent intravenous access are considered contraindications for PICC placement.

PICC lines are 1.1–3 Fr catheters of varying lengths, with the smallest single-lumen size being 1.1 Fr and the smallest double lumen being 2 Fr. According to the National Association of Neonatal Nurses (www.nann.org), 1.1–2 Fr catheters are used in infants <2.5 kg and 1.9–3 Fr in those >2.5 kg.

Recognized complications of PICCs include thrombosis, infection, catheter occlusion, phlebitis, chronic venous insufficiency, and pulmonary embolism.[40-43] Centrally placed catheter tips are associated with fewer

PICC LINE INSERTION TECHNIQUE

As for any central venous access, informed consent must be obtained. After sedation or induction of general anesthesia, the vein for PICC access is selected using ultrasound. Under sterile conditions and ultrasound guidance a thin metal needle or angiocatheter is used to enter the vein. A thin guidewire with a floppy tip is then inserted through the needle or catheter, into the vein, and the tourniquet is loosened. The needle is then removed and the thin PICC is advanced over the guidewire to the superior vena cava (SVC). The guidewire is then removed and an injection cap is attached to the catheter hub. Tip positioning into the SVC is driven by real-time fluoroscopy, if available, or by anatomic landmark and confirmed by x-ray.

complications than noncentrally placed catheter tip.[44] Peripherally inserted central catheters require frequent flushing and dressing change.

REFERENCES

1. Rupp SM, Apfelbaum JL, Blitt C, et al. Practice guidelines for central venous access: a report by the American Society of Anesthesiologists Task Force on Central Venous Access. *Anesthesiology.* 2012;116:539-573.
2. O'Grady NP, Alexander M, Burns LA, et al. Guidelines for the prevention of intravascular catheter-related infections. *Clinical Infectious Diseases.* 2011;52(9):e162-e193.
3. Reyes JA, Habash ML, Taylor RP. Femoral central venous catheters are not associated with higher rates of infection in the pediatric critical care population. *Am J Infect Control.* 2012;40:43-47.
4. Maecken T, Grau T. Ultrasound imaging in vascular access. *Crit Care Med.* 2007;35(5):S178-S185.
5. Denys BG, Uretsky BF. Anatomical variations of internal jugular vein location: impact on central venous access. *Crit Care Med.* 1991;19:1516-1519.
6. Alderson PJ, Burrows FA, Stemp LI, Holtby HM. Use of ultrasound to evaluate internal jugular vein anatomy and to facilitate central venous cannulation in paediatric patients. *Br J Anaesth.* 1993;70:145148.
7. Verghese ST, McGill WA, Patel RI, et al. Ultrasound-guided internal jugular venous cannulation in infants: a prospective

comparison with the traditional palpation method. *Anesthesiology.* 1999;91:71-77.

8. Sigaut S, Skhiri A, Stany I, et al. Ultrasound guided internal jugular vein access in children and infant: A meta-analysis of published studies. *Paediatr Anaesth.* 2009;19:1199-1206.

9. Sulek CA, Gravenstein N, Blackshear RH, et al. Head rotation during internal jugular vein cannulation and the risk of CA puncture. *Anesth Analg.* 1996;82:125-128.

10. Mimoz O, Pieroni L, Lawerence C, et al. Prospective, randomized trial of two antiseptic solutions for prevention of central venous or arterial catheter colonization and infection in intensive care unit patients. *Crit Care Med.* 1996;24:1818-1823.

11. Chaiyakunapruk N, Veenstra DL, Lipsky BA, et al. Chlorhexidine compared with povidone-iodine solution for vascular catheter care: a meta-analysis. *Ann Intern Med.* 2002;136(11):792-801.

12. Chuan WX, Wei W, Yu L. A randomized-controlled study of ultrasound prelocation vs anatomical landmark-guided cannulation of the internal jugular vein in infants and children. *Paediatr Anaesth.* 2005;15:733-738.

13. Rothschild JM. Ultrasound guidance of central vein catheterization. In: *On Making Health Care Safer: A Critical Analysis of Patient Safety Practices.* Rockville, MD: AHRQ Publications; 2001:chap. 21: 245–255. Available at http://www.ahrq.gov/clinic/ptsafety/chap21.htm.

14. National Institute for Clinical Excellence. Guidance on the use of ultrasound locating devices for placing central venous catheters. Technology Appraisal Guidance No. 49, September 2002. Available at www.nice.org.uk.

15. American College of Surgeons: Revised statement on recommendations for use of real-time ultrasound guidance for placement of central venous catheters. 2010. Available at http://www.facs.org/fellows_info/statements/st-60.html.

16. Troianos CA, Hartman GS, Glas KE, et al. Councils on Intraoperative Echocardiography and Vascular Ultrasound of the American Society of Echocardiography; Society of Cardiovascular Anesthesiologists: Special articles: Guidelines for performing ultrasound guided vascular cannulation: Recommendations of the American Society of Echocardiography and the Society of Cardiovascular Anesthesiologists. *Anesth Analg.* 2012;114:46-72.

17. Byron HJ, Lee GW, Park YH, et al. Comparison between ultrasound-guided supraclavicular and infraclavicular approaches for subclavian venous catheterization in children—a randomized trial. *Br J Anaesth.* 2013;111(5):788-792.

18. Pirotte T, Veyckemans F. Ultrasound-guided subclavian vein cannulation in infants and children: a novel approach. *Br J Anaesth.* 2007;98:509-514.

19. Saugel B, Scheeren TWL, Teboul J-L. Ultrasound-guided central venous catheter placement: a structured review and recommendations for clinical practice. *Critical Care.* 2017;21:225-235.

20. Alten JA, Santiago B, Gurley WQ, et al. Ultrasound-guided femoral vein catheterization in neonates with cardiac disease. *Pediatr Crit Care Med.* 2012;13:654-659.

21. Seda O, Bahattin KA, Seza A, et al. Left femoral vein is a better choice for cannulation in children: a computed tomography study. *Paediatr Anesth.* 2013;23:524-528.

22. Costello JM, Clapper TC, Wypij D. Minimizing complications associated with percutaneous central venous catheter placement in children: recent advances. *Pediatr Crit Care Med.* 2013;14:273-283.

23. Henderson JM, Spence DG, Komocar LM, et al. Administartion of nitrous oxide to pediatric patients provides analgesia for venous cannulation. *Anesthesiology.* 1990;72(2):269-271.

24. Witting MD. IV access difficulty: incidence and delays in an urban emergency department. *J Emerg Med.* 2012;42(4):483-487.

25. Linninger R. Pediatric peripheral IV insertion success rates. *Pediatr Nurs.* 2003;29:351-355.

26. Yen K, Riegert, Gorelick MH. Derivation of the DIVA Score: a clinical prediction rule for the identification of children with difficult intravenous access. *Pediatr Emerg Care.* 2008;24:143-147.

27. Kuhns L, Martin A, Gildersleeve S, et al. Intense transillumination for infant venipuncture. *Radiology.* 1995;116:734-735.

28. Katsogridakis Y, Seshadri R, Sullivan C, et al. Veinlite transillumination in the pediatric emergency department. *Pediatr Emerg Care.* 2008;24:83-88.

29. Hosokawa K, Kato H, Kishi C, et al. Transillumination by light-emitting diode facilitates peripheral venous cannulations in infants and small children. *Acta Anaesthesiol Scand.* 2010;54:957-961.

30. Heinrichs J, Fritze Z, Klassen T, et al. A systematic review and meta-analysis of new interventions for peripheral intravenous cannulation in children. *Peditr Emerg Care.* 2013;29:858-866.

31. de Graaff JC, Cuper NJ, Mungra RA, et al. Near-infrared light to aid peripheral intravenous cannulation in children: a cluster randomized clinical trial of three devices. *Anaesthesia.* 2013;8:835-845.

32. Kim MJ, Park JM, Rhee N, et al. Efficacy of VeinViewer in pediatric peripheral intravenous access: a randomized controlled trial. *Eur J Pediatr.* 2012;7:1121-1125.

33. The VeinViewer vascular system imaging system worsens first-attempt cannulation rate for experienced nurses in infants and children with anticipated difficult intravenous access. *Anesth Analg.* 2013;116(5):1087-1092.

34. Leyvi G, Taylor D, Reith E, et al. Utility of ultrasound-guided central venous cannulation in pediatric surgical patients: a clinical series. *Paediatr Anaesth.* 2005;15(11):953.

35. Kumar A, Chuan A. Ultrasound guided vascular access: efficacy and safety. *Best Pract Res Clin Anaesthesiol.* 2009;23:299-311.

36. Constantino TG, Parikh AK, Satz WA, et al. Ultrasonography-guided peripheral intravenous access versus traditional approaches in patients with difficult intravenous access. *Ann Emerg Med.* 2005;46:456-461.

37. Keyes LE, Frazee BW, Snoey ER, et al. Ultrasound-guided brachial and basilica vein cannulation in emergency department patients with difficult intravenous acess. *Ann Emerg Med.* 1999;34:711-714.

38. Egan G, Healy D, O'Neill, et al. Ultrasound guidance for difficult peripheral venous access: systematic review and meta-analysis. *Emerg Med J.* 2013;30:521-526.

39. Lamperti M, Bodenham AR, Pittiruti M, et al. International evidence-based recommendations on ultrasound-guided vascular access. *Intensive Care Med.* 2012;38:1105-1117.

40. Hogan MJ. Neonatal vascular catheters and their complications. *Radiol Clin North Am.* 1999;37:1109-1125.

41. Ryder MA. Peripheraly inserted venous catheters. *Nurs Clin North Am.* 1993;28:937-971

42. Kearns PJ, Coleman S, Wehner JH. Complications of long term arm-catheters: a randomized trial of central vs peripheral tip location. *J Parenter Enteral Nutr.* 1996;20:24.

43. Kossoff EH, Poirier MP. Peripherally inserted central venous catheter fracture and embolization to the lung. *Pediatr Emerg Care.* 1998;14:403-405.

44. Racadio J, Doellma D, Johnson ND, et al. Pediatric peripherally inserted central catheters: complication rates related to catheter tip location. *Pediatrics.* 2001;107:e28.

Arterial Access

Benjamin Kloesel and Viviane G. Nasr

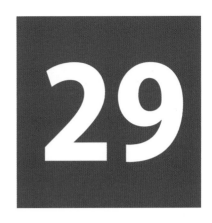

FOCUS POINTS

1. Arterial catheterization allows continuous blood pressure monitoring and facilitates arterial blood sampling.
2. Knowledge of anatomy, advantages/disadvantages of different cannulation sites, and pitfalls during placement and interpretation of the arterial waveform are crucial.
3. There are two approaches to arterial catheterization: through a technique in which a guidewire is used to thread a catheter into the vessel and through a direct puncture technique in which only one wall of the artery is punctured and the catheter is directly threaded into the vessel.
4. Ultrasound can facilitate arterial catheterization and has been shown to increase the chance for first-attempt success and reduce mean attempts to success.
5. Overdampening and underdampening of the transducer system cause incorrect blood pressure readings and should be evaluated with the "flush test."

INTRODUCTION

Monitoring of arterial blood pressure is often needed in critically ill adults and pediatric patients. Compared to adult anesthesia practice, arterial cannulation is performed less frequently in the pediatric population. As such, many procedures for which anesthesiologists would routinely perform arterial cannulations in adults are conducted in children with noninvasive blood pressure monitoring. In fact, arterial cannulation requires practice and becomes more challenging in younger and smaller size children. In this chapter, we will review the basic physiology, indications, contraindications, sites, and techniques for arterial cannulation.

BASIC PHYSIOLOGY

Invasive blood pressure monitoring via arterial catheterization is regarded as the "gold standard" for accurate hemodynamic assessment. The underlying physiology is based on pressure transduction via a fluid-filled catheter in the arterial blood vessel. Blood pressure fluctuations caused by cardiac ejections reach the arterial catheter, cause pulsations of the saline column that are transmitted to a diaphragm. The excursions of the diaphragm cause a change of resistance in the strain gauge transducer (Wheatstone bridge). This change in resistance is measured electronically, and processed, amplified, and converted into a visual display (waveforms).

Interpretation of the waveforms is presented below.

INDICATIONS

Arterial cannulation can theoretically be performed in any setting, but the need for monitoring equipment often limits the availability of arterial monitoring to the operating room, intensive care unit, or emergency department. While there are no absolute indications, most practitioners consider arterial cannulation if one or more of the following conditions apply:

- Tight blood pressure control (eg, resection of a secreting pheochromocytoma)
- Blood pressure monitoring during anticipated pharmacological or mechanical cardiovascular manipulation (eg, open heart surgery)

- Blood pressure monitoring in the setting of non-pulsatile blood flow (cardiopulmonary bypass, left ventricular assist device)
- Arterial blood sampling (eg, pH, gas, electrolyte, hemoglobin monitoring)
- Inability to acquire reliable blood pressure measurements via a noninvasive route
- Inability to use noninvasive blood pressure monitoring (eg, burns)

There is an increasing interest on ways to determine fluid responsiveness with changes in stroke volume, pulse pressure variation, and stroke volume variation. A large body of literature supports the use of pulse pressure variation in the adult population to predict fluid responsiveness, for example, in the intensive care unit and operating room, and some authors have even reported beneficial effects on outcomes.[1–3] In contrast, only few studies have been conducted in the pediatric population, and the available studies have been contradictory.[4–7]

CONTRAINDICATIONS

Specific contraindications for arterial cannulation include the presence of vascular malformations, pseudo-aneurysms, arteriovenous fistulas, and impaired collateral circulation (Table 29-1). Severe coagulopathy and local infection at the puncture site are considered relative contraindications. Coagulopathy can raise the likelihood for significant bleeding and hematoma, especially if multiple attempts are required.

The Allen test, described in 1929,[8] has been used to assess the collateral circulation of the hand prior to placement of an arterial line. It is important to note that a negative Allen test is not an absolute contraindication to arterial line placement. Slogoff et al showed no ischemic complications despite the presence of radial artery occlusion in 25% of the patients.[9]

Table 29-1. Indications and Contraindications of Arterial Line Placement

Indications	Contraindications
Blood pressure monitoring in acute hemodynamic changes and in patients supported with extracorporeal mechanical devices (extracorporeal membrane oxygenation, ventricular assist devices) Blood sampling (gases, electrolytes, etc.) Inability to use noninvasive blood pressure monitoring	Vascular malformations Pseudo-aneurysms Arteriovenous fistulas Severe coagulopathy (may lead to bleeding) Infection at site of placement

AVAILABLE CANNULATION SITES

▶ Upper Extremity

Radial Artery

This is the most common site of cannulation in pediatric anesthesia practice; it is easily accessible and palpable. It is considered safe, since the circulation of the hand is predominately supplied by the larger ulnar artery in most patients. In the past, the Allen's test was recommended for assessment of adequacy of the collateral circulation, but that has recently come into question.[10]

Ulnar Artery

The ulnar artery is a viable alternative to the radial artery. If an ultrasound-guided technique is used, it is worthwhile to scan both radial and ulnar artery prior to cannulation. For both the ulnar and radial locations, placement should be avoided on the side of an existing or planned systemic-to-pulmonary artery shunt (eg, modified Blalock-Taussig shunt) because the blood pressure readings may be erroneously low.

Brachial Artery

The brachial artery can be catheterized in the antecubital fossa. Although it is a large caliber vessel that can easily be palpated and visualized, there are concerns about the lack of sufficient (if any) collateral flow to the distal upper extremity especially if it is compromised by occlusion, thrombosis, or spasm. Schindler et al reviewed their institutional experience with arterial catheterization in neonates and infants and did not find permanent ischemic damage in their cohort of 385 patients who underwent brachial artery catheterization.[11]

Axillary Artery

If an upper extremity arterial catheter is needed and radial or ulnar cannulation is unsuccessful or not possible, the axillary artery may be an option. Compared to the brachial artery, the axillary artery has collaterals that can supply the distal aspects of the arm in case of an occlusion. Lawless and Orr reported a small number of axillary artery catheterizations in pediatric patients and no major complications were noted.[12]

▶ Lower Extremity

Femoral Artery

The femoral artery is often chosen for cannulation in neonates and small infants if initial attempts at other sites fail. From all available cannulation sites, the femoral artery has the largest diameter and is easily accessible by palpation or ultrasound-guided techniques. If the patient is vasoconstricted, more distal sites become increasingly difficult to cannulate. While collaterals are present, femoral artery occlusion can lead to serious adverse events including limb ischemia and loss. In addition, femoral artery catheters are at higher risk for infection due to their location in the inguinal crease and possible contamination with stool in infants wearing a diaper. Dumond et al reported the use of femoral artery catheters in 282 patients.[13] Twenty percent of patients were noted to have pedal pulse discrepancies between the catheterized extremity and the opposite limb, while 6.8% of patients lost pedal pulses by palpation and Doppler after catheter placement. All pulses recovered after femoral catheter removal and no patient suffered from ischemic complications, although four patients were treated with an intravenous vasodilator (papaverine). The group noted that predictors for loss of pedal pulses after femoral artery catheterization were catheter size greater than 2.5 Fr and duration of catheterization.

Dorsalis Pedis Artery and Posterior Tibial Artery

Both of these lower extremity arteries are accessible by palpation and ultrasound guidance and are part of a collateral network that supplies the foot. They are safe to access because of the available collaterals. Those sites are avoided in procedures involving cardiopulmonary bypass as the arterial pressure waveform may become inaccurate in the post-cardiopulmonary bypass period due to peripheral vasoconstriction.

Other Sites

Superficial Temporal Artery

The superficial temporal artery is the least frequently used site for arterial catheterization and its use is currently reported by only a limited number of centers.[14,15] While the site is easily accessible, concerns have been raised about the proximity to the cerebral vasculature and the potential for causing cerebral embolization and infarction with introduction of air or dislodgement of plaques during catheter flushing.[16] Nevertheless, it represents a back-up option in case catheterization attempts at other sites fail. Furthermore, Bhaskar et al suggested superficial temporal artery catheterization in patients presenting for repair of aortic coarctation or who require administration of anterograde cerebral perfusion in the presence of aberrant origin of the right subclavian artery.[17]

Umbilical Artery

Umbilical artery catheterization is frequently performed in neonates who require invasive blood pressure monitoring. As a result, pediatric anesthesiologists typically utilize those catheters but are often times not experienced in their placement. It is helpful to understand some unique aspects of umbilical artery catheters: (1) in emergency situations, they can be used to deliver resuscitation medications, fluids, and blood products (although application via an umbilical venous catheter is preferred); (2) these arteries

Table 29-2. Arterial Catheter Sizing

Age/Weight	Arterial Line Sizes
Infants <5 kg	24-gauge catheter for radial 2.5 Fr, 2.5 cm for radial 2.5 Fr, 5 cm for femoral
Infants/Toddlers <10 kg	22- or 24-gauge catheter for radial 2.5 Fr, 2.5 cm for radial 2.5 Fr, 5 cm for femoral
Preschool children <20–25 kg	20- or 22-gauge catheter for radial 3 Fr, 5 cm for femoral
Older children	20- or 22-gauge catheter for radial

can only be accessed within the first 3 to 4 days of life; (3) the catheter tip should be positioned "high" (ie, above the diaphragm at the T6–T9 level); and (4) the Center for Disease Control and Prevention (CDC) issued a recommendation that umbilical artery catheters should be left in place for a maximum of 5 days.[18]

Commonly used arterial catheter sizes are listed in Table 29-2. This should only serve as a guide and clinical judgment should be exercised with an individualized approach to each patient.

COMPLICATIONS

Multiple cannulation attempts with arterial wall puncture, especially in the setting of coagulopathy, may result in bleeding with local hematoma formation. A hematoma has the potential of compressing surrounding structures including blood vessels and nerves. Idiopathic pseudoaneurysms have also been reported with repeated cannulation attempts. Distal ischemia can occur due to placement of an arterial cannula that is too large in relation to the vessel diameter due to flow interruption.

Dislodgement of vascular plaques can occur during arterial cannulation. This causes distal embolization and may result in ischemia. A similar problem can arise if an arterial cannula in situ develops a thrombus that can dislodge and occlude the distal vascular bed.

One study reported an overall incidence of indwelling arterial catheter-related thrombosis of 3.25% primarily with femoral arterial catheters.[19]

Indwelling vascular catheters represent a possible nidus for bacterial colonization and infection; in comparison to central venous catheters, arterial catheters are less likely to become infected. One cohort analysis reported an incidence of 2.3% for catheter-related local infection and 0.6% for possible catheter-related septicemia.[20]

Accidental injection of drugs or solutions into the arterial catheter represents a preventable iatrogenic complication that can lead to severe ischemia and loss of a limb. That being said, no adverse events have been observed after accidental intraarterial injection of atropine, midazolam, fentanyl, succinylcholine, pancuronium, and vecuronium. In contrast, intraarterial injections of propofol, ketamine, diazepam, thiopental, meperidine, atracurium, and *cis*-atracurium have resulted in ischemia and/or necrosis.[21,22] Therefore, it is important to adequately label the arterial catheter and arterial pressure transducer system, especially around the various access points (eg, stopcocks). Attempts should be made to limit the number of access points to further reduce the risk of accidental injections.

Overall, the incidence of complications from arterial cannulation is low. This is supported by an analysis of the American Society of Anesthesiologists Closed Claims database in which only 13 out of 6894 claims (0.19%) were related to arterial cannulation.[23]

GENERAL APPROACH TO CANNULATION OF AN ARTERIAL BLOOD VESSEL

▶ Preparation

Based on the institutional policy, a verbal and/or written consent from the patient is needed after explaining the procedure as well as the risks and benefits of invasive arterial monitoring.

▶ Equipment

The equipment should include arm board, tape, chlorhexidine prep solution, sterile occlusive dressing, connector, arterial catheter, sterile gloves, sterile towels, saline flush, and the transducer system. Arterial cannulation in general should be conducted in a clean manner and it should be conducted in a sterile manner with gown and hat when central cannulation (axillary and femoral) is being used. One may use a standard peripheral angiocatheter or a commercially available specially designed arterial cannulation catheter. If a Seldinger technique is used, appropriately sized guidewires are also needed.

If the operator plans to utilize ultrasound, the following equipment should also be prepared: ultrasound machine with probe, sterile transducer sheath, and sterile transduction gel.

▶ Placement Using Palpation of the Arterial Pulsations

Standard Peripheral Angiocatheter

The operator holds the cannula with the dominant hand while palpating the radial pulse with the non-dominant hand using the index and middle fingertips. One should not press too firmly as this commonly compresses the radial artery so that no pulsation can be appreciated. After identification of the artery, the skin is punctured with the cannula. The cannula is then advanced slowly at a 45-degree angle toward the artery. Successful entry is noted by seeing blood return in the cannula lumen. At this juncture, the operator has two options. The first option is

to directly cannulate the vessel by carefully dropping to a shallower angle (10 to 20 degrees), advancing the cannula with the needle in place by another 1 to 2 mm and then threading off the cannula over the needle into the arterial vessel. The second option is to transfix the artery by advancing the cannula with needle through the anterior and posterior arterial wall. The needle is then removed. The operator then slowly withdraws the angiocatheter until the cannula's end is pulled through the posterior arterial wall into the vessel lumen at which point pulsatile blood immediately fills the catheter. The guidewire, held with the dominant hand, is then advanced through the cannula into the vessel. The guidewire should pass without resistance. If resistance is felt, it indicates that the catheter is malpositioned (eg, against the vessel wall, outside the vessel) and forcing the guidewire into the cannula against resistance can result in the creation of a false tract or pseudo-aneurysm. After successful placement of the guidewire, the operator can then advance the cannula into the vessel.

Butterfly Needle or Specialized Arterial Puncture Needle/Catheter System

A butterfly needle can be used to directly cannulate an arterial vessel, but it needs to be prepared by cutting off the tubing that extends from the needle end. With the butterfly needle or a dedicated arterial puncture needle, the same cannulation process as described in the previous paragraph. As soon as the artery is punctured, a guidewire can be advanced into the vessel lumen. The needle is then removed and an arterial cannula can be placed over the guidewire.

When using the Seldinger technique, it is imperative to ensure that the wire used fits the catheter planned. If a peripheral venous catheter is used, it can be moved forward and backward after the guidewire has been inserted to function as a dilator. When threading the arterial catheter, the dominant hand should grasp the catheter as close to the skin as possible to avoid dislodgement or malpositioning. Skin tension can be helpful while threading the catheter through the skin. The catheter can then be advanced over the guidewire into the vessel. Occasionally, a twisting motion of the catheter over the wire can help overcome skin resistance. The operator should never force the catheter into the skin as excessive pressure can create a false tract, damage the catheter, or bend the guidewire. If the catheter still cannot be advanced through the skin, a small skin incision can be performed with a scalpel. The incision has to be exactly at the guidewire entry site and care must be taken to not cut the guidewire.

▶ Placement with Ultrasound Guidance

As with all techniques, the successful use of ultrasound for arterial catheterization is operator-dependent and has a learning curve. Nevertheless, a recent systematic review and meta-analysis showed an increased chance for first-attempt success and significantly reduced mean attempts to success with ultrasound guidance.[24]

An out-of-plane ultrasound-guided technique is the preferred method and is performed as follows: The ultrasound probe is covered with a sterile sleeve. A sterile gel is applied inside the sleeve and on the skin. The ultrasound probe is applied to the skin gently to avoid compression of the artery and the depth is adjusted based on patient's size. In order to use the ultrasound-guided technique successfully, the operator should be able to manipulate the probe and the needle while looking at the ultrasound screen.

The artery is visualized by ultrasound and centered on the image on the screen. A 20–24G catheter (brand) based on the size of the patient is used. The catheter is placed close to the probe at a 15 to 30 degree angle in an out-of-plane technique. The catheter should be visualized above the center of the radial artery. If the position of the catheter is inadequate, it is withdrawn to the skin, and then reapplied aiming to the center of the artery. Fine adjustments are made with the needle until the tip is seen in contact with the anterior wall of the artery. At this point one of the following approaches can be taken:

- Use of a guidewire (Seldinger technique)

  The needle is advanced through the artery. Then the ultrasound probe is placed down. The metal stylet is removed and if there is a flash of blood, a wire is inserted through the catheter and advanced into the artery using the Seldinger technique. If there is no flash of blood after the stylet is removed, the cannula is withdrawn until blood flow is seen, and then a wire is inserted. The catheter is inserted inside the lumen, then the wire is removed while keeping proximal pressure to the artery to avoid bleeding from the catheter.

- Direct puncture

  The needle is slowly advanced into the artery while care should be taken to avoid puncturing the posterior wall. The ultrasound probe is adjusted to find the needle tip inside the artery. The needle orientation is then adjusted to position the tip in the middle of the artery and the needle is again advanced slightly under ultrasound guidance. This sequence (ultrasound probe adjustment, needle adjustment, needle advancement) is repeated until enough catheter length is within the blood vessel to allow threading off the catheter from the needle.

The monitoring tubing system is then connected to the catheter. In some instances, the catheter is replaced with a commercially available arterial catheter over the guidewire (please see the online video atlas section on arterial access).

Several advantages of using ultrasound-guided technique exist. Ultrasound pre-scanning allows the evaluation of vessel size at different potential access sites, vessel patency, and location and allows the exclusion of arterial thrombus, hematoma, or dissection. The use of ultrasound also helps visualize distortion or displacement of the artery caused by needle advancement. Furthermore, a lack of blood flashback during transfixation technique may occur frequently and is appreciated with the ultrasound-guided technique.

RADIAL ARTERIAL LINE CANNULATION

As mentioned earlier, the radial artery is common in adults and pediatrics and therefore a brief description of the landmarks and a video illustrating the arterial catheter placement are available (please see the online video atlas section on arterial access).

Anatomical Landmarks

Within the antecubital fossa, the brachial artery divides into the radial and ulnar artery. The radial artery runs anteriorly and laterally on the forearm. At the wrist, it passes between the radial collateral ligament and the tendons of the abductor pollicis longus and extensor pollicis brevis. In the hand, it crosses between the heads of the first dorsal interosseous muscle forming the deep palmar arch and joining the ulnar artery (Figure 29-1).

Although the radial artery is the most commonly used vessel for arterial cannulation, other possible upper and lower extremity sites include the ulnar artery, brachial artery, axillary artery, dorsalis pedis, posterior tibial, and femoral artery.

Positioning

The course of the radial artery is identified by palpation. The hand is dorsiflexed and immobilized. Mild dorsiflexion is applied to avoid injury to the median nerve and collapse of the artery. The skin is prepped with an antiseptic and draped.

Placement

Cannulation of the radial artery is described in the video. Studies looking at ultrasound-guided arterial cannulation attempts in pediatric patients have reported that trisomy 21 and depth of the artery (<2 mm and >4 mm) were independent predictors of catheterization difficulty. Subcutaneous artery depth of 2 to 4 mm showed a statistically significant better success rate for first-attempt and overall cannulation success. The subcutaneous saline injection for patients with artery depth of <2 mm can bring the vessel into the 2 to 4 mm depth range and has been used to improve overall catheterization success and catheterization time.[25]

WAVEFORM INTERPRETATION

With each heartbeat, the ventricles eject an amount of blood called stroke volume (SV). The contraction produces

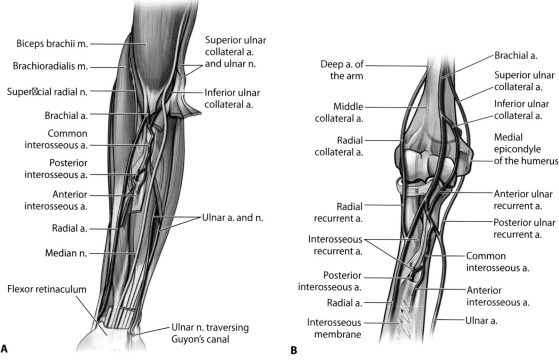

▲ **Figure 29-1.** Arterial anatomy. **A**. Arteries and nerves of the anterior forearm. **B**. Arteries of the elbow and forearm. (Reproduced with permission, from Morton DA, Foreman KB, Albertine KH: *The Big Picture: Gross Anatomy.* 2nd ed. 2019. https://accessmedicine.mhmedical.com. Copyright © McGraw Hill LLC. All rights reserved.)

a pressure wave that propagates throughout the vascular tree and is detected through an arterial catheter. It has a characteristic shape dependent on the sampling location. The shape of the pressure wave is further influenced by the speed of ejection of blood from the ventricle, the compliance of the vascular tree, and the rate at which the ejected blood can flow from the central arterial vascular compartment to the peripheral tissues.

When we break down the arterial pressure tracing itself, we can appreciate the following components:

- Systolic blood pressure (peak of the pressure tracing)
- Diastolic blood pressure (lowest point of the pressure tracing)
- Mean arterial blood pressure (area under the curve)
- Dicrotic notch (reflects aortic valve closure)
- Pulse pressure (difference between systolic and diastolic pressure)
- Anacrotic limb (initial upstroke of waveform, which reflects the rapid ejection of blood from ventricle through aortic valve)

- Dicrotic limb (downward slope of waveform after systolic peak has been reached, which reflects the distribution of blood into peripheral tissues)

Depending on the sampling location, blood pressures will vary slightly: at a more distal sampling site, systolic blood pressure is higher while diastolic blood pressure is lower, leading to an increase in pulse pressure. The contractility of the left ventricle is reflected by the slope of the upstroke (anacrotic limb). A steeper slope is associated with a quicker rise and a higher contractility. Pulse pressure reflects arterial compliance but is also influenced by stroke volume and contractility. Compliance is a major factor, which explains the differences in pulse pressure between elderly patients (arteriosclerosis leads to stiff vessels with low compliance = larger pulse pressure) and neonates (highly compliant vessels = smaller pulse pressure). Peripheral vascular resistance is reflected in the downslope of the waveform (dicrotic limb). Low peripheral vascular resistance, as encountered in sepsis, vasodilator therapy, or neurogenic shock, the waveform exhibits a sharp downslope. A shallow downslope can be

Table 29-3. Arterial Waveforms in Common Disease States

Aortic stenosis	• Blunted anacronic limb (Pulsus tardus) • Narrowed pulse pressure (Pulsus parvus) • Systolic peak may be lower • Dicrotic notch may disappear
Aortic regurgitation	• Steep rise of anacronic limb • Widened pulse pressure • Low diastolic blood pressure • Occurrence of second systolic peak (Pulsus bisferiens)
Hypertrophic cardiomyopathy	• Steep dicrotic limb, followed by second peak from reflected wave (Pulsus bisferiens)

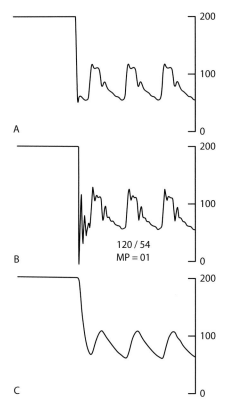

found in states with intense vasoconstriction.[26] Table 29-3 lists waveform findings that can be found in common disease states.

PROBLEMS DURING MONITORING

Dampening of the arterial pressure transducer system may result in incorrect blood pressure readings. An inverse relationship exists: overdampened systems will underestimate blood pressure, while under-dampened systems will overestimate blood pressure. To determine the dampening condition of the measurement system, the "flush test" is used: a small volume of normal saline is rapidly injected into the arterial pressure transducer system. Directly after the injection, oscillations are observed on the arterial waveform tracing (Figure 29-2).

One study examined arterial and noninvasive blood pressure monitoring in pediatric intensive care unit patients and noted several important findings:[28]

- Fifty-four percent of the examined arterial blood pressure monitoring systems were not optimally dampened, and neither demographic nor clinical variables predict the occurrence of optimal dampening; optimal dampening was dependent on the mechanical set-up of the system.
- There is much variability in the measured blood pressures (systolic, diastolic, and mean arterial blood pressures) between noninvasive and arterial blood pressure systems.
- Noninvasive blood pressure measurements may not be accurate enough in critically-ill children to guide management, especially when inotropes or vasodilators are being used.

▲ **Figure 29-2.** Fast-flush test demonstrates the harmonics of the pressure monitoring system. **A.** Optimally damped system: the pressure waveform returns to baseline after only one oscillation. **B.** Underdamped system: the pressure waveform oscillates above and below the baseline several times. **C.** Overdamped system: the pressure waveform returns to baseline slowly with no oscillations. (Reproduced with permission, from Kaplan JA, Reich DL, Lake CL, et al., eds. *Kaplan's Cardiac Anesthesia.* 5th ed. 2006. Copyright © Elsevier Saunders. All rights reserved.)

REFERENCES

1. Lopes MR, Oliveira MA, Pereira VO, Lemos IP, Auler JOJr, Michard F. Goal-directed fluid management based on pulse pressure variation monitoring during high-risk surgery: a pilot randomized controlled trial. *Crit Care.* 2007;11(5):R100.
2. Salzwedel C, Puig J, Carstens A, et al. Perioperative goal-directed hemodynamic therapy based on radial arterial pulse pressure variation and continuous cardiac index trending reduces postoperative complications after major abdominal surgery: a multi-center, prospective, randomized study. *Crit Care.* 2013;17(5):R191.
3. Yang X, Du B. Does pulse pressure variation predict fluid responsiveness in critically ill patients? A systematic review and meta-analysis. *Crit Care.* 2014;18(6):650.

4. Pereira de Souza Neto E, Grousson S, Duflo F, et al. Predicting fluid responsiveness in mechanically ventilated children under general anaesthesia using dynamic parameters and transthoracic echocardiography. *Br J Anaesth.* 2011;106(6):856-864.

5. Renner J, Broch O, Duetschke P, et al. Prediction of fluid responsiveness in infants and neonates undergoing congenital heart surgery. *Br J Anaesth.* 2012;108(1):108-115.

6. Renner J, Broch O, Gruenewald M, et al. Non-invasive prediction of fluid responsiveness in infants using pleth variability index. *Anaesthesia.* 2011;66(7):582-589.

7. Durand P, Chevret L, Essouri S, Haas V, Devictor D. Respiratory variations in aortic blood flow predict fluid responsiveness in ventilated children. *Intens Care Med.* 2008;34(5):888-894.

8. Allen E. Thromboangiitis obliterans: methods of diagnosis of chronic occlusive arterial lesions distal to the wrist with illustrative cases. *Am J Med Sci.* 1929;2:1-8.

9. Slogoff S, Keats AS, Arlund C. On the safety of radial artery cannulation. *Anesthesiology.* 1983;59(1):42-47.

10. Barone JE, Madlinger RV. Should an Allen test be performed before radial artery cannulation? *J Trauma.* 2006;61(2):468-470.

11. Schindler E, Kowald B, Suess H, Niehaus-Borquez B, Tausch B, Brecher A. Catheterization of the radial or brachial artery in neonates and infants. *Paediatr Anaesth.* 2005;15(8):677-682.

12. Lawless S, Orr R. Axillary arterial monitoring of pediatric patients. *Pediatrics.* 1989;84(2):273-275.

13. Dumond AA, da Cruz E, Almodovar MC, Friesen RH. Femoral artery catheterization in neonates and infants. *Pediatr Crit Care Med.* 2012;13(1):39-41.

14. McKay R, Johansson B, de Leval MR, Stark J. Superficial temporal artery cannulation in infants. *Thorac Cardiovasc Surg.* 1981;29(3):174-177.

15. Nobuo J, Tsunehiko S. Cannulation of the temporal artery in neonates and infants. *Paediatr Anaesth.* 2007;17(7):704-705.

16. Finholt DA. Superficial temporal artery cannulation is not benign. *Anesthesiology.* 1985;62(1):93.

17. Bhaskar P, John J, Lone RA, Sallehuddin A. Selective use of superficial temporal artery cannulation in infants undergoing cardiac surgery. *Ann Card Anaesth.* 2015;18(4):606-608.

18. O'Grady NP, Alexander M, Burns LA, et al. Guidelines for the prevention of intravascular catheter-related infections. *Clin Infect Dis.* 2011;52(9):e162-e193.

19. Brotschi B, Hug MI, Latal B, et al. Incidence and predictors of indwelling arterial catheter-related thrombosis in children. *J Thromb Haemost.* 2011;9(6):1157-1162.

20. Furfaro S, Gauthier M, Lacroix J, Nadeau D, Lafleur L, Mathews S. Arterial catheter-related infections in children. A 1-year cohort analysis. *Am J Dis Child.* 1991;145(9):1037-1043.

21. Joshi G, Tobias JD. Intentional use of intra-arterial medications when venous access is not available. *Paediatr Anaesth.* 2007;17(12):1198-1202.

22. Sen S, Chini EN, Brown MJ. Complications after unintentional intra-arterial injection of drugs: risks, outcomes, and management strategies. *Mayo Clin Proc.* 2005;80(6):783-795.

23. Bhananker SM, Liau DW, Kooner PK, Posner KL, Caplan RA, Domino KB. Liability related to peripheral venous and arterial catheterization: a closed claims analysis. *Anesth Analg.* 2009;109(1):124-129.

24. Gu WJ, Tie HT, Liu JC, Zeng XT. Efficacy of ultrasound-guided radial artery catheterization: a systematic review and meta-analysis of randomized controlled trials. *Crit Care.* 2014;18(3):R93.

25. Nakayama Y, Nakajima Y, Sessler DI, et al. A novel method for ultrasound-guided radial arterial catheterization in pediatric patients. *Anesth Analg.* 2014;118(5):1019-1026.

26. Esper SA, Pinsky MR. Arterial waveform analysis. *Best Pract Res Clin Anaesthesiol.* 2014;28(4):363-380.

27. Kaplan JA, et al, eds. *Kaplan's Cardiac Anesthesia.* 5th ed. Page 388. Figure 14-2.

28. Joffe R, Duff J, Garcia Guerra G, Pugh J, Joffe AR. The accuracy of blood pressure measured by arterial line and non-invasive cuff in critically ill children. *Crit Care.* 2016;20(1):177.

Regional Anesthesia: Head and Neck Blocks

Adrian T. Bosenberg and Nishanthi Kandiah

DEVELOPMENT OF THE SKULL[5]

A newborn's facial configuration differs from that of an adult. Ossification is incomplete and many bones are still in several elements united by fibrous tissue or cartilage. The face below the orbits, including the mandible, accounts for about one-half of the skull in adults. In the newborn the air sinuses are rudimentary, the mandible and maxillae are small, the teeth are absent, and thus the face below the orbit makes up only one-eighth of the skull.

The orbit in newborns is large and almost circular. The supra-orbital notch is near the middle of the supra-orbital margin in adults, whereas it lies more medial in the newborn. The maxilla is small, the distance between the alveolar ridges is short, and the infraorbital foramen is millimeters from the inferior orbital ridge.

The mandibular ramus also varies with age. At birth the angle of the mandible is small (obtuse) and develops with progressive growth of the mandible. In the child, before tooth eruption, the mental foramen is closer to the alveolar margin. When the teeth erupt the mental foramen descends to halfway between the margins, and in adults with the teeth preserved, the mental foramen is somewhat closer to the inferior border of the mandible.[6]

INNERVATION OF THE FACE

Briefly, the innervation of the head, face, and neck is best understood if one considers the embryological development as the face forms around the primitive mouth or stomodeum. Initially, the stomodeum is surrounded caudally by the mandibular arch (supplied by the mandibular division of the trigeminal nerve), laterally on each side by the maxillary processes (supplied by the maxillary division of the trigeminal nerve), and rostrally by the forebrain capsule, which develops the frontonasal process (supplied by the ophthalmic division of the trigeminal nerve) that eventually forms the nose. The two maxillary processes

341

grow inward and join together below the primitive nose to form the upper margin of the mouth.

Thus in the mature face, the forehead, eyebrows, upper eyelids, and nose are supplied by the ophthalmic division of the trigeminal nerve. The lower eyelids, cheek, and upper lip are supplied by the maxillary division, while the lower lip, chin, and mandibular and temporal regions are supplied by the mandibular division (Figure 30-1A). All these nerves may be blocked proximally to provide anesthesia in the sensory distribution of that particular nerve. Disproportionate growth of the cranial cavity in humans causes these dermatomal distributions to be distorted cranially, with the result that some skin innervated by the cervical plexus is drawn up over the angle of the mandible and posteriorly over the occipital area and the scalp as far as the vertex (Figure 30-1B).

Risks

Specific complications peculiar to regional anesthesia in this area are more likely to occur with deep blocks and usually involve damage to adjacent structures or spread to the central nervous system by direct or vascular injection.[7–9] Convulsions or extensive neuraxial anesthesia will require urgent resuscitation.

To date, complications have only been described in adults and include transient loss of consciousness, convulsions, and reversible blindness as a result of injection of small volumes of local anesthetic into the vertebral or carotid artery or one of their branches. Local anesthetic could also spread into the neuraxis by direct penetration of either the foramina of the skull or the dura to produce total brainstem anesthesia.[9]

Deep nerve blocks of the head and neck in children should only be attempted by experts for specific indications, preferably under imaging or radiological control. Superficial nerve blocks on the other hand are blocks of the terminal branches of these deep nerves. Although these blocks reduce the field of anesthesia, they are relatively simple to perform and carry a low risk.

Local anesthetic toxicity is dependent on the age of the patient, the agent used, the dose given, the use of a vasoconstrictor, and the site of injection: Maximum safe dose for commonly used local anesthetic agents have been described (lignocaine 3 mg/kg with epinephrine 6 mg/kg; bupivacaine 2 mg/kg; ropivacaine 3 mg/kg). Slow injection of fractionated doses with intermittent aspiration reduces the risk of toxicity. Most blocks of the head and neck can be achieved using less than 1.5 mL. The finest-gauge needle available should be used to reduce the risk of bruising and to avoid permanently marking the face.

Surgery of the Palate

The maxillary division of the trigeminal nerve (V2) provides sensory innervation to the hard and soft palate, upper jaw and maxillary sinus, back of the nasal cavity, and upper dental arch. Terminal branches of the maxillary

division include the greater and lesser palatine nerves and nasopalatine nerve that provides intraoral innervation to the hard and soft palate (Figure 30-2A).[10–16]

The maxillary division after leaving the foramen rotundum traverses the pterygopalatine fossa and passes forward and laterally to reach the floor of the orbit by the infraorbital fissure. The palate can be blocked proximally using a suprazygomatic approach,[12–15] or distally as it emerges from the greater palatine foramen as the greater palatine nerve on the hard palate.

With the patient supine and head in the neutral position, the needle is inserted perpendicular to the skin at the angle formed by the superior edge of the zygomatic arch and the posterior rim of the orbital ridge. The needle is advanced till bony contact with greater wing of sphenoid is made. This depth will vary from 15 to 25 mm depending on the size of the infant or child. Once bony contact is made the needle is redirected toward the philtrum and advanced 15 to 20 mm into the fossa after "walking off" the sphenoid. After a negative aspiration for blood 0.15 mL/kg local anesthetic can be injected. Ultrasound can be used to confirm correct placement within the fossa by directing an infrazygomatic-placed probe toward the fossa.[16]

Alternatively the *greater palatine nerve*, a terminal branch of the maxillary division, courses from the pterygoid ganglion through the greater palatine fossa and emerges from greater palatine foramen. The greater palatine foramen lies medial to the second molar or just anterior to the junction of the hard and soft palate in those infants who do not yet have molar teeth Figure 30-2B. Local anesthetic inserted superficially at this location will block the nerve as it emerges from the foramen. Advancing the needle into the foramen risks intraneural injection or nerve compression in the confined space.

SURGERY OF THE LIPS

Upper Lip

The *infraorbital nerve, also a branch of the maxillary division of the trigeminal nerve*, supplies sensory innervation to the skin and mucous membrane of the upper lip and lower eyelid, the cheek between them and to the alae of the nose (Figure 30-3A). Infraorbital nerve blocks have proved useful in neonates,[17] infants, and older children undergoing cleft lip repair.[18–21] Perioperative analgesia without risk of respiratory depression can be provided. Two approaches to the infraorbital nerve have been described in children: (i) the *intraoral approach* and (ii) the extraoral approach in neonates and infants.

In intraoral approach,[18–21] after lifting the upper lip and cleaning the mucosa, a fine needle is inserted under and into the gingivolabial fold at the level of the canine tooth (if present) and directed upward and outward toward the infraorbital foramen (Figure 30-3B). The infraorbital foramen, more easily palpable in older children, lies just below

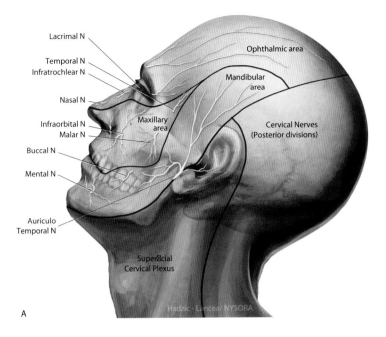

Lacrimal N
Temporal N
Infratrochlear N
Nasal N
Infraorbital N
Malar N
Buccal N
Mental N
Auriculo Temporal N

Ophthalmic area
Mandibular area
Maxillary area
Cervical Nerves (Posterior divisions)
Superficial Cervical Plexus

A

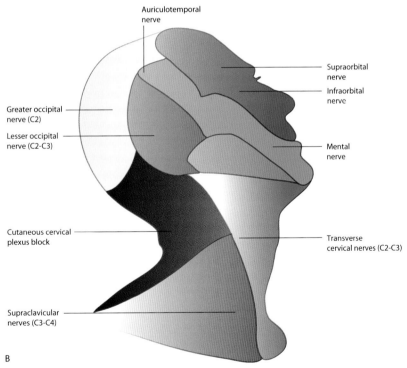

Auriculotemporal nerve
Supraorbital nerve
Infraorbital nerve
Greater occipital nerve (C2)
Lesser occipital nerve (C2-C3)
Mental nerve
Cutaneous cervical plexus block
Transverse cervical nerves (C2-C3)
Supraclavicular nerves (C3-C4)

B

▲ **Figure 30-1.** Innervation of the head and neck: (A) Distribution of the the branches of the trigeminal nerve (Reproduced with permission, from Hadzic A. *Hadzic's Textbook of Regional Anesthesia and Acute Pain Management*, 2nd ed. 2017. https://accessanesthesiology.mhmedical.com. Copyright © McGraw Hill LLC. All rights reserved). (B) Sensory distribution of the cervical plexus and innervation of the lateral aspect of the face and scalp (Reproduced with permission, from Hadzic A, eds. *Hadzic's Peripheral Nerve Blocks and Anatomy for Ultrasound-Guided Regional Anesthesia*, 2nd ed. 2012. https://accessanesthesiology.mhmedical.com. Copyright © McGraw Hill LLC. All rights reserved).

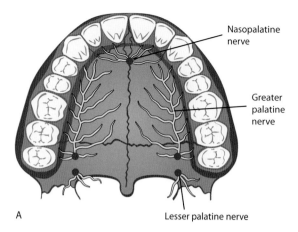

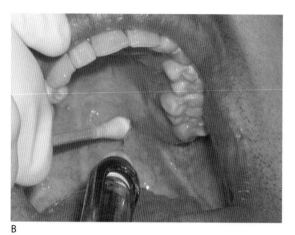

▲ **Figure 30-2.** (A) Terminal branches of the maxillary division of the trigeminal nerve and innervation of the soft and hard palate. (B) Needle insertion for the greater palatine nerve block is 1cm medial to the junction of the maxillary second and third molars (Reproduced with permission, from Hadzic A. *Hadzic's Textbook of Regional Anesthesia and Acute Pain Management*, 2nd ed. 2017. https://accessanesthesiology.mhmedical.com. Copyright © McGraw Hill LLC. All rights reserved).

the orbital rim on a line drawn caudad through the center of the pupil. When the tip of the needle is palpable in the area of the foramen, 0.5 to 1.5 mL of local anesthetic can be deposited at the foramen opening after prior aspiration. It is not necessary to enter the foramen as this may result in nerve damage by compression in the narrow infraorbital canal. Penetration of the flimsy orbital floor and damage to the orbital contents is another potential danger of entering the foramen.

Extraoral approach[17] will depend on whether the infra-orbital foramen is palpable or not. The foramen is palpable in older children and lies approximately 0.5 cm below the junction of the medial and middle thirds of the lower orbital rim. A fine needle is introduced vertical to the skin at this point until bone contact is made Figure 30-3C. A successful block can be achieved if the local anesthetic is placed in the vicinity of the foramen. The foramen is not easily palpable in neonates and small infants. In this age group a simple measurement made from the angle of the mouth to the palpebral fissure can be used. This is approximately 30 to 32 mm in term neonates. The infraorbital foramen will lie at the coordinates of half that distance (15 to 16 mm) from the palpebral fissure and quarter of that distance (7.5 to 8 mm) from the alae nasi.[17]

Lower Lip

The mandibular division of the trigeminal nerve V3 gives off several major branches: the buccal nerve, lingual nerve, inferior alveolar nerve, and the auriculotemporal nerves. The mental nerve, a terminal branch of the inferior alveolar nerve, emerges through the mental foramen in the mandible to provide sensory innervation to the lower lip and chin (Figure 30-4A). The position of the mental foramen varies with age. It lies more caudad on the mandibular ramus in children with teeth but is close to the alveolar margin in infants and neonates.[6] Retract the lower lip, and after cleaning over the midpoint of the mandible in a vertical line with the infraorbital foramen, the nerve can be blocked as it emerges from the mental foramen by infiltrating 0.5- to 1.0-mL local anesthetic (Figure 30-4B). The apex of the root of the second premolar can serve as an alternative landmark in children older than 2 years.

Surgery of the Ear

The nerve supply to the pinna is complex. The pinna is supplied by both the cervical plexus and the trigeminal nerve. Branches of the cervical plexus, the greater auricular nerve, and the lesser occipital nerve supply the posterior surface of the ear and the lower third of its anterior surface. The superior two-thirds of the anterior surface of the pinna is supplied by the auriculo-temporal branch of the mandibular division of the trigeminal nerve (Figure 30-5A).

Successful postoperative analgesia has been described for children undergoing otoplasties or surgical correction of "bat ears."[22–26] Blockade of the greater auricular, lesser occipital, and auriculo-temporal nerves provide more prolonged analgesia than local infiltration.

The cervical plexus supply to the ear can be blocked at various points; the more distal the block, the more localized the area of blockade. The choice of block may also be influenced by the ability to identify the landmarks in children of different ages. For example, in infants the posterior border of the sternocleidomastoid may be difficult

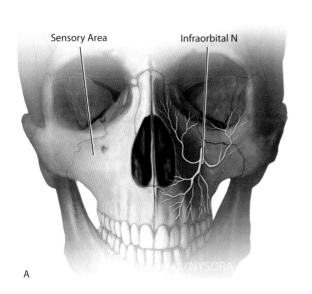

Sensory Area   Infraorbital N

A

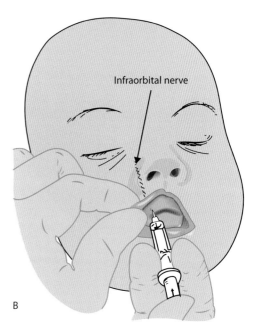

Infraorbital nerve

B

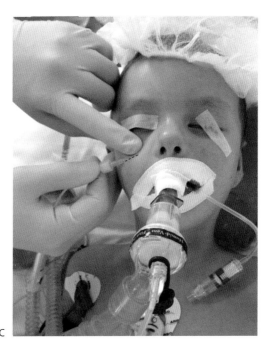

C

▲ **Figure 30-3.** (A) Sensory area of the intraorbital nerve (Reproduced with permission, from Hadzic A. *Hadzic's Textbook of Regional Anesthesia and Acute Pain Management*, 2nd ed. 2017. https://accessanesthesiology.mhmedical. com. Copyright © McGraw Hill LLC. All rights reserved). (B) Intraoral approach to the infraorbital nerve block. Needle insertion point is into the mucosa at the gingivolabial junction at the level of the canine tooth and directed toward the infraorbital foramen. (C) Extraoral approach to the infraorbital nerve block. The infraorbital foramen in palpated and the needle is introduced over this area until bony contact in achieved (Reproduced with permission, from Hadzic A. *Hadzic's Textbook of Regional Anesthesia and Acute Pain Management*, 2nd ed. 2017. https:// accessanesthesiology.mhmedical.com. Copyright © McGraw Hill LLC. All rights reserved).

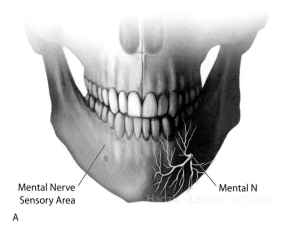

Mental Nerve
Sensory Area   Mental N

A

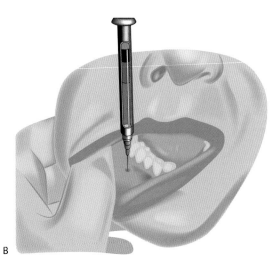

B

▲ **Figure 30-4.** (A) Sensory area of the mental nerve (Reproduced with permission, from Hadzic A. *Hadzic's Textbook of Regional Anesthesia and Acute Pain Management*, 2nd ed. 2017. https://accessanesthesiology.mhmedical.com. Copyright © McGraw Hill LLC. All rights reserved). (B) The mental nerve is blocked by inserting the needle into the buccal fold along the vertical line drawn from the intraorbital foramen or at the second premolar.

to identify in their relative short neck. A more peripheral block might be preferred in this age group. Irrespective of age the muscular landmarks should be delineated before sedating or anesthetizing the child to facilitate the accurate placement of the block.

The *auriculotemporal nerve* can be blocked by infiltration between the pinna and lateral corner of the eye as the nerve

ascends over the posterior aspect of the zygoma behind the superficial temporal artery (Figure 30-5B).

The *greater auricular nerve* and lesser occipital nerves can be blocked proximally as they emerge at the midpoint of the posterior border of the sternocleidomastoid (Figure 30-5C); more distally where the nerves lie more superficially by infiltration from the angle of the mandible to the mastoid process; or over the mastoid process posterior to the ear.

It is worth noting that the accessory nerve provides the motor innervation to the trapezius and lies very close to the cervical plexus (Figure 30-5D). It emerges at the junction of the upper and middle third of the posterior border of the sternocleidomastoid and may also be blocked when the more proximal approach is used, particularly in young children. The child (or parent) should be warned about the inability to shrug their shoulder after the block.

▶ Surgery to Eyelid

The sensory supply to the lower eyelid is provided by the infraorbital nerve. The upper eyelid is supplied medially by the supratrochlear nerve and laterally by the lacrimal and zygomaticofacial branches of the maxillary division of the trigeminal nerve.

▶ Surgery of the Forehead

The sensory innervation of the forehead and scalp to the vertex is provided by the supraorbital and supratrochlear nerves (Figure 30-6A).[27] These are terminal branches of the ophthalmic division of the trigeminal nerve (V1). The lateral aspect of the forehead and temporal region is supplied by the auriculotemporal (mandibular division) and zygomaticotemporal nerves (maxillary division of trigeminal nerve). Blockade of these nerves is simple and can be used for minor surgical procedures in this area (eg, removal of cysts, suture of lacerations, etc). When combined with blocks of other sensory nerves to the scalp (occipital, greater auricular), they provide excellent analgesia for craniofacial surgery.

The *supraorbital nerve* can be blocked as it emerges from the orbit through the supraorbital notch, although Beer et al have shown that this is not always true and the nerve may emerge a variable distance along and above the supraorbital rim.[27] The majority of exit points are asymmetrical. In older children the supraorbital notch lies in the same vertical plane as that of the pupil and infraorbital foramen but is slightly more medial in neonates and infants (Figure 30-6B).

The *supratrochlear nerve* emerges from the superomedial angle of the orbit and runs up the forehead parallel to the supraorbital nerve. The technique for blocking this nerve is the same except the needle is inserted in the medial portion of the orbital rim just lateral to the root of the nose. It is best to block these nerves by infiltrating 1 to 2 mL local anesthetic solution between skin and bone

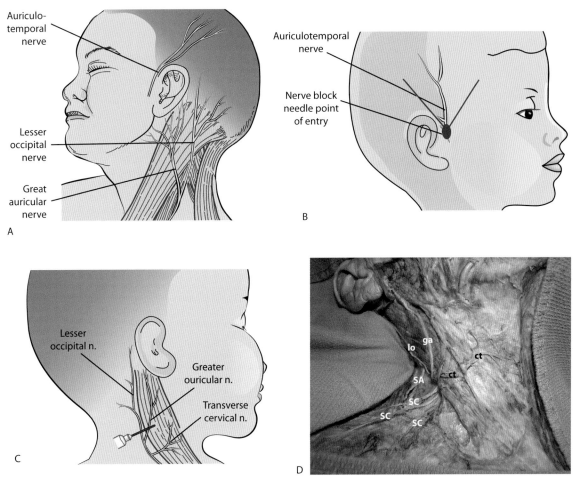

▲ **Figure 30-5.** (A) Nerve supply to the ear. (B) Lateral view of the head illustrating the course of the auriculotemporal nerve as well as needle entry point. (C) Lateral aspect of the head showing the location of the greater auricular and lesser occipital nerves proximally. The nerves can be blocked together at the midpoint of the posterior border of the sternocleidomastoid muscle. (D) Superficial cervical plexus branches (Reproduced with permission, from Hadzic A, eds. *Hadzic's Peripheral Nerve Blocks and Anatomy for Ultrasound-Guided Regional Anesthesia*, 2nd ed. 2012. https://accessanesthesiology.mhmedical.com. Copyright © McGraw Hill LLC. All rights reserved). Ct, transverse cervical; ga, greater auricular; lo, lesser occipital; sc supraclavicular. Note the spinal accessory nerve (SA) and its proximity to the proximal blockade of the greater auricular and lesser occipital nerves.

above the eyebrow to reduce the risk of periorbital hematoma formation. The two nerves can be blocked simultaneously using a single-needle insertion in midbrow above the root of the nose and infiltrating 1 to 2 mL local anesthetic laterally, along the supraorbital rim. Infiltration occurs over this location from lateral to medial (Figure 30-6B).

The *zygomaticotemporal nerve* can be blocked by subcutaneous infiltration as it emerges from the anterior aspect of the zygomatic arch.

Surgery of the Neck

The anterolateral aspect of the neck is supplied by the anterior primary rami of the cervical plexus (Figure 30-1B). These emerge as four distinct nerves from the posterior border of the sternocleidomastoid muscle at its midpoint. The lesser occipital and greater auricular nerves supply the ear and the skin over the angle of the mandible. The anterior cutaneous nerve supplies the skin from chin to suprasternal notch and the supraclavicular nerve supplies

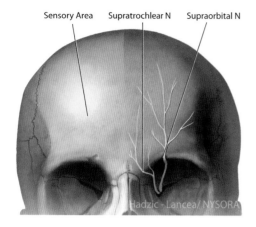

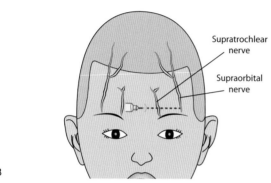

B

▲ **Figure 30-6.** (A) Sensory area of the supratrochlear and supraorbital nerves (Reproduced with permission, from Hadzic A. *Hadzic's Textbook of Regional Anesthesia and Acute Pain Management*, 2nd ed. 2017. https://accessanesthesiology.mhmedical.com. Copyright © McGraw Hill LLC. All rights reserved). (B) The supraorbital and supratrochlear nerves can be blocked using the single injection technique or by blocking each nerve individually as shown here.

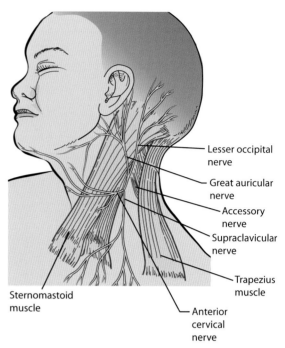

▲ **Figure 30-7.** Superficial cervical plexus emerges from the midpoint of the posterior border of the sternoicleidomastoid muscle. All four nerves can be blocked at this point.

the inferior aspect of the neck and clavicle as far as the second rib, laterally over the deltoid, and posteriorly to the spine of the scapula.

All four branches can be blocked by introducing a fine-gauge needle perpendicular to the skin and infiltrating 1 to 2 mL local anesthetic solution at the midpoint of the posterior border of the sternocleidomastoid and along the middle third of the posterior border of the sternocleidomastoid (Figure 30-7).[28,29] The depth of insertion, usually 0.5 to 1 cm, will vary according to the age of the patient and the extent of subcutaneous fat. Avoid puncturing the external jugular vein as it crosses the sternocleidomastoid close

to this point. Theoretically these nerves could be blocked individually but it is usual to block all four branches and also the accessory nerve if the deep fascia is penetrated.

Successful block of the superficial cervical plexus results in analgesia corresponding to the C2–4 dermatomes and can be used for both major and minor surgical procedures such as thyroid surgery and excision of thyroglossal cysts, branchial arch anomalies, or lymph node biopsy. In a recent report, it was considered a safer alternative than general anesthesia for a cervical lymph node biopsy in a child with a large mediastinal mass.[28] In the event of anatomical distortion by a large mass of nodes (lymphoma, tuberculosis) or cystic hygroma, the superficial cervical block is probably best avoided. Placement of internal jugular or subclavian venous catheters could also be made more comfortable for awake children by using a superficial cervical plexus block.

STELLATE GANGLION BLOCK

Indications for stellate ganglion block do not frequently arise in children, but the role of stellate ganglion block in chronic pain in children still needs to be defined.[29–35] Clinical syndromes unrelated to pain have been managed with stellate ganglion blockade. These include the Romano–Ward and Jervell–Lange–Nielson syndromes both characterized by prolonged QT interval and life-threatening cardiac dysrhythmias.[31,32]

The block is performed with the child in the supine position with the neck extended by placing an appropriate-sized towel or pillow beneath the shoulders. Chassaignac's tubercle, the anterior tubercle of the transverse process of the sixth cervical vertebra, is defined at the level of the cricoid cartilage and immobilized between the second and third fingers (Figure 30-4). With the same fingers the carotid artery is retracted laterally along with the anterior border of the sternocleidomastoid muscle. A fine-gauge needle can be inserted perpendicularly through the skin toward the sixth transverse process. After bony contact is made, the needle is withdrawn slightly and after negative aspiration 0.15 to 0.2 mL/kg local anesthetic can be injected slowly.

INFILTRATION

Local infiltration is most commonly used for minor surgery or when lacerations are sutured in the conscious child.[36–39] It sometimes involves multiple potentially painful injections. A simple nerve block such as those described earlier can reduce the number of injections, while increasing the field of anesthesia and reducing local tissue distortions.

However, there are a number of simple maneuvers that can make infiltration anesthesia less painful.[38,39] These include the use of fine-gauge needles, injecting warm buffered local anesthetic solution slowly into the sides of the laceration rather than through intact skin after the application of topical tetracaine.

Scalp infiltration is commonly used before craniotomy[35,36] to prevent the potentially detrimental hemodynamic response to scalp incision and reflection. A 0.125% concentration of bupivacaine with 1:400000 epinephrine is as effective as a 0.25% bupivacaine solution with 1:400000 epinephrine in reducing hemodynamic responses. The lower concentration produces lower blood levels and would therefore be safer to use for scalp lacerations if large volumes are required. Simple blocks to the nerves innervating the scalp would further reduce the risk.

CONCLUSION

Superficial nerve blockade of the face and neck is a relatively unexplored area in pediatric anesthesia. Regional anesthesia in this area of the body is challenging but a technically satisfying addition to the pediatric anesthesiologist's repertoire to provide excellent long-lasting analgesia for certain surgical procedures. Lack of knowledge or imagination should not put a limit on their potential benefit.

REFERENCES

1. Bosenberg AT. Blocks of the face and neck. *Tech Reg Anesth Pain Manag.* 1999;3(3):196-203.
2. Suresh S, Voronov P. Head and neck blocks in infants, children, and adolescents. *Paediatr Anaesth.* 2012;22(1):81-87.
3. Giaufre E, Dalens B, Gombert A. Epidemiology and morbidity of regional anaesthesia in children: a one year prospective survey of French Language Society of Paediatric Anesthesiologists. *Anesth Analg.* 1996;83:904-912.
4. Polaner DM, Taenzer AH, Walker BJ, et al. Pediatric Regional Anesthesia Network (PRAN): a multi-institutional study of the use and incidence of complications of pediatric regional anesthesia. *Anesth Analg.* 2012;115:1353-1364.
5. Osteology. In: Williams PL, Warwick R, Dyson M, et al, eds. *Gray's Anatomy.* (37th ed.). Edinburgh, UK: Churchill Livingstone; 1989:393.
6. Gershenson A, Nathan H, Luchansky E. Mental foramen and mental nerve: changes with age. *Acta Anat.* 1986;126:21-28.
7. Kozody R, Ready LB, Barsa JE. Dose requirement of local anaesthetic to produce grand mat seizure during stellate ganglion block. *Can Anaesth Soc J.* 1982;29:489.
8. Szeinfeld M, Laurencio M, Pollares VS. Total reversible blindness following stellate ganglion block. *Anesth Analg.* 1981;60:689-690.
9. Nique TA, Bennett CR. Inadvertant brainstem anaesthesia following extraoral trigeminal V2-V3 blocks. *Oral Surg.* 1981;51:468-470.
10. Doyle E, Hudson I. Anaesthesia for primary repair of cleft lip and palate: a review of 244 procedures. *Paediatr Anaesth.* 1992;2:139-145.
11. Peri G, Mondie JM. Blocks of the head, face and neck. In: Dalens B, ed. *Paediatric Regional Anaesthesia.* London, UK: Williams and Williams; 1995.
12. Mesnil M, Dadure C, Captier G, et al. A new approach for peri-operative analgesia of cleft palate repair in infants: the bilateral suprazygomatic maxillary nerve block. *Paediatr Anaesth.* 2010;20:343-349.
13. Captier G, Dadure C, Leboucq N, Sagintaah M, Canaud N. Anatomic study using three-dimensional computed tomographic scan measurement for truncal maxillary nerve blocks via the suprazygomatic route in infants. *J Craniofac Surg.* 2009;20:224-228.
14. Chiono J, Raux O, Bringuier S, et al. Bilateral suprazygomatic maxillary nerve block for cleft palate repair in children: a prospective, randomized, double-blind study versus placebo. *Anesthesiology.* 2014;120:1362-1369.
15. Prigge L, van Schoor AN, Bosman MC, Bosenberg AT. Clinical anatomy of the maxillary nerve block in pediatric patients. *Paediatr Anaesth.* 2014;24:1120-1126.
16. Sola C, Raux O, Savath L, Macq C, Capdevila X, Dadure C. Ultrasound guidance characteristics and efficiency of suprazygomatic maxillary nerve blocks in infants: a descriptive prospective study. *Paediatr Anaesth.* 2012;22:841-846.
17. Bosenberg AT, Kimble FW. Infraorbital nerve block in neonates for cleft lip repair: anatomical study and clinical application. *Br J Anaesth.* 1995;74:506-508.
18. Nicodemus HF, Ferrer MJR, Cristobal VC, et al. Bilateral infraorbital block with 0.5% bupivacaine as postoperative analgesia following cheiloplasty in children. *Scand J Plast Reconstr Hand Surg.* 1991;25:253-257.
19. Ahuja S, Datta A, Krishna A, et al. Infraorbital nerve block for relief of postoperative pain following cleft lip surgery in infants. *Anaesthesia.* 1994;49:441-444.

20. Mayer MN, Bennaceur S, Barrier G, et al. Bloc des nerfs sousorbitaires darts les cheiloplasties primaries precoces. *Rev Stomatol Chir Maxillofac.* 1997;98:246-247.

21. Kapetansky D, Warren R, Hawtof D. Cleft lip repair using intramuscular hydroxyzine sedation and local anaesthesia. *Cleft Palate Craniofac J.* 1992;29:481-483.

22. Cregg N, Conway F, Casey W. Analgesia after otoplasty: regional nerve blockade vs local anaesthetic infiltration of the ear. *Can J Anaesth.* 1996;43:141-147.

23. Burtles R. Analgesia for "bat ear" surgery. *Ann R Coil Surg Engl.* 1999;71:332.

24. Reeves G. Bat ears without tears. *Lancet.* 1989;I:1193, editorial.

25. Doyle M, Casey W, Pollard V, et al. Efficacy of local analgesia in postoperative pain for otoplasty. *Anesthesiology.* 1992;77:A1190.

26. Gleeson AP, Gray AJ. Management of retained ear rings using an ear block. *J Accid Emerg Med.* 1995;12:199-201.

27. Beer GM, Putz R, Mager K, et al. Variations in the frontal exit of the supraorbital nerve : an anatomic study. *Plast Reconstr Surg.* 1998;102:334-341.

28. Brownlow RC, Berman J, Brown REJr. Superficial cervical block for cervical node biopsy in a child with a large mediastinal mass. *J Ark Med Soc.* 1994;90:378-379.

29. Chauhan S, Baronia AK, Maheshwari A, et al. Superficial cervical plexus for internal jugular and subclavian venous cannulation in awake patients. *Reg Anesth.* 1995;20(5):459.

30. Parris WCV, Reddy BC, White HW, et al. Stellate ganglion blocks in pediatric patients. *Anesth Analg.* 1991;72:552-556.

31. Yanagida H, Kemi C, Suwa K. The effects of stellate ganglion block on 29. idiopathic prolongation of the Q-T interval with cardiac arrhythmia (the Romano-Ward syndrome). *Anesth Analg.* 1976;55:782-787.

32. Mesa A, Kaplan RF. Dysrhythmias controlled with stellate ganglion block in a child with diabetes and a variant of long QT syndrome. *Reg Anaesth.* 1993;18:60-62.

33. Lagade MR, Poppers PJ. Stellate ganglion block: a therapeutic modality for arterial insufficiency of the arm in premature infants. *Anesthesiology.* 1984;61:203-204.

34. Kageshima K, Wakasugi B, Hajiri H, et al. A 5 year old patient with allergic diseases responsive to stellate ganglion block. *Masui.* 1992;41:2005-2007.

35. Elias M, Chakerian MU. Repeated steltate ganglion blockade using a catheter for pediatric herpes zoster opthalmicus. *Anesthesiology.* 1994;80:950-952.

36. Bartfield JM, Lee FS, Raccio-Robak N, et al. Topical tetracaine attenuates the pain of infiltration of buffered lidocaine. *Acad Emerg Med.* 1996;5:1001-1005.

37. Hartley E J, Bisonnette B, St-Louis P, et al. Scalp infiltration with bupivacaine in pediatric brain surgery. *Anesth Analg.* 1991;73:29-32.

38. Palmon SC, Lloyd AT, Kirsch JR. The effect of needle gauge and lidocaine pH on pain during intradermal injection. *Anesth Analg.* 1998;86:378-381.

39. Bartfield JM, Sokaris S J, Raccio-Robak N. Local anaesthesia for lacerations: pain of infiltration vs outside the wound. *Acad Emerg Med.* 1998;5:100-104.

Regional Anesthesia: Upper and Lower Extremity Blocks

Tricia Vecchione

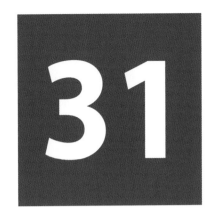

FOCUS POINTS

1. Contrary to adults, most pediatric peripheral nerve blocks are placed under general anesthesia.
2. Peripheral nerve block techniques in children are primarily used as an adjunct to general anesthesia for posteroperative analgesia.
3. The greatest immediate risk of peripheral nerve blocks is local anesthetic systemic toxicity from inadvertent intravascular injection.
4. The interscalene block is most optimal for procedures of the shoulder. It may not be ideal for procedures of the forearm and hand because of the chance of ulnar sparing.
5. The supraclavicular block provides a dense blockade from the humerus to the hand.
6. The infraclavicular block provides good analgesia from the humerus to the hand and is conducive for indwelling catheter placement.
7. The axillary approach to the brachial plexus is optimal for procedures distal to the elbow. It misses the musculocutaneous nerve, which needs to be blocked separately.
8. The femoral nerve block can be used for many surgical techniques involving the thigh and knee, such as skin grafts, mid to distal femur osteotomies, and knee arthroscopies. It can also serve as an adjunct to procedures distal to the knee requiring analgesia to the medial aspect, which is innervated by the saphenous nerve.
9. The sciatic nerve can be blocked at multiple locations along its course. It is useful for surgical procedures of the hip, thigh, and knee. It is very useful for procedures of the distal lower extremity but needs to be supplemented with a saphenous nerve block for complete analgesia.
10. The lumbar plexus provides coverage of three peripheral nerves (femoral, obturator, and lateral femoral cutaneous) at a very proximal location, making it a good block for proximal femur and hip procedures.

INTRODUCTION

The advancement in ultrasound technology and development of pediatric appropriate equipment have led to the increased use of regional anesthesia in infants and children. Additionally, the increased awareness of the potential neurotoxic effects of certain anesthetic agents on the developing brain has further prompted interest.[1] Although pediatric regional anesthesia is mostly used as an adjunct to general anesthesia or to provide postoperative analgesia, many techniques can be used as an alternative to general anesthesia when it may be difficult or dangerous. It can also be used in the treatment of a variety of acute and chronic pain conditions. The Pediatric Regional Anesthesia Network (PRAN), and the French-Language Society of Pediatric Anesthesiologist (ADARPEF) multi-institutional projects reporting the use and incidence of complications of pediatric regional anesthesia, has concluded that regional anesthesia can be commonly performed in children at a very low complication rate.[2–4]

INDICATIONS

The choice of anesthesia and regional anesthetic techniques are determined by the comorbidities of the patient and with in-depth consideration of the potential risks and benefits. Important considerations include the type of surgery, surgeon preference, the experience of the anesthesiologist, and the physical and cognitive state of the patient.[5] Peripheral regional nerve blockade can improve postoperative pain and patient and/or parent satisfaction. Additionally, it can reduce general volatile anesthetics requirements thereby potentially reducing neurotoxcity, providing benefits in patients with a history of postoperative nausea and vomiting, and improving intraoperative hemodynamic stability in patients with a tenuous hemodynamic status.[6]

CONTRAINDICATIONS

Absolute contraindications include patient or parental refusal, infection at the injection site, and an allergy to local anesthetics. Most other contraindications are relative and require weighing the risks and benefits to determine if the patient is a good candidate. Bleeding diatheses, resulting from genetic or acquired defects, increase the risks of hematomas with peripheral nerve blocks. Blood stream infections are also relative contraindications. Although most anesthesiologist may perform a single injection nerve block, catheter placement should generally be avoided in true bacteremia. Lastly, patients with preexisting peripheral neuropathies may be at increased risk for permanent nerve damage with nerve blockade.

SPECIFIC PEDIATRIC CONSIDERATIONS

There are distinct differences between adult and pediatric regional anesthesia. A major difference is that regional anesthesia is usually performed under general anesthesia or deep sedation. Anatomic structures are smaller and in closer proximity to each other and to vessels. Therefore, equipment should be appropriate for the patient size in order to increase safety. Also, there is a lower concentration of plasma protein binding in infants so meticulous attention to dosing is warranted to minimize the risk of local anesthetic toxicity.

CHOICE OF ANESTHETIC AND DOSING

The majority of pediatric regional anesthesia is performed with either 0.25% bupivacaine or 0.2% ropivacaine. At these concentrations, the degree of motor blockade is generally minimal while providing good sensory analgesia. For continuous infusions through a catheter, bupivacaine or ropivacaine concentrations of 0.1% to 0.125% are usually effective. In pediatric patients, the dose of local anesthetic is weight dependent. Higher concentrations of bupivacaine or ropivacaine (0.5%) can be used during surgical anesthesia where greater motor blockade is required, but with careful attention to patient size and toxic dosing limits. Since the greatest risk of regional anesthesia in children is local anesthetic toxicity, the total dose of bupivacaine should not exceed 3 mg/kg. The risk is highest during the initial bolus, thus the lowest effective volume and concentration should be used. For continuous infusions, it is recommended that the dose of bupivacaine be less than

0.3 to 0.4 mg/kg/h in children and less than 0.2 to 0.25 mg/kg/h in infants less than 6 months of age.[7,8] Late signs and symptoms of local anesthetic toxicity (seizures, arrhythmias, cardiovascular collapse) may be the only indication of a problem since most pediatric regional techniques are performed under general anesthesia. Treatment consists of airway management, seizure suppression, management of cardiac arrhythmias, and administration of intralipid. The initial bolus dose of 20% intralipid is 1.5 mL/kg followed by a continuous infusion started at 0.25 mL/kg/min, which can be doubled to achieve cardiac stability.[9]

UPPER EXTREMITY BLOCKS

The brachial plexus can be blocked at several sites. It originates from the C5 through T1 nerve roots and forms trunks, divisions, cords, and finally terminal nerves. The brachial plexus provides complete sensory and motor innervation of the arm, except the medial and posterior proximal upper arm, which is innervated by the intercostobrachial nerve (T2).[10]

Interscalene Brachial Plexus Block

Background and Indications

The interscalene brachial plexus block targets the roots and proximal trunks as they emerge between the anterior and middle scalene muscles at the level of the cricoid cartilage. It provides anesthesia to the upper arm and shoulder and is therefore useful for surgeries of the proximal humerus and shoulder. However, it may not consistently anesthetize the ulnar distribution of the upper extremity since the inferior roots are frequently missed.[11,12]

Patient Position

The patient is supine with the head turned away from the operative side (Figure 31-1).

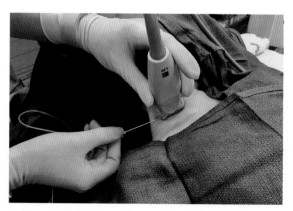

▲ **Figure 31-1.** Interscalene surface anatomy showing probe and needle positioning. (Used with permission, from Dr. Tricia Vecchione, Johns Hopkins University School of Medicine.)

Equipment

A high-frequency linear transducer (10 to 18 MHz) with a small footprint is recommended depending on the size of the patient. A 22–24G, 2-in., blunt needle can be used.

Technique

The transducer is placed in a transverse oblique orientation in the supraclavicular fossa. Once the subclavian artery and brachial plexus are identified, the ultrasound probe is then moved cephalad to the level of C6 where the brachial plexus roots and/or trunks can be visualized as hypoechoic circles between the anterior and middle scalene muscles (Figure 31-2). The needle is inserted in-plane with the probe and advanced from lateral to medial toward the roots. Once the needle is adjacent to the roots, local anesthetic is injected, after negative aspiration, in small 2- to 3-mL aliquots until circumferential spread around the plexus is achieved. Catheters can be placed via an insulated stimulating Tuohy needle and should be directed slightly more cephalad.

Local Anesthetic

Total volume is dependent on the size and weight of the patient. Typically, 0.2 to 0.3 mL/kg of 0.25% bupivacaine or 0.2% ropivacaine provides an effective analgesic block. The total dose should not exceed 3 mg/kg.

Complications

The interscalene block has multiple potential adverse effects. The close proximity of the vertebral artery increases the risk of intraarterial injection and seizures. Inadvertent intrathecal or epidural injection can occur due to the proximity of the vertebral column. Other side effects include blocking other nearby nerves such as the phrenic nerve, which can lead to hemidiaphragm paralysis and respiratory failure in patients with inadequate pulmonary reserve. Other nerves that can be blocked include the recurrent laryngeal nerve resulting in unilateral vocal cord paralysis (dyspnea and hoarseness), and sympathetic chain blockade leading to Horner's syndrome (ptosis, anhidrosis, and myosis).

Supraclavicular Brachial Plexus Block

Background and Indications

The supraclavicular approach targets the trunks and/or divisions where they pass between the first rib and clavicle. The plexus is tightly oriented at this level and blockade produces excellent anesthesia of the humerus, elbow, forearm, and hand. It is mostly used for surgical procedures distal to the shoulder.

Patient Position

The patient is supine with the head turned away from the operative side.

Equipment

A high-frequency linear transducer is recommended depending on the size of the patient. A 21–23G, 2-in., blunt, simulating needle can be used.

Technique

The transducer is placed in a transverse orientation in the supraclavicular fossa above the clavicle (Figure 31-3).

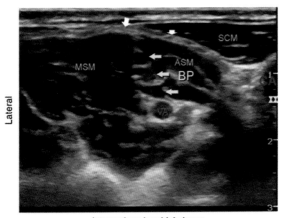

Interscalene brachial plexus

▲ **Figure 31-2.** Interscalene nerve block ultrasound image. (Reproduced with permission, from Hadzic A, eds. *Hadzic's Peripheral Nerve Blocks and Anatomy for Ultrasound-Guided Regional Anesthesia*, 2nd ed. 2012. https://accessanesthesiology.mhmedical.com. Copyright © McGraw Hill LLC. All rights reserved.)

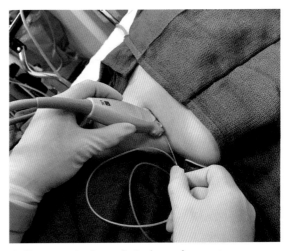

▲ **Figure 31-3.** Supraclavicular surface anatomy showing probe and needle positioning. (Used with permission, from Dr. Tricia Vecchione, Johns Hopkins University School of Medicine.)

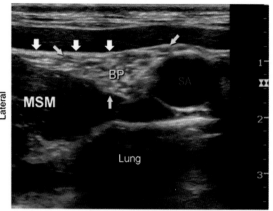

▲ **Figure 31-4.** Supraclavicular nerve block ultrasound image. (Reproduced with permission, from Hadzic A, eds. *Hadzic's Peripheral Nerve Blocks and Anatomy for Ultrasound-Guided Regional Anesthesia*, 2nd ed. 2012. https://accessanesthesiology.mhmedical.com. Copyright © McGraw Hill LLC. All rights reserved.)

Lateral to the subclavian artery and above the first rib and pleura, the brachial plexus is visible as a cluster of hypoechoic structures (Figure 31-4). The needle is advanced from the lateral end of the probe and directed in-plane toward the artery until the tip is deep to the plexus immediately above the first rib. After negative aspiration, injection of local anesthetic should lift the plexus superiorly off the first rib.

Local Anesthetic

Total volume is dependent on the size and weight of the patient. For most patients, 0.2 mL/kg of 0.25% bupivacaine or 0.2% ropivacaine is sufficient to produce an adequate block, whereas 0.5% concentrations can be used for surgical anesthesia and increased motor blockade.

Complications

Blockade of the plexus at this level can also cause recurrent laryngeal nerve and phrenic nerve paresis and Horner's syndrome. Given the proximity of the pleura and vascular structures, there is a risk of vascular puncture and pneumothorax.

▶ Infraclavicular Brachial Plexus Block

Background and Indications

The infraclavicular approach blocks the cords of the brachial plexus where the cords surround the axillary artery. It can be used for surgeries involving the proximal humerus, elbow, forearm, and hand. This location is more conducive than the supraclavicular approach to the placement of

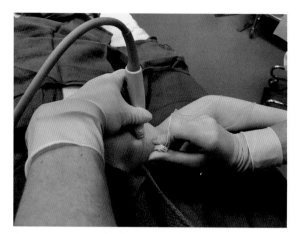

▲ **Figure 31-5.** Infraclavicular surface anatomy showing probe and needle positioning. (Used with permission, from Dr. Tricia Vecchione, Johns Hopkins University School of Medicine.)

catheters for postoperative analgesia, as the muscles provide a good anchor and has been shown to have reduced dislodgement rates.[13,14]

Patient Position

The patient is supine with the head turned away from the operative side. The arm is abducted and the elbow flexed at 90 degrees.

Equipment

A high-frequency 25-mm or 35-mm linear transducer is recommended depending on the size of the patient. A 21–23G, 2-in. or 4-in., blunt, stimulating needle can be used.

Technique

The transducer is oriented along the sagittal plane in the deltopectoral groove, medial and inferior to the coracoid process (Figure 31-5). The axillary artery is identified and if pleura is visualized, the probe can be moved laterally until pleura is no longer in view. The cords are hypoechoic structures located lateral, medial, and posterior to the artery (Figure 31-6). The needle is inserted in-plane at the cephalad border of the transducer and advanced caudally toward the cords. The needle should be advanced past the lateral cord to the posterior border of the artery where the posterior cord is located. Local anesthetic injection at this point will produce a U or horseshoe shape spread targeting all three cords of the brachial plexus. Upon withdrawing the needle, a second injection of local anesthetic anterior to the artery will ensure distribution of local anesthetic to all three cords. Catheters are best placed inferiorly to the plexus or between the lateral and posterior cords.

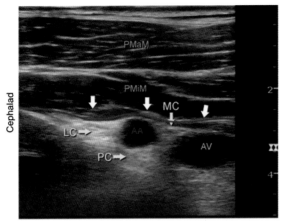

▲ Figure 31-6. Infraclavicular nerve block ultrasound image. (Reproduced with permission, from Hadzic A, eds. *Hadzic's Peripheral Nerve Blocks and Anatomy for Ultrasound-Guided Regional Anesthesia*, 2nd ed. 2012. https://accessanesthesiology.mhmedical.com. Copyright © McGraw Hill LLC. All rights reserved.)

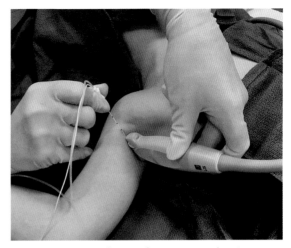

▲ Figure 31-7. Axillary surface anatomy showing probe and needle positioning. (Used with permission, from Dr. Tricia Vecchione, Johns Hopkins University School of Medicine.)

Local Anesthetic

Total volume is dependent on the size and weight of the patient. For most patients, 0.2 to 0.3 mL/kg of 0.25% bupivacaine or 0.2% ropivacaine is required to produce effective blockade.

Complications

Pneumothorax and chylothorax (with a left-sided block) are possible. Inadvertent vascular puncture is also a risk given the proximity of the cords around the axillary artery.

Axillary Brachial Plexus Block

Background and Indications

The axillary approach to the brachial plexus targets the terminal branches consisting of the ulnar, median, radial, and musculocutaneous nerves. The ulnar, median, and radial nerves have variable positions around the axillary artery but typical locations are as follows: the median nerve lies superior, the radial artery lies deep or posterior, and the ulnar nerve lies inferior or superficial. The nerves can be visualized as hyperechoic cirlcles around the artery. The musculocutaneous nerve exits the nerve sheath early, appearing as a hyperechoic structure between the biceps and coracobrachialis muscles, and needs to be blocked separately. The axillary nerve block can be used for surgeries of the elbow, forearm, and hand. It may need to be supplemented with blockade of the musculocutaneous nerve, which innervates the lateral aspect of the forearm.

Patient Position

The patient is supine with the arm abducted 90 degress, externally rotated and the elbow flexed at 90 degrees.

Equipment

A high-frequency, 25- or 35-mm transducer is recommend depending on the size of the patient. A 21–23G, 2-in., blunt, stimulating needle can be used.

Technique

The transducer is positioned transverse in the axilla, perpendicular to the axis of the humerus (Figure 31-7). First, the axillary artery and vein should be visualized and then small adjustments are made to see the terminal nerves (Figure 31-8). The needle is inserted in-plane in a superior to inferior orientation. Due to the presence of septae within the sheath at this location, each nerve may need to be targeted separately. The needle is initially directed posteriorly to the axillary artery toward the radial nerve and local anesthetic is injected. The needle is then withdrawn and injection of local anesthetic around the median nerve and then ulnar nerve is complete. The needle can be redirected to target the musculocutaneous nerve with the injection of a small amount of local anesthetic.

Local Anesthetic

Total volume is dependent on the size and weight of the patient. For postoperative analgesia, 0.2 to 0.3 mL/kg of 0.25% bupivacaine or 0.2% ropivacaine is adequate. Due to the precise targeting of individual nerves, only a small amount of local anesthetic is required at each nerve target. For the musculocutaneous nerve, 2 to 3 mL is sufficient.

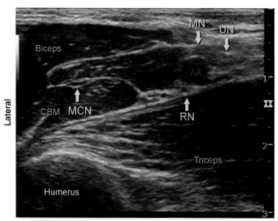

Axillary brachial plexus with anatomical structures labeled

▲ **Figure 31-8.** Axillary nerve block ultrasound image. (Reproduced with permission, from Hadzic A, eds. *Hadzic's Peripheral Nerve Blocks and Anatomy for Ultrasound-Guided Regional Anesthesia*, 2nd ed. 2012. https://accessanesthesiology.mhmedical.com. Copyright © McGraw Hill LLC. All rights reserved.)

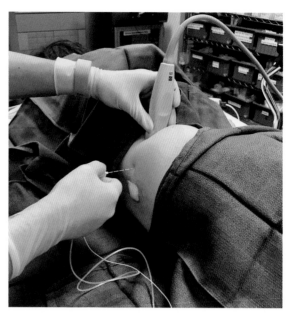

▲ **Figure 31-9.** Lumbar plexus positioning. (Used with permission, from Dr. Tricia Vecchione, Johns Hopkins University School of Medicine.)

Complications

The axillary approach is associated with a very low complication rate, provided intravascular injection is avoided.

LOWER EXTREMITY BLOCKS

There are several regional block techniques that can be used for surgeries of the hip, knee, foot, and ankle. Traditionally, the caudal approach was used to provide analgesia to the lower extremity. However, recent data supporting the efficacy and lower complication profile of peripheral nerve blocks versus the caudal block will most likely lead to the increasing use of peripheral nerve blocks.

▶ Lumbar Plexus Nerve Block

Background and Indications

The lumbar plexus is derived from L1–4. It provides anesthesia to three main nerves including the femoral, lateral femoral cutaneous, and obturator nerves. The lumbar plexus block can provide anesthesia to unilateral surgical procedures involving the hip, pelvis, and femur.[15] It can be combined with a sciatic nerve block to provide complete anesthesia to the lower extremity. It is also a suitable alternative for patients who have a contraindication to a neuraxial technique.

Patient Position

The patient is at lateral decubitus position with the side to block upright and the knees and hips flexed (Figure 31-9).

Equipment

Depending on the size of the patient and the depth needed to penetrate, a high-frequency linear probe or a curved intermediate frequency probe can be used. Usually, a 21G, 4-in. stimulating needle is used, but in toddlers and very small children, a 21G, 2-in. needle may be adequate. An 18G Tuohy needle can be used for catheter placement.

Technique

It is recommended to use nerve stimulation with ultrasound guidance for the lumbar plexus block with the goal of achieving twitches of the quadriceps muscle at a threshold of 0.5 mA. There are multiple ultrasound-guided approaches to the lumbar plexus. There are various techniques to this block but we describe this one specifically for brevity.

Local Anesthetic

The volume of local anesthetic depends on the age/weight of the patient and the concentration on the desired density and motor blockade. Generally, a volume a 0.2 to 0.4 mL/kg of 0.25% bupivacaine or 0.2% ropivacaine is used and the dose should not exceed the maximum toxic dose.

Complications

Due to the proximity of neuraxial structures, there is a risk of epidural or spinal blockade if the needle is directed too medially. Although rare, local anesthetic toxicity from intravascular injection and retroperitoneal hematomas have been reported.

Femoral Nerve Block

Background and Indications

The femoral nerve block can be used to provide analgesia to the anterior thigh and knee and is typically combined with a sciatic nerve block to achieve complete analgesia distal to the mid-thigh.[16] It is useful for surgical procedures including knee arthroscopy, mid to distal femur fractures or osteotomies, and skin grafts or muscle biopsies. The lateral femoral cutaneous nerve also needs to be blocked if the lateral thigh is within the surgical field.

Patient Position

The patient is supine with the hip slightly externally rotated.

Equipment

A high-frequency linear transducer and a 21–23G, 2-in., blunt, simulating needle is usually sufficient. An 18G insulated Tuohy needle can be used for catheter placement.

Technique

The transducer is placed in a transverse orientation in the inguinal crease (Figure 31-10). The femoral artery is identified and the nerve is lateral to the artery and deep to the fascia iliaca (Figure 31-11). The needle is inserted in-plane at the lateral end of the probe and advanced medially through the fascia iliaca toward the femoral nerve. A loss of resistance or "pop" may be felt as the needle passes through the fascia lata and fascia iliaca. The local anesthetic is injected and should be seen surrounding the nerve. If nerve stimulation is used, a quadriceps femoris muscle response is sought at a threshold of approximately 0.5 mA.

Local Anesthetic

The volume is dependent on the size of the patient and the concentration on the desired degree of motor blockade. Usually, 0.2 to 0.4 mL/kg of 0.25% bupivacaine or 0.2% ropivacaine is effective for postoperative analgesia.

Complications

Careful aspiration and incremental injection can help to avoid intravascular injection and local anesthetic toxicity. If an arterial puncture occurs, pressure should be held for 5 to 10 minutes to decrease the risk of a hematoma.

Saphenous Nerve Block

Background and Indications

The saphenous nerve is a purely sensory nerve. It provides cutaneous innervation to the medial side of the calf and foot. It can be used as an adjunct block to the sciatic nerve block for complete sensory blockade of the lower leg and foot. The saphenous nerve block is useful for surgeries of the medial aspect of the lower leg and ankle (when combined with the sciatic nerve block).[17]

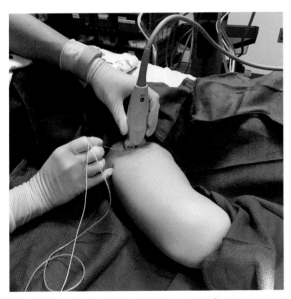

▲ **Figure 31-10.** Femoral nerve block surface anatomy showing probe and needle positioning. (Used with permission, from Dr. Tricia Vecchione, Johns Hopkins University School of Medicine.)

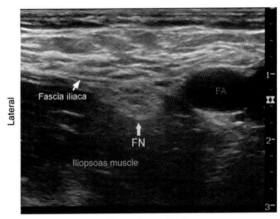

Femoral nerve block

▲ **FIGURE 31-11.** Femoral nerve block ultrasound image. (Reproduced with permission, from Hadzic A, eds. *Hadzic's Peripheral Nerve Blocks and Anatomy for Ultrasound-Guided Regional Anesthesia*, 2nd ed. 2012. https://accessanesthesiology.mhmedical.com. Copyright © McGraw Hill LLC. All rights reserved.)

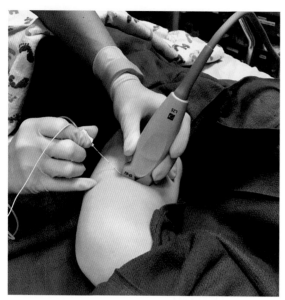

▲ **Figure 31-12.** Saphenous nerve block surface anatomy showing probe and needle positioning. (Used with permission, from Dr. Tricia Vecchione, Johns Hopkins University School of Medicine.)

Patient Position

The patient is supine with the hip slightly externally rotated.

Equipment

A high-frequency hockey stick or linear transducer and a 21-23G, 2-in., blunt, simulating needle are usually sufficient.

Technique

This block is performed approximately at the mid to distal third of the thigh (Figure 31-12). The transducer is placed in a transverse orientation over the mid to distal third of the thigh (Figure 31-12). The femur is located and probe moved medially until the superficial femoral artery is identified under the Sartorius muscle (Figure 31-13). The vastus medialis is anterolateral at this location. The saphenous nerve may be difficult to visualize on ultrasound, but it usually lies in the fascial plane between the sartorius and vastus medialis muscles (Figure 31-13). The needle is inserted in-plane until the needle tip is between the artery and the Sartorius muscle. Nerve stimulation is not needed since the saphenous nerve is purely sensory. Only a small volume of local anesthetic is necessary and results in expansion of the fascial plane between the Sartorius muscle and the vastus medialis muscle.

Local Anesthetic

Only a small volume of local anesthetic is required. Typically, 0.15 to 0.25 mL/kg (max 10 mL) of 0.25% bupivacaine or 0.2% ropivacaine is injected.

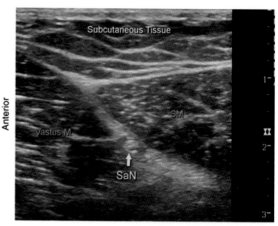

Saphenous nerve block above knee

▲ **Figure 31-13.** Saphenous nerve block ultrasound image. (Reproduced with permission, from Hadzic A, eds. *Hadzic's Peripheral Nerve Blocks and Anatomy for Ultrasound-Guided Regional Anesthesia*, 2nd ed. 2012. https://accessanesthesiology.mhmedical.com. Copyright © McGraw Hill LLC. All rights reserved.)

Complications

Nerve injury can occur if too much local anesthetic is injected due to increased pressure in the small compartment. There is also a risk of intravascular injection and local anesthetic toxicity.

▶ Sciatic Nerve Block

The sciatic nerve is formed by the nerve roots of L4–5 and S1–3. It provides motor innervation to the hamstrings and all of the lower extremity muscles distal to the knee. It also provides sensory innervation to the posterior thigh and knee as well as the lower extremity distal to the knee except for the anteromedial skin, which is innervated by the saphenous nerve. A sciatic nerve block can be used for procedures involving the posterior thigh/knee, fractures of the leg and ankle, foot surgery, and amputations. For certain surgical procedures, a femoral or saphenous nerve block may be needed as an adjunct to provide complete analgesia.[18,19] It can be blocked at multiple spots along its course. This demonstrates one of many various approaches to the sciatic nerve block. Nerve stimulation is recommended in addition to ultrasound guidance to enhance nerve localization due to the depth of the sciatic nerve at certain locations. Twitches of the hamstring, calf, and foot muscles can be elicited with the goal of achieving foot inversion or plantar flexion at 0.5 mA.

▶ Subgluteal Sciatic Block

Background and Indications

See Section "Sciatic Nerve Block."

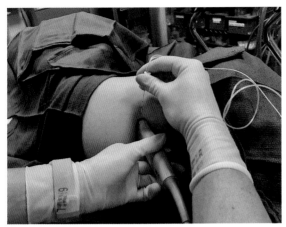

▲ **Figure 31-14.** Subgluteal nerve block surface anatomy showing probe and needle positioning. (Used with permission, from Dr. Tricia Vecchione, Johns Hopkins University School of Medicine.)

Patient Position

The patient is at lateral position with the legs flexed at the hip and knee or prone.

Equipment

The transducer choice is dependent on the size of the child and the anticipated depth of the nerve. A high-frequency linear probe can be used in children <30 kg, but an intermediate-frequency curvilinear probe may be needed to improve ultrasound penetration in larger patients, where the sciatic nerve is deeper. A 21–22G, 2-in. or 4-in. stimulating needle should be used depending on the size of the patient. An 18G Tuohy needle can be used for catheter placement.

Technique

The greater trochanter and ischial tuberosity can be palpated and the probe should be placed transverse between these two landmarks (Figure 31-14). The sciatic nerve appears as a hyperechoic, wide and flat structure deep to the gluteus maximus muscle (Figure 31-15). The needle is inserted in-plane at the lateral border of the probe and advanced medially. When the needle tip is positioned adjacent to the nerve, local anesthetic can be visualized surrounding the nerve.

Local Anesthetic

Typically, 0.1 to 0.2 mL/kg of 0.25% bupivacaine or 0.2% ropivacaine is used.

Complications

Neural damage from intraneural injection can occur. Color Doppler may be used to identify vessels to decrease the risk of vascular puncture.

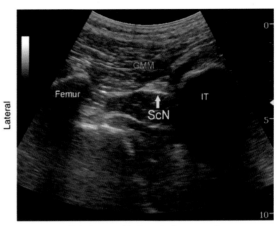

Sciatic nerve block-posterior approach

▲ **Figure 31-15.** Subgluteal sciatic nerve block ultrasound image. (Reproduced with permission, from Hadzic A, eds. *Hadzic's Peripheral Nerve Blocks and Anatomy for Ultrasound-Guided Regional Anesthesia*, 2nd ed. 2012. https://accessanesthesiology.mhmedical.com. Copyright © McGraw Hill LLC. All rights reserved.)

▶ Popliteal Sciatic Block

Background and Indications

The popliteal sciatic block is a popular approach for surgical procedures below the knee. At this location, the sciatic nerve bifurcates into the tibial and common peroneal nerves.[20]

Patient Position

The patient position is supine, lateral, or prone.

Equipment

A high-frequency linear probe and a 21G or 22G, 20-in. or 4-in. stimulating needle depending on the size of the patient should be used. An 18G Tuohy needle can be used for catheter placement.

Technique

The probe is placed transverse in the popliteal crease (Figure 31-16). The popliteal vessels are identified and the tibial nerve appears as circular hyperechoic structure superficial to the vessels. As the probe is moved cephalad, the tibial and common peroneal nerves join to form the sciatic nerve (Figure 31-17). When the birfurcation is identified, the needle is inserted in-plane at the lateral edge of the probe. When the needle is adjacent to the sciatic nerve, local anesthetic is injected and should be seen surrounding the nerve.

Local Anesthetic

Typically, 0.1 to 0.2 mL/kg of 0.25% bupivacaine or 0.2% ropivacaine is used.

Complications

Intravascular or intraneural injections are possible.

▶ Ankle Block

Background and Indications

There are five nerves that must be blocked to provide complete anesthesia for surgeries of the ankle or foot. The sural nerve, the superficial and deep peroneal nerves, and the posterior tibial nerve are branches of the sciatic nerve while the saphenous nerve is a branch of the femoral nerve. The ankle block provides analgesia for surgical procedures such as club foot repair, polydactyly reconstruction, foot osteotomies, and foreign body removals.

Patient Position

The patient is supine with a holster under the foot.

Equipment

A small footprint linear or "hockey stick" high-frequency transducer is optimal if performing the block under ultrasound guidance. A 22–25G, 3–5 cm needle is used.

Technique

Ultrasound guidance may be helpful when blocking the deep nerves such as the deep peroneal and the posterior tibial nerves. The deep peroneal nerve can be found between the extensor hallucis longus tendon and the extensor digitorum longus tendon. Inserting the needle lateral to the anterior tibial artery can block this nerve. The probe is placed in a transverse orientation at the anterior surface of the ankle and the nerve can be seen as a hyperechoic structure lateral to the artery (Figure 31-18). The posterior tibial nerve is located posterior to the medial malleolus adjacent to the posterior tibial artery. The needle is inserted between the medial malleolus and the Achilles tendon and directed posterior to the artery. For the ultrasound-guided technique, the probe is placed transverse posterior to the medial malleolus (Figure 31-19A). The

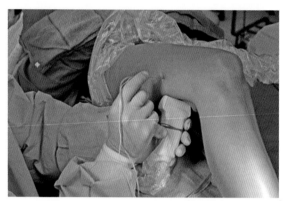

▲ **Figure 31-16.** Popliteal sciatic nerve block surface anatomy showing probe and needle positioning. (Reproduced with permission, from Hadzic A, eds. *Hadzic's Peripheral Nerve Blocks and Anatomy for Ultrasound-Guided Regional Anesthesia*, 2nd ed. 2012. https://accessanesthesiology.mhmedical.com. Copyright © McGraw Hill LLC. All rights reserved.)

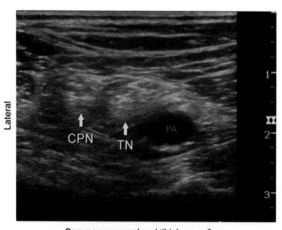

Common peroneal and tibial nerve-3 cm above popliteal crease, labeled

▲ **Figure 31-17.** Popliteal sciatic nerve block ultrasound image. (Reproduced with permission, from Hadzic A, eds. *Hadzic's Peripheral Nerve Blocks and Anatomy for Ultrasound-Guided Regional Anesthesia*, 2nd ed. 2012. https://accessanesthesiology.mhmedical.com. Copyright © McGraw Hill LLC. All rights reserved.)

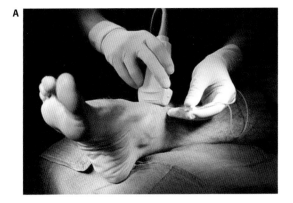

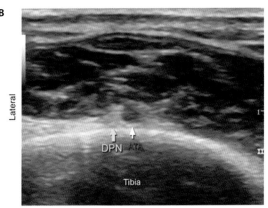

Ankle block-deep peroneal nerve

▲ **Figure 31-18. A.** Deep peroneal nerve block surface anatomy showing probe and needle positioning. **B.** Deep peroneal nerve block ultrasound image. (Reproduced with permission, from Hadzic A, eds. *Hadzic's Peripheral Nerve Blocks and Anatomy for Ultrasound-Guided Regional Anesthesia*, 2nd ed. 2012. https://accessanesthesiology.mhmedical.com. Copyright © McGraw Hill LLC. All rights reserved.)

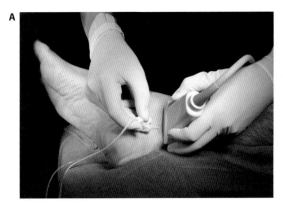

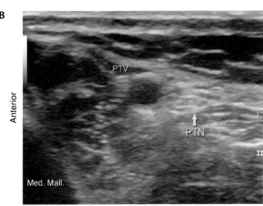

Ankle block-posterior tibial nerve

▲ **Figure 31-19. A.** Posterior tibial nerve block surface anatomy showing probe and needle positioning. **B.** Posterior tibial nerve block ultrasound image. (Reproduced with permission, from Hadzic A, eds. *Hadzic's Peripheral Nerve Blocks and Anatomy for Ultrasound-Guided Regional Anesthesia*, 2nd ed. 2012. https://accessanesthesiology.mhmedical.com. Copyright © McGraw Hill LLC. All rights reserved.)

nerve can be seen as a hyperechoic structure posterior to the artery (Figure 31-19B). The saphenous nerve is located adjacent to the vein anterior to the medial malleolus. It can be blocked by infiltrating the area anterior to the medial malleolus. The sural nerve is blocked by inserting the needle between the lateral malleolus and the calcaneus. The superficial peroneal nerve is blocked by injecting local anesthetic subcutaneously in a ring-like fashion from the medial to the lateral malleolus.

Local Anesthetic

The total volume of local anesthetic will depend on the size of the child. Typically, 0.1 mL/kg of 0.25% bupivacaine or 0.2% ropivacaine may be used. Generally, 1 to 3 mL is sufficient to anesthetize each nerve. Epinephrine should not

be added to the local anesthetic solution for the ankle block as this can lead to limb ischemia.

Complications

Vascular puncture is a risk; therefore, careful aspiration should be performed prior to injection of local anesthetic. Large volumes of local anesthetic may cause nerve damage from compression in this small, noncompliant space.

REFERENCES

1. Brown T. History of pediatric regional anesthesia. *Paediatr Anaesth*. 2012;22:3-9.
2. Giaufe E, Dalens B, Gombert A. Epidemiology and morbidity of regional anesthesia in children: a one-year prospective

survey of the French-Language Society of Pediatric Anesthesiologist. *Anesth Analg.* 1996;83:904-912.

3. Ecoffey C, Lacroix F, Giaufre E, et al. Epidemiology and morbidity of regional anesthesia in children: a follow-up one-year prospective survey of the French-Language Society of Pediatric Anesthesiologist (ADARPEF). *Paediatr Anaesth.* 2010;20:1061-1069.

4. Polaner D, Taenzer A, Walker B, et al. Pediatric Regional Anesthesia Network (PRAN): a multi-institutional study of the use and incidence of complications of pediatric regional anesthesia. *Anesth Analg.* 2012;115:1353-1364.

5. Tsui B, Suresh S. Ultrasound imaging for regional anesthesia in infants, children and adolescents: a review of current literature and its application in the practice of extremity and trunk blocks. *Anesthesiology.* 2010;112:473-492.

6. Bosenberg A. Benefits of regional anesthesia in children. *Pediatr Anesth.* 2012;22:10-18.

7. Berde C. Toxicity of local anesthetics in infants and children. *J Pediatr.* 1993;122:S14-S20.

8. Bosenberg AT, Thomas J, Cronje L, et al. Pharmacokinetics and efficacy of ropivacaine for continuous epidural infusion in neonates and infants. *Paediatr Anaesth.* 2005;15:739-749.

9. Neil JM, Mulroy MF, Weinberg GL. American Society of Regional Anesthesia and Pain Medicine checklist for managing local anesthetic system toxicity: 2012 version. *Reg Anesth Pain Med.* 2012;37:16-18.

10. Tobias JD. Brachial plexus anaesthia in children. *Paediatr Anaesth.* 2001;11:265-275.

11. Ganesh A, Wells L, Ganley T, et al. Interscalene brachial plexus block for post-operative analgesia following shoulder arthroscopy in children and adolescents. *Acta Anaesthesiol Scand.* 2008;52:162-163.

12. Devera HV, Furukawa KT, Scavone JA, et al. Interscalene blocks in anesthetized pediatric patients. *Reg Anesth Pain Med.* 2009;34:603-604.

13. De Jose MB, Banus E, Navarro EM, et al. Ultrasound-guided supraclavicular vs infraclavicular brachial plexus blocks in children. *Paediatr Aanesth.* 2008;18:838-844.

14. Marhofer P, Willschke H, Kettner SC. Ultrasound-guided upper extremity block-tips and tricks to improve clinical practice. *Paediatr Anaesth.* 2012;22:65-71.

15. Kirchmair L, Enna B, Mitterschiffthaler G, et al. Lumbar plexus in children. A sonographic study and its relevance to pediatric regional anesthesia. *Anesthesiology.* 2004;101:445-450.

16. Flack S, Anderson C. Ultrasound guided lower extremity blocks. *Paediatr Aanesth.* 2012;22:72-80.

17. Krombach J, Gray AT. Sonography for saphenous nerve block near the adductor canal. *Reg Anesth Pain Med.* 2007;32:369-370.

18. Dadure C, Capdevila X. Peripheral catheter techniques. *Pediatr Anesth.* 2012;22:93-101.

19. Oberndorfer U, Marhofer P, Bosenberg A, et al. Ultrasonographic guidance for sciatic and femoral nerve blocks in children. *Br J Anaesth.* 2007;98:797-801.

20. Simion C, Suresh S. Lower extremity peripheral nerve blocks in children. *Tech Reg Anesth Pain Manag.* 2007;11:222-228.

Regional Anesthesia: Truncal Blocks

Susan E. Eklund and Walid Alrayashi

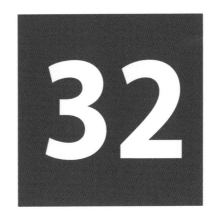

FOCUS POINTS

1. Most peripheral nerve blocks in children are performed under general anesthesia.
2. Transversus abdominus plane (TAP) blocks may provide analgesia for lower abdominal surgery (T10-L1).
3. Complications associated with TAP blocks include peritoneal or bowel injury.
4. Quadratus lumborum (QL) blocks can block a wide range of dermatomes of the anterior abdominal wall, roughly T7-L1. In addition, spread to the paravertebral space can provide analgesia for peritoneal or visceral pain.
5. Rectus sheath blocks provide analgesia to the anterior abdominal wall and are often used as complements to TAP or QL blocks, especially above the umbilicus.
6. Paravertebral (PV) blocks are primarily used for thoracic surgeries.
7. Complications associated with PV blocks are related to the proximity of this deep space to the pleura (pneumothorax). Other complications are inadvertent vascular puncture or intrathecal/epidural injection.

INTRODUCTION

As the name implies, truncal blocks deliver local anesthetic to nerve trunks, or bundles of nerves, rather than a specific, individual nerve. While trunks may form close to the spinal cord, they are bilateral rather than midline structures, and thus truncal blocks are unilateral. Also, since trunks are distal to the central nervous system, side effects of neuraxial blocks, such as urinary retention, nausea and vomiting, and bilateral motor blockade, can be avoided with truncal blocks.

Truncal blocks take advantage of tissue planes and allow for local anesthetics to spread within the plane to the intended neurovascular bundle or bundles. As with most regional blocks, the placement of truncal blocks is augmented using ultrasound, which has become the standard of care when performing most peripheral regional anesthetics.

LOCAL ANESTHETICS

The pediatric considerations, mechanisms, and metabolism of local anesthetics are covered in Chapter 8 and will not be repeated here. However, it is important to note that because truncal blocks are not targeting a specific nerve, but rather a plane, the spread of local anesthetic is crucial to the success of the block. Therefore, in smaller children and infants, it may be necessary to use a more dilute local anesthetic to increase the total volume of medication that may be delivered safely.[1] Dilute local anesthetic is usually effective in young, small children due to ongoing myelination at young ages that renders nerves susceptible to sodium channel blockade with lower concentrations.

BLOCK METHODOLOGY

As with many regional blocks, truncal blocks are often single-shot injections, but catheters may also be placed for continuous infusions or intermittent boluses. Equipment for truncal blocks is the same for other regional blocks: ultrasound with linear or curvilinear probe depending on target depth, sterile prep, drape, probe cover, short-beveled or Tuohy needle, catheter and supplies if applicable, sterile gloves, and local anesthetic.

As with many blocks performed in pediatric patients, truncal blocks in children are often performed with the patient under general anesthesia.[2,3] Most commonly, truncal blocks are performed with the needle in-plane with the ultrasound probe such that the needle may be visualized for the entire placement. To perform a single-shot block, a 22G short-bevel needle or similar is advanced to the plane where local anesthetic is to be deposited. Hydro-dissection with small aliquots of saline (0.5 to 1 mL) may be used to identify the potential space of the plane. If a catheter is to be placed, an 18G echogenic Tuohy needle is introduced, through which the initial dose of local anesthetic may be administered, followed by the catheter. In either case, the length of the needle and the type of ultrasound probe depend on the age and size of the patient; for an average-size adult, a medium-length needle is typically sufficient (80 mm) and a linear probe (10 to 15 Hz) provides enough depth to visualize the target plane.

TRANSVERSUS ABDOMINUS PLANE (TAP) BLOCK

Overview

Transversus abdominus plane (TAP) blocks are one of the most commonly performed truncal blocks for both pediatric and adult perioperative patients having abdominal surgery. Rafi first described the landmark technique in 2001,[4] and ultrasound guidance was then described by Hebbard et al in 2007.[5]

Anatomy

The classic landmark technique describes insertion of the needle in the lumbar triangle of Petit, posterior to the most superior aspect of the iliac crest. The internal oblique is the floor of the triangle and serves as a landmark for the neurovascular plane beneath which the T7-L1 neurovascular bundle travels. The correct plane is then identified by two "pops" through the fascial planes. With ultrasound guidance, the probe is initially positioned in the triangle of Petit. Using dynamic ultrasound scanning in the lateral-medial axis, the layers from superficial to deep can be identified as the adipose tissue, external oblique (EO), internal oblique (IO), and transversus abdominal muscle (TA) (Figures 32-1 and 32-2). The peritoneum can be identified by the presence of bowel loops seen below the transversus abdominus muscle.

Indications/Areas Covered/Surgery

TAP blocks may provide analgesia for lower abdominal surgery (T10-L1), including laparoscopic surgeries, colectomy or small bowel resection, ostomy creation or closure, and Pfannenstiel incisions. Oblique subcostal TAP blocks have been described,[6] and cover upper abdominal incisions' however, they are not commonly performed in pediatric patients.

Block Methodology

Most commonly, a TAP block is performed with the patient in the supine position, often post-operatively. For most patients, a linear probe provides adequate depth to visualize the plane between the internal oblique and transversus abdominus, where local anesthetic is deposited.

Specific Complications

Because of the depth of the internal oblique-transversus abdominus plane, peritoneal or bowel injury may occur with TAP blocks.

Considerations

Recent studies have called the efficacy of TAP blocks into question. While meta-analyses have shown some analgesic benefit overall, with reduced opiate consumption and pain scores, the effect sizes are small, the data both scant and heterogeneous, and clinical benefit still unclear.[7,8]

A posterior approach to the TAP block, which aims for local deposition closer to the quadratus lumborum, where the transversus abdominus muscle terminates at the thoracolumbar fascia, has been described to have more reliable analgesia up to T9 in a small group of children.[9]

QUADRATUS LUMBORUM BLOCK

Overview

The quadratus lumborum (QL) block deposits local anesthetic between the quadratus lumborum and the psoas major. It was first described by Blanco and McDonnell,[10] then modified as the "shamrock sign" technique by Sauter et al.[11] The QL block is a posterior extension of the TAP block, and allows for more reliable plane dosing of local anesthetic.

Anatomy and Indications/Areas Covered/Surgery—Surface, Nerves

Like TAP blocks, QL can block a wide range of dermatomes of the anterior abdominal wall, roughly T7-L1. Additionally, due to spread of local anesthetic to the paravertebral space, QL blocks can provide analgesia for peritoneal or visceral pain.[12,13]

QL blocks were initially described for superficial surgeries,[10] and unilateral surgeries,[13,14] but have been also described for laparotomies,[12,15] and hip and femur surgeries in both adults and children,[13,16] as well as Cesarean sections in adult women (Figure 32-3).[17]

Block Methodology

Local anesthetic is deposited with short-beveled single-shot needle or a 22G Tuohy needle.

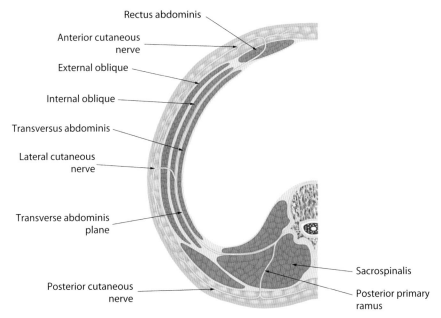

▲ **Figure 32-1.** Transverse section of abdominal wall. (Reproduced with permission, from Karmakar MK, Soh E, Chee V, et al., eds. *Atlas of Sonoanatomy for Regional Anesthesia and Pain Medicine.* 2018. https://accessanesthesiology. mhmedical.com. Copyright © McGraw Hill LLC. All rights reserved.)

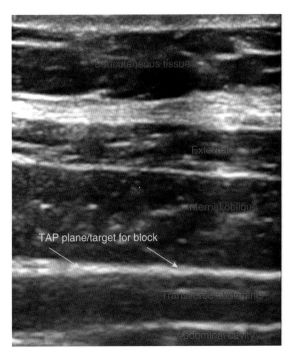

▲ **Figure 32-2.** Ultrasound image for transversus abdominus plane (TAP) block. (Reproduced with permission, from Atchabahian A, Gupta R. *The Anesthesia Guide.* 2013. https://accessanesthesiology.mhmedical. com. Copyright © McGraw Hill LLC. All rights reserved.)

The patient may be positioned prone or lateral for the posterior approaches, or supine with an ipsilateral hip wedge ("sloppy lateral") for an anterior approach. For the posterior approach, a curvilinear probe provides optimal ultrasonographic imaging "shamrock" landmarks characteristic of QL block: the QL as it meets L4 transverse process (superficial), the erector spinae (posterior), and the psoas major (anterior).[11]

For the anterior approach, a linear probe is usually sufficient. The QL is identified in the posterior axillary line, where the thoracolumbar fascia joins the anterior surface of the QL. From this position, scanning anteriorly shows the TAP planes, which can be used to confirm position. Typical of many regional blocks, the needle is introduced in-plane.

The QL can be performed with three different approaches: QL1, QL2, and QL3 (Figure 32-4).

QL1

The needle is advanced anterior to posterior to the point where the abdominal muscles taper together and the QL muscle begins. LA is deposited at this junction, medial to the QL and lateral to the EO/IO/TAP muscles.

QL2

The needle is introduced in a similar fashion and location to the QL1. However, the local anesthesia is deposited more posterior and superficial, between the QL and the EO/erector spinae.

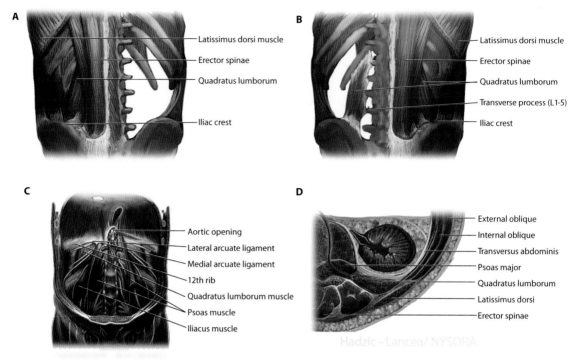

▲ **Figure 32-3.** The quadratus lumborum (QL) muscle in four views: **A.** QL muscle from the back covered by the erector spinae and latissimus dorsi muscles. **B.** QL muscle from the back, with ES and LD muscles removed to show the origin and insertion of the QL muscle. **C.** QL muscle from the front, on the left side the psoas muscle is cut, showing the ventral rami of the spinal nerve roots pass in front of the QL. **D.** QL muscle cross-section showing the surrounding muscles and the QL relation to the kidney. (Reproduced with permission, from Hadzic A. *Hadzic's Textbook of Regional Anesthesia and Acute Pain Management*, 2nd ed. 2017. https://accessanesthesiology.mhmedical. com. Copyright © McGraw Hill LLC. All rights reserved.)

QL3

The QL3 uses a posterior approach, going through the paravertebral muscle, through the posterior-medial portion of the QL, and depositing local at the anterior thoracolumbar fascia, just superficial to the psoas major.

▷ Considerations

As with TAP blocks, there is a risk of injury to the peritoneum and bowel. The kidney lies just anterior and deep to the QL beneath the perinephric fat bilaterally. The liver and spleen are near the block sites, particularly in small children where overall anatomy is small. The local vasculature includes lumbar branches from the aorta.

RECTUS SHEATH (RS) BLOCK

▷ Overview

Rectus sheath (RS) blocks provide analgesia to the anterior abdominal wall and are often used as complements to TAP or QL blocks for the upper portion of the abdomen, often above the umbilicus. Its use was first described in children in 1996 by Ferguson et al.[18]

▷ Anatomy/Block Technique—Surface, Nerves

While the anterior abdominal wall has innervation from T6-L1, the anterior rami of T8-11 contribute to periumbilical sensation and are the main target of the RS block. With the patient supine, local anesthesia is deposited between the posterior aspect of the rectus sheath and the anterior portion of the rectus abdominus muscle (Figure 32-5). The linea alba is a midline structure that can be identified with ultrasound to aid in placement of bilateral blocks. As with other blocks, catheter placement is feasible.[19]

▷ Indications/Areas Covered/Surgery

Typically, the peri- and supra-umbilical trunks are targeted by RS blocks, while lower abdominal incisions are blocked with QL blocks (see Section "Quadratus Lumborum Block"). Candidates for RS blocks often include

A

B

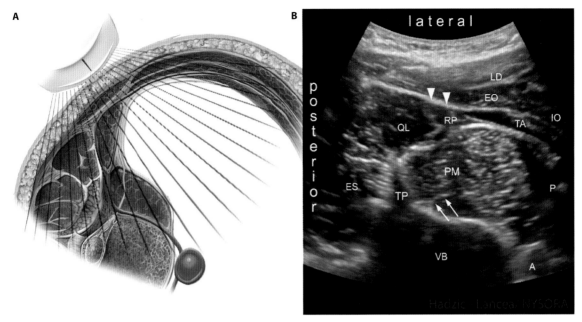

▲ **Figure 32-4. A.** Lateral abdominal wall with ultrasound probe. **B.** Ultrasound image of the lateral abdominal wall. QL, quadratus lumborum; PM, psoas major; ES, erector spinae; TP, transverse process; VB, vertebral body (L4); TA, transverse abdominis; IO, internal oblique; EO, external oblique; LD, latissimus dorsi; RP, retroperitoneal space; P, peritoneal space; A, aorta; arrows, lumbar plexus; arrow heads, transversus abdominis aponeurosis. (Reproduced with permission, from Hadzic A. *Hadzic's Textbook of Regional Anesthesia and Acute Pain Management*, 2nd ed. 2017. https://accessanesthesiology.mhmedical.com. Copyright © McGraw Hill LLC. All rights reserved.)

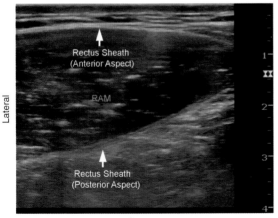

Rectus sheath block

▲ **Figure 32-5.** Rectus sheath block. Labeled ultrasound anatomy of the rectus abdominis sheath. RAM, rectus abdominis muscle. (Reproduced with permission, from Hadzic A, eds. *Hadzic's Peripheral Nerve Blocks and Anatomy for Ultrasound-Guided Regional Anesthesia*, 2nd ed. 2012. https://accessanesthesiology. mhmedical.com. Copyright © McGraw Hill LLC. All rights reserved.)

midline laparotomy with extension above the level of the umbilicus, certain subcostal incisions for liver surgery, and incisions above level of umbilicus.

Considerations

A meta-analysis of five studies by Hamill et al in 2016 showed benefit of RS block in children, although the researchers noted heterogeneous data.[7]

PARAVERTEBRAL (PV) BLOCK

Overview

The PV block was initially described in children by Lonnqvist in 1992.[20] Since that time, it has become a mainstay of pediatric regional anesthesia for a wide range of surgical procedures.[21] While initially it was performed using a landmark technique, use of ultrasound is now common practice.[22]

Anatomy

The PV block targets spinal nerves just lateral to the neuraxiom, before the formation of the intercostal and

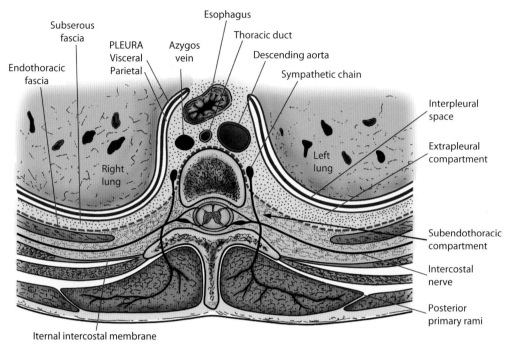

Esophagus
Subserous
fascia
Thoracic duct
PLEURA
Visceral
Parietal
Azygos
vein
Descending aorta
Endothoracic
fascia
Sympathetic chain
Interpleural
space
Right
lung
Left
lung
Extrapleural
compartment
Subendothoracic
compartment
Intercostal
nerve
Posterior
primary rami
Iternal intercostal membrane

▲ **Figure 32-6.** Paravertebral region. (Reproduced with permission, from Karmakar MK, Soh E, Chee V, et al., eds. *Atlas of Sonoanatomy for Regional Anesthesia and Pain Medicine.* 2018. https://accessanesthesiology.mhmedical.com. Copyright © McGraw Hill LLC. All rights reserved.)

thoracoabdominal nerves (Figure 32-6). To perform the block, the patient is positioned in the lateral position with the operative side up. In the landmark technique, the transverse process is identified, and the paravertebral space is found by "walking off" the needle in the caudal direction until a loss of resistance is appreciated. While Marhofer and colleagues initially described an out-of-plane ultrasound-guided placement of PV block in adults in 2010,[23] Boretsky and colleagues described in-plane ultrasound-guided technique in children in 2013.[22] In the in-plane technique, the ultrasound is positioned over the spinous process, then moved just lateral to show the transverse process and pleura (Figure 32-7). The needle is continuously visualized as it is advanced in-plane lateral to medial through the erector spinae and intercostal muscles toward the lower portion of the transverse process. Just beyond the internal intercostal membrane, small aliquots of normal saline are used to assess depression of the pleura to confirm needle tip position in the paravertebral space. Once confirmed, local anesthetic may be administered and a catheter placed, if desired.

▶ Indications/Areas Covered/Surgery

PV blocks are primarily used for thoracic surgeries; however, they have been used in wide-ranging surgeries in the entire thoracoabdominal region, including laparotomy;

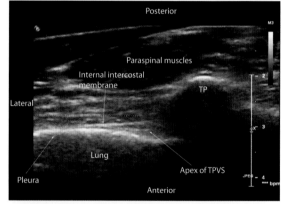

Posterior
Paraspinal muscles
Internal intercostal
membrane
TP
Lateral
Lung
Apex of TPVS
Pleura
Anterior

▲ **Figure 32-7.** Ultrasound thoracic paravertebral region. Transverse sonogram of the right thoracic paravertebral region using a high-frequency linear transducer with the ultrasound beam being insonated over the transverse process. Note how the acoustic shadow of the transverse process (TP) obscures the thoracic paravertebral space (TPVS). The hypoechoic space posterior to the parietal pleura and anterolateral to the TP is the apex of the TPVS, or the medial limit of the posterior intercostal space. (Reproduced with permission, from Karmakar MK, Soh E, Chee V, et al., eds. *Atlas of Sonoanatomy for Regional Anesthesia and Pain Medicine.* 2018. https://accessanesthesiology.mhmedical. com. Copyright © McGraw Hill LLC. All rights reserved.)

ostomy creation and take-down; liver, kidney, and lung transplantation; periacetabular osteotomy; ventral and inguinal hernia repair; and several others.[24]

Specific Complications/ Contraindications

As the paravertebral space is a deep potential space, bleeding concerns are similar to that of neuraxial anesthetics. In the thoracic region, pneumothorax is a concern.[24]

ERECTOR SPINAE PLANE (ESP) BLOCK

Overview

Erector spinae plane (ESP) blocks are an emerging regional anesthetic modality first described in 2016,[25] which deposits local anesthetic between the erector spinae muscle and the underlying transverse process. Thus far, ESP blocks have been predominately described in case series and case reports; however, initial data for analgesia for several types of surgery are promising.[25–31]

Anatomy

The erector spinae muscles lie along each side of the spine, superficial to the transverse processes (TPs). ESP blocks are hypothesized to anesthetize the dorsal and ventral rami of thoracic nerves and the sympathetic chain.[29,31]

Indications/Areas Covered/Surgery

ESP blocks have been described for surgeries at all thoracoabdominal dermatomes (cervical, thoracic, lumbar), with a predominance in thoracotomies or rib fractures as well as hip and femur surgeries.[29]

Block Methodology

ESP blocks are often performed with the patient in the lateral position, with the surgical or block side up. Prone positioning is another option. The ultrasound transducer is placed over the TP and the needle is introduced in-plane, through the erector spinae muscle to the TP. Local anesthetic is deposited such that the erector spinae muscle is hydro-dissected away from the TP. A catheter may be introduced during placement of the initial block for subsequent intermittent boluses or continuous infusion.

Considerations

Data about the safety and efficacy of ESP blocks are limited. Unlike PV blocks and neuraxial anesthetics, ESP blocks are placed in a more superficial plane, so there is theoretically enhanced safety in terms of bleeding risk; however, this has yet to be born out in the literature.

OTHER TRUNCAL BLOCKS

The serratus anterior, PECS I and II, and ilioinguinal blocks are also truncal blocks. While their use is more common in adults, use in pediatric patients is limited. In the case of ilioinguinal blocks, the ease of caudal blocks in infants and young children likely skews regional anesthetics toward caudal instead of truncal blocks.

REFERENCES

1. Suresh S, De Oliveira GSJr. Blood bupivacaine concentrations after transversus abdominis plane block in neonates: a prospective observational study. *Anesth Analg.* 2016;122(3):814-817.
2. Walker BJ, Long JB, De Oliveira GS, et al. Peripheral nerve catheters in children: an analysis of safety and practice patterns from the pediatric regional anesthesia network (PRAN). *Br J Anaesth.* 2015;115(3):457-462.
3. Walker BJ, Long JB, Sathyamoorthy M, et al. Complications in pediatric regional anesthesia: an analysis of more than 100,000 blocks from the pediatric regional anesthesia network. *Anesthesiology.* 2018;129(4):721-732.
4. Rafi AN. Abdominal field block: a new approach via the lumbar triangle. *Anaesthesia.* 2001;56(10):1024-1026.
5. Hebbard P, Fujiwara Y, Shibata Y, Royse C. Ultrasound-guided transversus abdominis plane (TAP) block. *Anaesth Intensive Care.* 2007;35(4):616-617.
6. Hebbard PD, Barrington MJ, Vasey C. Ultrasound-guided continuous oblique subcostal transversus abdominis plane blockade: description of anatomy and clinical technique. *Reg Anesth Pain Med.* 2010;35(5):436-441.
7. Hamill JK, Rahiri JL, Liley A, Hill AG. Rectus sheath and transversus abdominis plane blocks in children: a systematic review and meta-analysis of randomized trials. *Paediatr Anaesth.* 2016;26(4):363-371.
8. Charlton S, Cyna AM, Middleton P, Griffiths JD. Perioperative transversus abdominis plane (TAP) blocks for analgesia after abdominal surgery. *Cochrane Database Syst Rev.* 2010(12):CD007705.
9. Hernandez MA, Vecchione T, Boretsky K. Dermatomal spread following posterior transversus abdominis plane block in pediatric patients: our initial experience. *Paediatr Anaesth.* 2017;27(3):300-304.
10. Blanco R, McDonnell JG. Optimal point of injection: the quadratus lumborum type I and II blocks. *Anaesthesia.* 2013;68(4).
11. Sauter AR, Ullensvang K, Niemi G, et al. The shamrock lumbar plexus block: a dose-finding study. *Eur J Anaesthesiol.* 2015;32(11):764-770.
12. Kadam VR. Ultrasound-guided quadratus lumborum block as a postoperative analgesic technique for laparotomy. *J Anaesthesiol Clin Pharmacol.* 2013;29(4):550-552.
13. Chakraborty A, Goswami J, Patro V. Ultrasound-guided continuous quadratus lumborum block for postoperative analgesia in a pediatric patient. *A A Case Rep.* 2015;4(3):34-36.
14. Chakraborty A, Khemka R, Datta T. Ultrasound-guided truncal blocks: a new frontier in regional anaesthesia. *Indian J Anaesth.* 2016;60(10):703-711.
15. Oksuz G, Bilal B, Gurkan Y, et al. Quadratus lumborum block versus transversus abdominis plane block in children undergoing low abdominal surgery: a randomized controlled trial. *Reg Anesth Pain Med.* 2017;42(5):674-679.

16. Blanco R, Ansari T, Riad W, Shetty N. Quadratus lumborum block versus transversus abdominis plane block for postoperative pain after cesarean delivery: a randomized controlled trial. *Reg Anesth Pain Med*. 2016;41(6):757-762.

17. Parras T, Blanco R. Randomised trial comparing the transversus abdominis plane block posterior approach or quadratus lumborum block type I with femoral block for postoperative analgesia in femoral neck fracture, both ultrasound-guided. *Rev Esp Anestesiol Reanim*. 2016;63(3):141-148.

18. Ferguson S, Thomas V, Lewis I. The rectus sheath block in paediatric anaesthesia: new indications for an old technique? *Paediatr Anaesth*. 1996;6(6):463-466.

19. Tsui BC, Green JS, Ip VH. Ultrasound-guided rectus sheath catheter placement. *Anaesthesia*. 2014;69(10):1174-1175.

20. Lonnqvist PA. Continuous paravertebral block in children. Initial experience. *Anaesthesia*. 1992;47(7):607-609.

21. Bhalla T, Sawardekar A, Dewhirst E, Jagannathan N, Tobias JD. Ultrasound-guided trunk and core blocks in infants and children. *J Anesth*. 2013;27(1):109-123.

22. Boretsky K, Visoiu M, Bigeleisen P. Ultrasound-guided approach to the paravertebral space for catheter insertion in infants and children. *Paediatr Anaesth*. 2013;23(12):1193-1198.

23. Marhofer P, Kettner SC, Hajbok L, Dubsky P, Fleischmann E. Lateral ultrasound-guided paravertebral blockade: an anatomical-based description of a new technique. *Br J Anaesth*. 2010;105(4):526-532.

24. Vecchione T, Zurakowski D, Boretsky K. Thoracic paravertebral nerve blocks in pediatric patients: safety and clinical experience. *Anesth Analg*. 2016;123(6):1588-1590.

25. Forero M, Adhikary SD, Lopez H, Tsui C, Chin KJ. The erector spinae plane block: a novel analgesic technique in thoracic neuropathic pain. *Reg Anesth Pain Med*. 2016;41(5):621-627.

26. Darling CE, Pun SY, Caruso TJ, Tsui BCH. Successful directional thoracic erector spinae plane block after failed lumbar plexus block in hip joint and proximal femur surgery. *J Clin Anesth*. 2018;49:1-2.

27. Elkoundi A, Bentalha A, Kettani SEE, Mosadik A, Koraichi AE. Erector spinae plane block for pediatric hip surgery. *Korean J Anesthesiol*. 2018;72(1):68–71.

28. Munshey F, Caruso TJ, Wang EY, Tsui BCH. Programmed intermittent bolus regimen for erector spinae plane blocks in children: a retrospective review of a single-institution experience. *Anesth Analg*. 2018.

29. Tsui BCH, Fonseca A, Munshey F, McFadyen G, Caruso TJ. The erector spinae plane (ESP) block: A pooled review of 242 cases. *J Clin Anesth*. 2018;53:29-34.

30. Tulgar S, Ermis MN, Ozer Z. Combination of lumbar erector spinae plane block and transmuscular quadratus lumborum block for surgical anaesthesia in hemiarthroplasty for femoral neck fracture. *Indian J Anaesth*. 2018;62(10):802-805.

31. Ueshima H, Otake H. Clinical experiences of erector spinae plane block for children. *J Clin Anesth*. 2018;44:41.

Regional Anesthesia: Neuraxial

Donna LaMonica, Ingrid Fitz-James Antoine, and Veronica Carullo

FOCUS POINTS

1. Local anesthetics are the primary medication utilized in regional and neuraxial anesthesia or analgesia, with or without other adjuvants.
2. The local anesthetics most commonly utilized are the amino-amides, bupivacaine, and lidocaine. However, given the decreased metabolism and clearance of amino-amides and resultant increased risk of local anesthetic toxicity in infants less than 6 months, chloroprocaine is preferred particularly for infusions administered for greater than 48 hours.
3. Adjuvant analgesics are used in combination with local anesthetics to improve the quality of neuraxial analgesia and at the same time decrease the concentration of local anesthetic agent needed to achieve adequate analgesia.
4. The single-shot caudal technique is the most commonly utilized neuraxial technique for ambulatory surgeries involving the truncal or lower extremity dermatomes.
5. Spinal anesthesia can be particularly useful when used as the sole anesthestic in ex-premature and term infants in an attempt to avoid intubation and/or exposure to general anesthesia.
6. Continuous epidural anesthesia/analgesia is primarily utilized for surgeries involving bilateral lower extremities, open thoracic surgeries, major intra-abdominal surgeries with visceral dissection, or spinal surgeries.

LOCAL ANESTHETICS AND DEVELOPMENTAL CONSIDERATIONS

Local anesthetics are the primary medication utilized in regional and neuraxial anesthesia or analgesia, with or without other adjuvants. The main mechanism of action regardless of chemical structure is the blockage of sodium channels with resultant blockade of neuronal impulse. As in adults, in order to prevent a neuronal impulse, three nodes of Ranvier must be blocked. The pharmacodynamic and pharmacokinetic differences in neonates and infants are imperative to understanding dosage administration. Local anesthetics largely exist in the ionized form and are therefore distributed to the extracellular body water compartment. In neonates and children, this space is nearly double that in adults and therefore results in lower peak plasma concentrations with initial bolus dosing due to the larger volume of distribution. However, due to synthetic liver function immaturity, infants under 6 months of age have decreased serum levels of both albumin and alpha-1-glycoprotein.[1] The lower concentrations of these serum proteins allow for higher free or unbound local anesthetics, placing these patients at higher risk of local anesthetic systemic toxicity with repeated doses or continuous infusions. Luz et al. reported that free plasma bupivacaine concentrations were significantly higher in infants than in older children receiving continuous epidural anesthesia.[2] Furthermore, the ability of the liver to clear and metabolize local anesthetics is greatly reduced in neonates, infants, and children under the age of 4.[3] The amino-amide local anesthetics rely on the cytochrome p450 system in the liver for metabolism which is also not yet fully developed in the neonate and infant. The ability to conjugate is not reached until approximately 3 to 6 months of age.[3] Due to the impaired hepatic clearance of the amino-amide local anesthetics, the elimination half-lives of these drugs are prolonged and the doses should be decreased for this group of patients.

The local anesthetics most commonly used are bupivacaine and lidocaine, both of which are amino-amides. Other amino-amides include levobupivacaine, ropivacaine, and mepivacaine. Levobupivacaine and ropivacaine offer a similar analgesic profile to racemic bupivacaine with lower affinity for cardiac myocytes and is less likely to cause fatal toxicity.[4] The other group of local anesthetics is of the ester-type local anesthetics including chloroprocaine, tetracaine, and procaine. These are quickly hydrolyzed by plasma cholinesterase. Though the activity of plasma cholinesterase is decreased in infants younger than 6 months of age, studies have not shown increased toxicity with use of chloroprocaine and it should be considered for infusions that will last longer than 48 hours in order to avoid the systemic toxicity associated with the amino-amides such as bupivacaine.[5]

NEURAXIAL TECHNIQUES

The choice of neuraxial technique and pharmacological agents utilized is largely dependent on the type of surgery and whether and how long the patient is being admitted to the inpatient setting. For ambulatory surgeries involving the lower extremities or truncal dermatomes, spinal anesthesia or single-shot caudal anesthesia or analgesia is commonly used. Epidural catheters are less commonly used in the ambulatory setting and are typically reserved for surgeries involving bilateral lower extremities, open thoracic surgeries, major intra-abdominal surgeries with visceral dissection, or spinal surgeries.[6]

Spinal

Intrathecal anesthesia has been shown to be beneficial, particularly in the neonatal period. When used as a sole anesthetic, it has been shown to decrease the use of opioids and therefore the attendant respiratory depression, apneic episodes, and bradycardia in the postoperative setting.[3] Regardless, apnea in the infant should be monitored until post 60 weeks' conceptual age.[3] The limitation of spinal anesthesia includes both time constraints (approximately 1 to 2 hours) as well as surgical location. These procedures are largely for incisions below the T10 dermatome, ie, inguinal hernia repair, hypospadias correction, circumcision, or lower extremity surgeries, and can be particularly useful in ex-premature and term infants in an attempt to avoid the risk of prolonged intubation or apnea post general anesthesia.

The physical spinal space differs in adults and infants considerably. Most importantly, the extent to which the spinal cord extends is lower in infants than in adults. Specifically, the conus medullaris extends to L3 in infants and does not move cephalad to the adult level of L1 until after 1 year of age.[3] For this reason, access to the spinal canal is performed at the L5-S1 level in this age group using a midline approach. Typically, a 1.5-inch styletted 22-gauge spinal needle is used, although a variety of pediatric sizes and types of needles are available. Furthermore, the spinal space can be reached at approximately 1.5 cm rather than the average 5 cm in adults. Consideration for dosing on a per kilogram basis for the infant can be 5 to 10 times greater than for adults. This can be explained by the greater percentage of CSF versus body weight in an infant. Additionally, the turnover of CSF is higher in infants than in adults. With this in mind, the duration of surgical anesthesia is also much lower in infants than in adults, thereby limiting the surgical time to approximately 1 to 2 hours.

The typical local anesthetics for spinal anesthesia include tetracaine and bupivacaine. The baricity of either can be altered with the use of dextrose, though the duration of action of either seems to be nearly equivalent.[7] Lidocaine is not commonly used in the spinal space secondary to the potential for transient neurological symptoms that have been documented with its use.

Dosing guidelines can be found in Table 33-1.

Epidural

Caudal

The caudal epidural technique remains the most popular choice for postoperative analgesia in the infant to achieve opioid sparing in the operative theater. The incomplete fusion of the sacral vertebrae allows for epidural access via the sacral hiatus which is found between the two sacral cornu at the level of the fifth sacral vertebra. The sacrococcygeal ligament covers the sacral hiatus and the dural sac extends down to the level of S3. The proximity of the dural sac, as well as the ease of passing a needle through bone in an infant, poses significant risks for dural puncture and incorrect needle placement. The use of ultrasound to visualize caudal anatomy can increase successful needle placement as well as minimize the risk of dural puncture.

A single-shot technique is indicated for procedures below T10 dermatome, whereas a caudal catheter can be used for higher level dermatomal coverage. A single-shot technique is commonly used for ambulatory procedures in those children who are not yet walking, as leg weakness

Table 33-1. Local Anesthetics for Spinal Anesthesia

Anesthestic Agent	Dose Range (mg/kg)
Bupivacaine 0.5% (isobaric) with epinephrine 1:200,000	0.5–1 mg/kg
Bupivacaine 0.75% in 8.25% dextrose (hyperbaric)	0.5–1 mg/kg
Tetracaine 0.5% in 5% dextrose (hyperbaric)	0.4–0.8 mg/kg

secondary to motor blockade may be a scary occurrence for those now accustomed to being mobile. That being said, some institutions will routinely place a caudal block for analgesia even in school-aged children, thereby necessitating parental education to avoid unassisted weight-bearing for 6 to 12 hours status post administration.

The continuous caudal epidural technique can be used for procedures as high as a T4 dermatomal level. Those catheters intended for a higher dermatomal blockade are inserted at the caudal level with cephalad advancement to the appropriate thoracic dermatome. When advanced blindly, radiographic determination of the catheter is recommended as it is difficult to ascertain the final tip location otherwise.[8] Alternatively, the use of electrical stimulation, otherwise known as the Tsui test, or the use of ultrasound can obviate the need for radiographic confirmation and minimize unnecessary exposure to radiation.[9,10]

Procedurally, a caudal block can be successfully completed quite easily. At our institution, we place the patient in the lateral decubitus position after the monitors, airway, and intravenous line are secured. The knees should be flexed to the chest, as this facilitates palpation of the sacral cornu. Sterile preparation can be achieved using either chlorhexidine, alcohol, or betadine solution. After proper positioning and using a sterile technique, the sacral cornu is usually identified quite easily by palpating for two bony prominences at the sacral hiatus approximately 0.5 to 1 cm apart. Using a 22-gauge angiocatheter, at approximately a 45-degree angle to the skin, the needle is inserted in between the sacral cornu and advanced into the sacral canal. Once the sacrococcygeal ligament is pierced, which is indicated by a very slight "pop" with the catheter tip, the catheter angle is dropped to about 15 degrees to the skin and the catheter and needle advanced approximately 3 mm together, after which the catheter alone is advanced over the needle into the caudal space. The needle is then removed and the catheter examined for cerebrospinal fluid (CSF) or blood leakage. A syringe with the caudal medication can be connected directly to the catheter. Gentle aspiration should be negative for blood or CSF prior to injection. Injection should be performed with fingers over the skin to detect unintentional extravasation into the subcutaneous tissue. If this is the case, a palpable wheal will be felt with injection. Injection should occur without encountering resistance and should be done in a slow, incremental manner, carefully watching the EKG monitor for changes, most specifically, for QRS changes or peaking of T waves.

The dosage of drug varies depending on the dermatomal level and density of the block desired. Higher volumes of local anesthetic are necessary to achieve a higher level of blockade. Higher concentrations of local anesthetic are needed to achieve anesthesia versus analgesia. In general bupivacaine 0.25% or lower concentrations is used for caudal analgesia. Two commonly used formulas to determine

volume are those described by Armitage and Takasaki and colleagues. Armitage recommends using 0.5 mL/kg for procedures involving lumbosacral dermatomes, 1 mL/kg for procedures involving thoracolumbar dermatomes, and 1.25 mL/kg for procedures involving mid-thoracic dermatomes.[11] Takasaki and colleagues suggest a volume of 0.05 mL/kg dermatome to be blocked.[12] Preservative-free formulations should always be utilized when delivering drug to the neuraxial space.

Lumbar/Thoracic

Placement of epidural catheters in infants and children is distinctly different than in adults, largely because the placement of the catheter is done after the child is anesthetized. Though there is a level of safety concern regarding the placement of epidurals under general anesthesia, a large case-series by Krane et al. has reported that the risk of performing these procedures in the anesthetized child is not increased.[13]

In addition to caudal epidural placement, placement in lumbar or thoracic locations may be utilized for procedures involving higher dermatomal levels.[3] Examples include major abdominal surgery, open thoracic surgery, spinal surgery, and chronic pain management in life-limiting diseases.[6] Potential benefits of epidural catheter placement in the lumbar or thoracic levels include a lower risk of fecal contamination, catheter placement closer to the desired level of analgesia, and a smaller volume of drug for a more cephalad dermatomal level.[3]

Suggested dosing for the epidural local anesthetics is as follows:

Epidural infusions:

  Neonates:

  Term neonates: Bupivacaine $\leq$0.2 mg/kg/h for no more than 48 hours, then change to choloroprocaine 1.5% at a rate of 0.2 to 0.8 mL/kg/h

  Infants:

  1–6 months: Bupivacaine 0.2 mg/kg/h

  >6 months: Bupivacaine 0.4 mg/kg/h

Pediatric patient-controlled epidural analgesia (PCEA)— thoracic:

  Bupivacaine 0.125% + Fentanyl 2 mcg/mL or Bupivacaine 0.1% + Fentanyl 2 mcg/mL

  Continuous rate: 0.2 mg/kg/h

  Demand dose: 0.04mL/kg

  Lockout 20 minutes

Pediatric patient-controlled epidural analgesia (PCEA)— lumbar:

  Bupivacaine 0.1% + Fentanyl 2 mcg/mL

  Continuous rate: 0.25 mL/kg/h

  Demand dose: 0.05 mL/kg

  Lockout 20 minutes

ADJUVANT ANALGESICS

Adjuvant analgesics are used in combination with local anesthetics to improve the quality of neuraxial analgesia and at the same time decrease the concentration of local anesthetic agent needed to achieve adequate analgesia. In addition to improving onset of neural blockade they also improve the quality and duration of the blockade while limiting the density of motor blockade, which would be likely to occur if local anesthetics were used alone.

The most commonly utilized adjuvants for neuraxial analgesia are opioids (ie fentanyl, sufentanil, morphine, and hydromorphone). Opioids act primarily on pre- and post-synaptic mu-opioid receptors in the substantia gelatinosa of the dorsal horn of the spinal cord. The most important determinant of onset and duration of analgesia is lipid solubility. Lipophilic opioids (ie fentanyl, sufentanil) produce rapid onset of analgesia with limited cephalad spread, whereas hydrophilic opioids (ie morphine, hydromorphone) have a much slower onset with prolonged duration of analgesic effects and greater cephalad spread. Accordingly, there is an increased risk of delayed respiratory depression with hydrophilic opioids as compared to lipophilic opioids. However, given the narrow therapeutic index of amino-amide local anesthetics, it is often necessary to rely on hydrophilic opioids to improve dermatomal coverage for epidural analgesia when the tip of the epidural catheter is not optimally positioned to cover the distribution of pain.

The other common adjuvant drug utilized in neuraxial analgesia is the centrally acting partial alpha-2 adrenergic agonist, clonidine. A recent meta-analysis by Schnabel et al. suggested its efficacy in increasing the duration of analgesia when given with local anesthetics and improved safety profile given the low incidence of adverse effects including respiratory depression.[14] This makes clonidine an ideal adjuvant agent for neonatal and infant neuraxial analgesia.

Ketamine has also been successfully used as an adjuvant in caudal analgesia,[15] but a preservative-free formulation is not available in the United States, which limits its application in this circumstance. Furthermore, given the expression of neuronal toxicity in translational animal models, ketamine's safety profile has been controversial particularly when considering its use in developing organisms.

PLACEMENT TECHNIQUES

Thoracic and lumbar epidural catheters may be placed safely in anesthetized infants and children. Despite concern in the adult literature about risk of neural injury in the deeply sedated or anesthetized patients, no studies have validated this to be the case in clinical practice. The vast majority of regional and neuraxial anesthetic techniques in infants and children are performed under general anesthesia and large-scale prospective studies in the United States

and Europe have found the risk of complications to be very low.[16–19]

▶ Direct Injection

The technique for placement of lumbar or thoracic epidural catheters is similar to that in adults, but with several important exceptions. Most commonly, a midline approach is utilized. However, it is important to note that the ligamentum flavum is thinner and less dense in infants when compared to older children and adults and perception of engagement in ligament may be more difficult. This necessitates slower and more careful passage of the needle to prevent inadvertent subarachnoid puncture. It may take experience to perceive the more subtle differences in the characteristics of the tissue planes in small children. Additionally, the angle of approach may be more perpendicular in infants and children due to the angle of the spinous processes in this age group. Another important consideration is the use of saline with loss of resistance technique as the use of loss of resistance with air has been associated with venous air embolism in infants and children.[20] Similar to the concept of a hanging drop technique, an IV infusion may be connected to the epidural Tuohy needle, and when the epidural space is entered the IV infusion begins to drip.[3]

Most pediatric epidural kits available in the United States contain 17- to 18-gauge, 4.5- to 6-cm Tuohy needles. Authors report better control with the use of a short 5-cm needle in infants and children in comparison to an adult sized 9- to 10-cm needle. Additionally, most kits contain 20- to 21-gauge catheters as there is a higher incidence of kinking and high resistance with smaller catheters, ie, 24 gauge.[3]

▶ Fluoroscopy/Epidurograms

Ease of epidural catheter advancement is not a reliable indicator of successful placement in the epidural space, and successful advancement from caudal to thoracic or lumbar to thoracic levels is variable. For this reason, fluoroscopic confirmation via an epidurogram was recommended to ascertain tip position of epidural catheters advanced to the thoracic level in order to avoid the potential for respiratory compromise if a catheter is inadvertently advanced too cephalad and to avoid the potential for inadequate analgesia in the event of catheter coiling or malposition.[8] Alternative methods to limit radiation exposure, including the Tsui test and the use of ultrasound technology, have been developed and are more commonly used in current clinical practice.

▶ Tsui Test

The Tsui test consists of using a nerve stimulator on epidural nerve roots at low voltages in order to confirm epidural placement via visual confirmation of muscle twitch.[9] Generally speaking, this direct method of epidural catheter placement (ie, at the dermatomal level of the surgical intervention) is favored for children greater than 10 kg. Goobie et al. prospectively looked at 30 pediatric patients to assess the direct placement of epidural catheters via Tsui test and found that though the positive predictive value of the test was 82%, it was not clinically advantageous over the "blind stick" method via landmarks and test dosing.[9] Despite this, the educational utility of this method still persists.

The method of the Tsui test/stimulation catheter placement is like that of the direct stick with the additional use of a nerve stimulator that has a grounding anode and a stimulating cathode. Normal saline serves as the conducting fluid. Muscle twitch should typically be elicited between 1 and 10 mA and any muscle twitch less than 1mA should raise suspicion of intravascular or intrathecal location. Greater than 10 mA should also be considered a misplaced epidural.

The technical aspect of placing the epidural with the use of Tsui epidural stimulation is like that of standard epidural placement with a Tuohy needle. The epidural catheter itself is more successfully advanced with the use of a metal stylette that is within the catheter. This metal stylette allows for passing of the catheter over long distances in the pediatric patient, as the stiffness circumvents the troublesome kinking or coiling of the soft tip catheters.[9]

Ultrasound

It is becoming increasingly common to use ultrasound during preprocedural assessment of the spinal anatomy prior to performing neuraxial procedures in infants and children. The advent of ultrasound technology has allowed clinicians to visualize anatomical structure with clarity, as well as perform guided procedures with greater precision. Rapp et al described the use of ultrasound for lumbar and thoracic epidurals as a valuable tool in those greater than one year of age.[21] This can be useful to predict skin-to-dura distance, improve first-pass success rate, and decrease the risk of complications.[22,23] The detailed images are possible in infants less than 9 months of age due to absence of vertebral ossification; therefore, the application of ultrasound is particularly useful in this high-risk population. In older infants and children, vertebral ossification impedes transmission resulting in more limited acoustic windows.[24]

CONCLUSIONS

Regional neuraxial anesthesia/analgesia is a well-established and safe practice that is being routinely applied in the pediatric perioperative setting with the accessibility of appropriate equipment, instrumentation, well-established guidelines for administration of neuraxial analgesics, and the availability of ultrasound guidance. The addition of regional techniques to the clinical armamentarium of pediatric anesthesia not only limits opioid usage, which permits the restoration of the child's pre-anesthetic emotional and intellectual awareness, but

also affords parents the opportunity to resume their role in providing the emotional safety in an environment of comfort, which is effectively accomplished by guiding parental expectation through education. These skills are unique to the pursuit of our subspecialty, and well worth the extra time and effort.

REFERENCES

1. Anand KJS, Stevens BJ, McGrath PJ. *Pain in Neonates and Infants*. Edinburgh: Elsevier; 2007.
2. Luz G, Weiser CH, Innerhofer P, Frischhut B, Ulmer H, Benzer A. Free and total bupivacaine plasma concentrations after continuous epidural anaesthesia infants and children. *Paediatr Anaesth*. 1998;8:473-478.
3. Suresh S, Polaner D, Cote CJ. Regional anesthesia. In: Coté CJ, Lerman J, eds. *A Practice of Anesthesia for Infants and Children*. Philadelphia, PA: Elsevier Saunders; 2013:835-853.
4. Burlacu CL, Buggy DJ. Update on local anesthetics: focus on levobupivacaine. *Ther Clin Risk Manag*. 2008;4(2):381-392.
5. Veneziano G, Iliev P, Tripi J, Martin D, Aldrink J, Bhalla T, Tobias J. Continuous chloroprocaine infusion for thoracic and caudal epidurals as a postoperative analgesia modality in neonates, infants, and children. *Paediatr Anaesth*. 2016;26:84-91.
6. Moriarty A. Pediatric epidural analgesia. *Paediatr Anaesth*. 2011;22:51-55.
7. Rice L, Demars P, Crooms J, Whalen T. Duration of spinal anesthesia in infants under one year of age: comparison of three drugs. *Anesth Analg*. 1987;66:S148.
8. Valairucha S, Seefelder C, Houck C. Thoracic epidural catheters placed by the caudal route in infants: the importance of radiographic confirmation. *Paediatr Anaesth*. 2002;12:424-428.
9. Goobie SM, Montgomery CJ, Basu R, McFadzean J, O'Connor G, Poskitt K, Tsui BCH. Confirmation of direct epidural catheter placement using nerve stimulation in pediatric anesthesia. *Anesth Analg*. 2003;97:984-988.
10. Tsui BCH. Innovative approaches to neuraxial blockade in children: the introduction of epidural nerve root stimulation and ultrasound guidance for epidural catheter placement. *Pain Res Mgmt*. 2006;11(3):173-180.
11. Armitage EN. Regional anesthesia in paediatrics. *Clin Anesthesiol*. 1985;3:553.
12. Takasaki M, Dohi S, Kawabata Y, Takahashi T. Dosage of lidocaine for caudal anesthesia in infants and children. *Anesthesiology*. 1977;47:527-529.
13. Krane EJ, Dalens BJ, Murat I, Murell D. The safety of epidurals placed during general anesthesia. *Reg Anesth Pain Med*. 1998;23:433-438.
14. Schnabel A, Poepping DM, Pogatzki-Zahn EM, Zahn P. Efficacy and safety of clonidine as additive for caudal regional anesthesia: a quantitative systematic review of randomized controlled trials. *Paediatr Anaesth*. 2011;21:1219-1230.
15. Lee HM, Sanders GM. Caudal ropivacaine and ketamine for postoperative analgesia in children. *Anaesthesia*. 2000;55:806-810.
16. Giaufre E, Dalens B, Gombert A. Epidemiology and morbidity of regional anesthesia in children: a one-year prospective survey of the French-Language Society of Pediatric Anesthesiologists. *Anesth Analg*. 1996;83:904-912.
17. Llewellyn N, Moriarty A. The national pediatric epidural audit. *Paediatr Anaesth*. 2007;17:520-533.

18. Ecoffey C, Lacroix F, Giaufre E, Orliaguet G, Courreges P. Epidemiology and morbidity of regional anesthesia in children: a follow-up one-year prospective survey of the French-Language Society of Paediatric Anaesthesiologists (ADARPEF). *Paediatr Anaesth.* 2010;20:1061-1069.

19. Polaner DM, Taenzer AH, Walker BJ, et al. Pediatric Regional Anesthesia Network (PRAN): a multi-institutional study of the use and incidence of complications of pediatric regional anesthesia. *Anesth Analg.* 2012;115(6):1353-1364.

20. Ames WA, Hayes JA, Petroz GC, Roy L. Loss of resistance to normal saline is preferred to identify the epidural space: a survey of Canadian pediatric anesthesiologists. *Can J Anesth.* 2005;52:607-612.

21. Rapp HJ, Folger A, Grau T. Ultrasound-guided epidural catheter insertion in children. *Anesth Analg.* 2005;101:333-339.

22. Tsui B, Suresh S. Ultrasound imaging for regional anesthesia in infants, children, and adolsecents: A review of current literature and its application in the practice of extremity and trunk blocks. *Anesthesiology.* 2010;112:473-492.

23. Kelleher S, Boretsky K, Alrayashi W. Images in anesthesiology: Use of ultrasound to facilitate neonatal spinal anesthesia. *Anesthesiology.* 2017;126:561.

24. Vecchionne T, Boretsky K. Ultrasound images of the epidural space through the acoustic window of the infant. *Anesthesiology.* 2017;126:562.

Special Considerations

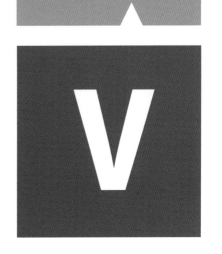

Intraoperative Complications and Crisis Management

Erik B. Smith and Joann Hunsberger

FOCUS POINTS

1. Complications can occur even when we provide excellent care to patients.
2. Successful anesthesia complication and crisis management requires a structured team-based approach.
3. Simulation helps teams practice crisis scenarios in a protected, safe environment. Simulation helps improve performance when actual crisis situations occur. Simulation is especially helpful for situations not commonly encountered in routine practice.
4. Cognitive aids can help prevent complications before they occur and also help manage active crises. Such aids include checklists, protocols, guidelines, and smartphone applications.
5. Complications and bad outcomes must always be discussed fully and honestly with patients and their families.
6. Malpractice lawsuits can arise from complications; therefore, risk managers and attorneys may provide guidance to involved parties.
7. Delivery of bad news must be joint effort between involved surgeons and anesthesiologists. The SPIKES protocol discussed within provides a family-centered framework for bad news discussions.
8. Complications encountered in pediatric anesthesia practice include medication errors, cardiac events, aspiration, laryngospasm, dental injury, and malignant hyperthermia.

INTRODUCTION

Complications and crises occur during anesthetic care even with meticulous attention to clinical detail. The best complication and crisis management strategies rely on forward thinking and planning rather than unorganized or reactionary behavior. Thus, training, simulation, and resource mobilization are hallmarks of effective crisis management. This preemptive approach embodies the ideal anesthesiologist mindset. With preparation and planning an anesthesiologist can successfully manage a full spectrum of complications from routine to rare.

Precise complication rates in pediatric anesthesiology are difficult to quantify; most are minor and quickly resolved with appropriate management, and therefore are not uniformly documented or transferred to complication registries. Laryngospasm, for example, is common in pediatric anesthesia practice. Many practitioners do not document or database laryngospasm when resolved quickly by positive pressure ventilation. However, major complications like cardiac arrest are nearly universally documented, and often are databased in registries. Therefore, we have anecdotal data on statistics of minor complications and more concrete data regarding frequency of major complications.

This chapter examines crisis management topics including simulation, cognitive aids, discussion of bad news, and legal issues. It will then explore common complications and select uncommon complications, along with their respective management.

CRISIS MANAGEMENT PRINCIPLES

Conceptual framework for anesthesiology crisis management has been adapted from strategies found in commercial aviation. This is not surprising, as aviation shares many attributes with anesthesiology including periods of "smooth sailing" punctuated by potential crisis events that the lay public (and even other medical practitioners) never know of, appreciate, or understand.

Structured crisis management training in medicine had at one point been nearly nonexistent. Anesthesiologists made major efforts in the 1990s to incorporate formalized crisis training into residency education, with efforts focused on simulation.[1] In fact, anesthesiology as a field has pioneered crisis management within medicine. Our efforts have spread into nearly every other field of medicine and even into governmental health policy efforts.

Crisis resource management principles guide effective team-based responses. These principles are as follows: establish and support a leader, establish followers, engage in effective communication, seek global assessments, seek support, and use available human and physical resources.[2] In conjunction with these principles nontechnical crisis management skills must be developed to enable effective management. These skills include decision making, situational awareness, teamwork, task management, information exchange, and assertiveness.[3]

Team building is crucial in successful crisis management. When anesthesia emergencies occur, team members frequently have never worked together. Similarly, they may have never managed the emergency at hand. Repeated exposure to simulation will orient team members to each other's roles and illustrate how they can function best on a team. Note that available operating room staff typically includes anesthesiologists, surgeons, nurses, and technologists; ideal simulations should involve members of each aforementioned field.[2]

SIMULATION

Simulation is a modern tool that provides crisis education to trainees and experienced practitioners. It provides exposure to both common and uncommon emergencies. High-fidelity simulation is available via commercially available mannequins, often complemented by human actor interactions. Also common are computer-based simulations such as those seen with pediatric advanced life support (PALS) and advanced cardiac lice support (ACLS) training websites. Other simulation experiences include standardized patients and task training exercises.[4] Simulation is of particular value in pediatric anesthesiology, as there are key differences between pediatric and adult populations. These differences are often not fully appreciated by those who less commonly manage pediatric patients.[4]

Simulation provides real-time assessment, feedback, remediation, and support Moreover, this practice is done without exposure to risk, as there are no real patients involved. Simulation done in one's workplace can reveal system failures within that institution, and can therefore provide rich opportunities for internal quality improvement.[4]

Standardized patient simulation gives trainees an opportunity to work with real patients in a protected setting. It allows trainees to practice a variety of skills including performing a physical exam, obtaining informed consent, and delivering bad news.

Physical task training stations allow for exposure to airway management tools, neuraxial anesthesia, ultrasound scanning, and difficult intravenous line placement. Some of these topics may include less frequently used emergency devices including cricothyrotomy kits, intraosseous line devices, and chest tube kits.[4]

High-fidelity simulation is key to development of non-technical crisis management skills. Successful development of these skills requires focused debriefing and assessment of these skills. Effective debriefing includes feedback from all members of the team (not just the anesthesiologist) and intended focus on the aforementioned crisis resource management principles and nontechnical crisis management skills.[2] Focused nontechnical skills assessment may benefit from a systematized approach rather than less structured discussion.[3]

COGNITIVE AIDS

Cognitive aids are tools that provide structured tangible assistance during crisis situations. As opposed to perioperative checklists, protocols, and guidelines, they are meant to be used while a situation is occurring.[4] Their inherent benefit is that they provide steps a clinician can take during crisis while allowing that clinician to have concise guidance on clinical management steps, differentials to consider, and tasks that must be delegated.[5] Note that many crisis situations, such as malignant hyperthermia (MA), are rare events; therefore, anesthesiologists may not have complex working knowledge of such issues.[5] Cognitive aids augment and supplement provider knowledge in these situations.

Cognitive aids take many forms including mnemonics, checklists, information sheets, and electronic applications. Effective cognitive aids contain information most relevant to the crisis at hand without extemporaneous information or distraction. For example, a cognitive aid on laryngospasm should include immediate management techniques while excluding risk factors or preoperative workup suggestions. Familiarity and agreed-upon validation of cognitive aids are essential for utility in a crisis scenario. Therefore, hospital administration and staff should review cognitive aids before their implementation.

When well-designed cognitive aids are used, evidence suggests improved crisis management performance and improved outcomes.[6] For example, a study of anesthesiology resident management of MA showed that use of the Malignant Hyperthermia Association of the United States (MHAUS) cognitive aid correlated with improved MH management performance. In that study providers who did not use the cognitive aid scored the worst in MH treatment performance, and those who did use the aid scored the best in MH treatment.[6] Similarly, a seminal study assessed central-line placement checklists in ICUs, and found that use of this cognitive aid reduced hospital mortality.[7]

While the aforementioned evidence highlights the potential benefits of cognitive aids, consider that not every cognitive aid is well designed or useful. Even the best-intentioned aid may unintentionally cause confusion or misinformation.[5] The U.S. Food and Drug Administration (USFDA), for example, provided a machine checkout cognitive aid, which many regard as confusing and not useful.[6] Adequate assessment of cognitive aids is therefore essential before their dissemination and use. Assessment tools include the Cognitive Aids in Medicine Assessment Tool, which is a derivative of assessment tools used in commercial aviation.[8]

We recommend referencing the following well-regarded pediatric anesthesiology cognitive aids:

- Pedi Crisis App
- Pedi Crisis Cards
- ACLS and PALS training, including flow cards
- MHAUS Malignant Hyperthermia Poster and Hotline

LEGAL ASPECTS OF COMPLICATIONS

Some patients and their families pursue malpractice lawsuits when complications occur. Given this reality in our healthcare system, we strongly recommend discussing anesthesia complications with your risk management department and with a qualified attorney. Risk managers offer risk-based post-indecent management advice, and may also be available to discuss strategies for discussing events with patients and family. Note, however, that risk managers have a duty to their employer, whether that is a hospital legal department, an insurer, or a private physician group. You should, therefore, consider speaking with your own attorney, as your legal interests may at times differ from other defendant parties.

The American Society of Anesthesiologists Closed Claims Project analyzes and catalogs liability claims made against anesthesiologists. Their most recent pediatric anesthesia liability study found that between the years 1970 and 2001 children between 0 and 3 years of age made up 53% of claims. Death and brain death have been the most common claim types.[9] Other claims included, in order of frequency, burns, cardiac arrest, nerve injury, airway injury, skin inflammation, and other medical related issues. Note that lawsuits related to respiratory-related issues have decreased markedly since the 1990s due to the widespread use of pulse oximetry and capnography.[9] Similarly, claims for cardiac issues have decreased due to decreased use of halothane, which is arythmogenic.[9]

Malpractice insurance has decreased in cost from $39,303 in 1985 to $19,594 in 2013 for a $1 million per incident/$3 million per year policy (the most common policy type). This reduction in cost is likely due to the aforementioned implementations of pulse oximetry and capnography. Both of these life-saving quality improvements were pioneered by anesthesiologists.[10]

DELIVERING BAD NEWS

Pediatric anesthesiologists care for children with the intent of delivering safe, complication-free care. But complications and bad outcomes are unavoidable, and all practicing anesthesiologists will need to at some point deliver bad news to patients' families and patients themselves.

The SPIKES protocol (Table 34-1) is a mnemonic that outlines mindful presentation of bad news.[11] The SPIKES protocol was originally developed by oncologists to deliver challenging news to oncology patients, but has since been adapted by those in many other specialties including anesthesiology.[11]

Ideally the anesthesiologist and surgeon should together deliver bad news to parents. The providers should set the stage with an appropriate environment for this discussion, ideally a private room. Care should be taken to be seated and to be at eye level of parents. The providers should introduce themselves to the parents, and remind the parent of each provider's respective roles. Note that in emergency procedures the anesthesiologist may not have met the parent in person prior to the procedure. Similarly, parents meet several healthcare professionals in the perioperative period, and may not remember the role of all involved parties.

The next step is to ascertain parent's perception including the level of understanding the parents have of the current situation and to assess their medical knowledge and ability to understand complex situations.

Table 34-1. SPIKES Protocol

S	Setting up the stage	Introduce yourself and state your role in medical team Ensure a private, comfortable location for discussion
P	Perception	Assess understanding and knowledge
I	Invitation	Allow patient to request information
K	Knowledge	Explain events timeline Use appropriate language without euphemisms Allow for reaction to news and questions
E	Emotions	Show concern for patient and validate emotions Show empathy
S	Strategy summary	Discuss plan for future care

At the parent's invitation, the anesthesiologist and surgeon can then inform the parents of the timeline of events, using plain language avoiding medical jargon. Once the parents have heard the news, the anesthesiologist should allow them time to react to the information and a chance to have all their questions answered.

Being prepared with a mindset of empathy to a parent's emotional response can help ease one of the biggest challenges of delivering unfavorable information. At the conclusion of the conversation, providers should summarize the situation and determine the next steps of care.[11] The anesthesiologist should be honest in his or her presentation of the facts and provide assurance of availability in the future. Note that the purpose of this protocol is not to determine guilt, nor is it a legal briefing.

When using the SPIKES protocol as a tool for delivering bad news, it is important to remember that it was developed initially for oncologists whose clinical situation is very different from the anesthesiologist. The anesthesiologist will need to communicate effectively and use a patient and family-centered approach to delivering bad news.[12-14] Communication characteristics that are necessary for a patient-centered approach include that the provider be friendly, supportive, nonintimidating, available (not distracted or rushed), and informative.[14,15]

As in other medical specialties such as emergency medicine, this can be difficult because of the stressfulness of the situation. The anesthesiologist may have just emerged from a code situation after performing Pediatric Advanced Life Support (PALS) or possibly a massive resuscitation effort. A healthy child may have suffered a devastating and unexpected complication during an elective surgery. An anesthesiologist may feel sadness, guilt, and inadequacy along with stress and anxiety so he or she may need to take a few moments alone, with a trusted colleague, or in discussion with legal counsel prior to starting the conversation with the patient's parents. The provider may feel inadequate or unprepared to deliver bad news,[12,14,16] so this time can be used to calm the provider and rehearse the information to be delivered to the parents. Because of the need to practice adequate communication of bad news, training opportunities for anesthesia fellows and residents have gone beyond the classroom into simulation education[12,16] using protocols like SPIKES to improve communication skills and physician comfort with this difficult task.

MEDICATION ERRORS

Medication errors are potentially catastrophic events in pediatric anesthesia practice. Pediatric anesthesiologists frequently dilute drugs by factors of 10 or 100 and also dose most drugs based on weight. Thus, there is potential for very large dosing errors. Other error types include drug swaps, drug misidentification, and inadvertent dosing of drugs to which the patient is allergic.

Determining frequency of medication error is challenging because many errors go unreported or are subjectively under-interpreted.[17] Adverse outcomes may therefore be difficult to link to said errors.[17] The overall frequency of drug administration error depends on study techniques, and estimates of drug errors vary quite widely. One large study of three South African hospitals (combining pediatric and adult practice) suggested the error rate is one in 245 anesthetics. The rate of error at the examined pediatric hospitals was 1 in 329 anesthetics.[18] Note that these studies exclude near-miss events, which are likely much more common than the aforementioned statistics.

In assessing adult and pediatric anesthesiology practice overall, the most common errors are drug substitutions or swaps followed by dosing errors.[17,18] Overall the most common drug swap error involved administering muscle relaxants instead of reversal agents.[17] Ampule or vial misidentification was also a major issue.[18]

When examining the pediatric anesthesia practice specifically, drug dosing errors were as common as drug swaps. This is likely due to increased potential for error inherent in diluting drugs and weight-based dosing of drugs.[18,19]

Treatment of medication error depends on the exact drug given and is beyond the scope of this chapter. More important is discussion of medication error prevention. Suggested safety measures include systematic management, storage, and labeling of drugs (including color coding).[18] Drug syringes should be legibly labeled and all ampules or vials should be read before drugs are drawn up—examination of drug name and concentration are both key.[19] When possible, a second provider should verify drug dilutions and labels.[19] Ideally, premade pediatric formulations of medications should be available to avoid dilution and dosing errors. Note also that widespread lack of precise pharmacokinetic data and lack of appropriate formulations make pediatric medication administration challenging even with otherwise appropriate checks and balances on dosing.[19]

CARDIAC EVENTS AND CARDIAC ARREST

The Pediatric Perioperative Cardiac Arrest (POCA) registry follows causes of perioperative cardiac arrest. Its current evidence suggests 49% of perioperative cardiac arrests are related to anesthesia. Of these events, causes included cardiovascular (79%), respiratory (53%), medication (35%), and equipment (9%). Cardiovascular causes included hemorrhage-associated hypovolemia, electrolyte imbalance, and nonhemorrhage-associated hypovolemia being the most common causes. Respiratory causes included laryngospasm, airway obstruction, and other forms of inadequate oxygenation and ventilation. Medication causes included first halothane-induced cardiovascular depression, followed by sevoflurane-induced cardiovascular depression, then other medication-induced issues. Equipment issues included central-line complication, followed by kinked or plugged endotracheal tubes, then peripheral intravenous line issues.[20,21]

Cardiac event management is issue specific and often follows the PALS pathways. Please refer to Chapter 39 for more information on cardiopulmonary resuscitation (CPR).

ASPIRATION

Perioperative pulmonary aspiration occurs when contents from the stomach, esophagus, mouth, or nose pass into the respiratory tract after induction of anesthesia, during a procedure or surgery or in the immediate postoperative period, including during extubation. Aspirated materials can include particulate matter such as food particles or other foreign objects. Aspirated material may also include nonparticulate matter such as stomach acid, saliva, blood, or gastrointestinal contents. The American Society of Anesthesiologists (ASA) compiled guidelines for preoperative fasting based on currently available clinical data and practitioner opinion.

One way to prevent aspiration is to recognize which patients are at highest risk of aspiration during the preoperative assessment. The preoperative assessment should evaluate the patient's adherence to preoperative fasting guidelines, comorbidities, and physical assessment. The preoperative fasting guidelines summarized below have been established to reduce the risk of aspiration during anesthesia for an elective procedure on a healthy patient.[22] A more in-depth discussion of the fasting guidelines is available in Chapter 10.

Risk factors of aspiration that are particularly important for children include:[23,24]

- Emergency surgery, especially abdominal surgery
- Recent ingestion of food
- Trauma
- Decreased consciousness
- Neuromuscular diseases especially those which decreased ability to protect trachea
- Delayed gastric emptying, bowel obstruction, ileus
- Difficult airway
- Increased ASA physical status
- Young age

Timing Before Surgery	Guidelines
8 hours	Stop fatty food
6 hours	Stop light meals, infant formula, and nonhuman milk
4 hours	Stop breast milk
2 hours	Stop clear liquids

Included in the preoperative assessment should be an evaluation of patient's teeth as loose deciduous teeth are a common occurrence in pediatric anesthesia and should be electively removed after induction of anesthesia to prevent aspiration. Removal of the loose tooth should be discussed with parents or guardians during the preoperative evaluation. Nonpermanent orthodontic hardware should also be removed prior to induction. Gastric decompression with a nasogastric or an oral gastric tube may be necessary in patients with bowel obstruction prior to induction of anesthesia. A rapid sequence induction with cricoid pressure is preferred if the patient is at risk for aspiration and is not a difficult airway. Even after a seemingly minor trauma (broken arm) and adherence to preoperative fasting guidelines, peristalsis may be delayed due to the traumatic nature of the incidence and use of opioids for preoperative analgesics, requiring rapid sequence induction.

If a patient has a difficult airway and is at risk of aspiration, the anesthesiologist must carefully consider the risks prior to induction and intubation. In general, children do not tolerate awake intubations, making it difficult to keep a child spontaneously breathing and able to protect his or her airway during an awake intubation. Likewise, regional anesthetic techniques without general anesthesia are not tolerated by children. It is important to remember that even with an endotracheal tube in place, aspiration prevention is not guaranteed.

Prior to extubation after emergency procedures, examples of which include bleeding tonsils (evacuate blood), trauma (delayed gastric emptying), and appendectomy (ileus), the patient's stomach should be suctioned to remove residual gastric contents. At the end of procedures for children at risk of aspiration, the provider should also ensure that the patient is fully awake to maximize airway protection prior to extubation.

Signs and symptoms of aspiration include coughing, wheezing, cyanosis, and hypoxia with increased oxygen requirements. Fever and tachypnea may also develop, while radiographic changes may be delayed. Aspiration can occur silently without visualization of gastric contents in the oropharynx.

Aspiration contents can be divided into three categories, each with different clinical effects: acidic fluid, nonacidic fluid, and particulate. Acidic fluid aspiration first causes a chemical pneumonitis when the lung tissue reacts to the acid, and then a second phase being an inflammatory response to the original pneumonitis. Nonacidic fluid aspiration causes atelectasis and alveolar collapse, but is generally less severe than with acidic fluid aspiration. Particulate matter aspiration causes a physical obstruction of airway which results in hypoxia and hypercapnia with radiographic findings of hyperinflation and atelectasis.

Treatment for aspiration is supportive.[25] Suctioning of any visualized gastric contents should be implemented immediately. The provider may choose to leave the endotracheal tube in place and delay extubation or reintubate if there is concern for severe aspiration and the patient may require ventilator support in an ICU setting. Some cases may respond to positive end expiratory pressure which can help decrease atelectasis and alveolar collapse. For the less severe cases, only supplementary oxygen may be required. Neither antibiotics nor steroids should be routinely administered. Antibiotics may be considered in the case of aspiration of bowel contents. Bronchoscopy may be required in the case of aspiration of large particulates which cause obstruction of airway passages. Lung lavage is discouraged as it can push particulates further down into the lungs.

Pediatric patients regurgitate or vomit in approximately 1 in 200 procedures,[26] but the incidence of perioperative pulmonary aspiration of gastric contents is much lower, approximately 4 to 10 in 10,000 pediatric anesthetics[23,25] and death occurring from perioperative aspiration is very rare.[26] However, compared to adults, the risk of aspiration in children is double.[25]

LARYNGOSPASM

Laryngospasm is a potentially life-threatening complication that involves reflex closing of the laryngeal muscles and inability to ventilate the patient. It can be either partial or complete. It is caused by a combination of uninhibited reflex pathways associated with inadequate depth of anesthesia and stimulation. Inciting stimulation includes direct laryngoscopy or suctioning, secretions or blood hitting the glottic opening, or airway adjunct inadvertently irritating the glottis opening.[27] Major risk factors for perioperative laryngospasm include presence of upper respiratory infection, airway anomalies,[28] light anesthesia, and use of Desflurane.[29]

Laryngospasm is far more common in pediatric populations as compared to adults, with a rate of approximately 17 in 1000 anesthetics delivered in pediatric populations, as compared to 8.7 per 100 anesthetics in the general population. Of note, laryngospasm is the leading respiratory cause of cardiac arrest in children.[21] In addition to cardiac arrest, laryngospasm can cause hypoxia, bradycardia, and pulmonary edema.

Laryngospasm is a clinical diagnosis that necessitates prompt treatment even if this diagnosis is not entirely clear. It presents with loss of end-tidal carbon dioxide, paradoxical chest movement, and chest or neck retractions, and a stridorous noise in the case of partial laryngospasm.[27] Prolonged laryngospasm symptoms include oxygen desaturation, bradycardia, and potential cardiac arrest.

Treatment of laryngospasm includes first administering 100% oxygen with continuous positive airway pressure. Next, intravenous agents such as propofol at 0.5 mg/kg to 0.8 mg/kg and succinylcholine 1 to 2 mg/kg with atropine 0.02 mg/kg should be administed.[27] Note that a smaller dose of succinylcholine may be equally effective with fewer

side effects. If hypoxia or bradycardia is present, propofol should be avoided due to its myocardial depressant activity. If intravenous access is lost or not established, it is recommended to administer intramuscular succinylcholine 4 mg/kg and atropine at 0.02 mg/kg.[27,29]

DENTAL INJURY

Pediatric patients are at risk for dental injury during intubation, especially during their transition from primary to secondary teeth. Children's primary teeth emerge between 8 months for central incisors all the way through 33 months for secondary incisors. These primary teeth are replaced by permanent teeth starting at 6 years old for primary incisors through 12 years old for secondary incisors. The highest incidence of dental injury in children is between ages 7 and 8 years old.[30]

Incidence of dental injury during pediatric anesthetics occurs at a rate of approximately 0.05% per anesthetic.[30] This study found a relationship between inaccurate preoperative dental history and examination, and dental injury. Many cases were due to inadequate anesthesiologist history and exam; some were also due to children having loose teeth that parents were unaware of. Studies are conflicted on whether emergency surgery or difficulty during intubation are associated with dental injury.[30]

If dental injury occurs, it is recommended to have a pediatric dentist perform an intra-oral exam to determine the extent of the injury and to determine whether any immediate repair or reimplantation is appropriate. If there is any question of lost tooth fragments, a chest X-ray is indicated to rule out tooth aspiration or ingestion.[31] Tooth aspiration is an emergency, and tooth or fragment retrieval may require bronchoscopy or gastroscopy for retrieval.[30]

Uncomplicated avulsion of primary teeth does not require further intervention. Avulsion of permanent teeth may require reimplantation, and these teeth should be stored in normal saline or cold milk. Reimplantation within 30 minutes is associated with a good dental prognosis.[31]

MALIGNANT HYPERTHERMIA

Malignant hyperthermia (MH) is an autosomal dominant genetic disorder of the RYR1 or DHP receptor that clinically manifests as increase in metabolic rate after exposure to a triggering agent such as succinylcholine or a volatile anesthetic. Individuals who are MH susceptible have an abnormal muscle receptor that allows intracellular calcium accumulation from the sarcoplasmic reticulum after exposure to a triggering agent, which in turn leads to sustained muscle contraction, muscle breakdown leading to rhabdomyolysis, anaerobic metabolism, and acidosis.[32]

Early clinical signs of MH include hypercarbia and mixed respiratory/metabolic acidosis. These signs occur when aerobic metabolism provides energy for the muscle, resulting in oxygen and adenosine triphosphate consumption and carbon dioxide production. The switch to anaerobic metabolism increases acidosis and lactate production. Rhabdomyolysis occurs with subsequent hyperkalemia and myoglobinuria. Hyperthermia occurs because the sustained muscle contraction generates heat that the body is not able to eliminate, which in turns causes increased carbon dioxide production and oxygen usage.

Hyperthermia is actually a later sign in MH, with hypercarbia that is resistant to modifications in ventilator settings being a more important early clinical sign. Another early clinical sign is generalized muscle rigidity when neuromuscular blockade is in use. Abnormal laboratory findings include a mixed metabolic/respiratory acidosis and then subsequent hyperkalemia, elevated creatine kinase, and myoglobinuria, which may all be especially pronounced in muscular patients.[33] In children, the most common clinical sign in the presentation of MH is tachycardia.[34]

The diagnosis of MH is made based on clinical signs (as noted above) while laboratory findings will also support the diagnosis, but are not necessary to initiate treatment of MH. Supporting laboratory studies include an arterial blood gas (ABG) with acidosis, elevated creatine kinase, elevated serum and urine myoglobin and potassium. Of note, MH can rarely occur postoperatively, with the onset generally within 40 minutes of stopping the anesthetic.[35]

Even while initiating treatment of MH, the anesthesia provider should consider other potential differential diagnoses including fever, sepsis, transfusion reaction, neuroleptic malignant syndrome, pheochromocytoma, thyroid storm, serotonin syndrome, inadequate ventilation, carbon dioxide absorption from laparoscopy, and allergic reactions.

If MH is suspected, the institution's MH protocol should be initiated. Request the MH treatment cart or tray, which should include emergency medications including dantrolene—the only known treatment for MH. Additional assistance should be requested in the operating room for help in assessing and treating the patient. Triggering agents should be stopped and the surgery halted or concluded as soon as possible. If additional support is needed, the MHAUS hotline (1-800-644-9737) is always available for help in managing the MH crisis. Acidosis, hyperkalemia, and hyperthermia caused by the MH should be treated. Below is the list of steps to be taken for treatment of MH, which has been summarized on the Pedi-Crisis Mobile Application.[36]

1. Obtain the MH Kit.

2. Notify surgeon/proceduralist and conclude procedure.

3. Stop triggering agents (volatile anesthetic agents and/or succinylcholine). Start non-triggering anesthetic.

4. Place charcoal filters on the anesthesia circuit and increase oxygen flows to 10 L/min.

5. Intubate if not already. Hyperventilate patient to decrease $EtCO_2$.

6. Administer dantrolene at 2.5 mg/kg IV, every 5 minutes until resolution of symptoms.

7. Maintain pH 7.2 using sodium bicarbonate 1 to 2 mEq/kg IV for metabolic acidosis.

8. Cool patient if >39°C to goal temperature of 38°C with ice to axilla, groin, and around head, cold saline infusion, or cold water NG lavage.

9. Treat hyperkalemia with calcium gluconate 30 mg/kg IV or calcium chloride 10 mg/kg IV, sodium bicarbonate 1 to 2 mEq/kg IV and regular insulin 0.1 U/kg with dextrose 0.5 g/kg.

10. For ventricular tachycardia or atrial fibrillation, do not use calcium channel blocker; treat with amiodarone 5 mg/kg.

11. Send Labs: arterial blood gas (ABG)/venous blood gas (VBG), electrolytes, serum creatine kinase, serum/urine myoglobin, coagulation profile.

12. Place urinary catheter to monitor urine output. Place large-bore IV and arterial line.

13. Call ICU and arrange bed.

14. Be prepared in case of cardiac arrest to perform advanced life support/CPR/extracorporeal membrane oxygenation (ECMO).

REFERENCES

1. Holzman RS, Cooper JB, Gaba DM, Philip JH, Small SD, Feinstem D. Anesthesia crisis resource management: real-life simulation training in operating room crises. *J Clin Anesth.* 1995;7(8):675-687.

2. Murray WB, Foster PA. Crisis resource management among strangers: principles of organizing a multidisciplinary group for crisis resource management. *J Clin Anesth.* 2000;12(8):633-638.

3. Yee B, Naik VN, Joo HS, et al. Nontechnical skills in anesthesia crisis management with repeated exposure to simulation-based education. *Anesthesiology.* 2005;103(2):241-248. Available at http://www.ncbi.nlm.nih.gov/pubmed/16052105. Accessed June 11, 2017.

4. Fehr JJ, Boulet JR, Waldrop WB, Snider R, Brockel M, Murray DJ. Simulation-based assessment of pediatric anesthesia skills. *Anesthesiology.* 2011;115(6):1.

5. Marshall S. The use of cognitive aids during emergencies in anesthesia. *Anesth Analg.* 2013;117(5):1162-1171.

6. Harrison TK, Manser T, Howard SK, Gaba DM. Use of cognitive aids in a simulated anesthetic crisis. *Anesth Analg.* 2006;103(3):551-556.

7. Lipitz-Snyderman A, Steinwachs D, Needham DM, Colantuoni E, Morlock LL, Pronovost PJ. Impact of a statewide intensive care unit quality improvement initiative on hospital mortality and length of stay: retrospective comparative analysis. *BMJ.* 2011;342.

8. Evans D, Mccahon R, Barley M, Norris A, Khajuria A, Moppett I. Cognitive Aids in Medicine Assessment Tool (CMAT): preliminary validation of a novel tool for the assessment of emergency cognitive aids. *Anaesthesia.* 2015;70(8):922-932.

9. Jimenez N, Posner KL, Cheney FW, Caplan RA, Lee LA, Domino KB. An update on pediatric anesthesia liability: a closed claims analysis. *Anesth Analg.* 2007;104:147-153.

10. Lam T, Nagappa M, Wong J, Singh M, Wong D, Chung F. Continuous pulse oximetry and capnography monitoring for postoperative respiratory depression and adverse events: A systematic review and meta-analysis. *Anesth Analg.* 2017;125(6):2019-2029.

11. Baile WF, Buckman R, Lenzi R, Glober G, Beale EA, Kudelka AP. SPIKES-A six-step protocol for delivering bad news: application to the patient with cancer. *Oncologist.* 2000;5(4):302-311.

12. Park I, Gupta A, Mandani K, Haubner L, Peckler B. Breaking bad news education for emergency medicine residents: A novel training module using simulation with the SPIKES protocol. *J Emerg Trauma Shock.* 2010;3(4):385-388.

13. Fine RL. Keeping the patient at the center of patient—and family—centered care. *J Pain Symptom Manage.* 2010;40(4):621-625.

14. Schmid Mast M, Kindlimann A, Langewitz W. Recipients' perspective on breaking bad news: how you put it really makes a difference. *Patient Educ Couns.* 2005;58(3):244-251.

15. Shaw J, Dunn S, Heinrich P. Managing the delivery of bad news: an in-depth analysis of doctors' delivery style. *Patient Educ Couns.* 2012;87(2):186-192.

16. Chumpitazi CE, Rees CA, Chumpitazi BP, Hsu DC, Doughty CB, Lorin MI. Creation and assessment of a bad news delivery simulation curriculum for pediatric emergency medicine fellows. *Cureus.* 2016;8(5):e595.

17. Wheeler SJ, Wheeler DW. Medication errors in anaesthesia and critical care. *Anaesthesia.* 2005;60(3):257-273.

18. Llewellyn RLGP. Drug administration errors . *Anaesth Intens Care J.* Available at http://www.aaic.net.au.ezp.welch.jhmi.edu/document/?D=20080179. Accessed June 7, 2017.

19. Merry AAB. Medication errors—new approaches to prevention. *EBSCOhost.* Available at http://eds.b.ebscohost.com.ezp.welch.jhmi.edu/ehost/pdfviewer/pdfviewer?sid=e8f86338-e4fc-4f05-b61e-163fea12d6cf%40sessionmgr103&vid=1&hid=126. Accessed June 7, 2017.

20. Gonzalez L, Pignaton W, Kusano P, Modolo N, Braz J, Braz L. Anesthesia-related mortality in pediatric patients: a systematic review. *Clinics.* 2012;67(4):381-387.

21. Bhananker SM, Ramamoorthy C, Geiduschek JM, ct al. Anesthesia-related cardiac arrest in children: update from the Pediatric Perioperative Cardiac Arrest Registry. *Anesth Analg.* 2007;105(2):344-350.

22. Practice guidelines for preoperative fasting and the use of pharmacologic agents to reduce the risk of pulmonary aspiration: application to healthy patients undergoing elective procedures. *Anesthesiology.* 2011;114(3):495-511.

23. Warner MA, Warner ME, Warner DO, Warner LO, Warner JE. Perioperative pulmonary aspiration in infants and children. *Anesthesiology.* 1999;90:66–71. Available at http://anesthesiology.pubs.asahq.org/article.aspx?articleid=1946967. Accessed August 31, 2017.

24. Manchikanti L, Colliver JA, Marrero TC, Roush JR. Assessment of age-related acid aspiration risk factors in pediatric, adult, and geriatric patients. *Anesth Analg.* 1985;64(1):11-17.

25. Borland LM, Sereika SM, Woelfel SK, et al. Pulmonary aspiration in pediatric patients during general anesthesia: incidence and outcome. *J Clin Anesth.* 1998;10(2):95-102.

26. Cravero JP, Beach ML, Blike GT, Gallagher SM, Hertzog JH, Pediatric Sedation Research Consortium. The incidence and nature of adverse events during pediatric sedation/anesthesia with propofol for procedures outside the operating room: a report from the Pediatric Sedation Research Consortium. *Anesth Analg.* 2009;108(3):795-804.

27. Hampson-Evans D, Morgan P, Farrar M. Pediatric laryngospasm. *Paediatr Anaesth.* 2008 Apr;18(4):303-307.

28. Flick RP, Wilder RT, Pieper SF, et al. Risk factors for laryngospasm in children during general anesthesia. *Pediatr Anesth.* 2008;18(4):289-296.

29. Orliaguet GA, Gall O, Savoldelli GL, Couloigner V. Case scenario. *Anesthesiology.* 2012;116(2):458-471.

30. Yi T, Tan S, Lim SL, et al. Peri-anaesthetic dental injury in children: a retrospective audit in a tertiary paediatric centre. 2015;24(2). Available at http://journals.sagepub.com/doi/pdf/10.1177/201010581502400203. Accessed May 21, 2017.

31. Sowmya B, Raghavendra P. Management of dental trauma to a developing permanent tooth during endotracheal intubation. *J Anaesthesiol Clin Pharmacol.* 2011;27(2):266-268.

32. Louis CF, Zualkernan K, Roghair T, Mickelson JR. The effects of volatile anesthetics on calcium regulation by malignant hyperthermia-susceptible sarcoplasmic reticulum. *Anesthesiology.* 1992;77(1):114-125. Available at http://www.ncbi.nlm.nih.gov/pubmed/1609985. Accessed August 31, 2017.

33. Larach MG, Gronert GA, Allen GC, Brandom BW, Lehman EB. Clinical presentation, treatment, and complications of malignant hyperthermia in North America from 1987 to 2006. *Anesth Analg.* 2010;110(2):498-507.

34. Nelson P, Litman RS. Malignant hyperthermia in children. *Anesth Analg.* 2014;118(2):369-374.

35. Litman RS, Flood CD, Kaplan RF, Kim YL, Tobin JR. Postoperative malignant hyperthermia. *Anesthesiology.* 2008;109(5):825-829.

36. Pedi Crisis: Mobile App for healthcare providers. Children's Hospital of Philadelphia. Available at http://www.chop.edu/health-resources/pedi-crisis-mobile-app-healthcare-providers. Accessed August 31, 2017.

Pediatric Ambulatory Anesthesia: What is New and Safe?

Steven Butz

Ambulatory surgery exploded in the 1990s. The most recent survey by the Centers for Disease Control and Prevention (CDC) in 2009 indicated that there were 53,329,000 ambulatory surgeries in the United States. Of these, 3,266,000 were carried out on patients under the age of 15 years and were evenly split between freestanding and hospital-based facilities. The pediatric cases were largely adenotonsillectomies, ear tube placements, fracture reductions/fixations, circumcisions, and diagnostic procedures such as endoscopies.[1] Community providers performed most of these cases without specialty training in pediatric anesthesia.

Ambulatory surgery centers (ASCs) are defined by the Centers for Medicare and Medicaid Services (CMS) as any distinct entity that operates exclusively for the purpose of providing surgical services to patients not requiring hospitalization and in which the expected duration of services would not exceed 24 hours following an admission.[2] This limits some procedures, but much of what a pediatric anesthesia practice covers meets these rules. A robust ASC can accommodate subspecialty cases from otolaryngology, orthopedics, general surgery, urology, ophthalmology, plastic surgery, dermatology, dentistry, gastroenterology, and even neurology, radiology, and physiatry.

The success of an ASC depends on being prepared for the cases with not only correct staffing and instrumentation, but also patient selection. Ambulatory surgery depends on cases that are predictable with defined risks that can be accounted for. Predictability results not only from routine surgical and anesthesia care but also from patients with well-controlled medical issues. The common ailments seen in pediatric care that are capable of serious disruption to a surgical schedule are asthma, respiratory infections, congenital heart disease, congenital syndromes, sickle cell anemia, prematurity, and family history of MH.

Asthma is the leading chronic disease in children. Patients with reactive airway can certainly tolerate anesthesia, but screening for active disease is important. Asthma is marked by an inflammatory reaction of the airway leading to bronchoconstriction in response to triggers. Common triggers are respiratory infection, exercise, or allergies.

The history should elicit a baseline for treatments and control. Medication history can give an idea of how severe the disease is. Just using albuterol as needed suggests a milder disease than being on maintenance steroids and leukotriene inhibitors with frequent beta-agonist use. Be aware that the medication history may better reflect the care by the caregivers than the disease severity. It is not uncommon to get a history of asthma triggered by respiratory infection in someone that shows up with an obvious respiratory illness. When asked about last inhaler use, the parents tell you it has been months! Eliciting a good history on medication compliance is very important.

A conservative approach to caring for these children begins with the surgical procedure and airway management planned. If the child is having airway surgery and/or planned intubation, giving a nebulizer treatment preoperatively can be beneficial. Patients that have been identified as having active disease on a preoperative phone call or have been recently cancelled for illness would likely benefit from a short course of steroid therapy preoperatively leading up to the day of surgery. Otherwise, if the patient has an asthma plan with "sick day" care, he or she can follow that leading up to the day of surgery. Be mindful that if a child arrives ill or with active wheezing, a dose of IV steroids won't have effects until hours afterward and may be of little use in managing the patient in the recovery area after a short procedure.[3]

It has been author's experience that if patients with asthma show up with wheezing, they can proceed with surgery if it can be cleared with a nebulizer treatment. If they show up with a fever, unabated wheezing, and/or oxygen saturations below 95% on admission, they tend to be the patients that have desaturations in recovery and require aggressive respiratory therapy to get them stable enough to leave. These patients make up the majority of patient transfers at the author's center.

A practice controversy is what to tell the canceled patient about how soon he or she can return for surgery.

A poll of anesthesiologists revealed that they wait 2 to 4 weeks with most at 4 weeks. Studies have supported the fact that the bronchiole tree remains irritated for 4 to 6 weeks after a respiratory illness and 6 weeks is a better choice. Of course, this all presumes that this is a single illness and that the patient will not get ill again immediately following. For example, otolaryngology patients have pathology inherent to their disease that puts them at risk for continued nasal congestion and respiratory illness.

The following is a guideline from Tait and Malviya for the approach to a child with a respiratory illness. First assessment is to see if surgery is emergent or if the upper respiratory symptoms are from a noninfectious etiology. If either is yes, proceed to the next step. Severe symptoms should be delayed. The need for general anesthesia requires a risk/benefit assessment. Things to consider are asthma history, invasive airway management including tracheal intubation, time pressure, opportunity pressure, or experience of team caring for the child. If the risk assessment is suggestive of a poor outcome, the case should be canceled. A case with favorable risk assessment may proceed, but the guardians (and patient when appropriate) should be informed of the risks.[4]

It was the year 1983 in which pediatric providers were made aware of the risks of anesthetizing infants with a history of prematurity. There were deaths among premature infants that experienced apnea postoperatively. A flurry of papers helped define what children were at risk, but there were small cohorts and used inconsistent definitions of apnea. Post-conceptual age (PCA) is an important concept and is defined by the weeks of gestation plus weeks in age. In summary, apnea was defined as 15 to 20 seconds long and the oldest infants with apnea had a PCA of 41 weeks in the study by Liu et al.[5] The group headed by Welborn found apnea in infants under 45 weeks PCA and Kurth's group found apnea in an infant 55 weeks PCA.[6,7] In 1995, Dr. Cote combined 8 studies to create a cohort of 255 premature infants. He determined that risk factors for apnea were related to gestational age, post-conceptual age, and anemia (hematocrit <30%). He also found that most apnea occurred within 2 hours of an anesthetic; however, it may be as long as 10 to 12 hours afterward.[8]

Fortunately, there is little that would be considered surgically appropriate on a premature infant to be done on an ambulatory basis. However, cases of ankyloglossia, extra-digits, and eye exams are possible. One should keep in mind that using 60 weeks PCA as a minimum would exceed all recommendations in the literature for premature infants. Furthermore, using 45 weeks PCA for full-term infants would be prudent. For anyone doing cases on a population this young, it would be wise to have pediatric specialists available and evaluate the entire facility for appropriateness.

A pediatric cardiac patient with heart failure, poor general health (failure to thrive), cyanotic heart disease, or

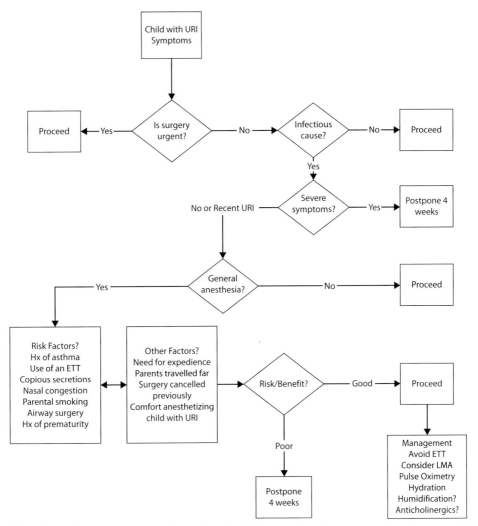

▲ **Figure 35-1.** (Decision flow chart for assessement of a child presenting for surgery with an upper respiratory infection. (Adapted with permission, from Tait AR, Malviya S. Anesthesia for the Child with an Upper Respiratory Tract Infection: Still a Dilemma? *Anesth Analg.* 2005;100 (1): 59-65. https://journals.lww.com/anesthesia-analgesia.)

Table 35-1. Summary of Premature Infant and Apnea Studies

	Liu et al[5]	Welborn et al[6]	Kurth et al[7]	Gregory and Steward[18]
Year	1983	1986	1987	1983
No. of infants (preterm)	214 (41)	86 (38)	47 (49) (2 infants twice)	Editorial in same issue as Liu et al[5]
Def. of apnea	20 seconds	15 seconds	15 seconds (less if bradycardia)	
Oldest with apnea	Under 41 weeks PCA, under 4 months old	PCA <45 weeks	55 weeks PCA (in group 55–60 weeks PCA)	
Take home message	Anesthesia may unmask ventilatory defect in preterm infants 41–46 weeks PCA	Only preterm infants less than PCA 45 weeks had post-op apneic episodes. Full-term infants had none.	Premies <45 weeks PCA need monitoring 36 hours post-op, those 45–60 weeks PCA need 12–24 hours	Monitor premies <45 weeks PCA for 18 hours. Delay surgery if possible. Be prepared with ventilator.

pulmonary hypertension has been shown to be at higher risk for postoperative mortality. Assessing a former cardiac patient can be challenging in regard to fitness for ambulatory surgery. A strong rule of thumb is to not attempt to anesthetize a child with single-ventricle physiology as an ambulatory patient. The complex physiology of these patients does not tolerate positive-pressure ventilation well and once these patients begin to decompensate, it requires elements typically found in a high-level pediatric ICU or advanced pediatric cardiology team to resuscitate them. Diagnoses that are associated with this type of physiology include hypoplastic left heart syndrome, tricuspid atresia, or pulmonary valve atresia. They also may have a history of a Norwood, Fontan, or Hemi-Fontan (Glenn) procedure.

The rules for giving prophylactic antibiotics to prevent subacute bacterial endocarditis (SBE) have been simplified as of 2009. They are required only in patients with unrepaired cyanotic lesions, completely repaired congenital heart defects (CHDs) with prosthetic material or device during the first 6 months after the procedure, repaired CHD with residual defects at the site or adjacent to the site of a prosthetic patch or prosthetic device (which inhibit endothelialization), or previous endocarditis.[9]

Congenital syndromes can be very troubling especially if the provider is not familiar with the condition. Fortunately, there are many sources either online or in print detailing congenital and genetic syndromes far too numerous to list here and their anesthetic implications. Part of teasing out the implications of a syndrome, it helps to figure out if it has a genetic etiology or is due to an error in development. For example, a patient with gastroschisis may be similar to one with an omphalocele. However, the omphalocele occurs due to a problem with developmental steps that the gut does not return to the abdominal cavity after rotating in the umbilical stalk. A gastroschisis occurs when the abdominal wall becomes damaged or weakened such as during an ischemic event. The omphalocele has implications for other genetic errors that are usually not seen in gastroschisis patients. Examples of developmental issues that are typically in isolation are amniotic band syndrome, fetal alcohol syndrome, and intrauterine strokes.

The genetic syndromes are either inherited or from a spontaneous mutation. Many are quite familiar and represent classic cases in pediatric anesthesia' such as cystic fibrosis, tetralogy of Fallot, Down syndrome, CHARGE syndrome, and glycogen storage diseases. However, some patients with these syndromes may still be appropriate for ambulatory surgery. The key is to recognize the potential issues and assess if the facility is capable of handling them from a staffing and resource point of view. For instance, a Down syndrome patient with adenotonsillar hypertrophy coming for procedure is a common occurrence. Recognize that obstruction may be multilevel and obstruction from a relatively large tongue may occur in recovery. You want a capable recovery nursing staff that can recognize and manage that issue. These patients may have difficult IV access, atlantoaxial subluxation, cardiac disease, developmental delay, and perhaps sleep apnea. A competent surgeon and an anesthesiologist are required, but the facility, too, must be able to accommodate this patient and his/her special needs. As with all of ambulatory surgery, anticipating problems and being proactive will be the best practice to avoid poor patient outcomes.

Malignant hyperthermia is a topic that deserves some special attention. Children are no more at risk than adults except that they usually do not have a history of a prior anesthetic or may not be old enough to demonstrate some of the more subtle manifestations. The disease is autosomal dominant and has been mapped to the RYR1 and CACNA1S genes that code for skeletal muscle proteins involved in calcium transport. Although some mutations have been mapped thanks to tissue donations from people diagnosed with MH, there are many more possible. There are blood tests for some of the common genes, but not having a common gene does not mean a person does not have *any* gene making them susceptible.

An article by Gurnaney et al. detailed muscular dystrophies and their link to MH. The authors concluded that three types of muscular dystrophy were definitely at risk for MH. The other types still were associated with hyperkalemic arrests and postoperative respiratory failure, but the risk of MH was considered baseline with the general population. The three types identified are rare and are King–Denborough syndrome, central core myopathy, and multi-minicore disease with RYR1 mutation. Keep in mind that treatment of MH in the form of dantrolene has been available for many years, and yet, there are still deaths from this disease.[10]

The Malignant Hyperthermia Association of the United States has created teaching aids to assist in a MH crisis and staff a 24-hour hotline. It also has definite recommendations for equipment an ASC should have available and how susceptible patients should be managed. Part of that is having complete treatment of dantrolene available (36 vials) or the newer formulations and keeping monitoring of a susceptible patient for 12 hours following the anesthetic. With these thoughts in mind, it is easier to establish a policy for allowing MH-susceptible patients in an appropriately staffed and equipped facility. A single crisis in a freestanding ASC will quickly use all of the facility's resources of staff and supplies and will have a large disruption in care given to other patients.

The risk of an adverse event is very real and needs to be actively prevented. As noted above, the best way to prevent one is to be able to predict it. In the adult world, some of these risks have been well studied. It has been just starting in the pediatric realm. One such article by

Table 35-2. Multivariable Model Predicting Occurrence of Postoperative Adverse Event from the Derivation Cohort and the Risk Scores

Patient Characteristic	β	OR (95% CI)	P-value	Risk Score
Age (years)				
>3 (reference)	0.00	1.00		0
<3	0.55	1.73 (1.36–2.21)	<0.0001	1
ASA physical status				
I	0.00	1.00		0
II	0.50	1.65 (1.24–2.21)	0.0006	1
III	0.79	2.20 (1.48–3.28)	<0.0001	2
Pre-existing pulmonary disease	1.01	2.75 (2.06–3.66)	<0.0001	2
Morbid obesity	0.95	2.57 (1.36–4.87)	0.004	2
Type of procedure				
Radiology	1.00	1.00		0
Surgery	1.37	3.95 (2.56–6.08)	<0.0001	3

CI, confidence interval; OR, odds ratio.
Reproduced with permission, from Subramanyam R, et al. Perioperative respiratory adverse events in pediatric anesthesia. *Anesth Analg*. 2016; 122(5): 1578-85. https://journals.lww.com/anesthesia-analgesia.

Subramanyam et al, in 2016, used almost 9000 charts to develop risk criteria and then validated it in over 10,000 more charts. This group was looking at airway adverse events that they defined. The risks identified were as follows: age <3 years, ASA class II or III (no IV in study), pre-existing pulmonary disease, morbid obesity, and having a surgical procedure (as opposed to radiologic procedure). A grading scale was also developed along with giving an overall risk of respiratory event as 2.8% for all comers (see Table 35-2).[11]

Another study from 2016 by Whippey et al looked at risks for transferring pediatric patients from an ASC. The reasons were loosely grouped into anesthesia-related, surgical, social, and medical. The univariate analysis included age <2 years, prescription medication use, gastroesophageal reflux disease (GERD), obstructive sleep apnea, and

other comorbidities. A multivariate analysis included age <2 years, ASA class III or IV, surgery >1 hour, procedure complete after 1500 hours, obstructive sleep apnea (OSA), orthopedic surgery, dental surgery, ENT surgery, or an intra-operative event occurring.[12]

Univariate Analysis	Multivariate Analysis
• Age <2 years • Prescription medication use • GERD • OSA • Other comorbidities	• Age <2 years • ASA class III or IV • Surgery >1 hour • Procedure complete after 1500 hours • OSA • Orthopedics, dental, ENT surgery • Intra-operative event

Source: Data from Whippey A, Kostandoff G, Ma HK, et al. Predictors of unanticipated admission following ambulatory surgery in pediatric population. *Paediatr Anaesth* 2016;26(8):831-7.

Obstructive sleep apnea has been large concern in the adult ambulatory world. The STOP-BANG grading system for OSA has become a regular part of pre-admission screening for adult ambulatory surgery reflecting the work of Francis Chung's group in Toronto. Part of the irony with pediatric patients is that tonsil surgery has sleep-disordered breathing as a primary diagnosis, accounts for one of the most frequent outpatient surgeries in children. In fact, data support that the more severe a child's OSA is, the more likely the child is to be transferred. The leading diagnosis that precipitates transfer is hypoxia. To address this concern, Tait and Malviya, developed a pediatric OSA scoring system known as STBUR.

The STBUR score asks about snoring, trouble breathing, and feeling unrefreshed after sleeping. The following five questions are as follows:

1. Does the child snore more than half the time?
2. Can snoring be heard through a closed door?
3. Does the patient have pauses in his breathing at night?
4. Does the patient have gasps in her breathing at night?
5. Is the child difficult to wake up in the morning or fall asleep during school?

The score is out of 5. Patients scoring 3 out of 5 have a three times greater chance of respiratory complications. A score of 5 out of 5 indicates a 10 times greater risk. The definition of respiratory complications can be as mild as desaturations postoperatively so a score of 5/5 may not mean the patient will need to be transferred, but it can focus a provider's attention on the most at-risk patients.[13]

Other conditions seen following surgery are emergence delirium, postoperative nausea and vomiting, and readiness for recovery. Each episode of postoperative nausea and vomiting (PONV) can delay a discharge by 30 minutes. Likewise, emergence delirium can tie up nursing resources over what is planned and delay a patient leaving by an hour or more. Lastly, having solid criteria for going home can keep the path to leaving better defined and more regular.

Every pediatric anesthesia provider or recovery room nurse has likely experienced emergence delirium. It is defined as a motor agitation state without awareness of surroundings. Classically, children suffering this will not engage their favorite toy or television show. They also may alternate quickly between parents trying to comfort them. The pathology is poorly understood, but there are strong associations (see Table 35-3). One of the minor issues is being able to explain this to the parents and what it means for going home and future anesthetics. This situation can be quite upsetting to a family.[14]

Somewhat related is the issue of developing post-traumatic stress disorder following an anesthetic. Taking a screaming child back to the operating room can have negative sequela. There can be bedwetting, temper tantrums, sleep disturbances, attention-seeking behaviors, or a new fear of loneliness. The risks are very similar to emergence delirium and may appear in a child that has suffered delirium postoperatively. Any of these may appear even months after the attributing anesthetic.

The next logical question is typically how to prevent emergence delirium. There is a frequent reaction to blame preoperative midazolam. However, there are about as many articles that implicate as exonerate midazolam as a cause. Without a clear answer that way, anesthesia providers must weigh the benefit of the preoperative sedation and amnesia versus the possible risk of delirium. Table 35-4 gives recommendations for prevention, but not treatment of delirium. This means you need to screen your patients for their risks or history of having it after previous anesthetics. Clinically, effective treatment is with a combination of propofol and dexmedetomidine. This can be achieved with boluses of dexmedetomidine under 0.5 mcg/kg to avoid hemodynamic depression. Usually, a combination of 0.25 mcg/kg of dexmedetomidine IV and 0.5 mg/kg propofol IV gives good results such as unconsciousness

with patent airway lasting 20 to 40 minutes. After that the patient wakes much more clearly. Other drugs in the literature used singly in treatment are fentanyl, sufentanil, propofol, dexmedetomidine, ketamine, midazolam, and clonidine.[14]

Pediatric PONV has a different set of risk factors than adult patients. It tends to be fairly rare in the very young and more associated with a specific procedure. TJ et al. published a risk factor protocol in 2007 that still holds true. (see Figure 35-2).[15]

The treatments follow a similar trend from the adult world. Patients with two or more risk factors should receive two drugs from different classes for prophylaxis. Treating everyone without regard to risk of PONV may only increase the incidence of side effects seen from the drugs without significantly altering the rate if PONV. As in adults, choices for antiemetics are based on appropriate receptor choice and not simply reusing the same type. In very young patients, the anticholinergic anti-emetics may not be appropriate. Propofol is still a good anesthetic choice to decrease the incidence of PONV. However, the risk of narcotics triggering PONV does not seem to be as important in pediatrics as it is in adult patients. Figure 35-2 reinforces this.

Discharge times for patients can be highly variable. A couple of large studies shed some light on keeping them predictable and safe. A group in France led by Moncel looked at over 1600 ASA class I and II patients from 6 months old to 16 years old. They scored their patients at 1 and 2 hours postoperatively and found that over 97% met criteria at 1 hour and 99.8% met them at 2 hours. They used a scoring system that looked at hemodynamics, balance/ambulation, pain scores, PONV rating, respiratory status, and surgical bleeding. They also asked if family had questions for anesthesia provider. The two scores most often associated with delay were respiratory status and questions for the anesthesia provider. Compared to historical control, they were able to consistently reduce discharge times by 69 minutes with less than 1% unexpected admission rate.[16]

Armstrong et al published a Canadian study that combined a scoring using post-anesthetic discharge scoring system (PADSS) and Aldrete scores. The group found that physiologic-based criteria improved discharge times over simple, time-based criteria. Approximately 75% we discharged 15 to 45 minutes sooner. About 20% showed no difference. The score used is listed in Table 35-5.[17]

Pediatric anesthesia certainly has a place in the ambulatory world. There are a great many cases that can be performed in a free-standing center with few risks of complications. As always, the secret to a successful pediatric ambulatory surgery center is based on wise patient selection, well-trained staff, and the ability to predict and treat complications. It can be a rewarding practice but can be very labor-intensive and challenging even if patients are ASA class I or II.

Table 35-3. Associations with Emergence Delirium

Preschool-aged patients
Sevoflurane or desflurane anesthetics
Patient preoperative anxiety
ENT surgery
May be unrelated to pain

Table 35-4. Pharmacologic Prevention of Emergence Delirium in Children

Agent	Route and Timing of Administration	Efficacy	Doses
Midazolam	OR, IV, IR	No	OR: 0.5 mg/kg
	Preoperative		IV: 0.1 mg/kg
			IR: 0.5 mg/kg
Midazolam	IV, end of surgery	Yes	IV: 0.1 mg/kg
Hydroxyzine combined to midazolam	OR, preoperative	Yes	1 mg/kg
Propofol	Continuous intraoperative	Yes	Induction 2–3 mg/kg
			Maintenance: 3–12 mg/kg/h
Propofol	End of surgery	Yes	1 mg/kg
Ketamine	IV, preoperative	Yes	0.25 mg/kg
	IV, end of surgery	Yes	0.25 mg/kg
	OR, preoperative	Yes	6 mg/kg
α2 Adrenoceptors: Clonidine	OR or IR, preoperative	Yes	2, 3 or 4 µg/kg
α2 Adrenoceptors: Clonidine	IV after induction	Yes	2, 3 or 4 µg/kg
α2 Adrenoceptors: Clonidine	CAU	Yes	3 µg/kg
α2 Adrenoceptors: Dexmedetomidine	IV, preoperative	Yes	0.2 µg/kg
α2 Adrenoceptors: Dexmedetomidine	IV, intraoperative	Yes	0.3 µg/kg
α2 Adrenoceptors: Dexmedetomidine	IV, intraoperative	Yes	1 µg/kg
α2 Adrenoceptors: Dexmedetomidine	IV, intraoperative	Yes	0.5 µg/kg
α2 Adrenoceptors: Dexmedetomidine	Caudal	Yes	1 µg/kg
Fentanyl	IV, intraoperative	Yes	2.5 µg/kg
			1 µg/kg
Transcutaneous fentanyl	Preoperative	Yes	10–15 µg/kg
			100 µg/kg
Intranasal fentanyl	Intraoperative after induction	Yes	2 µg/kg
Nalbuphine	IV, end of surgery	Yes	0.1 mg/kg
Intraoperative nonopioids analgesia: Ketorolac	IV, during surgery	Yes	1 mg/kg
Caudal analgesia	After induction	Yes	1 mL/kg Bupivacaine (0.25%)
Gabapentin	Preoperative	Yes	15 mg/kg
Magnesium infusion	Intraoperative	Yes	30 mg/kg bolus and continuous infusion of 10 mg/kg/h
Dexamethasone	Preoperative	Yes	0.2 mg/kg

IR, intrarectal; IV, intravenous; OR, oral; PACU, postoperative care unit; PONV, postoperative nausea and vomiting.
Source: Reproduced with permission, from Dahmani S, Delivet H, Hilly J. Emergence delirium in children: an update. *Curr Opin Anesthesiol.* 2014; 27(3): 309-315. https://journals.lww.com/co-anesthesiology.

Risk Factors	Points
Surgery ≥ 30 min.	1
Age ≥ 3 years	1
Strabismus surgery	1
History of POV or PONV in relatives	1
Sum =	0 . . . 4

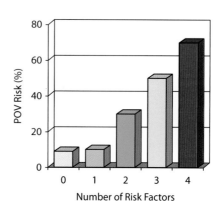

▲ **Figure 35-2.** Simplified risk score for POV in children. Simplified risk score from Eberhart et al. *Anesth Analg.* 2004;99:1630-1637 to predict the risk for POV in children. When 0, 1, 2, 3, or 4 of the depicted independent predictors are present, the corresponding risk for PONV is approximately 10%, 10%, 30%, 55%, or 70%. (Reproduced with permission, from Gan TJ, Meyer TA, Apfel CC, et al. Society for Ambulatory Anesthesia guidelines for the management of postoperative nausea and vomiting. *Anesth Analg.* 2007; 105(6): 1615-28. https://journals.lww.com/anesthesia-analgesia.)

Table 35-5. Physiological Criteria-Based Discharge Scoring System Was a Combination of the Scoring Systems Reported by Aldrete[a] and Chung[b]

Discharge Criteria		Score
Conscious level and activity	Awake and orientated, appropriate movements	2
	Rousable with minimal stimulation, weak movements	1
	Responsive only to tactile stimulation, no movement	0
Respiratory stability	Able to cough, deep breathe or cry	2
	Hoarseness with crying or coughing	1
	Stridor, dyspnea, or wheeze	0
Oxygen saturation	Maintains >95% on room air	2
	90–95% on room air	1
	Requires O_2 to maintain >90%	0
Hemodynamic stability	HR and systolic BP within 15% of baseline value	2
	HR and/or systolic BP within 15–30% of baseline	1
	HR and/or systolic BP outside 30% of baseline, mottled	0
Post-op pain	None, or mild discomfort	2
	Moderate to severe, controlled with intravenous analgesia	1
	Persistent severe pain	0
Post-op nausea or vomiting	None, or mild nausea with no vomiting	2
	Transient vomiting or retching	1
	Persistent moderate to severe nausea and vomiting	0
Surgical site	No blood or fluid loss	2
	Minimal loss, no intervention required	1
	Ongoing losses, dressing changes required	0

[a]Aldrete JA. The post-anesthesia recovery score revisited. *J Clin Anesth.* 1995;7:89-91.
[b]Chung F. Discharge criteria–a new trend. *Can J Anaesth.* 1995;42:1056-1058.
BP, blood pressure; HR, heart rate.
Source: Reproduced with permission, from Armstrong J, et al. A prospective observational study comparing a physiological scoring system with time-based discharge criteria in pediatric ambulatory surgical patients. *Can J Anesth.* 2015; 62:1082–1088. www.springer.com/journal/12630.

REFERENCES

1. Cullen KA, Hall MJ, Golosinskiy A. Ambulatory surgery in the United States, 2006. *Natl Health Stat Report.* 2009;(11):1-25.
2. Rules and regulations. *Federal Register.* 2011;76(205). October 24, 2011.
3. Maxwell LG, Yaster M. Perioperative management issues in pediatric patients. *Anesthesiol Clin North Am.* 2000;18(3):601-632.
4. Tait AR, Malviya S. Anesthesia for the child with an upper respiratory tract infection: still a dilemma? *Anesth Analg.* 2005;100(1):59-65.
5. Liu LM, Cote CJ, Goudsouzian NG, et al. Life-threatening apnea in infants recovering from anesthesia. *Anesthesiology.* 1983;59(6):506-510.
6. Welborn LG, Ramirez N, Oh TH, et al. Postanesthetic apnea and periodic breathing in infants. *Anesthesiology.* 1986;65(6):658-661.
7. Kurth CD, Spitzer AR, Broennie AM, Downes JJ. Postoperative apnea in preterm infants. *Survey Anesthesiol.* 1987;31(5):298.
8. Coté CJ, Zaslavsky A, Downes JJ, et al. Postoperative apnea in former preterm infants after inguinal herniorrhaphy: a combined analysis. *Anesthesiology.* 1995;82(4):809-822.
9. Cannesson M, Earing MG, Collange V, Kersten JR. Anesthesia for noncardiac surgery in adults with congenital heart disease. *Anesthesiology.* 2009;111:432-440.
10. Gurnaney H, Brown A, Litman RS. Malignant hyperthermia and muscular dystrophies. *Anesth Analg.* 2009;109(4):1043-1048.
11. Subramanyam R, Yeramaneni S, Hossain MM, Anneken AM, Varughese AM. Perioperative respiratory adverse events in pediatric anesthesia. *Anesth Analg.* 2016;122:1578-1585.
12. Whippey A, Kostandoff G, Ma HK, Cheng J, Thabane L, Paul J. Predictors of unanticipated admission following ambulatory surgery in pediatric population. *Paediatr Anaesth.* 2016;26(8):831-837.
13. Tait AR, Voepel-Lewis T, Christensen R, O'Brien LM. The STBUR questionnaire for predicting perioperative respiratory adverse events in children at risk for sleep-disordered breathing. *Paediatr Anaesth.* 2013;23(6):510-516.
14. Dahmani S, Delivet H, Hilly J. Emergence delirium in children: an update. *Curr Opin Anaesthesiol.* 2014;27:309-315.
15. Gan TJ, Meyer TA, Apfel CC, et al. Society for Ambulatory Anesthesia guidelines for the management of postoperative nausea and vomiting. *Anesth Analg.* 2007;105(6):1615-1628, table of contents.
16. Moncel JB, Nardi N, Wodey E, Pouvreau A, Ecoffey C. Evaluation of the pediatric post anesthesia discharge scoring system in an ambulatory surgery unit. *Ped Anaesth.* 2015;25:636-641.
17. Armstrong J, Forrest H, Crawford MW. A prospective observational study comparing a physiological scoring system with time-based discharge criteria in pediatric ambulatory surgical patients. *Can J Anesth.* 2015;62:1082-1088.
18. Gregory G and Steward D. "Life-threatening perioperative apnea in the Ex-"premie"". *Anesthesiology.* 1983;59:495-498.

Anesthesia at Pediatric Offsite Locations

Amy Henry

INTRODUCTION

The topic of "Offsite Anesthesia" or "Non-Operating Room Anesthesia" (NORA) is becoming increasingly common in the pediatric anesthesiology world. With the rising number of imaging modalities and non-invasive procedures being performed outside of the traditional operating room, anesthesiologists will be increasingly asked to provide care to pediatric patients—often times, in unfamiliar locales. Providing safe care is of top priority, and requires an in-depth knowledge of the patient, procedure, and an understanding of the logistics and limitations of the location itself.

GENERAL CONSIDERATIONS

Children or infants may require procedures and imaging exams at sites outside of the usual operating room environment. Imaging exams on non-movable equipment (MRI and CT), rare disease processes that require specialized treatment (radiation therapy) or providers with subspecialty skills and procedures requiring specialized equipment (interventional radiology), will require a traveling anesthesia provider. A qualified provider who is *comfortable with being uncomfortable* is ideal, as problems not typically experienced in the familiar operating room setting are likely. This traveling provider must pay the utmost attention to details, preferably have a good rapport with team members, and be prepared for adverse events which will inevitably occur.

▶ Preoperative Evaluation

The ability to provide safe anesthetic care to a child begins with a thorough preoperative evaluation and a clear understanding of the patient's disease. This includes, in particular, assessment of the patient's airway, respiratory, and cardiovascular systems. A note from the referring physician is helpful in ascertaining why the procedure or imaging exam is being performed. The patient's family should be contacted a day or two before the procedure by telephone, to review any changes in the medical history, discuss day-of-procedure medication administration, and ensure an understanding of non-profit organization (NPO) guidelines. For unfamiliar parents, a brief description of what to expect on the day of the procedure can be helpful in allaying any pressing concerns.

Patients scheduled for procedures and imaging exams as an outpatient may have recently seen their primary care physician, who may mark them "cleared for anesthesia." This "clearance" needs to be taken with caution, as it is ultimately at the discretion of the anesthesiologist whether or not the patient is truly ready on the day of the anesthetic. To avoid confusion and potential frustration by the patient, family, and ordering provider, it can be recommended that patients with a significant past medical history have an appointment in a pre-anesthesia clinic to compile any relevant history, results of tests, and labs, to perform a physical exam, and to assess their readiness for anesthesia. Patients with complex medical histories and/or preterm infants may also need arrangements for admission with observational status.

For patients with less complex past medical histories, and/or patients having simple imaging exams or procedures, the responsibility of the history and physical rests exclusively on the shoulders of the anesthesiologist. Performing a chart review of previous anesthetics is useful. In particular, it is important to look at prior intraoperative airway information, vital signs, drugs used, any pertinent intraoperative notes, as well as the immediate postoperative documentation in the Post-Anesthesia Care Unit. For returning patients, talking with them about prior anesthetics can help guide current anesthetic plans, basing technique upon past successes and failures.

▶ Location Set-up Requirements

The American Society of Anesthesiologists (ASA) has published *Standards, Guidelines, and Practice Parameters*, which can be found on the ASA Web site.[1] Its "Statement on Non-operating Room Anesthetizing Locations"

updated in October 2013, includes minimal guidelines for all anesthesia personnel providing care to patients outside of the operating room. These guidelines include the following:

- A reliable source of oxygen available for the entire procedure (centrally-piped oxygen source strongly encouraged), as well as a backup oxygen supply, which should include the equivalent of, at a minimum, a full E-cylinder.
- A reliable and adequate suction source (one that meets operating room standards is strongly encouraged), with appropriate suction tubing and apparatus
- A reliable and adequate scavenging waste system during the use of inhalational anesthetic gases
- A self-inflating hand resuscitator bag able to deliver at least 90% oxygen and positive-pressure ventilation
- Adequate anesthetic drugs, supplies, and equipment to care for the patient
- Adequate monitoring equipment to adhere to the ASA "Standards for Basic Anesthetic Monitoring" (Table 36-1)

Additionally, the guidelines include minimal requirements with respect to electrical outlets and the provision of emergency power supply; adequate illumination of the patient, machine, and equipment, as well as a backup battery-powered source of illumination (other than a laryngoscope); sufficient space to accommodate the patient, equipment, and caregivers; and pediatric emergency equipment and drugs to provide cardiopulmonary resuscitation.

▶ Personnel

As with caring for any patient, but particularly with offsite pediatric anesthesia, there should be adequate staff trained to assist the anesthesia provider, and a means to request further assistance. This includes trained personnel to assist

Table 36-1. ASA Standard Basic Anesthetic Monitoring Guidelines

1. Qualified anesthesia personnel shall be present in the room throughout the conduct of all general anesthetics, regional anesthetics, and monitored anesthesia care.
2. During the conduct of all anesthetics, the patient's oxygenation [inspired gas (oxygen analyzer) and blood oxygenation (pulse oximeter and color)], ventilation (continuous observation, $ETCO_2$ analysis, circuit disconnect alarm), circulation (continuous ECG, BP, and HR measured at least every 5 minutes), and temperature (when clinically significant changes are expected) shall be continually evaluated.

transporting the patient from one location to another, and a continuation of appropriate basic anesthetic monitoring. It should be strongly recommended that personnel involved in caring for patients during an anesthetic (including transporting the patient during emergence) be Pediatric Advanced Life Support (PALS) certified.

Choice of Sedative Medications/ Anesthetic Plan

The anesthetic plan will vary depending upon patient characteristics, past medical history, and the type of procedure or imaging modality. Patients may or may not require a peripheral intravenous line for the procedure and/or imaging exam, which may alter the anesthetic plan. This will also vary based upon the specific offsite location. For example, a volatile agent cannot be administered in a location with no available scavenging system. Common anesthetics and their reversal agent (when applicable) should be immediately available and easily administered.

As with any anesthetic, a back-up (and a secondary back-up) plan should be considered. While providing offsite anesthesia, preparation is crucial. An anesthesiologist may need to allow for significant additional time for the delivery of drugs, equipment, or even emergency help.

Postoperative Care

Like the anesthetic plan, the exact location of the postoperative care of the patient will vary depending upon patient characteristics, past medical history, and type of procedure or imaging exam. Certain patients and procedures will necessitate the care and monitoring provided in an intensive care unit. Others may require the commonly used Phase 1 recovery in the Post-Anesthesia Care Unit. Still others may emerge quickly enough from their anesthetic that they may bypass Phase 1 and go directly to Phase 2 care.

Transportation of the patient after conclusion of the procedure can be risky, especially if the procedure and recovery area are separated by distance and include the use of elevators. The patient should have standard monitors in place, and the provider should bring a mask, anesthesia bag, and full E-cylinder oxygen tank. The provider should also consider bringing any emergency medications that may be necessary to administer during the transport.

The length of stay following a procedure will be based upon the surgical procedure and/or imaging exam, as well as patient and anesthetic variables. Overnight admission as an observational status for airway monitoring, cardiopulmonary monitoring, and pain control is reasonable. Another indication for overnight observation would be young gestational age, with infants <60 weeks post-conceptual age qualifying based upon their increased risk for apnea and bradycardia. This is particularly important in formerly premature infants, and especially in those receiving opioids. In the general anesthesia spinal (GAS) study, which compared infants aged 60 weeks or younger receiving either general anesthesia or spinal anesthesia for inguinal herniorrhaphy, the infants were monitored for apnea up to 12 hours postoperatively. The overall rate of apnea in this trial was 3%, with a greater risk of apnea (6%) in premature infants.[2] A conservative approach would be to monitor patients younger than 60 weeks post-conceptual age for at least 12 hours post-procedurally for apnea and bradycardia. This time period can be altered at the discretion of the supervising anesthesiologist, especially for extremely short anesthetics, or those in which opioids were not administered.

RADIOLOGY IMAGING LOCATIONS AND CONSIDERATIONS

Radiological imaging modalities are used for diagnostic and therapeutic purposes in children of all ages with widely varying systemic illnesses. An understanding of the physics of radiation and imaging modalities will better prepare the anesthesiologist to keep themselves, and their patient, safe. The anesthesia provider can learn basic fluoroscopy safety, by textbook or journal review, or by completion of a fluoroscopy safety course, available on the Internet.

MRI

Children that require MRI will often require anesthesia, due to the length and enclosing nature of the scanner. The high magnetic field present in the MRI environment poses challenges to the anesthesia provider, as completion of the scan requires normally functioning equipment that will not cause image-altering electrical interference.

MRI-compatible anesthesia machines, monitors, and infusion pumps are all available and will be required to safely administer anesthesia, as will equipment including laryngoscopes and their batteries, stethoscopes, and IV poles. MRI-compatible equipment can be safely used outside of the 50-gauss line, which is usually marked on the floor of most MRI rooms, but should be verified with the hospital's biomedical department.[3] ASA Standard Basic Anesthesia Monitoring guidelines should be followed, which will require magnet-safe pulse oximetry probes and cables, electrocardiogram leads, and temperature probes. Respiratory and end-tidal CO_2 monitoring can be accomplished by using a nasal cannula, and is extremely important in a patient that is distant from the anesthesia provider. Care providers are required to follow safety measures and remove all metal from themselves, including pagers, scissors, and even hair clips, as they can act as missiles as they are attracted into the magnet.

The length of the MRI will vary, with a usual range of 45 to 90 minutes. Several techniques can be used to provide safe and effective anesthetic care—all will ideally create an immobile, spontaneously breathing patient, who will have minimal postoperative nausea and vomiting, a rapid emergence, and be ready for a quick discharge. For young patients without a peripheral IV (PIV), the author either induces anesthesia with sevoflurane to allow placement of a PIV while the patient is unconscious, or uses a needle-free, subcutaneously injected buffered lidocaine system, the J-tip, to anesthetize the skin prior to PIV placement. For extremely anxious patients, oral midazolam, 0.3 to 0.5 mg/kg, can be given to allow a smoother induction. TIVA (total intravenous anesthetic) is then followed by one of two techniques. One effective technique is the use of a continuous propofol infusion. Most pediatric patients require an infusion rate of approximately 200 mcg/kg/min to assure immobility, assuming a non-instrumented airway.[3] Frankville and colleagues describe a similar technique, however, using a loading dose of 2 mg/kg of propofol, followed by a continuous infusion of 100 mcg/kg/min.[4] The author of this chapter uses a combination of the two techniques, giving a propofol bolus dose of 1 to 2 mg/kg, followed by an infusion of 100 to 200 mcg/kg/min, titrated to vital signs while maintaining an unobstructed, spontaneous airway.

The use of dexmedetomidine as a sole anesthetic agent for MRI has been employed and studied in the pediatric population. In 2005, Koroglu et al described the use of IV dexmedetomidine providing adequate sedation in children ages 1 to 7 years for MRI, without adverse hemodynamic or respiratory effects.[5] In 2006, they compared dexmedetomidine (1 mcg/kg initial dose, followed by 0.5 mcg/kg/min continuous infusion) versus propofol (3 mg/kg initial dose, followed by continuous infusion of 100 mcg/kg/min), finding dexmedetomidine to be a reliable sedative drug in certain patients.[6] Similarly, Mason et al described their high-dose technique of using a 10-minute IV bolus of 3-mcg dexmedetomidine followed by a continuous infusion of 2 mcg/kg/h, which allowed for adequate sedation without significant adverse sequelae.[7]

Another effective method commonly used at the author's institution involves a combination of dexmedetomidine and propofol. An IV bolus dose of 1 mcg/kg of dexmedetomidine over 10 minutes, combined with a single-bolus of 1 to 2 mg/kg of propofol, is used to induce anesthesia. Careful attention to the airway and vitals during this induction phase is important, as commonly described bradycardia may occur with administration of dexmedetomidine, particularly in children less than 12 months of age.[8] This regimen will occasionally require intermittent propofol bolus doses (0.5 to 1 mg/kg) for scans requiring table movement, patient repositioning, or when the radiology nurse manipulates the PIV for contrast injection, especially as the 45-minute mark approaches. While slightly more involved, this technique has the potential benefit of a wide-awake patient at the conclusion of the scan, who bypasses the extended recovery phase of anesthesia and is ready for a prompt discharge.

Patients may occasionally require placement of an oropharyngeal or nasopharyngeal airway to maintain an unobstructed airway. A supraglottic airway or endotracheal tube might also be placed for airway obstruction or airway protection. Both cardiac MRI and MRI angiography may require intermittent breath-holding during certain image sequences. This necessitates not only a secure airway, but commonly the administration of a muscle relaxant. It will also require the anesthesia provider to be physically in the scanning room during specific imaging sequences, to pause mechanical ventilation and/or administer medications (e.g. propofol) to temporarily induce apnea, while closely monitoring the patient.

CT

Children require computed tomography (CT) imaging for the evaluation of many disease processes. Children from the ages of a few months old through ages 3 or 4 will often require some type of anesthesia to allow scan completion. It is reasonable for skilled pediatric CT technicians and nurses to first attempt short scans without sedation (the practice at the author's institution). The importance of distraction techniques and a friendly disposition cannot be overemphasized at this point. A child-life specialist, or "professional distractor," can be extremely useful during this attempt.

If the child and/or parent is unwilling to attempt the scan without sedation, and/or fails the nonsedated attempt, an anesthesia provider may be necessary. A brief, but thorough history and physical should be performed, and the anesthetic plan discussed with the parent or guardian. In the case of scheduled scans, the anesthesia provider ideally has access to the proposed scans ahead of time, allowing for a complete review of the medical record.

Types of anesthetics may vary for these scans, depending upon the length of the scan, patient comorbidities, or need for IV access (for injection of iodinated contrast and angiogram imaging). The type of anesthetic commonly used at the author's institution for short CT scans is a mask induction with volatile agent. For brief scans without contrast injection, it may be possible to perform the scan quickly following completion of the induction phase. For longer scans, anesthetic maintenance can be achieved using volatile agent or TIVA. A continuous technique using the anesthesia mask and careful placement of a mask-strap keeps the anesthetic depth constant and simultaneously allows for monitoring of $ETCO_2$ in a spontaneously ventilating patient. Alternatively, once an adequate depth of general anesthesia is achieved following mask induction, volatile agent can be administered intermittently by mask, with use of a nasal cannula to monitor $ETCO_2$. This requires the anesthesia provider and CT technician to be in close communication with one another, as the timing of the scans could interfere with the need for patient intervention, for example, deepening the anesthetic or airway manipulation. Patient histories, physical characteristics and history of snoring or sleep apnea may influence the anesthetic plan, and placement of a supraglottic airway or endotracheal tube is sometimes necessary. Total IV anesthesia with propofol can also be used successfully, by either intermittent injection or continuous infusion, and is perfect for the short duration of most CT scans. In rare cases, the anesthesiologist may have to wear lead protection and remain present during the scan, usually for airway monitoring.

If a peripheral IV is required, as is in the case for injection of iodinated contrast and angiography, the IV anesthesia can be placed in the holding area, preferably using a local anesthetic vapo-coolant (freeze spray) or local anesthetic via jet-injector (J-tip lidocaine). Alternatively, it can be placed after inhalation induction by mask. It should be noted that while some patients may tolerate placement of the PIV, they may have a difficult time tolerating the physical injection of the intravenous contrast media. The feeling of IV contrast being injected by bolus has been described as a mild, warm flushing at the site of injection, which spreads over the body and may be particularly intense in the perineum. Patients may also experience nausea, headache, flushing, itching, and/or a metallic taste.[9]

Fluoroscopy

The anesthesia provider will occasionally be contacted to assist with imaging exams in the General Fluoroscopy Department. Commonly encountered exams in this area include barium enemas, as well as simple radiographs of extremities, the head and neck, and chest. Autistic patients with developmental delays or physically stronger patients (often adolescents or young adults) may require sedation for even the briefest of exams. Utilization of an oral anxiolytic, such as diazepam, prescribed by the patient's primary care physician, can be given to patients described as "difficult to get into the hospital without getting upset," and may be sufficient to allow exam completion. If insufficient, intramuscular injection with ketamine and/or midazolam, or inhalational volatile anesthetic technique can be employed. The latter technique will require a scavenging system for exhaled gases, and therefore may be less feasible. Additional assistants, care providers, or security personnel may be required with older (and heavier) patients who are combative.

Nuclear Medicine

Nuclear medicine technology is used for patient requiring diagnostic scans for various disease processes, including bone abnormalities (infection, tumor, or fracture), metastatic tumors (PET—positron emission tomography), urologic abnormalities (Lasix–Rena scan), gastrointestinal bleeding, brain, heart and lung function, and others. A peripheral IV is usually required for injection of a radioactive agent. After injection, a specified amount of time is required to pass until a body scan is performed. For most scans, there is zero stimulation during the scan itself, similar to other radiographic imaging. For all scans, it is a requirement that the patient is motionless, in part due to the very narrow scanner dimensions, but also because

excessive movement may require the scan to be recompleted in its entirety. The scanner itself emits no radiation; therefore, the anesthesia provider may be present in the room during the entire scan.

Like other imaging procedures described in this chapter, the anesthetic technique will vary depending upon patient characteristics, and type and length of the scan. Most scans will be 45 minutes to an hour in length. Any provider skilled in peripheral IV placement can place the line. The child may be allowed to temporarily leave the Nuclear Medicine Department following injection of radioactive material if the scan requires a time delay, but adherence to strict NPO guidelines must be stressed, as well as ensuring the PIV is safely secured and will not be removed, either inadvertently or intentionally by the child. When the patient returns for the scan, anesthesia is commonly maintained at the author's institution using propofol (by continuous infusion) or dexmedetomidine. As described in the MRI section of this chapter, a bolus dose of 1 mcg/kg of dexmedetomidine over 10 minutes, combined with a single-bolus of 1 to 2 mg/kg of propofol at induction, is usually sufficient to complete the 45- to 60-minute painless scan. The patient may require an intermittent propofol bolus (0.5 to 1 mg/kg), especially as the 45-minute mark approaches. This technique has the potential benefit of a wide-awake patient at the conclusion of the scan, who may bypass the extended recovery phase of anesthesia and is ready for a prompt discharge.

Nuclear medicine bladder scans require placement of a urinary catheter to monitor elimination of radioactively detected urine. The radioactive material is injected *after* securement of the PIV and urinary catheter and the scan begins immediately. If a scavenging system is available, this could allow induction of general anesthesia by inhalational technique to facilitate PIV and urinary catheter placement, which are both painful and anxiety-provoking. The maintenance of anesthetic can be with propofol and/or dexmedetomidine, as described above.

Interventional Radiology

Procedures in the interventional radiology suite can vary from simple peripherally inserted central catheter (PICC) lines to interventions for patients with complex medical problems. Commonly performed procedures in this offsite location include diagnostic and therapeutic cerebral angiography, venography, sclerotherapy of lymphatic and vascular malformations, soft-tissue, bone, and organ biopsies, drain and tube placements, lumbar punctures, placement of larger intravenous catheters (tunneled central lines), joint steroid injections, and placement of nasogastric and nasojejunal feeding tubes. The variability of patient comorbidities and status can be dramatic. The proceduralists may vary from physicians, to physician assistants, to nurse practitioners. The anesthesia provider in this area should be flexible, communicate well, and expect the unexpected.

The anesthetic plan in the interventional radiology suite widely varies. Length of procedure, patient age, comorbidities, and maturity level will naturally affect the anesthetic choice.

Sedation, ranging from light to moderate, may suffice for simple procedures such as placement of PICC lines, peripheral joint aspirations/steroid injections, lumbar punctures, and placement of nasogastric and nasojejunal feeding tubes. Oral (benzodiazepines) or intravenous (benzodiazepines, opioids, ketamine, propofol, dexmedetomidine) medications are reasonable choices. Deeper sedation, and potentially general anesthesia, may be required for more painful procedures, such as bone and organ biopsies, tunneled central lines, and drain placements for abscesses.

Spontaneous versus controlled ventilation, and anesthesia with or without an airway will be determined by procedure type, length, and patient factors. Airway anatomy and physiology, patients with a full stomach, or those that are vomiting may necessitate placement of an endotracheal tube. An endotracheal tube is also necessary during procedures requiring manipulation of the end-tidal CO_2, such as cerebral angiograms and neurointerventions, which may require vasoconstriction or vasodilation of cerebral vessels. Angiography may additionally require intermittent breath-holds, necessitating controlled ventilation. This can be achieved with administration of either a muscle relaxant or a bolus of propofol.

During certain cerebral embolization procedures, as with injection of glue for arterial-venous malformations, the interventionalist may ask for a brief complete cessation of blood flow. The goal is to slow the flow through arteriovenous malformation feeding artery and to prevent systemic embolization of glue.[10] It is reasonable to first attempt this with a bolus of propofol to cause temporary hypotension and reduced blood flow. Use of sodium nitroprusside has also been described by Sinha and colleagues. If these techniques are insufficient, it may be required to administer incremental doses of intravenous adenosine to cause transient asystole. Cutaneous pacemaker should be readily available. Some advocate placement of cutaneous pacemaker pads prior to adenosine administration. While arterial line placement is not necessary for all interventional radiological procedures, it is absolutely recommended in cases requiring controlled hypotension.

It is common for larger pediatric hospitals to have a dedicated interventional radiology suite. The specialty though has diverse training and subspecialties, and a particular pediatric interventional radiology physician may not have subspecialty training in a particular disease process. While relatively uncommon, an example of this would be a child presenting with an acute thrombotic stroke requiring angiographic thrombus–directed tPA administration. At the author's institution, the adult interventional radiologist travels to the pediatric hospital to provide emergency intervention. The anesthetic care of an emergent procedure such as this will require an established plan and critical communication, as multiple systems interact during the care of the patient, all while under time pressure.

Anesthetic emergence of patients at the interventional radiology suite may differ from those commonly cared for in the operating room. Placement, and subsequent removal, of large-bore sheaths for the procedure leaves puncture sites that are at increased risk of bleeding. Both intravenous and intra-arterial techniques are utilized, making bleeding risk variable, but nonetheless introduce the potential risk for significant postoperative hematoma and limb ischemia. Sheath sites and peripheral pulses will need to be monitored in the postoperative phase of care. Patients will need to remain flat and immobile for an extended period of time, occasionally for up to 4 to 6 hours. For the young and high-risk patients, it can be helpful to use dexmedetomidine, by either bolus or continuous infusion, to maintain post-procedural sedation at least for the first hour, when bleeding risk is greatest. A continuous infusion of dexmedetomidine will require continuous one-on-one monitoring by an experienced care provider, usually in an intensive care unit.

OTHER OFF-SITE ANESTHETIC LOCATIONS

Radiation Therapy

In all but the largest of pediatric hospitals, radiation therapy for oncologic diseases will occur at offsite locations, usually at adult hospitals. Targeted therapy for brain and brainstem tumors as well as intra-abdominal and pelvic tumors (neuroblastoma and sarcoma) are common. Conventional radiotherapy, shaped-beam radiotherapy, gamma knife, and high-energy proton beam therapy (cyclotron) have all been used in children, and have similar monitoring and anesthetic requirements.[3] The imaging and treatment, while non-stimulating and brief, can be accompanied by potential adverse events, as oncologic patients can be some of the most critically ill cared for by anesthesiologists.

Treatments are performed daily, often over a period of 4 to 6 weeks. The treatment itself may only last 5 to 10 minutes, but the patient will be required to be immobile during its entirety. Patients will have long-term intravenous access in situ, usually a tunneled central line or port. Adherence to sterile techniques with manipulation of these lines is of critical importance, due to the patient's likely immunocompromised state. Anesthetics are generally intravenous based, as there are rarely scavenging systems in radiation therapy locations. Propofol, by either continuous infusion or intermittent bolus, is commonly utilized. For patients presenting with depressed mental status but still requiring some form of sedation to remain still, an intravenous midazolam or dexmedetomidine bolus may suffice.

A unique consideration in patients having radiation therapy is the requirement that all personnel must be evacuated from the radiation room during the treatment phase.

This will require continuous live video monitoring of the patient and vital signs. Minimal monitoring guidelines, established by the American Society of Anesthesiologists (ASA) in the "Statement on Non-operating Room Anesthetizing Locations," must be followed at all times.

Magnetoencephalography (MEG) Scans

This imaging technique is used to produce a magnetic source image to pinpoint seizure focus in patients with a refractory seizure disorder. Used in conjunction with MRI, the MEG scan allows a more accurate mapping of seizure foci. Compared to electroencephalography (EEG), the scan allows better spatial resolution in epilepsy foci localization.[11] The scanner is used to detect and amplify magnetic signals produced by the brain without emitting radiation or magnetic fields as do CT and MRI.

Children requiring MEG scans may require anesthesia for portions of the scan to allow completion. Propofol, which would be a natural choice, can produce high-frequency artifacts, making interpretation of the data by the neurologist difficult. A case series of patients reported in *Pediatric Anesthesia* by König from Cincinnati Children's Hospital describes a successful anesthetic technique using dexmedetomidine, which minimizes the interfering interictal activity.[11] They report using dexmedetomidine as the primary technique, either after sevoflurane induction to allow PIV placement or with an existing PIV line. Loading doses of 1.5 to 2 mcg/kg followed by infusions of 0.8 mcg/kg/h are reported in their case series. A similar technique is utilized at the author's institution, with good success.

Anesthetizing on the Wards

Anesthesia providers will occasionally be asked to provide sedation for children requiring procedures such as lumbar puncture, nasogastric tubes, and dressing changes. Some procedures may be considerably painful, and some patients may have repeated procedures on sequential days. The goal for these procedures should be to complete them with the minimal amount of stress as possible while keeping the patient safe. Anesthetic choice should be tailored to the procedure and any relevant patient comorbidities.

Critical Care Unit

Postoperative patients being managed in the critical care setting often require further procedures but may not be stable enough for transfer to the operating room. Cardiac patients requiring cardioversion, or those with an open chest requiring closure, may be best suited to have a bedside procedure. Neonatal patients can have specialized management strategies, including high-frequency oscillation ventilation (HFOV), which make transportation difficult.

Neonatal emergency surgery may also require bedside procedures, which will require a mobile anesthesiologist.

Space is often limited and time is crucial. Communication is vital when this occurs, as there will be many providers involved—surgeons, surgical technicians, anesthesiologists, nurses, anesthesia technicians and possibly trainees.

REFERENCES

1. *Standards, Guidelines, and Practice Parameters.* Available at www.asahq.org.
2. Davidson AJ, Morton NS, Arnup SJ, et al. Apnea after awake regional and general anesthesia in infants: the general anesthesia compared to spinal anesthesia study—comparing apnea and neurodevelopmental outcomes, a randomized controlled trial. *Anesthesiology.* 2015;123(1):38-54.
3. Holzman RS, Mancuso TJ, Polaner DM. *A Practical Approach to Pediatric Anesthesia.* 2008; Philadelphia, PA: Wolters Kluwer Health/Lippincott Williams & Wilkins.
4. Frankville DD, Spear RM, Dyck JB. The dose of propofol required to prevent children from moving during magnetic resonance imaging. *Anesthesiology.* 1993;79:953-958.
5. Koroglu A, Demirbilek S, Teksan H, Sagir O, But AK, Ersoy MO. Sedative, haemodynamic and respiratory effects of dexmedetomidine in children undergoing magnetic resonance imaging examination: preliminary results. *Br J Anaesth.* 2005;94(6):821-824.
6. Koroglu A, Teksan H, Sagir O, Yucel A, Toprak HI, Ersoy OM. A comparison of the sedative, hemodynamic, and respiratory effects of dexmedetomidine and propofol in children undergoing magnetic resonance imaging. *Anesth Analg.* 2006;103(1):63-67.
7. Mason KP, Zurakowski D, Zgleszewski SE, et al. High dose dexmedetomidine as the sole sedative for pediatric MRI. Pediatric *Anesthesia.* 2008;18(5):403-411.
8. Estkowski LM, Morris JL, Sinclair EA. Characterization of dexmedetomidine dosing and safety in neonates and infants. *J Pediatr Pharmacol Ther.* 2015;20(2):112-118.
9. Singh J, Daftary A. Iodinated contrast media and their adverse reactions. *J Nucl Med Technol.* 2008;36(2):69-74.
10. Sinha PK, Neema PK, Rathod RC. Anesthesia and intracranial arteriovenous malformation. *Neurol India.* 2004;52:163-170.
11. König MW, Mahmoud MA, Fujiwara H, Hemasilpin N, Lee KH, Rose DF. Influence of anesthetic management on quality of magnetoencephalography scan data in pediatric patients: a case series. *Pediatric Anesthesia.* 2009;19:507-512.

Post-Anesthesia Care Unit

Jeannette Kierce

Preparation for recovery begins long before the child arrives on the unit; there are a number of things that can be done starting in the preoperative area that will influence emergence and wakeup. There is some evidence that a quiet induction in a calm child is more likely to result in a quieter wakeup.[1,2] It also appears to be the case that slower, more gradual emergence combined with minimal stimulus during that emergence may also decrease agitation in the PACU.[3] Preemptive pain management will decrease pain as an element, and PONV prophylaxis, including avoidance of risks factors and medications, can also be valuable especially in those at higher risk.

PACU SETUP

Physical Space Requirements

The PACU should ideally be located in close proximity to the operating room (OR); both to decrease transport times and to ensure readily availability of personnel and support in case of emergency. An open plan is frequently employed to facilitate monitoring, but provision should be made for either separation of spaces (ie, curtain) or physical movement to a different area to provide some privacy for child and parents in the later stages of recovery.

Personnel Requirements

Nursing staff must be competent in recognizing and initiating treatment for commonly encountered issues and recognizing when assistance is desirable/necessary. They should have experience and training in pediatric resuscitation, including airway management and cardiovascular support, in recognizing and assessing pain, and good interpersonal ability to manage parents. Skills should be frequently assessed and updated to maintain competency; practice sessions or simulations can be invaluable. Clear delineation of physician supervision must be established and a clear policy of whom to call for assistance known to all staff. Also clearly indicated must be handoff and signout protocols.

Equipment Requirements

The recovery space must be equipped to handle all potential issues that may arise during the recovery process. Oxygen (O_2) should be provided with humidification and a blender for titration. A second O_2 source with an attached self-inflating bag ready for use is desirable. Tubing for blow-by O_2 and a variety of masks, nasal cannulas, and oral and nasal airways of different sizes should be immediately at hand. Suction must be present and functioning with appropriate size catheters for use in the child. This equipment may be present in the room but out of sight to decrease anxiety in the child and his or her family.

Full cardiopulmonary monitoring should be performed with noninvasive blood pressure (NIBP), electrocardiogram (EKG), pulse oximetry (SpO_2), respiratory rate (RR), and temperature (T). End-tidal carbon dioxide ($EtCO_2$) monitoring should be available and certainly used, at minimum, in the instrumented airway to monitor adequacy of ventilation. Nasal cannulas with capability for $EtCO_2$ monitoring along with O_2 provision are available and compatible with many monitors. The capability to monitor invasive pressure lines (when present) should be available.

Commonly used medications for the treatment of pain, PONV, and respiratory distress should be readily accessible but secure in the environment—as should medications for the reversal of narcotics, benzodiazepines, and neuromuscular blockers.

Emergency equipment, possibly most readily organized in the form of a code cart, should be present on the unit and periodically checked for completeness and expiration. This should include medications, airway management equipment, and (possibly) invasive line kits with all equipment needed for placement.

TRANSPORT TO PACU

The laryngeal mask airway or endotracheal tube, if present, can be removed deep or awake according to the judgment and preference of the provider. Once the airway is judged to be stable, the patient may be transported to the PACU. The child is placed in the stretcher in the lateral position with the neck moderately extended to decrease airway obstruction. This position also protects against oropharyngeal secretions falling onto the vocal cords and against vomiting resulting in aspiration. Guardrails should be up and padding considered to prevent a fall or injury resulting from the sudden motion of the child; keeping a hand on the child can also help in this regard. Oxygen is generally recommended for transport as children are more likely to desaturate on the way to the PACU. How the oxygen is delivered may be dependent upon acceptance by the child; nasal cannulas may work well in the older child, but "blow-by" may be the only form tolerated in younger children. Provider monitoring of respirations during transportation can be accomplished with precordial stethoscope or direct detection of exhalation on a hand under the chin. At a minimum, pulse oximetry monitoring is frequently employed for transport for any but the shortest trip to the PACU. For the more critical patient, full cardiorespiratory monitoring is recommended along with drugs and equipment for emergent reintubation. If the child is intubated, a ventilator should be confirmed to be present in the PACU before transport is undertaken, and ventilation supported or provided with a self-inflating bag. The child should be covered with a blanket during transport to keep him or her warm when traveling through a less regulated temperature environment.

PACU MANAGEMENT

Initial Care and Handoff

Upon arrival in the PACU, nursing staff should arrive immediately at the bedside. First priority should be to confirm patency of airway and adequacy of ventilation, and ensure the presence and application of O_2. Monitors should be applied and initial vitals including heart rate (HR), NIBP, SpO_2, T, and RR recorded. Etiology of agitation, if present, should be assessed and treated. Initial assessment of pain and nausea or vomiting should be made and treatment given if needed. Formal report should be given to nursing personnel once initial assessment is complete. The report should include preoperative information such as age and weight, allergies, comorbidities, and premedication given. Intraoperative information should include surgery performed, type of anesthesia and medications administered, airway management, lines, and fluids. Drips, blood products transfused, latest labs, and complications should also be included as applicable. Medications of relevance to the PACU and postoperative course of care should be reported along with time of administration. These might include antibiotics, steroids, analgesics, anticonvulsants, and sedatives. Regional, peripheral nerve blocks or local infiltration should be reported when performed.

The Road to Recovery

Once care is turned over to the PACU staff, the child is monitored on a continuous basis until he or she is fully recovered from the anesthetic. Vitals are recorded every 15 minutes at minimum with interventions applied as needed. In the initial recovery phase, minimal stimulation is frequently applied when possible as it can result in a less agitated return to consciousness. Depending on the unit, parents may be brought to the bedside immediately upon arrival, after initial assessment and report, or when the child awakens. In all cases, it is good if they have been prepared for what they will see. If the child remains unconscious, reassurance that this is normal and that the child will wake up calmer if allowed to do so on their own should be stressed. If the child is awake and agitated, parents should be informed that this, too, is not unusual and enlist their help in calming the child.

PACU PROBLEMS

Agitation

It is essential to try to determine the etiology of agitation, as many conditions may manifest in this way. Obviously, it is easiest if the child can communicate this information themselves, but this is not always possible, especially in preverbal or neurologically challenged children. Some of the things that may present as agitation include hypoventilation with hypoxia and/or hypercarbia, pain, metabolic issues, preexisting neurological and/or behavioral conditions, and separation anxiety. Knowledge of the child's pre-op baseline, and parental presence, may help distinguish some of these, but a high degree of suspicion must be kept for the others. When no other cause of the agitation can be identified and the degree of agitation is profound, the child may be experiencing emergence delirium (ED). This is a dissociated state of consciousness with inconsolability, thrashing, and incoherence. The characteristic feature of the phenomenon is that child does not seem to be aware of its surroundings and does not recognize even his or her parents. It is generally brief in duration and self-limited, but intervention may be needed to prevent the child from injuring himself or herself or others. Complications of uncontrolled ED include increased bleeding and pain, increased medication use, increased need for staffing, increased infectious risk from pulling at dressings and drains, loss of intravenous access, and a longer PACU stay.

There are a number of theories as to the etiology of this condition, but no definitive answers. Some of the proposed causes include rapid awakening in a strange environment, variable recovery of central nervous system (CNS) function, precipitous withdrawal of agent from GABA receptors, psychomotor side effects of potent agents, and inadequately treated pain.[4] While pain may be a partial answer, the condition is also seen in pain-free settings in which anesthesia has been given.[5] Independent risk factors that have been determined or proposed include age <5 years, head and neck cases, use of inhalational agents as opposed to total intravenous anesthesia, rapid emergence, anxious child and/or parents, poor socialization, and low adaptability scores in the child.[6] Depth of anesthesia as measured by bispectral index scores (BIS) does not seem to be predictive of incidence.[7] There is some evidence that the level of anxiety on induction has a significant impact on the severity of agitation on emergence.[8] Decreasing that anxiety can be accomplished in a number of ways including sedative premedication, parental presence at induction, or distraction. If the rapidity of emergence or drug metabolism contributes to the severity of ED, then it would logically follow that slowing the emergence might mitigate some of the symptoms,

and this does indeed appear to be the case. When combined with minimal stimulation as the child emerges from the anesthetic, the improvement can be significant.[9]

Among the tools that have been developed to evaluate ED, the Pediatric Anesthesia Emergence Delirium Scale (PAEDS) has high specificity and sensitivity. This tool consists of five descriptors scored on a 0–4 scale (with 4 being most abnormal):

1. The child makes eye contact with the caregiver;
2. The child's actions are purposeful;
3. The child is aware of his/her surroundings;
4. The child is restless;
5. The child is inconsolable.[10]

A wide variety of therapies have been reported to be efficacious both as prophylaxis and as treatment for ED; most medications have indeed been proposed for both.[11] Nonpharmacological management can include swaddling. Parental presence can be reassuring; allowing the parent to hold the child or get up into the stretcher with it can be very calming. These may be enough as this is a self-limited condition and is generally of short duration.

Some treatments focus on the use of analgesic strategies either preemptively or in the PACU to mitigate the severity of emergence agitation by removing the component that may be attributable to pain. Narcotics given prophylactically in the OR decrease the incidence of ED, and also work as treatment—probably through combination of analgesia and sedation.[12,13] Other analgesic agents may or may not have any impact: nonsteroidal anti-inflammatory drugs (NSAIDs)[14] and acetaminophen[15] may or may not have any consistent impact in studies on ED although they contribute to better post-op analgesia. Local infiltration, peripheral nerve blocks, and regional anesthesia done prophylactically have been shown to be effective.[16]

The other approach to treatment (with much overlap) primarily seeks to sedate the child and/or slow the wakeup from anesthesia (Table 37-1). Propofol used during the case either alone or in combination with decreased minimum alveolar concentration (MAC) of potent agent decreases incidence of ED. Propofol may be given in the form of an infusion, or as a single dose at the end of case alone to be effective.[17] A single bolus for induction does not seem to have the same prophylactic effect. As treatment in the PACU, it is very short acting, but may interrupt the agitation long enough to mitigate severity.[18] Ketamine and nalbuphine have both been successfully given prophylactically to decrease the risk of developing ED in the PACU.[19–21] Dexmedetomidine or clonidine given pre- or intraoperatively has also been shown to decrease the incidence. As a treatment in PACU, they can suffer from relatively longer durations of action and higher degree of sedation which may delay discharge, particularly in the outpatient setting.[22–24] Midazolam given as a premedication or in the OR may act as prophylaxis although reports

Table 37-1. Selected Medication Dosing for Emergence Delirium in PACU

Fentanyl	1 mcg/kg
Propofol	1 mg/kg
Dexmedetomidine	0.25–0.5 mcg/kg
Clonidine	2 mcg/kg
Midazolam	0.025 mg/kg
Ketamine	0.25mg/kg to 0.5 mg/kg IV
Nalbuphine	0.1 mg/kg IV

are mixed; this may depend on the severity of preoperative anxiety and the length of the case.[25] Many other reports indicate that it increases incidence rather than decreases it. It has been given as treatment of ED in the PACU with mixed results; the level of sedation produced has led to prolonged PACU times.[26,27]

Desaturation and Respiratory Distress

A large percentage of otherwise normal children will develop desaturation during transport or during their stay in PACU if no supplemental O_2 is provided. It occurs sooner, is more pronounced, and lasts longer than in adults. The cause is usually atelectasis, but upper airway problems such as obstruction, croup, laryngospasm, bronchospasm, and apnea are also more common in children.

Atelectasis is common in the PACU and is due to loss of FRC from the combination of supine position and residual general anesthesia. This results from abdominal pressure being transmitted to the thoracic cavity via the cranially displaced diaphragm in the spontaneously breathing patient; muscle relaxant residual and narcotic administration may accentuate this effect.[28] Other factors such as mucus plugging, less well-developed diaphragmatic musculature causing easier fatigue, and absorption atelectasis due to high FiO_2 may also contribute. Closing volume is also greater in young children in whom the elastic supporting structure of the lung is incompletely developed. This puts the infant at greater risk for atelectasis because airway closure can occur even during tidal breathing.[29]

Decreased hypopharyngeal and tongue muscle tone causing mechanical obstruction of the upper airway is present as a residual effect of anesthesia with potent agents; sedative agents, narcotics, and residual neuromuscular blockade (NMB) will exaggerate this effect. Airway manipulation consisting of chin lift and/or jaw thrust may relieve the obstruction, or bag-mask ventilatory assistance may be needed. Train-of-four monitoring can be employed as in adults to assess the degree of NMB and need for additional reversal. Naloxone and flumazenil can be given to reverse narcotic and benzodiazepines, respectively. If none of the above is effective, the child can be reintubated and ventilated until his or her ability to spontaneously maintain an adequate airway is regained.

Laryngospasm in the PACU is most frequently caused by secretions contacting the vocal cords in a heavily sedated child. It can be recognized by the presence of respiratory effort in the absence of actual air movement. Treatment includes positive pressure delivered via bag/mask for milder cases or pharmacological release with sedation, and/or succinylcholine and intubation if necessary.

Croup resulting from airway edema will most frequently present, at least early on, as adequate air movement with increased effort and high-pitched inspiratory stridor. Treatment is humidified O_2 and nebulized racemic epinephrine to decrease swelling. Steroids will not help acutely, but can be given as they will help in the longer term to decrease the swelling.

Bronchospasm is seen in the PACU not only in children with asthma and seasonal allergies, but also in those with an (known or unsuspected) upper respiratory infection, and in those exposed to cigarette smoking (or marijuana smoke). This will frequently not present initially as desaturation, but as increased work of breathing. The treatment includes albuterol nebulization treatment, O_2, and steroid for longer term stabilization.

Obstructive sleep apnea (OSA) is most commonly due to adenotonsillar hypertrophy in children; although with the increasing amount of childhood obesity, more children are presenting with a mixed form. A pre-op history of snoring, frequent arousal during sleep, daytime hyperactivity or poor attention, or bedwetting can alert one to the possible existence of this disease process.

Neonatal apnea comes in a variety of forms with different etiologies and implications. Apnea of prematurity is correlated with the degree of prematurity and corrected gestational age (CGA), as well as hemoglobulin levels. Post-anesthetic apnea rates approach normal sometime after 55 to 60 weeks CGA.[30] As the name suggests, the phenomenon is rarely seen in full-term infants and is most likely related to immaturity of brainstem respiratory control in the premature brain.[31] There does seem to be less frequent occurrence with subarachnoid blocks (SABs) as opposed to general anesthesia (GA), although this benefit is lost if sedation is given.[32] Periodic breathing can be seen in both premature infants and full-term infants as a normal pattern; pauses in breathing rarely last more than about 12 seconds and are not accompanied by bradycardia, although mild desaturations that resolve spontaneously with resumption of breathing can occur.[33] Premature infants have a biphasic response to hypercarbia on their ventilation; initially the TV increases, then the RR decreases. This response can be blunted in the presence of increased FiO_2.[31]

Central hypoventilation syndrome is related to neurological disease processes (congenital vs acquired), and is a manifestation of dysfunctional autonomic regulation of ventilation. The ventilatory response to hypercarbia is blunted, and supplemental oxygen may cause apnea. These children can be exquisitely sensitive to the central nervous syndrome depressant effects of sedatives, narcotics, hypnotics, and obviously GA. In disease of long-standing and/or poor control, significant degrees of pulmonary hypertension and heart failure may be present. The autonomic regulation of other organ systems may also be impaired leading to decreased gastric motility with increased aspiration risk, or dysfunction of cardiac rate control with bradycardia or heart block.[34]

Postoperative pulmonary edema (POPE) can be seen after tonsillectomy and adenoidectomy, or other obstructive airway mass excision such as airway papilloma. Removal of the obstructing mass causes relief of the increased end-expiratory pressure that has been ongoing and results in pulmonary edema. This is usually mild and self-limited, but may occasionally require treatment with diuretic and positive end-expiratory pressure (PEEP); occasionally a brief period of ventilation is needed while waiting for it to resolve.[35]

Hemodynamic Instability

Compared to the adult patient, cardiovascular events in the pediatric post-op population are far less common.

Bradycardia is essentially hypoxia until proven otherwise. If the saturation is adequate, other causes that may cause bradycardia, such as medication effects (narcotic), should be sought. There is not generally any need to treat the bradycardia other than addressing the cause, unless it is combined with hypotension.

Tachycardia in the recovery room may be due to hypovolemia, hyperthermia, pain, or agitation. Carefully assessing the child and his or her other vital signs can frequently direct attention to the correct cause; this should be addressed to reduce the HR.

Hypotension in the post-op period should raise concerns for hypovolemia and/or hemorrhage. Hypovolemia should be suspected in cases in which the child was NPO for a prolonged period before surgery or in which large volume shifts or blood losses were seen. A crystalloid fluid bolus is a reasonable first step in treatment of hypotension. In cases where significant blood loss occurred in the OR, or could potentially be happening in a disguised fashion in the PACU (bleeding tonsils), checking a hemoglobin level to rule out significant anemia would be appropriate.[36]

Hypertension is almost always due to pain and/or agitation, but rarer conditions should be kept in mind and ruled out if the hypertension persists despite treatment.

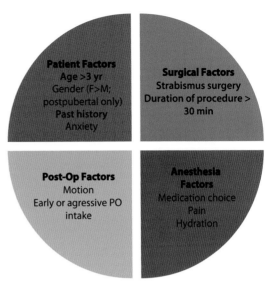

▲ **Figure 37-1.** Risk factors for PONV.

Postoperative Nausea and Vomiting

The incidence of PONV in young patients is generally held to be about double that of the adult population. In many studies only POV is measured due to the difficulty in identifying nausea in pediatric patients, so this rate may actually be significantly higher. In pediatric patients POV incidences are lowest below age 3 and highest in the range of 11 to 14 years with female preponderance after reaching puberty.[37] This is generally identified by both parents and the child as being one of the least satisfactory parts of their PACU experience and can contribute to unanticipated admission if uncontrolled.[38] Many of the other risk factors (Figure 37-1) identified in adults are true for children as well.[39]

Treatment

There is considerable debate about the desirability of prophylaxis for PONV as opposed to treatment; much of the conversation focuses on cost-effectiveness versus patient satisfaction. Given that there are readily identifiable risk factors for this complication, a prudent approach may be to use prophylaxis in those children identified to be at least at moderate risk (see Figure 37-2). This prophylaxis can take a multitiered approach of using regional anesthesia where possible, considering the use of nonpharmacological interventions, eliminating as many of the modifiable risk factors as possible in the OR, and antiemetic medication administration.[40-42]

Preoperative measures that can be used to influence the frequency and severity of PONV include attention to the state of hydration and catabolic state. Prolonged NPO times should be avoided if at all possible, and IV hydration

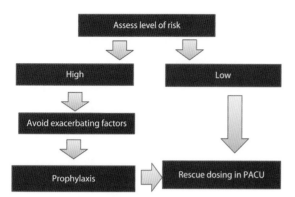

▲ Figure 37-2. An approach to PONV management.

Table 37-2. Selected Antiemetic Dosing

Ondansetron	0.10 to 0.15 mg/kg to 4 mg
Dexamethasone	0.25 mg/kg to 10 mg
Diphenhydramine	0.5 to 1 mg/kg
Dolasetron	0.35 mg/kg to 12.5 mg
Granisetron	10 mcg/kg
Droperidol	10–15 mcg/kg

given to compensate when it does occur. Recent research is showing benefit to carbohydrate-containing drinks on the morning of surgery in the adult population; similar studies on children are currently lacking.[43] A nonpharmacological approach to PONV prophylaxis that is attracting increased interest is that of acupressure, acupoint injection, and/or acupuncture. Acupressure and acupuncture can be performed with or without electrical stimulus to intensify the effect. In adults, the stimulus is usually performed prior to induction of general anesthesia. Since needles for acupuncture are not well tolerated by younger children awake, it has been questioned whether this modality is realistically available in the pediatric population. P6 acupoint injection has proved to be as effective as droperidol even when performed under GA in children for prevention of early PONV.[44] Scopolamine in patch form at a dose of 1.5 mg is approved for use in children over 12 years old and weighing at least 40 kg. There are few studies specifically addressing the use of scopolamine in younger children. Because of the relative lack of data, scopolamine is most commonly reserved for use in adolescents who suffer from motion sickness or have a history of intractable PONV with previous surgery. The patch is ideally placed at least 2 hours preoperatively. It has the advantage of being able to provide continuous treatment into the postoperative/post-discharge period.[45]

Intraoperative choices can also affect the incidence and severity of PONV in the susceptible patient. Use of potent agent and >50% N_2O are very strong risk factors for PONV in the susceptible patient, so avoiding their use is indicated when feasible.[46] Propofol, used exclusively or as an adjunct to decreased MAC of potent agent, is very efficacious in preventing PONV; even a single bolus at the end of the case (although not solely on induction) is shown to be beneficial.[47] While pain treatment should be provided prior to emergence, decreasing the dose of, or eliminating the use of, narcotics for prophylactic analgesia and replacing them with nonsteroidal anti-inflammatory drugs (NSAIDs) and/or acetaminophen, combined with aggressive use of local infiltration or regional blocks where possible, will also contribute to decreasing PONV incidence.[46,47] For patients at moderate to high risk of PONV, recommendation has been made to use dual antiemetic prophylaxis. Ondansetron, a serotonin receptor (5HT3) antagonist, and others of its class have been shown to be more effective as a group in the prevention of vomiting than nausea and have a very good safety profile. It is for this reason they are frequently the drugs of first choice for prophylaxis in children.[48] Dexamethasone is a steroid medication with anti-inflammatory and antiemetic properties. It is effective as compared to placebo for prophylaxis of both early- and late-phase POV with no clinically significant adverse effects in otherwise healthy patients.[49] For moderate- to high-risk patients, the recommendation is for dual antiemetic prophylaxis prior to the end of surgery; dexamethasone and ondansetron are the most common combination with increased efficacy compared to the use of either alone.[50] Droperidol has been demonstrated to be effective in treating both early and late PONV. However, increased sedation, delayed emergence, and other minor CNS side effects such as anxiety and agitation have been observed. In addition, the Food and Drug Administration has added a black-box warning after some cases of arrhythmia resulting from prolonged QT were identified. The recommendations for EKG monitoring as well as the other CNS side effects have largely caused a decrease of use of this agent as a first-line agent.[51]

When the child suffers from PONV in the PACU, the approach to treatment differs depending on whether prophylactic medications had previously been used. In the previously untreated child, a dose of ondansetron is a first-line treatment, with dexamethasone often being the second choice. In the child who has been previously given antiemetics, a different class of medication should be given unless more than 6 hours have passed since the time of initial dosing (see Table 37-2).

Temperature Instability

Hypothermia is a frequent finding in the postanesthesia recovery unit. This is not only a concern from a comfort standpoint, but also a concern because of decreased metabolism of certain drugs, and slower awakening as well as evidence of poorer wound healing and increased risk of postoperative wound infections.[52] The best treatment is prevention by paying close attention in the OR to temperature preservation strategies. If present in the PACU, covering the child with warm blankets is efficacious in milder cases; the application of a forced-air warming blanket may be needed in more severe cases.

Hyperthermia can also be a concern because while it may merely be a result of overaggressive warming, it can also be an indicator of inflammation or infection. Overaggressive warming can usually be managed simply by removing some of the covering blankets. Inflammation may respond to antipyretics, while infection may require antibiotics. More serious concerns such as malignant hyperthermia should always be considered, especially if conservative measures fail to result in a decrease in temperature (or if it keeps increasing).

Pain and Discomfort

Measurement/assessment of pain in children can be challenging due to variation in individual manifestations and communication ability, and the difficulty of differentiating from anxiety, fear, agitation, and disorientation. Cultural factors, and cognitive delay or preexisting psychological and/or social effects also contribute to the difficulty.[53]

There are a number of validated tools including the observational tools such as Premature Infant Pain Profile (PIPP);[54] Face, Legs, Activity, Cry, Consolability Scale (FLACC);[55] and Children's Hospital of Eastern Ontario

Pain Scale (CHEOPS);[56] and the self-report tools such as Faces Pain Scale,[57] Visual Analogue Scale,[58,59] and the Numerical Rating Scale[60] among many others. These are geared to different ages and developmental stages.[61] It should be noted that measurement of pain in the post-anesthetic state can be even more challenging than usual due to residual drug effects.

When managing postoperative pain in children, the most common approach is to use a multimodal approach including behavioral interventions, local anesthetic infiltration, peripheral nerve block as single or continuous infusion, NSAIDs, acetaminophen, adjuncts such as dexmedetomidine or dexamethasone, opioids, and possibly antispasmodics (Figure 37-3).[62,63]

Preparing both the child and the parents ahead of time for discomfort and or numbness (in the case of local anesthetic usage) when the child awakens can significantly decrease the distress in the PACU, as can distraction and parental comforting. Having the parent at the bedside to comfort them and calm them when they awaken from anesthesia can help with the fear. Distraction methods such as TV or tablet use can also be useful.

Regional analgesia can be a very effective way of preventing pain in the PACU. Placing blocks in the pre-op area or in the PACU is often not as successful as in adult patients due to inability of children to tolerate or cooperate by holding still; older adolescents may allow placement with sufficient sedation. An alternative is to place the nerve block/regional anesthesia in the OR under GA either at the start of the case or prior to emergence. There have been concerns raised about safety of placing blocks under GA,

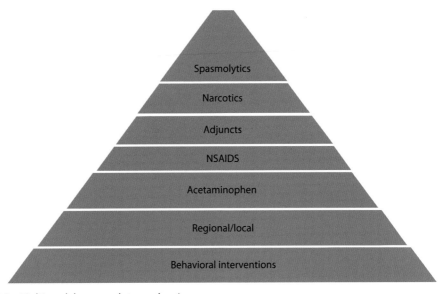

▲ **Figure 37-3.** Multimodal approach to analgesia.

but there does not seem to be any difference in complication rates when compared with awake placement.[64] It also allows extending the benefits of regional to children who would not otherwise be eligible. Placement at the beginning of the case can decrease the amount of medications needed in the OR and potentially decrease the incidence of PONV and other medication adverse effects.

Nonsteroidal anti-inflammatory drugs, most commonly ketorolac or ibuprofen, can be used throughout the perioperative period. Ibuprofen can be given orally either in the preoperative area prior to induction, particularly for shorter cases, or in the PACU. Ketorolac can be given in the OR or PACU via the intravenous route. There have been concerns raised about increased bleeding, renal risk, and orthopedic healing with the use of ketorolac, which have led some to limit its use in the perioperative period.[65]

Paracetamol and its prodrug acetaminophen can be given throughout the perioperative period in oral, intravenous, or rectal form. The rectal form of administration is more effective in the infant than in older children, but suffers from variable absorption. Numerous studies have demonstrated safety with higher rectal doses, but concern remains for hepatotoxicity if the cumulative dose exceeds 100 mg/kg/day.[66]

Several medications potentiate analgesic effects of other medications allowing lower doses to be effectively used (see Table 37-3). Perioperative systemic administration of alpha-2 antagonists (dexmedetomidine, clonidine) is associated with a useful potentiation of both systemic analgesics (particularly opioids) and local anesthetic sensory block in neuraxial and perineural routes.[67] Patients treated with dexamethasone have been found to experience less postoperative pain, require less postoperative opioids, have longer time to first analgesic dose, need less rescue analgesia, and have shorter PACU stays. The effect of dexamethasone is believed to be attributable to the anti-inflammatory properties of the medication. Although this effect is small, it tends to be stronger with earlier dosing.[68] Ketamine, a phencyclidine derivative, is useful as an adjunct analgesic that can prevent the development of opioid tolerance and hyperalgesia by inhibition of the NMDA receptors.[69]

Narcotics can be given in either the PO or IV form. The most commonly used narcotics in pediatric perioperative period are fentanyl, morphine, and hydromorphone in the IV form, and oxycodone or hydromorphone (in older children) in oral preparations. Due to variable metabolism leading to increased risk in some children (particularly after tonsillectomy), most pediatric practitioners now avoid codeine.

A number of procedures, such as ureteral reimplantation, dorsal rhizotomy, some orthopedic procedures, and posterior cervical decompression, can result in significant amounts of muscle spasm contributing to post-op pain. Children undergoing these procedures may benefit from spasmolytic medications such as diazepam.[70]

Discharge from PACU

Appropriateness for discharge from PACU is most often assessed using a postanesthesia recovery score. The most commonly used is the modified Aldrete Score which measures BP, respiration, consciousness, O_2 saturation, and motor activity on a 0–2 scale for a total maximum score of 10.[71] These scores are best combined with individual assessment of fitness for discharge with allowances being made for such considerations as preoperative baseline condition and whether the child is an inpatient or being discharged home into parental care. Recovery is usually divided into two stages: Stage I and Stage II (see Table 37-4).

Table 37-3. Selected Analgesic Dosing for Pediatric Patients

Acetaminophen	10–15 mg/kg (PO, IV, PR)
Ketamine	0.5–1 mg/kg IV
Ibuprofen	5–10 mg/kg PO
Ketorolac	0.5–1 mg/kg IV or IM
Morphine	50–100 mcg/kg IV
Oxycodone	0.1 mg/kg PO

Table 37-4. Sample Criteria for Discharge from PACU

Stage I (discharge to Stage II or floor)	Stage II (discharge home)
Awake or easily aroused	Intact gag reflex, swallowing, and cough allowing for oral intake
Airway maintained with intact protective reflexes	Ambulation/movement baseline/appropriate for development
SpO$_2$ >95% (room air) or stable at preoperative level (with or without supplemental O$_2$)	If regional anesthesia used, must demonstrate returning motor function
Normothermia	Minimal nausea or vomiting
Pain controlled	No signs of respiratory distress
Nausea/vomiting controlled	Oriented for developmental stage
No active bleeding	Voiding not necessary, but helpful
Hemodynamically stable within 20% of baseline	Hemodynamically stable within 20% of baseline

When the child is deemed ready for discharge, parents should be given instructions regarding fluid intake, pain and PONV management, as well as any special instructions in regard to the surgical procedure such as developments to be concerned about, wound care, and bathing. These should be provided verbally with time given for questions and for clarification. The instructions should then also be provided in written form for the parents to refer to when home; it can be helpful if a time schedule for pain medications is included. In the case of a foreign language–speaking family, if possible it can be very helpful to provide written instructions in their native language.

Unplanned Admission

A large proportion of pediatric surgeries are scheduled as outpatient cases; a significant concern with such cases is the unanticipated admission. This may be a result of unmanageable pain, PONV, inadequate oral intake, respiratory complications, surgical complications such as bleeding, or social reasons. The frequency of such admissions is a quality measure in addition to having significant familial implications. It also frequently results in prolonged PACU stay while waiting for a bed to become available. Common strategies to minimize the number of unanticipated admissions are more aggressive prophylaxis for PONV, generous use of regional anesthesia, and the use of non-narcotic analgesics whenever possible.[72]

Follow-Up Phone Call or Visit

Part of the practice of anesthesia is keeping track of complications. The post-op visit or phone call allows follow-up on issues such as recall, PONV, and pain-control/regional function as well as satisfaction with care.

REFERENCES

1. Yip P, Middleton P, Cyna AM, Carlyle AV. Nonpharmacological interventions for assisting the induction of anaesthesia in children. *Cochrane Database Syst Rev.* 2009;CD006447.
2. Kain ZN, Caldwell-Andrews AA, Mayes LC, et al. Family-centered preparation for surgery improves perioperative outcomes in children: a randomized controlled trial. *Anesthesiology.* 2007;106:65-74.
3. Bong CL, Lim E, Allen JC, et al. A comparison of single-dose dexmedetomidine or propofol on the incidence of emergence delirium in children undergoing general anaesthesia for magnetic resonance imaging. *Anaesthesia.* 2015;70:393-399.
4. Mohkamkar M, Farhoudi F, Alam-Sahebpour A, Mousavi SA, Khani S, Shahmohammadi S. Postanesthetic emergence agitation in pediatric patients under general anesthesia. *Iran J Pediatr.* 2014;24(2):184-190.
5. Cravero J, Surgenor S, Whalen K. Emergence agitation in paediatric patients after sevoflurane anaesthesia and no surgery: a comparison with halothane. *Paediatr Anaesth.* 2000;10(4):419-424.
6. Voepel-Lewis T, Malviya S, Tait AR. A prospective cohort study of emergence agitation in the pediatric postanesthesia care unit. *Anesth Analg.* 2003;96:1625-1630.
7. Frederick HJ, Wofford K, de Lisle DG, Schulman SR. A randomized controlled trial to determine the effect of depth of anesthesia on emergence agitation in children. *Anesth Analg.* 2016;122(4):1141-1146.
8. Kain ZN, Caldwell-Andrews AA, Maranets I, et al. Preoperative anxiety and emergence delirium and postoperative maladaptive behaviors. *Anesth Analg.* 2004;99:1648.
9. da Silva LM, Braz LG, Modolo NSP. Emergence agitation in pediatric anesthesia: current features. *J Pediatr (Rio J) Porto Alegre.* 2008;84(2):107-113.
10. Sikich N, Lerman J. Development and psychometric evaluation of the pediatric anesthesia emergence delirium scale. *Anesthesiology.* 2004;100(5):1138-1145.
11. Dahmani S, Delivet H, Hilly J. Emergence delirium in children: an update. *Curr Opin Anaesthesiol.* 2014;27(3):309-315.
12. Cohen IT, Finkel JC, Hannallah RS, Hummer KA, Patel KM. The effect of fentanyl on the emergence characteristics after desflurane or sevoflurane anesthesia in children. *Anesth Analg.* 2002;94(5):1178-1181.
13. Abdelhalim AA, Alarfaj AM. The effect of ketamine versus fentanyl on the incidence of emergence agitation after sevoflurane anesthesia in pediatric patients undergoing tonsillectomy with or without adenoidectomy. *Saudi J Anaesth.* 2013;7(4):392-398.
14. Kim D, Doo AR, Lim H, Son JS, Lee JR, Han YJ, Ko S. Effect of ketorolac on the prevention of emergence agitation in children after sevoflurane anesthesia. *Korean J Anesthesiol.* 2013;64(3):240-245.
15. Sajedi P, Baghery K, Hagibabie E, Mehr AM. Prophylactic use of oral acetaminophen or iv dexamethasone and combination of them on prevention emergence agitation in pediatric after adenotonsillectomy. *Int J Prev Med.* 2014;5(6):721-727.
16. Aouad MT, Kanazi GE, Siddik-Sayyid SM, Gerges FJ, Rizk LB, Baraka AS. Preoperative caudal block prevents emergence agitation in children following sevoflurane anesthesia. *Acta Anaesthesiol Scand.* 2005;49:300-304.
17. Aouad MT, Yazbeck-Karam VG, Nasr VG, El-Khatib MF, Kanazi GE, Bleik JH. A single dose of propofol at the end of surgery for the prevention of emergence agitation in children undergoing strabismus surgery during sevoflurane anesthesia. *Anesthesiology.* 2007;107(5):733-738.
18. van Hoff SL, O'Neill ES, Cohen LC, Collins BA. Does a prophylactic dose of propofol reduce emergence agitation in children receiving anesthesia? A systematic review and meta-analysis. *Paediatr Anaesth.* 2015;25(7):668-676.
19. Dalens BJ, Pinard AM, Létourneau DR, Albert NT, Truchon RJ. Prevention of emergence agitation after sevoflurane anesthesia for pediatric cerebral magnetic resonance imaging by small doses of ketamine or nalbuphine administered just before discontinuing anesthesia. *Anesth Analg.* 2006;102(4):1056-1061.
20. Abu-Shahwan I, Chowdary K. Ketamine is effective in decreasing the incidence of emergence agitation in children undergoing dental repair under sevoflurane general anesthesia. *Paediatr Anaesth.* 2007;17(9):846-850.
21. Khattab AM, El-Seify ZA. Sevoflurane-emergence agitation: effect of supplementary low-dose oral ketamine premedication in preschool children undergoing dental surgery. *Saudi J Anaesth.* 2009;3(2):61-66.
22. Shukry M, Clyde MC, KalarickalL PL, Ramadhyani U. Does dexmedetomidine prevent emergence delirium in children

after sevoflurane-based general anesthesia? *Pediatr Anesth.* 15:1098-1104.

23. Kulka PJ, Bressem M, Tryba M. Clonidine prevents sevoflurane-induced agitation in children. *Anesth Analg.* 2001;93(2):335-338.

24. Malviya S, Voepel-Lewis T, Ramamurthi RJ, Burke C, Tait AR. Clonidine for the prevention of emergence agitation in young children: efficacy and recovery profile. *Paediatr Anaesth.* 2006;16(5):554-559.

25. Bae JH, Koo BW, Kim SJ, Lee DH, Lee ET, Kang CJ. The effects of midazolam administered postoperatively on emergence agitation in pediatric strabismus surgery. *Korean J Anesthesiol.* 2010;58(1):45-49

26. Breschan C, Platzer M, Jost R, Stettner H, Likar R. Midazolam does not reduce emergence delirium after sevoflurane anesthesia in children. *Paediatr Anaesth.* 2007;17(4):347-352.

27. Ko YP, Huang CJ, Hung YC, et al. Premedication with low-dose oral midazolam reduces the incidence and severity of emergence agitation in pediatric patients following sevoflurane anesthesia. *Acta Anaesthesiol Sin.* 2001;39(4):169-177.

28. Ray K, Bodenham A, Paramasivam E. Pulmonary atelectasis in anaesthesia and critical care. *Brit J Anaesth.* 2014;14(5):236-245.

29. Duggan M, Kavanagh BP. Pulmonary atelectasis: a pathogenic perioperative entity. *Anesthesiology.* 2005;102(4):838-854.

30. Taneja B, Srivastava V, Saxena KN. Physiological and anaesthetic considerations for the preterm neonate undergoing surgery. *J Neonatal Surg.* 2012;1(1):14.

31. Zhao J, Gonzalez F, Mu D. Apnea of prematurity: from cause to treatment. *Eur J Pediatr.* 2011;170(9):1097-1105.

32. Frumiento C, Abajian JC, Vane DW. Spinal anesthesia for preterm infants undergoing inguinal hernia repair. *Arch Surg.* 2000;135(4):445-451.

33. Kelly DH, Stellwagen LM, Kaitz E, Shannon DC. Apnea and periodic breathing in normal full-term infants during the first twelve months. *Pediatr Pulmonol.* 1985;1(4):215-219.

34. Baum VC, O'Flaherty JE. *Anesthesia for Genetic, Metabolic & Dysmorphic Syndromes of Childhood.* 2nd ed. Philadelphia, PA: Lippincott, Williams & Wilkins. 2007:277-278.

35. Udeshi A, Cantie SM, Pierre E. Postobstructive pulmonary edema. *J Crit Care.* 2010:25(3):538.e1-e5.

36. Pawar DK. Common post-operative complications in children. *Indian J Anaesth.* 2012;56(5):196-501.

37. Bourdaud N, Devys JM, Bientz J, et al. Development and validation of a risk score to predict the probability of postoperative vomiting in pediatric patients: the VPOP score. *Paediatr Anaesth.* 2014;24(9):945-952.

38. Chatterjee S, Rudra A, Sengupta S. Current concepts in the management of postoperative nausea and vomiting. *Anesthesiol Res Pract.* 2011;2011:748031.

39. Eberhart LHJ, Geldner G, Kranke GP, et al. The development and validation of a risk score to predict the probability of postoperative vomiting in pediatric patients. *Anesth Analg.* 2004;99:1630-1637.

40. Gan TJ, Meyer T, Apfel CC, et al. Consensus guidelines for managing postoperative nausea and vomiting. *Anesth Analg.* 2003;97:62-71.

41. Gómez-Arnau JI, Aguilar JL, Bovaira P, et al. Postoperative nausea and vomiting and opioid-induced nausea and vomiting: guidelines for prevention and treatment. *Rev Esp Anestesiol Reanim.* 2010;57(8):508-524.

42. Kovac AL. Management of postoperative nausea and vomiting in children. *Paediatr Drugs.* 2007;9(1):47-69.

43. Yilmaz N, Çekmen N, Bilgin F, Erten E, Özhan MO, Coşar A. Preoperative carbohydrate nutrition reduces postoperative nausea and vomiting compared to preoperative fasting. *J Res Med Sci.* 2013;18(10):8277.

44. Wang S-M, Kain ZN. P6 acupoint injections are as effective as droperidol in controlling early postoperative nausea and vomiting in children. *Anesthesiology.* 2002;97(8):359-366.

45. Transderm Scopolamine. Package Insert. Baxter.

46. Horn CC, Wallisch WJ, Homanics GE, Williams JP. Pathophysiological and neurochemical mechanisms of postoperative nausea and vomiting. *Eur J Pharmacol.* 2014;722:55-66.

47. Rose JB, Watcha MF. Postoperative nausea and vomiting in paediatric patients. *Br J Anaesth.* 1999;83(1):104-117.

48. Tramèr MR, Reynolds DJM, Moore RA, McQuay HJ. Efficacy, dose-response, and safety of ondansetron in prevention of postoperative nausea and vomiting: a qualitative systematic review of randomized placebo-controlled trials. *Anesthesiology.* 1997;87:1277-1289.

49. Subramaniam B, Madan R, Sadhasivam S, et al. Dexamethasone is a cost-effective alternative to ondansetron in preventing PONV after paediatric strabismus repair. *Br J Anaesth.* 2001;86(1):84-89.

50. Henzi I, Walder B, Trame'r MR. Dexamethasone for the prevention of postoperative nausea and vomiting: a quantitative systematic review. *Anesth Analg.* 2000;90:186-194.

51. Henzi I, Sonderegger J, Tramer MR. Efficacy, dose response, and adverse effects of droperidol for prevention of postoperative nausea and vomiting. *Can J Anaesth.* 2000;47:537-551.

52. Reynolds L, Beckmann J, Kurz A. Perioperative complications of hypothermia. *Best Pract Res Clin Anaesthesiol.* 2008;22(4):645-657.

53. Cohen LL, Lemanek K, Blount RL, et al. Evidence-based assessment of pediatric pain. *J Pediatr Psychol.* 2008;33(9):939-955.

54. Stevens B, Johnston C, Petryshen P, Taddio A. Premature infant pain profile: development and initial validation. *Clin J Pain.* 1996;12:13-22.

55. Merkel SI, Voepel-Lewis T, Shayevitz JR, Malviya S. The FLACC: a behavioral scale for scoring postoperative pain in young children. *Pediatr Nurse.* 1997;23(3):293-297.

56. McGrath P, de Veber L, Hearn M. Multidimensional pain assessment in children. *Adv Pain Res Ther.* 1985;9:387-393.

57. Hicks CL, von Baeyer CL, Spafford PA, van Korlaar I, Goodenough B. The Faces Pain Scale—Revised: toward a common metric in pediatric pain measurement. *Pain.* 2001;93:173-183.

58. Shields BJ, Cohen DM, Harbeck-Weber C, Powers JD, Smith GA. Pediatric pain measurement using a visual analogue scale: a comparison of two teaching methods. *Clin Pediatr (Phila).* 2003;42:227-227.

59. Shields BJ, Palermo TM, Powers JD, Grewe SD, Smith GA. Predictors of a child's ability to use a visual analogue scale. *Child Care Health Dev.* 2003;29(4):281-290.

60. Pagé MG, Katz J, Stinson J, Isaac L, Martin-Pichora AL, Campbell F. Validation of the numerical rating scale for pain intensity and unpleasantness in pediatric acute postoperative pain: sensitivity to change over time. *J Pain.* 2012;13(4):359-369.

61. von Baeyer CL. Children's self-reports of pain intensity: scale selection, limitations and interpretation. *Pain Res Manag.* 2006;11(3):157-162.

62. Lönnqvist PA, Morton NS. Postoperative analgesia in infants and children. *Br J Anaesth.* 2005;95(1):59-68.

63. Lee JY, Jo YY. Attention to postoperative pain control in children. *Korean J Anesthesiol.* 2014;66(3):183-188.

64. Taenzer AH, Walker BJ, Bosenberg AT, et al. Asleep versus awake: does it matter? Pediatric regional block complications

by patient state: a report from the Pediatric Regional Anesthesia Network. *Reg Anesth Pain Med*. 2014;39(4):279-283.

65. Michelet D, Andreu-Gallien J, Bensalah T, et al. A meta-analysis of the use of nonsteroidal antiinflammatory drugs for pediatric postoperative pain. *Anesth Analg*. 2012;114(2):393-406.

66. Bajwa SJS, Haldar R. Pain management following spinal surgeries: an appraisal of the available options. *J Craniovertebr Junction Spine*. 2015;6(3):105-110.

67. Grosu I, Lavand'homme P. Use of dexmedetomidine for pain control. *F1000 Med Rep*. 2010;2:90.

68. Waldron NH, Jones CA, Gan TJ, Allen TK, Habib AS. Impact of perioperative dexamethasone on postoperative analgesia and side-effects: systematic review and meta-analysis. *Br J Anaesth*. 2013;1(2):191-200.

69. Lee SK. The use of ketamine for perioperative pain management. *Korean J Anesthesiol*. 2012;63(1):1-2.

70. Geiduschek JM, Haberkern CM, McLaughlin JF, Jacobson LE, Hays RM, Roberts TS. Pain management for children following selective dorsal rhizotomy. *Can J Anaesth*. 1994;41(6):492-496.

71. Aldrete JA, Droulik D. A post anesthesia recovery score. *Anesth Analg*. 1970;49:924-934.

72. Awad IT, Moore M, Rushe C, Elburki A, O'Brien K, Warde D. Unplanned hospital admission in children undergoing daycase surgery. *Eur J Anaesthesiol*. 2004;21(5):379-383.

Pediatric Critical Care Medicine

Proshad Nemati Efune and Blake Nichols

INTRODUCTION

The field of pediatric critical care medicine is relatively young, having been established in the 1980s.[1] Prior to its formalization, many different types of physicians cared for critically ill children, including pediatric anesthesiologists. The focus on physiology, pharmacology, resuscitation, bedside care, life-sustaining technology, and procedural interventions is a shared focus between the two fields. This chapter will introduce the pediatric anesthesiologist to common disease states and management strategies undertaken in the pediatric intensive care unit (PICU), to allow for a common language and understanding between the pediatric anesthesiologist and intensivist.

THE RESPIRATORY SYSTEM

Modes of Ventilation

Noninvasive Ventilation

Noninvasive positive pressure ventilation (NPPV) is a management strategy for children with respiratory failure that provides respiratory support via a noninvasive facemask. It avoids complications associated with intubation, namely the need for sedation and airway clearance mechanisms. NPPV maintains small airway patency, increases end-expiratory lung volumes, and improves compliance. Continuous positive airway pressure (CPAP) provides a constant end-expiratory pressure to achieve the aforementioned goals, whereas bilevel positive airway pressure also provides an inspiratory pressure that further helps to support fatigued respiratory muscles. The NPPV can be used to support pediatric patients with respiratory failure due to upper airway pathology by maintaining upper airway patency and preventing apnea and hypopnea.

High-flow nasal cannula (HFNC) provides heated and humidified gas at levels that may meet or exceed a patient's spontaneous inspiratory flow rate. HFNC improves oxygenation and reduces dead space through washout of upper airway CO_2, effectively increasing ventilation. HFNC also likely generates some positive pressure, the degree of which is unknown. HFNC is used in a variety of situations in the PICU, most frequently in the management of bronchiolitis. While it is widely used, few studies exist on its clinical utility. A multicenter randomized controlled trial of 142 infants <6 months of age with bronchiolitis admitted to the PICU actually showed nasal CPAP of 7-cm H_2O to be superior to HFNC at a rate of 2 L/kg/min. However, only two patients in the entire study cohort required eventual intubation.[2]

Adaptive Pressure-Control Ventilation

A relatively newer mode of ventilation is adaptive pressure-control ventilation. This mode combines the advantages of a decelerating flow pattern typical of pressure-controlled ventilation with a guaranteed delivered tidal volume characteristic of volume-controlled ventilation. The first breath the ventilator delivers is a volume-limited breath. The measured plateau pressure is then used by the ventilator to pressure-limit the following breath. This pattern is continued with the ventilator automatically adjusting the minimal inspiratory pressure required to deliver the guaranteed tidal volume for each subsequent breath. If the tidal volume delivered is higher than the preset volume, the ventilator adjusts to deliver the next breath with a lower pressure. Adaptive pressure-control ventilation is known by various names depending on the brand of ventilator.

Commonly it is known as pressure-regulated volume control (PRVC). The pediatric literature comparing adaptive pressure-control ventilation to conventional modes is scant. This mode of ventilation does seem to decrease peak inspiratory pressures,[3] but its impact on clinical outcomes in pediatrics is unclear.

Airway Pressure Release Ventilation

Airway pressure release ventilation (APRV, Figure 38-1) is a pressure-limited, time-triggered, time-cycled mode of ventilation that allows for spontaneous breathing throughout all phases of the respiratory cycle. An elevated baseline pressure (P_{hi}) is maintained with short deflations to a lower pressure (P_{lo}).

In a randomized crossover pediatric trial performed in 2001 by Schultz et al., APRV provided similar ventilation, oxygenation, mean airway pressure, hemodynamics, and patient comfort as synchronized intermittent mechanical ventilation in patients with mild to moderate lung injury with lower inspiratory airway pressures.[4]

High-Frequency Oscillatory Ventilation

High-frequency oscillatory ventilation (HFOV) is a piston-driven ventilator that delivers low tidal volumes (ie, less than physiological dead space) at high frequencies and eliminates the need for bulk gas flow in the lungs for effective carbon dioxide (CO_2) clearance. A high distending

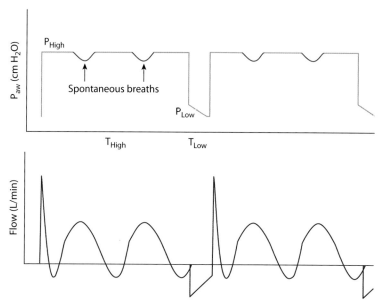

▲ **Figure 38-1.** Airway pressure release ventilation (APRV). Pressure high = P_{high}; pressure low = P_{low}; time high = T_{high}; time low = T_{low}. The spontaneous breaths seen are without pressure support; therefore, they appear concave. If with pressure support, the spontaneous breaths appear as convex. (Reproduced with permission, from Go RC: *Critical Care Examination and Board Review.* 2019. https://accessanesthesiology.mhmedical.com. Copyright © McGraw Hill LLC. All rights reserved.)

pressure is continuously supplied with small volume oscillatory vibrations superimposed. This high distending pressure maintains alveolar recruitment, while the small tidal volumes limit sheer injury and cyclic stretch of the lungs from repeated opening and closing of alveoli. Thus, HFOV is uniquely poised to prevent further lung injury in severe lung disease such as acute respiratory distress syndrome. Withdrawal of the piston provides a pressure gradient for active CO_2 removal, allowing alveolar ventilation to occur despite the use of sub-physiological tidal volumes.

Operator-controlled variables in HFOV include mean airway pressure (P_{aw}), frequency (f), amplitude of oscillation (ΔP), and ratio of inspiratory time to expiratory time ($I:E$). CO_2 elimination in HFOV is proportional to the frequency and the square of the tidal volume. Tidal volume is directly proportional to ΔP and *inversely* proportional to f. A lower frequency lengthens the cycle time which increases tidal volume and lengthens inspiratory time. Adjustments in frequency seem to affect CO_2 clearance to a greater degree than adjustments in ΔP. Partial endotracheal tube cuff deflation may be necessary for effective CO_2 clearance in severe lung disease. Alveolar recruitment (and thereby oxygenation) is directly proportional to P_{aw} and $I:E$. So long as the P_{aw} is set above the lungs opening pressure, HFOV results in improved oxygenation and higher lung volumes compared to conventional ventilation at a similar P_{aw}.

HFOV was initially popularized in preterm neonates with respiratory distress syndrome, where it has been shown to reduce length of mechanical ventilation and the need for supplemental oxygen at 36 weeks' postmenstrual age.[5] It also seems to be beneficial in the preoperative stabilization of infants with congenital diaphragmatic hernia, perhaps even improving survival,[6,7] in the treatment of persistent pulmonary hypertension of the newborn,[8] in air leak syndromes where it provides satisfactory gas exchange at a lower pressure cost, and in pediatric acute respiratory distress syndrome (see Section "Acute Respiratory Distress Syndrome").

Adjuncts

Inhaled Nitric Oxide

Nitric oxide (NO) results in relaxation of smooth muscle through an increase in intracellular cGMP. Inhaled NO (iNO) is a pulmonary vasodilator that has been shown to decrease the need for extracorporeal membrane oxygenation (ECMO) in neonates with persistent pulmonary hypertension of the newborn.[9–11] It has also been shown to reduce the incidence of pulmonary hypertensive crises and to decrease the time until extubation criteria are met in patients at risk for pulmonary hypertension following repair of congenital heart disease.[12] Rapid withdrawal of iNO should be avoided, particularly after prolonged therapy, as rebound pulmonary hypertension may occur due to down-regulation of endogenous NO synthesis.

Heliox

Heliox is a helium-oxygen gas mixture with an excellent safety record, that can be delivered both invasively and non-invasively and is used in the management of obstructive airway disease, particularly in life-threatening fixed or dynamic upper airway obstructive disease, such as croup, subglottic stenosis, and laryngotracheomalacia. Heliox creates conditions of laminar flow, which reduces the extent to which airway radius affects airway resistance (Poiseuille's law: airway resistance is inversely proportional to the radius to the fifth power with turbulent air flow versus to the fourth power with laminar flow). The addition of helium to the gas mixture also reduces density and increases viscosity, both of which reduce the Reynolds number and act to change a turbulent flow pattern to a laminar one.

$$Re = 2Vr\rho/\eta$$

where Re = Reynolds number, V = velocity of air flow, r = airway radius, ρ = density of air, and η = viscosity of air.

Premixed Heliox cylinders typically contain helium-oxygen ratios of 80:20 or 70:30, which limits its applicability to patients without severe hypoxemia. Studies on its use in post-extubation stridor and croup indicate clinical utility.[13] Heliox can also be utilized for lower airway obstructive disease such as asthma, where there may be a benefit when utilized for severely ill patients and when used early in the disease course.[13]

ACUTE RESPIRATORY DISTRESS SYNDROME

Acute respiratory distress syndrome (ARDS) is a clinical syndrome involving inflammation of the lung leading to increased permeability of the alveolar-capillary interface, translocation of fluid into the alveolar and interstitial space, decreased lung compliance, mismatch of ventilation and perfusion, and subsequent impairments in gas exchange. To meet the definition of pediatric ARDS (PARDS), a known clinical insult needs to have occurred within 7 days of symptom onset, the respiratory failure cannot be fully explained by cardiac failure or fluid overload, and chest imaging needs to show new infiltrate(s) consistent with acute pulmonary parenchymal disease.[15] The "Berlin criteria"[14] were developed in 2012 to further standardize the diagnosis. The criteria define severity of ARDS by degree of hypoxemia:

ARDS	PaO_2/FiO_2 (mm Hg)	Oxygenation Index (OI)
Mild	200–300	4–8
Moderate	100–200	8–16
Severe	≤100	≥16

The definitions were found to have a better predictive validity for mortality as compared to older criteria (ARDS definition task force). The oxygenation index (OI) ([$FiO_2 \times 100 \times$ mean airway pressure]/PaO_2) is another metric of lung disease and has been recommended over the *P/F* ratio to assess severity of PARDS in patients who are mechanically ventilated.[15]

There are a variety of pulmonary and extra-pulmonary causes of ARDS, including pneumonia, aspiration, drowning, trauma, sepsis, pancreatitis, and blood product transfusion (Table 38-1).

The initial phase is commonly called the *acute* or *exudative phase* and is characterized by bilateral patchy pulmonary infiltrates on chest radiograph, severe hypoxemia, decreased pulmonary compliance, and alveolar epithelial cell damage. Patients may recover after this phase or may enter a second phase also known as the *fibroproliferative phase*, which is characterized by refractory hypoxemia, distorted lung architecture, and prominent interstitial infiltration by fibroblasts and inflammatory cells. The final or *recovery phase* consists of gradual clinical improvement as type II pneumocytes begin to repopulate healthy alveoli.

Mortality of PARDS ranges from 18% to 35%[16,17] with immunodeficient patients having a higher risk of mortality, up to 70%.[18-20] Many studies have shown multi-organ dysfunction to be the single most important independent clinical risk factor for mortality in PARDS.[17,18,21-23] Small case series of survivors of PARDS demonstrate persistent

Table 38-1. Treatable Precipitating Causes of Acute Lung Injury (ALI) and Acute Respiratory Distress Syndrome (ARDS)

Infectious etiologies
Bacterial or other sepsis responsive to antimicrobial therapy
Diffuse bacterial pneumonias (eg, *Legionella* species)
Diffuse viral pneumonias (eg, cytomegalovirus, influenza A)
Diffuse fungal pneumonias (eg, *Candida* and *Cryptococcus* spp.)
Pneumocystis jirovecii (carinii) pneumonia
Other diffuse lung infections (eg, miliary tuberculosis)
Noninfectious etiologies
Diffuse alveolar hemorrhage post–bone marrow transplant
Diffuse alveolar hemorrhage due to vasculitis (eg, Goodpasture syndrome)
Acute eosinophilic pneumonia
Lupus pneumonitis
Toxic drug reactions (eg, aspirin, nitrofurantoin)

abnormalities in lung function as evidenced by spirometry up to several years after hospital discharge.[24-29]

Therapy is largely supportive in the management of PARDS. Mild ARDS can be treated with NPPV, with the caveat that the patient be very closely monitored for failure and the need for intubation. Few studies exist on the use of NPPV in PARDS. In a randomized study of children with acute hypoxemic respiratory failure, Yanez et al. found that the incidence of intubation was significantly lower in patients treated with NPPV versus usual care.[30] The use of NPPV is particularly appealing in the management of immunocompromised patients who are at higher risk of acquiring ventilator-associated pneumonia while intubated. When intubation is required, to avoid ventilator-induced lung injury, with the recognition that volutrauma is more injurious than barotrauma,[31] mechanically ventilated patients should have tidal volumes limited to 3 to 6 mL/kg, particularly in patients with more severely limited pulmonary compliance.[18,32,33] Plateau pressure should be limited to 28-cm H_2O,[18,33] but may need to be increased to 32 cm H_2O in more severe disease to achieve adequate tidal volumes. Positive end-expiratory pressure (PEEP) should be titrated to oxygenation, and levels up to 15-cm H_2O may be required. Meta-analyses have shown higher levels of PEEP, as part of a lung protective strategy may be associated with lower hospital mortality in adults with moderate to severe ARDS.[34,35] When conventional ventilation fails to support oxygenation, particularly when plateau pressures more than 28-cm H_2O are needed, HFOV may be used. HFOV has been shown to improve gas exchange in children, but with no effect on survival without chronic respiratory support.[36,37] In patients with moderate to severe ARDS, permissive hypercapnia and low tidal volume ventilation may improve outcome;[38,39] a pH > 7.15 is generally acceptable; however, the lower limit of pH is debated. Permissive hypercapnia should be avoided in patients with intracranial hypertension, pulmonary hypertension, severe hemodynamic instability, and select congenital heart diseases (ie, single ventricle lesions). Because improved oxygenation has not been linked to improved outcomes,[32] the concept of permissive hypoxemia has also been established, whereby SpO_2 of 88% to 92% is acceptable in patients with severe ARDS to reduce ventilator-induced lung injury. Systemic oxygen delivery should be closely monitored during this approach, and the risks and benefits should be weighed closely as the long-term effects of permissive hypoxemia have yet to be elucidated.

iNO acts as a selective pulmonary vasodilator, which may improve perfusion to well ventilated areas of lung and improve oxygenation. Studies of both pediatric and adult patients with ARDS have demonstrated improvement in oxygenation with the use of iNO, but no improvements in mortality, duration of mechanical ventilation, or ICU or hospital length of stay.[40] The use of iNO can be considered in cases of PARDS with documented pulmonary hypertension, or as a bridge to extracorporeal life support in severe

PARDS, but should not be used routinely.[41] The intratracheal instillation of surfactant has been extensively studied in PARDS. While early studies were promising, most recently a randomized controlled trial of 110 pediatric patients with ARDS was stopped early due to futility. No reduction in mortality or improvement in oxygenation was seen with the use of exogenous surfactant versus placebo.[42]

Prone positioning, like iNO, has been shown to improve oxygenation in PARDS. In a multicenter, randomized controlled trial, Curley et al examined the impact of prone positioning in children with a PaO_2/FiO_2 ratio < 300 mm Hg. The study was terminated early based on futility as no difference could be detected between the prone and supine treatment arms in terms of ventilatory free days, mortality, or a host of other secondary outcomes.[43] However, further study is warranted in children, as a large randomized controlled trial of prone positioning in adults with severe ARDS (PaO_2/FiO_2 ratio < 150 mm Hg) showed a statistically significant 50% reduction in all-cause mortality at 28 days.[44] At this time, routine prone positioning is not recommended in PARDS management.[41]

Glucocorticoids have been studied extensively in adults, but no randomized controlled trials have been conducted in PARDS. Adult studies have yielded conflicting results[45,46] and at this time routine use is not recommended. There is also insufficient evidence to support the routine use of inhaled beta-adrenergic receptor agonists or chest physiotherapy.[41]

Additional, nonpulmonary therapy for PARDS includes minimal, yet effective, sedation to facilitate mechanical ventilation, neuromuscular blockade if sedation proves inadequate, prioritization of nutritional support, and goal-directed fluid and red blood cell transfusion with an aim to prevent positive fluid balance following initial stabilization.[47]

THE CARDIOVASCULAR SYSTEM

The cardiovascular system features prominently in multiple disease processes encountered in the PICU such as shock, hypertensive crises, and post-cardiac arrest syndrome.

Shock

While shock is often perceived as inadequate perfusion to maintain end-organ function, it is better defined as inadequate oxygen supply to provide for the demands of various tissues in the body, which can lead to cellular metabolic dysfunction and cellular death.[48] There are several different classifications of shock that are caused by varied pathophysiological states (Table 38-2).

Early recognition of shock can be difficult, but is critical in the management of patients to prevent cardiovascular collapse.[49-51] Shock should be suspected any time two or more of the pediatric SIRS criteria are present (see discussion in the section "Infectious Disease")—one of which must include abnormal temperature or white blood cell count.[51,52] While septic shock is the most common form, other forms of shock occur regularly in the PICU. The clinician must be prepared to recognize shock quickly and treat it aggressively. Children often present with components of several different types of shock—ie, a patient with septic shock will likely also have a component of cardiac dysfunction.[53]

Shock is most often divided into warm and cold states. Warm shock manifests as bounding pulses, warm extremities to palpation, and flash capillary refill (<1 second) and is commonly seen with the distributive etiologies. Cold shock manifests as cold extremities to palpation with severely decreased capillary refill and diminished pulses and is often seen with cardiogenic, obstructive, or hypovolemic etiologies of shock.

Table 38-2. Classification and Physiology of Shock

Classification of Shock Types	Causes	Pathophysiology
Distributive	Sepsis Anaphylaxis Neurogenic	Disruption of vascular integrity leads to redistribution of oxygen delivery away from essential tissues and to pooling of blood into interstitium
Hypovolemic	Hemorrhagic GI/Renal losses	Inadequate oxygen delivery caused by decreased intravascular volume; cardiac output decreased secondary to inadequate preload
Cardiogenic	Primary or acquired heart disease Dysrhythmias	Inadequate oxygen delivery caused by inadequate cardiac contractility and stroke volume
Obstructive	Physical obstruction of cardiac output (eg, tension pneumothorax, pulmonary embolus, cardiac tamponade, etc.)	Obstruction of cardiac output causes inadequate oxygen delivery by severely reducing both preload and stroke volume
Dissociative	Carbon monoxide Cyanide	Inability of hemoglobin to release oxygen at the tissue level secondary to changed affinity of heme molecule for oxygen

Shock can also be divided into compensated and uncompensated states. A compensated shock state is often more difficult to recognize as the body maintains a normal blood pressure for age. In a decompensated state, cardiac output is not maintained and hypotension develops. Patients in a decompensated state require immediate and rapid resuscitation as they are at acute risk for cardiorespiratory arrest. In a decompensated state, there is rapid progression of tissue hypoxia, cellular acidosis, and cellular death.[54,55]

Organ dysfunction is often the earliest indicator of shock. Nervous system dysfunction may manifest as confusion, alterations in mental status, lethargy, headache, or inconsolability. Cardiac dysfunction may manifest as tachycardia, capillary refill time >3 seconds, and/or hypotension. Often, the first system to be injured is the renal system, manifested by urine output less than 1mL/kg/h. Potential laboratory abnormalities include metabolic acidosis, hyperlactatemia, increased hepatic function enzymes, and/or elevations in the blood urea nitrogen and creatinine values—all from inadequate oxygen supply and resultant tissue damage. This delineation of derangements in physical and laboratory findings is by no means exhaustive. The existence of hyperlactatemia from a free-flowing sample should alert the clinician that anaerobic metabolism is occurring due to lack of oxygen supply, although may be secondary to poor performance of the liver causing an inability to metabolize the lactate.[56,57]

Treatment of Shock

Treatment of shock is based on the principles of restoration of intravascular volume, optimizing tissue oxygen delivery (DO$_2$), and decreasing oxygen demand. The Surviving Sepsis Campaign guidelines developed by the Society for Critical Care Medicine recommends crystalloid for the initial restoration of intravascular volume in the setting of septic shock.[58] In the setting of hemorrhagic shock, crystalloid should likely be limited in favor of blood products.[59,60] While fluid resuscitation is necessary in the treatment of distributive shock, it may worsen cardiogenic shock. It is also important to remember that intravascular volume may be low in cardiogenic shock and fluid resuscitation is often required to restore preload and optimize cardiac output. An appropriate strategy when cardiogenic shock is suspected involves giving smaller aliquots of volume, 5 mL/kg or 10 mL/kg (maximum of 500 mL total), and then assessing for liver enlargement below the right costal margin and listening to the lung fields for crackles, a sign of lung fluid overload secondary to cardiac dysfunction.

To maximize oxygen delivery, a patient in shock should be placed on noninvasive oxygen support. A nonrebreather is sometimes necessary to increase the dissolved oxygen in the blood. In the setting of anemia, giving packed red blood cells for volume resuscitation is the most efficient therapeutic strategy to increase oxygen delivery.

Another important strategy for treating shock of any type is to decrease the metabolic demands of the body. This requires aggressive treatment of fever with antipyretics and often the use of external cooling measures. External cooling measures should be used with caution because it can cause shivering placing a great metabolic demand on the body and can often worsen hyperthermia. Measures should be taken to prevent shivering. In an intubated and sedated patient, this may require medical paralysis. Intubation and sedation greatly reduce metabolic demands, but it is important to realize that intubating a patient in shock can acutely decrease preload to the heart and cause cardiovascular collapse. During spontaneous respiration, inspiration creates negative intrapleural pressure, which increases blood flow to the right heart from the body. Intubation abruptly changes the intrapleural pressure to positive and may severely decrease preload.

Inotropic and Vasoactive Medications

In the case of fluid refractory shock, inotropic or vasoactive support is often required. Inotropic medications improve cardiac contractility in a depressed heart, whereas vasopressor medications augment systemic vascular resistance. Many medications have both effects. Dopamine or epinephrine can be initiated through a peripheral venous line or an intraosseous line without hesitation.[58] Epinephrine and other inotropic medications are superior in the case of cold shock, when inotropy and increased cardiac output are required. Norepinephrine and other vasoactive agents are superior in the case of warm shock when systemic vascular resistance is low, and a stronger vasopressor effect is required to augment afterload. When the patient requires higher level of support or the addition of norepinephrine, central venous access should be obtained. The most recent Surviving Sepsis Campaign guidelines recommend the utilization of norepinephrine as a firstline vasopressor for patients in septic shock.[58] If inotropic and vasopressor support proves to be inadequate for the resuscitation of severe shock, then additional therapies may be necessary.

Mechanical Circulatory Support—Extracorporeal Membrane Oxygenation

When cardiorespiratory failure occurs that is not tempered by inotropes and vasoactive medications, additional support may be required to provide oxygenated blood to the distal tissues in the form of venoarterial ECMO (VA ECMO). VA ECMO requires surgical placement of intravascular cannulas and a specialized team to manage the extracorporeal circuit. In VA ECMO, a venous cannula drains blood from the right side of the heart, often at the level of the superior and/or inferior vena cava. Blood is then circulated with a pump through an oxygenator and warmed to body temperature prior to being delivered to the patient beyond the left side of the heart, often at the level of the aortic arch. The flow of the extracorporeal circuit can be titrated to achieve a cardiac output necessary for the demands of the body. Maximal cardiac output may be limited by cannula size and the inability to drain blood from the right side of the heart. In this case, cannulas can be changed to central locations, or an additional draining cannula can be added.[61] While there are many risks and nuances to ECMO, it can often be used to provide full cardiac and respiratory support to a patient in a state of cardiorespiratory dysfunction as a bridge to recovery or as a bridge to definitive surgical therapy.[62,63] VA ECMO can also be successfully used in refractory cardiac arrest where patients are cannulated during ongoing, high-quality cardiopulmonary resuscitation.[62] Major risks of ECMO include the need for anticoagulation, and the prospect of hemorrhage that comes with anticoagulation, stroke, infection, inability to detect fever as temperature is controlled by the circuit, and the need for heavy sedation and/or paralysis. At times, extubation on ECMO allows for speedier recovery.[64]

Hypertensive Crises

Hypertension in children is a systolic blood pressure greater than the 95th percentile for age, height, and sex.[65] There are two major types of acute hypertension in children that require rapid recognition and treatment: hypertensive urgency, an acute elevation in mean arterial pressure without end-organ damage, and hypertensive emergency, an acute elevation in mean arterial pressure with end-organ damage.[65] Hypertensive crises can lead to severe end-organ failure and potentially death. Children can present with a wide array of symptoms with acute hypertension including, but not limited to, headache, visual changes, seizures, acute hemorrhage, heart failure, or acute kidney injury.[65] Intravenous medications with rapid onset that are easily titratable offer the best solution for treating acute hypertension. Monitoring arterial blood pressure continuously via a peripheral arterial line during an infusion of antihypertensive medications is paramount to treatment. It is extremely important to remember that if the hypertension is chronic, mean arterial pressure should be lowered gradually. The regulatory mechanisms of the tissues may be accommodating for high pressures and an acute drop in pressure can lead to organ ischemia.[65]

Post-Cardiac Arrest Syndrome

Post-cardiac arrest patients require special attention in the PICU. Return of spontaneous circulation (ROSC) following cardiac arrest causes a systemic inflammatory response that may lead to hyperthermia and refractory hypotension.[66] The recent Therapeutic Hypothermia After Pediatric Cardiac Arrest (THAPCA) trial showed no advantage to using therapeutic hypothermia after cardiac arrest, but there is likely a distinct advantage to maintaining therapeutic normothermia.[67] Clinicians should use medications and external cooling measures as necessary to keep the patient

from developing fever. If the patient does develop fever, it should be treated aggressively with intravenous antipyretics and external cooling measures as fever requires a substantial metabolic demand. From a ventilatory standpoint, patients with normoxia have been shown to have improved outcomes compared with hypoxia or hyperoxia.[68] Patients who experience cardiac arrest are also at risk of developing PARDS and may benefit from lung-protective ventilator management as described previously.[69] Additional issues following cardiac arrest may include glucose abnormalities, seizures, and acute kidney injury, all of which must be monitored closely and supported as necessary in an intensive care unit.

NUTRITION

Nutritional Support

Nutritional support is an extremely important aspect of the management of critically ill children. Many barriers exist to optimal delivery of nutrition, including inaccurate estimates of energy expenditure and macronutrient requirements and interruptions in nutrition delivery. Malnutrition may increase hospital mortality and length of stay in children.[70] Providing adequate nutritional support should be an important goal for all members of a critically ill child's healthcare team.

Enteral Feeding

Early enteral feeding is preferred over parenteral nutrition whenever possible, as it is more physiological and cost-effective. The European Society for Clinical Nutrition and Metabolism (ESPEN) and the American Society for Parenteral and Enteral Nutrition recommend early enteral nutrition over parenteral nutrition unless there are significant contraindications to enteral feeding.[71,72]

The optimal route of enteral feeding (gastric versus post-pyloric) remains unclear. While gastric feeding is typically easier due to a higher likelihood of successful placement of the feeding tube, post-pyloric feeds may be considered in children at high risk for aspiration (ie, due to depressed mental status, GERD, history of aspiration, or delayed gastric emptying).

Many barriers exist to providing optimal enteral nutrition in the PICU. Fluid restriction, interruptions for procedures, and perceived intolerance are just a few examples. As expected, avoidable interruptions in feeding lead to a decreased chance of reaching caloric goals.[73]

When possible, non-nutritive sources of fluids should be restricted before restricting enteral nutrition in fluid-overloaded patients. The American Society of Anesthesiologists does not provide clear guidelines on NPO times for children receiving post-pyloric enteral feedings prior to anesthesia, nor do they provide guidelines on the need for a fasting state when patients are already intubated.[74] Generally, it is felt that 2 to 4 hours of NPO time following cessation of post-pyloric feeds is reasonable prior to an anesthetic. The practice regarding patients who are already intubated is widely variable, with many anesthesiologists maintaining standard NPO times, and some not requiring a fasting state at all. The risk of aspiration likely varies depending on the type of procedure, with ENT and intra-abdominal procedures possibly contributing the greatest risk. In patients receiving vasoactive medications there are also concerns, and while there is no clear literature to guide the decision, feeding patients who are hemodynamically stable on a single vasoactive is likely safe.[75] The definition of feeding intolerance is widely variable, and clear protocols and feeding algorithms may help to standardize feeding practices and increase the likelihood of achieving nutritional goals in critically ill children. When feasible, enteral feeding interruptions should be avoided in critically ill children.

Total Parenteral Nutrition

Total parenteral nutrition (TPN) is provided when enteral feeding will not be feasible or is not tolerated after several days of critical illness. It typically requires central venous access for administration but can be given peripherally if the dextrose concentration is limited (below 10% to 12.5%). Carbohydrate is administered in the form of dextrose and comprises 60% to 75% of nonprotein calories. The dextrose concentration is gradually increased to avoid hyperglycemia. In addition to the delivery of carbohydrates and protein, essential fatty acids are delivered in the form of intravenous lipid emulsion. Thirty percent to 40 percent of calories are delivered as fat and the withholding of fat can lead to free fatty acid deficiency. IV lipid emulsion is safely delivered peripherally. Multivitamins and trace minerals are also delivered via TPN.

Common complications of TPN include liver dysfunction, cholestasis, hyperglycemia, hypertriglyceridemia, and line-associated infection. Patients on high concentrations of dextrose are at risk for hypoglycemia upon withdrawal of TPN.

A large (>4000 adult patients) multicenter trial showed that patients randomized to late initiation of parenteral nutrition (after day 8) had an increased chance of being discharged earlier from the ICU and from the hospital and had fewer ICU infections as compared to patients with early initiation of parenteral therapy (within 48 hours of ICU admission).[76] However, a subsequent large multicenter study of >2000 mechanically ventilated adults with septic shock failed to show a difference in ICU-acquired infections between patients randomized to receive enteral nutrition versus parenteral nutrition in the first 3 days of mechanical ventilation. The authors did find an increased incidence of vomiting, diarrhea, bowel ischemia, and acute colonic pseudo-obstruction in patients receiving enteral nutrition.[77] Finally, a large multicenter trial of >1400 critically ill children showed that patients randomized to late parenteral nutrition (day 8 of ICU admission) had lower rates of infection, shorter length of ICU stay, shorter duration of ventilatory support, fewer patients requiring renal replacement therapy, and lower hospital stay.[78]

▶ Glycemic Control in the PICU

The pendulum has swung several times over the past few decades regarding glycemic control in adult ICUs, initially with little regard to the impact of blood glucose management on outcomes, to "tight glycemic control," and finally to glycemic control with a more liberal target (ie, 150 to 180 mg/dL). Each of these shifts in management came after large randomized studies supporting an improvement in outcome measures with the various techniques.

The incidence of hyperglycemia in the PICU depends on patient population, with patients who are more ill with more organ injury generally at higher risk. When insulin infusions are used to manage hyperglycemia, a protocol-driven approach may be preferable.[79] Blood glucose is ideally measured from an arterial catheter. In a dual-site randomized study of post-cardiac surgery patients <36 months of age, there was no difference in the primary outcome of rate of health care–associated infections between the tight glycemic control group (target 80 to 110 mg/dL) or conventional therapy. There was also no difference in mortality, length of stay, organ failure, or hypoglycemia. Importantly, the investigators used continuous glucose monitoring to detect impending hypoglycemia.[80] In a subsequent post hoc analysis, the investigators discovered that there was an increased rate of health care–associated infections in the patients <60 days old who were randomized to tight glycemic control.[80,81] A multicenter study of 1369 children examined children admitted to the PICU and expected to require mechanical ventilation and vasoactive drugs for at least 12 hours; 60% of these patients were recovering from cardiac surgery. Patients randomized to the tight glycemic control group had a target blood glucose of 72 to 126 mg/dL and the conventional group had a target <216 mg/dL. The investigators found no difference in the primary outcome of number of days alive and free from mechanical ventilation between the two groups with an increased incidence of hypoglycemia in the intensive insulin arm. There was also no difference when the subgroup of cardiac surgery patients was examined. While health care–associated infections were not explicitly addressed as an outcome, there was no difference in blood stream infections between the two treatment arms.[82]

▶ Electrolyte Derangements

Electrolyte derangements are extremely common in critically ill children, usually secondary to organ injury, medication administration, and various ICU therapies. While an exhaustive review of electrolyte disorders is outside the scope of this chapter, it is worth noting that even mild disruptions in homeostasis can be ill-tolerated in very sick children and can lead to death. Electrolyte abnormalities should be anticipated and prevented whenever possible. A list of commonly encountered electrolyte disorders and possible causes is presented in Table 38-3. Of note, chronic sodium derangements should be corrected slowly and carefully, as severe neurological sequelae can result if corrected rapidly.

Table 38-3. Common Electrolyte Derangements and Potential Causes in Critically Ill Children

Electrolyte Disturbance	Causes, Associated Derangements
Hyponatremia	Hypovolemia Syndrome of inappropriate antidiuretic hormone release Hypothyroidism Glucocorticoid insufficiency Cerebral salt wasting Diuretic usage Renal tubular acidosis Cirrhosis Congestive heart failure Nephrotic syndrome Excess water intake
Hypernatremia	Hypovolemia Diabetes insipidus Diuretic usage Hyperglycemia
Hypokalemia	Diabetic ketoacidosis Hyperaldosteronism Alkalosis Hypothermia Renal tubular acidosis Hypomagnesemia Osmotic diuresis Gastrointestinal losses Medications: diuretics, beta-agonists, insulin, cisplatin
Hyperkalemia	Hemolyzed sample Prolonged tourniquet application Severe thrombocytosis or leukocytosis Acidosis Cell necrosis/lysis Renal failure Adrenal insufficiency Hypoaldosteronism Medications: angiotensin-converting enzyme inhibitors, nonsteroidal anti-inflammatories, cyclosporine, potassium sparing diuretics
Hypomagnesemia	Malabsorption Renal tubular acidosis Medications: diuretics, aminoglycosides, cyclosporine, amphotericin B, tacrolimus, sirolimus, pentamidine, foscarnet, cisplatin, mannitol, acetazolamide, ticarcillin
Hypermagnesemia	Magnesium-containing drugs in the presence of renal failure
Ionized hypocalcemia	Hypoparathyroidism Vitamin D deficiency Sepsis Pancreatitis Toxic shock syndrome Alkalosis Increased chelation secondary to blood transfusion, contrast administration, hyperphosphatemia
Hypercalcemia	Iatrogenic Hyperparathyroidism Thyrotoxicosis Prolonged immobilization Vitamin D or A intoxication Thiazide diuretics

(Continued)

Table 38-3. Common Electrolyte Derangements and Potential Causes in Critically Ill Children (*Continued*)

Electrolyte Disturbance	Causes, Associated Derangements
Hypophosphatemia	Malabsorption Vitamin D deficiency Renal losses due to hyperparathyroidism, chronic corticosteroid use, diuretics, renal tubular disease, hypomagnesemia, diabetic ketoacidosis, renal transplantation, chemotherapeutics Intracellular shift due to respiratory alkalosis, insulin, hypothermia, refeeding syndrome, burns, massive fluid resuscitation, beta-agonist use
Hyperphosphatemia	Renal failure Cell lysis Iatrogenic Hypoparathyroidism

RENAL

The kidneys perform several major functions including the delicate balance of fluid and electrolytes. When the kidneys are unable to perform these duties, they often require assistance in the form of renal replacement therapy (RRT), but the first step lies in recognition of acute kidney injury (AKI).

Acute Kidney Injury

Acute kidney injury (AKI) and total body fluid overload are common findings in critically ill children with a widely variable incidence up to 89%.[83–86] Critically ill children who experience AKI and fluid overload have significantly increased mortality and ICU length of stay.[83,87] The first sign of AKI in children is a decrease in urine production, and providers in the PICU must monitor urine output closely. Many clinicians practice by measuring creatinine levels to assess for AKI, but creatinine elevations often occur later in the course of AKI and the levels can be altered by diet, hydration status, and skeletal muscle composition.[88] Several other biomarkers have been studied to find a superior marker for AKI, such as cystatin C, a molecule secreted by all cells. Cystatin C has a half-life much shorter than creatinine, allowing for the detection of AKI up to 48 hours sooner than by creatinine elevations.[88] AKI has been assigned multiple definitions over the years, most of which are based on the pediatric modification of the adult RIFLE (Risk, Injury, Failure, Loss, End-stage renal disease) criteria originally developed in 2004 and modified for pediatrics in 2007.[84,89] These criteria define different stages of renal injury based on decreasing urine output and estimated creatinine clearance index. The pRIFLE criteria have been externally validated to provide prognostic value for children with AKI.[90,165]

Once AKI has been diagnosed, the decision must be made whether to utilize RRT to support the renal system. Common indications for RRT include volume overload, intoxications, azotemia, and significant electrolyte derangements.[91,92] Fluid restriction and diuresis should be trialed aggressively at the first sign of volume overload but may be inadequate. RRT is an important therapy for use in critically ill children to ameliorate the fluid and electrolyte derangements associated with critical illness, but does come with its own inherent risks, such as the need for anticoagulation and risk of infection. There are no definitive criteria of when to initiate RRT, but many have suggested initiation when urine output has decreased and the patient has 10% fluid overload.[93,94]

Renal Replacement Therapy

The basic principles of RRT involve the movement of solutes or volume through a semi-permeable membrane. Particles can pass through a semi-permeable membrane via either a concentration gradient or a pressure gradient. Diffusion refers to solutes passing through the membrane down a concentration gradient. Diffusion requires a dialysate fluid on the opposite side of the semi-permeable membrane, and it increases with increasing gradient differential. Convection occurs when solutes pass through the membrane secondary to a pressure gradient and it increases with increasing pressure differential. Diffusion and convection are dependent on the relative size of the solute particles and the pores in the semipermeable membrane. Ultrafiltration follows the same principle as convection, but simply refers to the movement of a solvent down a pressure gradient through the semipermeable membrane.

Peritoneal Dialysis

Peritoneal dialysis (PD) operates on the principle that the visceral peritoneum can function as a semi-permeable dialysis membrane. A catheter is usually placed surgically, although it can be placed at the bedside using the Seldinger technique, and allows for the instillation of dialysate directly into the peritoneal cavity.[95] Fluids can be instilled directly into the peritoneum and dwell there for a specified time to allow for the diffusion of solutes and fluids across the membrane. After the dwell time is complete, the dialysate and waste can be removed, and a new dialysate fluid can be instilled. PD is relatively easy to perform and does not cause significant hemodynamic compromise in most cases. It can be used to remove fluid and/or solutes by simply modifying the composition of the instilled dialysate. Catheters are often placed at the time of complex abdominal or cardiovascular surgeries when a prolonged and difficult recovery period is expected.[96–98] Major advantages to PD are that central venous access and systemic anticoagulation are not required.[99] The major complications of PD are the associated risk of peritonitis from the instillation of dextrose-containing fluids through a port from the external environment, hyperglycemia from the absorption of dextrose-containing fluids, and mechanical malfunction of the PD catheter.[95] Certain PD catheters may require up to 2 weeks for granulation to take place to fully secure the catheter. If the PD catheter is used prior to healing, fluid may leak from around the catheter and lead to the inability to perform meaningful dialysis. No studies have demonstrated a difference in overall mortality between PD or continuous veno-venous hemofiltration/hemodialysis (CVVH/D),[86] but CVVH has been shown to provide better solute removal. It should be noted that these findings are based on observational studies.

Intermittent Hemodialysis

Intermittent hemodialysis (HD) offers several distinct advantages including the rapid correction of metabolic derangements and rapid fluid removal.[100] For patients with critical hyperkalemia or acute tumor lysis syndrome that is life threatening, HD is the clear choice.[101] Major complications associated with the use of HD include central venous access requirement and rapid fluid shifts, which may lead to hemodynamic compromise in critically ill children. HD is less often used for critically ill children who require RRT for renal failure with volume overload because these patients often already have hemodynamic compromise.

Continuous Renal Replacement Therapy

Continuous renal replacement therapy (CRRT) is often the preferred modality in critically ill children due to the ability to gently remove volume and electrolytes and have minimal effect on hemodynamic status. From a recent study, CRRT is required in approximately 5% of all PICU admissions and is associated with a mortality rate of 60%—this likely reflects the underlying severity of illness and multi-organ dysfunction in children requiring CRRT.[102]

CRRT is most commonly performed via the use of a central venous catheter, although it can be performed using continuous movement of fluids in PD as well. Central venous access for CRRT comes with the inherent risks of placing a large-bore venous catheter including bleeding, trauma, thrombus formation, and infection. The most ideal placement is the internal jugular vein to allow for consistent and reliable catheter patency and circuit flow. Femoral access has been associated with more interruptions in circuit flow secondary to thrombus formation and/or catheter kinking. Subclavian catheter placement is associated with more serious complications such as hemo- or pneumothoraces.[103]

The methods of clearance using CRRT through a continuous veno-venous circuit can employ either continuous veno-venous hemofiltration (CVVH), which operates under the principles of convective solute removal, continuous veno-venous hemodialysis (CVVHD), which operates using the principle of diffusion with a counter-current dialysate flow through the circuit, or a combination of both—hemodiafiltration (CVVHDF). The dialysate can be modified in order to improve the diffusion capacity of the membrane, and, likewise, the flow through the circuit can be adjusted to improve the efficiency of solute removal via convection.

Complications

All forms of CVVH require anticoagulation, either systemically with heparin, or regionally using citrate that can be added as the blood enters the circuit. Citrate works by binding calcium, which is necessary as a cofactor to activate clotting factors. It is a good alternative to systemic anticoagulation, but calcium must be infused in the circuit prior to the blood re-entering the systemic circulation to maintain appropriate coagulation in the remainder of the body and protect against hypotension. Citrate should be used with caution in patients with liver failure as they have a decreased ability to metabolize it, and citrate may accumulate and bind calcium in the body. This may result in a phenomenon known as citrate lock or citrate toxicity—the accumulation of calcium–citrate complexes leading to elevated total calcium to ionized calcium ratio. Associated ionized hypocalcemia leads to depressed myocardial function, prolonged QT interval, potentially fatal dysrhythmias, and severe vasoplegia. Citrate toxicity must be treated rapidly by stopping the citrate infusion and aggressively replenishing ionized calcium.[104] Citrate toxicity is thought to be more common in patients with liver failure, given the decreased ability to metabolize citrate. Many clinicians perform CVVH in patients with liver failure without any form of anticoagulation, but it has recently been shown that regional citrate anticoagulation is safe in pediatric patients with liver failure extending the CVVH circuit life over no anticoagulation at all.[105] Heparin anticoagulation requires close monitoring to maintain anticoagulation within a therapeutic range.

Medication clearance will also be altered with the initiation of CVVH. Dosing adjustments will likely be necessary for many medications especially ones with narrow therapeutic windows and are best performed with the assistance of a specialized clinical pharmacist.

HEMATOLOGICAL AND INFECTIOUS DISEASE CONSIDERATIONS IN THE PICU

Transfusion Practices

Anemia

Anemia is a prevalent problem in critically ill children. The various causes include blood loss, decreased production, decreased red blood cell survival, and underlying chronic disease. Iatrogenic anemia due to blood draws is perhaps the most common etiology of anemia in the PICU, particularly in neonates and infants. Chronic blood loss is more likely to be tolerated as compared to acute blood loss. The signs and symptoms of anemia differ based on the chronicity of development, but may include tachycardia, pallor, fatigue and in severe cases, elevated lactate levels, metabolic acidosis, and low central venous oxygen saturations. Fetal hemoglobin represents a proportion of hemoglobin in infants in the first few months of life and has a higher oxygen affinity, resulting in decreased unloading of oxygen to the tissues. In addition, neonates have a limited ability to compensate for anemia, as their stroke volumes are somewhat fixed as compared to older children and adults due to a relative reduction in contractile elements of the immature myocardium.

Transfusion triggers have been the subject of many studies in critically ill adults. In a landmark study in 2007 (Transfusion Strategies for Patients in Pediatric Intensive Care Units or TRIPICU), 637 stable, critically ill children without cyanotic heart disease were randomized to a restrictive strategy with a hemoglobin threshold of 7 g/dL versus a liberal strategy group with a threshold of 9.5 g/dL. Hemoglobin concentration was maintained at a mean level of 2.1 g/dL lower in the restrictive strategy group, with that group receiving 44% fewer transfusions. There was no difference in the primary outcome of new or progressive multiple-organ dysfunction syndrome, indicating that a restrictive strategy is safe in stable, critically ill children.[106]

Different transfusion strategies apply in children with heart defects. In a subgroup analysis of children with non-cyanotic heart disease in the TRIPICU study, no significant difference was noted in the incidence of new or progressive multiple-organ dysfunction, suggesting that a threshold hemoglobin of 7 g/dL is safe in this patient population.[106] In a randomized controlled trial of 107 children with non-cyanotic congenital heart disease following corrective surgery on cardiopulmonary bypass, length of hospital stay (the primary outcome) was lower in the restrictive strategy group (transfusion threshold 8 g/dL) than in the liberal group (threshold 10.8 g/dL) with no difference in the secondary outcomes.[107] The data is less robust in children with cyanotic congenital heart disease. In a randomized trial of 60 children (33 status post Glenn procedure and 27 status post Fontan), a restrictive transfusion threshold of 9 g/dL did not result in different lactate levels as compared to a liberal threshold of 13 g/dL. There was a slightly higher oxygen extraction rate in the restrictive group, but its clinical significance is likely low (31% vs 26%, $p = 0.013$).[108] Most recently, the Pediatric Critical Care Transfusion and Anemia Expertise Initiative (TAXI) recommends transfusion when the hemoglobin is less than 5 g/dL and gives no specific recommendations if the hemoglobin is 5 g/dL to 7 g/dL. When hemoglobin is >5 g/dL, transfusion should be guided by physiological derangements.[109]

Transfusion-Associated Risks

The three main causes of mortality secondary to transfusions include transfusion-related acute lung injury (TRALI), transfusion-associated circulatory overload (TACO), and hemolytic transfusion reactions.[110] Previous reports have estimated the incidence of adverse outcome to be 18:100,000 red blood cell units issued for children less than 18 years and 37:100,000 for infants. Most adverse events are related to incorrect blood component transfused, followed by acute transfusion reactions and TRALI.[111] A less commonly recognized risk of blood product transfusion is transfusion-related immunomodulation, in which blood transfusions modulate the inflammatory response, increasing the risk of developing infections, sepsis, multi-organ dysfunction, and cancer recurrence.[112] Considering the risks of transfusion, the risk-to-benefit ratio of each transfusion should be weighed carefully in critically ill children.

Disseminated Intravascular Coagulation

Disseminated intravascular coagulation (DIC) occurs as a result of the abnormal and uncontrolled upregulation of thrombin generation pathways. Abnormal thrombin generation ultimately leads to formation of microthrombi in the vasculature, end-organ dysfunction, and a bleeding diathesis secondary to the consumption and down-regulation of prohemostatic drivers. DIC occurs in the setting of many different diffuse inflammatory processes, the most widely recognized one being sepsis. Tissue factor expression, particularly on damaged endothelial cells or activated monocytes and macrophages, appears to be the driving force for thrombin generation in DIC. Therapy for DIC remains supportive, with replacement of prohemostatic factors as necessary to control bleeding complications. There is some concern that administration of these factors may worsen uncontrolled thrombin generation. Thromboelastography-guided replacement may be of some value and has been used extensively in trauma.

Sepsis

Sepsis is frequently encountered by pediatric intensivists. Despite advancements in care, sepsis remains a leading cause of mortality in pediatric ICUs, in the United States, and certainly worldwide.[113,114]

Sepsis Definitions

Sepsis is defined as "life-threatening organ dysfunction caused by a dysregulated host response to infection."[115] A 2005 international pediatric sepsis consensus conference defined pediatric systemic inflammatory response syndrome (SIRS, a nonspecific inflammatory process occurring in response to a variety of insults) as the presence of at least two of the following, one of which must be abnormal temperature or white blood cell count: core temperature >38.5°C or <36°C, unexplained tachycardia (or bradycardia in children <1 year old), tachypnea, or white blood cell count elevated or depressed for age. The consensus conference proceeded to define pediatric sepsis as *SIRS* in the presence of a suspected or proven infection, severe sepsis as sepsis plus one of the following: cardiovascular organ dysfunction or ARDS or two or more other organ dysfunctions, and *septic shock* as sepsis plus cardiovascular organ dysfunction.[116] The Third International Consensus Definitions for Sepsis and Septic Shock (Sepsis-3) is a task force that updated the adult definitions of sepsis in 2016. They concluded that SIRS may often actually reflect an appropriate host response to infection, and so is unhelpful in many cases, while sepsis is always associated with organ dysfunction, thereby making the term "severe sepsis" redundant. Organ dysfunction was defined as an increase in sequential organ failure assessment (SOFA) score by ≥2 points consequent to an infection. They found a change in SOFA score to perform better than or similarly to SIRS for the predictive validity of hospital mortality. They also found the "quick SOFA," or qSOFA, score to perform similarly to the SOFA score outside the ICU. The qSOFA score criteria include respiratory rate ≥22 breaths/min, altered mentation, or systolic blood pressure ≤100 mm Hg, with the presence of two of the three variables indicating likelihood of sepsis. Septic shock was defined as vasopressor requirement to maintain a mean arterial pressure ≥65 mm Hg and/or a serum lactate level >2 mmol/L in the absence of hypovolemia.[115] Most recently in 2017, the Sepsis-3 definitions were evaluated in a large cohort of critically ill children. In this study, pediatric SOFA (pSOFA) score was adapted from the original SOFA score using age-adjusted cutoffs and including noninvasive surrogates of lung injury in the respiratory criteria.[117] The pSOFA score was found to have excellent discrimination for in-hospital mortality, with an area under the curve of 0.94 (95% CI, 0.92–0.95). Those patients in their study cohort classified as having sepsis and septic shock according to the Sepsis-3 definitions had a mortality rate of 12.1% and 32.3%, respectively. In comparison, the total cohort had an in-hospital mortality rate of 2.6%. The authors concluded that the Sepsis-3 definitions are feasible and potentially valid in children.[117]

Treatment

While most adults in septic shock present with high cardiac output and low systemic vascular resistance (SVR), most children will present with a low cardiac output and high SVR, often requiring inotropes and vasodilators to improve perfusion.[118] It is also common for children with septic shock to have several different underlying pathophysiological mechanisms for their shock. For example, children with septic shock are often hypovolemic secondary to capillary leak, insensible losses, and venodilation leading to an effective decrease in circulating blood volume, can have myocardial depression from bacterial toxins and inflammatory mediators, and can have reductions in SVR, all contributing to a state of malperfusion.

The three pillars of pediatric sepsis management are (1) early recognition, (2) early source control, and (3) early reversal of the shock state. Early recognition is difficult,

even for the most experienced physicians. A high index of suspicion is required, and the signs and symptoms can often be subtle and difficult to distinguish from simple infection. Additionally, there are no available lab tests that are highly sensitive or specific for the diagnosis.

The Surviving Sepsis Campaign guidelines were updated in 2016 for adults,[119] with a formal update to the pediatric guidelines yet to be published. The major differences between these updated adult guidelines and previous pediatric guidelines include the following recommendations/suggestions:

- The use of dynamic (ie, pulse pressure/stroke volume variation, passive leg-raise) variables over static variables to predict fluid responsiveness
- Resuscitation guided to normalize lactate
- Narrowing of broad-spectrum antimicrobial therapy as soon as possible
- The use of crystalloid during resuscitation with the addition of albumin when substantial amounts of crystalloids are required
- Norepinephrine as the first-choice vasopressor with the addition of vasopressin or epinephrine infusions when necessary
- Dopamine reserved for highly selected cases
- RBC transfusions reserved for when hemoglobin is <7 g/dL in the absence of extenuating circumstances (severe hypoxemia, acute hemorrhage)
- The avoidance of parenteral nutrition in the first 7 days in patients for whom early enteral feeding is not feasible

Kawasaki provided a review of the pediatric sepsis literature that has been published since the Surviving Sepsis Campaign pediatric-specific considerations were last formulated in 2012.[120] Table 38-4 highlights guidelines for pediatric patients in septic shock.

NEUROCRITICAL CARE

Many neurological abnormalities in children warrant intensive care management and often require a team approach between the intensivist, neurologist, and neurosurgeon. One vulnerability of the pediatric brain is the higher metabolic rate compared with the adult.[121] The cerebral oxygen supply is typically tightly regulated by the innate ability of the cerebral blood vessels to vasodilate and allow higher flow, or vasoconstrict to dampen flow, based on both mean arterial blood pressure and metabolic demands. Discrete areas of the brain can independently modulate blood flow based on their metabolic demands. Many insults can interrupt this ability to self-regulate, placing the brain at risk for injury based on too much flow, leading to vasogenic edema and increased intracranial pressure (ICP), or too little flow, leading to ischemic injury and cellular death. This physiological disruption during

Table 38-4. 2012 Surviving Sepsis Guidelines with Special Considerations for Pediatric Patients with Additional Updates Based on Kawasaki's Review

Therapeutic end points of resuscitation	Initial: Capillary refill <2 seconds Normal blood pressure for age Normal pulses Warm extremities Urine output >1mL/kg/h Normal mental status After initial resuscitation: Central venous O_2 saturation >70% Cardiac index between 3.3 and 6 L/min/m² (typically not feasible to monitor in pediatric patients, and more recent data indicate this may not be necessary) Consider guiding resuscitation to normalize lactate Consider transthoracic echo to further guide fluid and vasoactive therapy
Treatment of infection	Antibiotics within 3 hours of the identification of sepsis Blood cultures to be drawn before administration whenever feasible Early source control, if possible
Fluid resuscitation	Fluid boluses of either crystalloid or colloid over 5 to 10 minutes—titrate to therapeutic end points Fluid resuscitation should cease if hepatomegaly or rales develops—transition to inotropic support Consider dynamic variables to predict fluid responsiveness
Inotropes	Initiate inotropes in fluid nonresponders Epinephrine may be preferable over dopamine Add vasodilator therapies in patients with low cardiac output and high SVR Consider norepinephrine in "warm shock"
Hydrocortisone	Consider stress dose hydrocortisone in refractory patients with suspected adrenal insufficiency
Blood transfusion	Hemoglobin target 10 g/dL in patients with low central venous O_2 saturations Target 7 g/dL following stabilization
Mechanical ventilation	Employ lung protective strategies
Glycemic control	Control hyperglycemia with insulin infusions as necessary to maintain blood sugar levels <180 mg/dL; monitor closely for hypoglycemia
Extracorporeal life support	Institute in patients who remain refractory to standard therapies
Fluid removal	Utilize diuretic therapy or continuous renal replacement therapy to reverse fluid overload once shock has resolved
Nutrition	Employ enteral nutrition in children who can be fed enterally and parenteral nutrition in those who cannot

brain injury requires close monitoring by an intensivist and aggressive management to prevent secondary injury to the non-injured brain matter. Many neurological insults including status epilepticus, meningitis, traumatic brain injury (TBI), cerebral ischemia, or hemorrhage require intensive care management. In addition to these injuries, the neurological system also requires close attention during post-cardiac arrest syndrome or medical sedation and may be implicated in the often underrecognized issue of delirium in the pediatric critically ill population.

Traumatic Brain Injury in Children

Traumatic brain injury (TBI) is a public health burden with up to 691 per 100,000 population for youth aged 0 to 20 years being seen in the emergency department per year.[122] The most common cause of TBI in children under the age of 5 years is falls, and for teens motor vehicle collisions.[122]

The intensivist should assess young children who experience falls for signs of abusive trauma. The severity of TBI at the outset has important prognostic implications for both immediate treatment and long-term outcomes. It is often divided into mild, moderate, and severe based on the Glasgow Coma Scale (GCS) of 13–15, 9–12, and <8, respectively.[122–125] While the GCS has been shown to be less sensitive with more severe TBI or in patients with polytrauma, it should still be used as a guide.[124,126] TBI is often associated with intracranial hemorrhage, vasogenic edema, and/or cytotoxic edema, all of which can lead to disruption of cerebrovascular autoregulation and intracranial hypertension.

Definition of Intracranial Hypertension

Intracranial hypertension can be difficult to recognize. The Monro–Kellie Doctrine states that the cerebrospinal fluid (CSF), brain, and cerebral blood content all exist in a defined volume. A disruption of one volume should lead to opposite disruptions of the other two volumes to maintain the overall intracerebral volume at a constant state. If one of the volumes is disrupted beyond the ability of the other two volumes to accommodate, intracranial hypertension results. Signs and symptoms of increased intracranial pressure (ICP) may be non-specific and can include headache, nausea, vomiting, and visual disturbances or pupillary changes, to name a few. The Cushing reflex entails systemic hypertension, reflex bradycardia in response to hypertension, and disorganized breathing. It is a well-recognized sign of intracranial hypertension but occurs late and often represents impending herniation.[127]

Etiologies of Increased ICP

Typical etiologies of intracranial hypertension may include tumors, spontaneous hemorrhage, or traumatic brain injury. It has become more recognized recently that children with bacterial meningitis are also at risk for increased ICP.[128] Patients most at risk for intracranial hypertension are those with severe TBI (GCS < 8) and a CT scan showing cerebral edema. However, head CTs may be unreliable for the diagnosis of cerebral edema. When less obvious, such as in the sedated patient, intracranial hypertension can be measured directly by a surgically placed, invasive monitor, and is more easily defined by the objective criterion of ICP >20 mm Hg.[125,129]

Monitoring

The question of whether to monitor should be a joint decision with the neurosurgeon, but monitoring allows the clinician to tailor ICP lowering therapies that will likely lead to improved outcomes.[129] Patients with severe TBI and an abnormal CT scan of the head should have a monitor placed. Monitors allow for direct measurement of the ICP and some (external ventricular drains) provide the ability to remove CSF.

Treatment

The goal of TBI treatment is to minimize the amount of secondary injury to the remaining cerebral tissue that has not been affected by the primary injury.[125] Secondary injury can be caused by hyperthermia, seizures, hypoxia, ischemia, hypotension, glucose disturbances, and increased ICP. Cerebrovascular autoregulation is no longer intact in severe TBI, so the intensivist must be vigilant in maintaining the appropriate supply of oxygen for the brain's metabolic demands. A good measure of this is to calculate a cerebral perfusion pressure (CPP) which is equal to the difference between the mean arterial pressure (MAP) and the intracranial pressure (CPP = MAP – ICP). The appropriate CPP is dependent on the child's age, with a goal of >40 mm Hg for infants and up to 55 to 60 mm Hg for children over 7 years.[129] Alternatively, the clinician should attempt to optimize the cerebral metabolic rate of oxygen by decreasing the brain's metabolic demands while still maintaining oxygen supply.

First-Tier Therapies

In children with severe TBI, it is paramount to achieve initial restoration of euvolemia, maintenance of the airway, and reduction of cerebral metabolic demand with sedation and control of fever. Children with brain injury should not be allowed to become hyperthermic. Fever should be treated aggressively with intravenous antipyretics and/or external cooling measures to maintain therapeutic normothermia. Intracranial pressure monitors can be placed at the bedside or in the operating room by a neurosurgeon if warranted. First-tier therapies should be employed as soon as possible and include maintenance of an arterial partial pressure of CO_2 of 35 to 39 mm Hg to avoid cerebral vasodilation and thus control cerebral blood flow, drainage of CSF from the ICP monitor if present, and treatment of seizures with anti-epileptic medications.[130] Sedated patients may still experience sub-clinical seizures and electroencephalography is often necessary.[131] These patients may also benefit from prophylactic anti-epileptic medications.[132] When first-tier therapies fail to control elevated ICP, second tier therapies need to be employed.

Second-Tier Therapies

Second-tier therapies focus on more dramatic actions to acutely lower ICP and typically include hyperventilation to a partial pressure of CO_2 of 30 to 34 mm Hg, hyperosmolar therapy to reduce cerebral edema, and barbiturate therapy to induce therapeutic coma and decrease metabolic demand.[130] These second-tier therapies are not without risks. Moderate hyperventilation risks ischemia secondary to cerebral vasoconstriction, and barbiturate therapy may cause significant hypotension, leading to a risk of ischemia secondary to decreased CPP. Hyperosmolar therapy with mannitol or 3% hypertonic saline has been shown to reduce ICP effectively.[130,133–135] Mannitol acts as an efficient diuretic in addition to reducing cerebral edema. If diuresis is extensive post mannitol infusion, additional fluid resuscitation may be required in order to maintain age-appropriate CPP.

Third-Tier Therapies

When second-tier therapies fail to address the elevated ICP, an additional CT scan should be obtained to assess for new or worsening bleeding and/or increased swelling. Therapeutic hypothermia to 32 to 34°C may be used with the goal of reducing cerebral metabolic demand. Therapeutic hypothermia risks increased shivering, which adds significantly to the body's metabolic demands, and should be controlled medically with sedation and/or paralysis. More severe hyperventilation to a partial pressure of CO_2 <30 mm Hg has been suggested as a temporary therapy, but this should be used with great caution given the risk of causing secondary ischemic injury. Finally, decompressive craniectomy should be considered as a therapeutic maneuver to decrease ICP.[134,136] Decompressive craniectomy has been shown to ameliorate acute neurological deterioration and impending herniation secondary to increased ICP.[130]

Sedation

Sedation is often necessary in the PICU for children who are intubated or having painful procedures. Some of the most commonly used drugs to assist with sedation are a combination of narcotics and benzodiazepines.[130] Achieving the appropriate level of sedation in an intubated child is often difficult. Children are often over-sedated, rather than under-sedated, which can lead to prolonged PICU and hospital stays, decreased ability to initiate rehabilitation, and other morbidities such as higher rates of extubation failure.[137,138]

Appropriate sedation titration requires clear sedation goals. The State Behavioral Scale (SBS) was developed as a standardized method of assessing a patient's level of sedation versus agitation while on sedatives and provides a clear goal for bedside staff to assess and affect sedation.[139] Moreover, it has been shown in the landmark RESTORE (Randomized Evaluation of Sedation Titration for Respiratory Failure) trial that nursing-driven sedation titration leads to less overall opioid exposure, need for fewer sedative classes, and more time awake and calm while intubated compared with non-nursing driven protocols.[140] Providing an appropriate sedation goal allows the bedside staff to have a positive impact on the patient's level of sedation.

Delirium

Delirium is a common, and often underrecognized, condition in critically ill children. Children at highest risk are those younger than 3 years of age with critical illness and any history of behavioral issues. Many of the common practices in the PICU increase the risk of delirium, such as turning down the lights, or darkening the room by closing the blinds, which can disrupt normal circadian rhythm. Likewise, many of the drugs that are used for sedation, such as ketamine and benzodiazepines, may also contribute to delirium.[141] The Cornell Assessment of Pediatric Delirium (CAP-D) score was developed and externally validated as a sensitive and rapid assessment tool to diagnose children with delirium.[142] Delirium should be recognized and treated aggressively to minimize morbidity and length of stay. Common treatments include environmental measures such as re-establishing a normal day-night cycle and surrounding the patient with familiar objects and people from home.[141] Atypical antipsychotics, dexmedetomidine, and melatonin have all been shown to be effective pharmacological treatments for pediatric delirium.[141,143]

Prevention of delirium by performing these environmental practices and utilizing fewer sedative medications should be practiced by all intensive care providers.

Post-Arrest Care

Cardiac arrest may also lead to disruption of cerebral vascular autoregulatory mechanisms. Neurological outcomes of post-cardiac arrest are difficult to predict, but EEG has been shown to be a useful prognosticator.[144] Intensive care management should focus on minimizing secondary injury by aggressively treating fever, minimizing glucose excursions, treating seizures, fine-tuning ventilator management, and treating electrolyte disturbances.[145] It is also important to maintain appropriate CPP for age following cardiac arrest when cardiac dysfunction is common, and the brain is at risk for ischemia. This often includes the addition of an inotropic medication to support cardiac output and maintain normal mean arterial pressure, which can prevent secondary brain injury.

HOSPITAL-ACQUIRED CONDITIONS

With the complexity of care required for critically ill children, hospital-acquired conditions are frequent. Prevention is of paramount importance and should not be overlooked.

Health care–Associated Infections

Health care–associated infections are a major source of morbidity and mortality in critically ill children. Risk factors for their acquisition include operative status, illness severity score, device utilization ratio, antimicrobial therapy, parenteral nutrition, and length of stay before onset of infection.[146] In a publication of the 2013 National Healthcare Safety Network (NHSN) report, the ventilator-associated pneumonia (VAP) rate was 0.7 per 1000 ventilator days for PICU patients, with an even higher rate in neonatal ICU (NICU) patients.[147] A national database of pediatric trauma victims identified the following risk factors for hospital-acquired pneumonia: any mechanical ventilation, with longer time on the ventilator increasing risk, increased injury severity, older age, and presence of multiple comorbid conditions.[148] The diagnosis of VAP in children between the ages of 1 and 12 years includes radiological changes and three of the following: (1) fever or hypothermia, (2) leukopenia or leukocytosis, (3) new onset purulent sputum, (4) new onset or worsening cough, dyspnea, apnea, or tachypnea, (5) rales or bronchial breath sounds, and (6) worsening gas exchange. For infants <1 year of age, in addition to radiological findings, worsening gas exchange must be present and three of the following: (1) temperature instability, (2) leukopenia or leukocytosis, (3) new onset purulent sputum, (4) tachypnea, apnea, nasal flaring, retractions, or grunting, (5) wheezing, rales, or rhonchi, (6) cough, and (7) bradycardia or tachycardia.[149]

In the NHSN 2013 data, the catheter-associated urinary tract infection (CAUTI) rate for PICU patients was 2.5 per 1000 urinary catheter days.[147] A CAUTI is generally defined as the presence of a urinary catheter within the last 48 hours plus fever, urgency, frequency, dysuria, or suprapubic tenderness and $>10^5$ microorganisms per milliliter of urine with no more than two species of microorganisms, or between 10^3 and 10^5 organisms if symptoms are present and there is an abnormal urinalysis.[149] CAUTI prevention strategies include insertion using aseptic technique, use of a closed drainage system, ensuring dependent drainage, and utilizing intermittent catheterization if a longer duration of catheterization is anticipated.[150]

According to the NHSN 2013 report, the central line–associated bloodstream infection (CLABSI) rate for PICU patients was 1.2 per 1000 central-line days. NICU patients, particularly extremely low-birth-weight infants, appear to be at even higher risk of CLABSI, with a pooled mean of 2.1 infections per 1000 central-line days. Adult studies have shown femoral catheterization to increase the risk of infectious complications as compared to subclavian catheterization,[151] but have not shown a difference in catheter-related bloodstream infection when comparing jugular to femoral vein cannulation.[152] A retrospective pediatric study did not show a difference in central venous catheter (CVC) infection rates between the internal jugular, subclavian, and femoral sites.[153] Tunneling central lines appears to reduce the rate of bacterial colonization in pediatric patients.[154] Peripherally inserted central catheters (PICCs) are also an attractive option for central access as they are relatively easy to place, have a low rate of catheter related bloodstream infections,[155] and can be left in place for extended amounts of time. A definitive diagnosis of CLABSI requires that the same organism grow from at least one percutaneous blood culture and from a culture of the catheter tip, or that a blood sample each from the catheter hub as well as a peripheral vein are positive.[156] The 2011 Centers for Disease Control and Prevention (CDC) guidelines[157] for the prevention of intravascular catheter-related infections recommend the following as applicable to pediatric patients:

2011 CDC guidelines for the prevention of intravascular catheter-related infections
Use of ultrasound guidance to place CVCs to reduce the number of cannulation attempts and mechanical complications
Use of a CVC with the minimum number of ports or lumens essential for the management of the patient
Prompt removal of any intravascular catheter that is no longer essential
Replacement as soon as possible of a CVC that was not inserted under aseptic technique
Performance of hand hygiene (with soap and water or with alcohol based hand rub) before and after inserting, replacing, accessing, repairing, or dressing a catheter
Use of max sterile barrier precautions (cap, mask, sterile gown, sterile gloves, and sterile full-body drape for insertion or guidewire exchange)
Use of chlorhexidine preparations to clean skin, replacement of CVC site dressing if the dressing becomes damp, loosened, or visibly soiled
Avoidance of topical antibiotic ointment on insertion sites
Avoidance of chlorhexidine-impregnated dressings at the site of short-term, non-tunneled CVCs for premature neonates
Use of 2% chlorhexidine wash for daily skin cleansing
Avoidance of guidewire exchanges to replace non-tunneled CVCs suspected of infection

Central to all device-associated infection prevention strategies is minimizing the duration of device use and minimizing entry into/handling of the device.

Venous Thromboembolism

Venous thromboembolism (VTE) typically presents as deep venous thrombosis (DVT) in the PICU. Unlike in adults, VTE is usually associated with underlying medical conditions such as malignancy, obesity, surgery, trauma, congenital heart disease, or congenital thrombophilia. CVCs are present in approximately one-third of patients with VTE.[158] DVT should be suspected if there is extremity swelling, plethora, or pain. VTE related to CVC is most often asymptomatic but should be suspected if there is repeated occlusion of the CVC. The most common diagnostic tool is compression ultrasonography with Doppler.

Thromboprophylaxis should be considered in patients with the following risk factors: age >14 years, malignancy, previous VTE, prolonged immobility, thrombophilic condition, recent trauma or surgery, and receipt of estrogen-containing medications.[159,160] Pharmacological thromboprophylaxis is not frequently utilized in the PICU, unless several risk factors are present, and the risk of severe bleeding is low. Mechanical thromboprophylaxis techniques include pneumatic compression boots and compression stockings. Early ambulation is also of paramount importance.

Stress Ulcer Prophylaxis

In critically ill patients, the gastric mucosa is exposed to ischemic challenges, which can lead to a breach in the protective barrier, causing gastric enzymes and acid to directly injure the gastric tissue and lead to ulcer formation and gastrointestinal bleeding. Commonly cited risk factors include mechanical ventilation, anticoagulation, head injury, multi-organ failure, corticosteroid, and nonsteroidal anti-inflammatory medication use. Histamine-receptor blockers and proton pump inhibitors are frequently used for prophylaxis and decrease the incidence of stress ulcers in critically ill children.[161] While some studies show that absence of stress ulcer prophylaxis increases the risk of VAP,[162] there is also literature that raising the gastric pH increases the risk of VAP.[163] Early introduction of enteral feeds has been shown to be protective against stress ulcer development in adults.[164]

Hospital-Associated Pressure Ulcers

Special attention should be paid to the development of hospital-associated pressure ulcers (HAPU) in patients at risk for prolonged immobility. Frequent turning, careful padding and routine inspection of pressure points, and early ambulation are important strategies to mitigate risk. Pressure damage can also occur secondary to facemask use during noninvasive positive pressure ventilation, highlighting the importance of periodic removal of the facemask and assessment of the skin, as well as rotating different types of masks (ie, nasal vs full facemask).

Post–Intensive Care Syndrome

As post-intensive care unit (PICU) mortality has drastically declined over the past several decades, increasing attention is being placed on long-term morbidity. The recently coined "post–intensive care syndrome" refers to the long-term clinical, psychological, and functional disruptions that survivors and their families experience after discharge from the ICU. PICU survivors are at risk for neurocognitive dysfunction, behavior problems, post-traumatic stress disorder, and reduced quality of life in general. High-quality research is necessary to further elucidate the epidemiology, risk factors, and preventive strategies for post-intensive care syndrome.

REFERENCES

1. Rosenberg DI, Moss MM; the Section on Critical Care and Committee on Hospital Care. Guidelines and levels of care for pediatric intensive care units. *Pediatrics.* 2004;114(4):1114-1125.
2. Milesi C, Essouri S, Pouyau R, et al. High flow nasal cannula (HFNC) versus nasal continuous positive airway pressure (nCPAP) for the initial respiratory management of acute viral bronchiolitis in young infants: a multicenter randomized controlled trial (TRAMONTANE study). *Intensive Care Med.* 2017;43:209-216.
3. Kocis KC, Dekeon MK, Rosen HK, et al. Pressure-regulated volume-control vs volume-control ventilation in infants after surgery for congenital heart disease. *Pediatr Cardiol.* 2001;22:233-237.
4. Schultz TR, Costarino AT, Durning SM, et al. Airway pressure release ventilation in pediatrics. *Pediatr Crit Care Med.* 2011;2(3):243-246.
5. Courtney SE, Durand DJ, Asselin JM, Hudak ML, Aschner JL, Shoemaker CT. High-frequency oscillatory ventilation versus conventional mechanical ventilation for very-low birth-weight infants. *N Engl J Med.* 2002;347(9):643-652.
6. Bohn D. Congenital diaphragmatic hernia. *Am J Respir Crit Care Med.* 2002;166:911-915.
7. Ng GYT, Derry C, Marston L, Choudhury M, Holmes K, Adamson Calvert S. Reduction in ventilator-induced lung injury improves outcome in congenital diaphragmatic hernia? *Pediatr Surg Int.* 2008;24:145-150.
8. Kinsella JP, Truog WE, Walsh WF, et al. Randomized, multicenter trial of inhaled nitric oxide and high-frequency oscillatory ventilation in severe, persistent pulmonary hypertension of the newborn. *J Pediatr.* 1997;131:55-62.
9. The Neonatal Inhaled Nitric Oxide Study Group. Inhaled nitric oxide in full-term and nearly full-term infants with hypoxic respiratory failure. *N Engl J Med.* 1997;336(9):597-604.
10. Roberts JD, Fineman JR, Morin FC III, et al. Inhaled nitric oxide and persistent pulmonary hypertension of the newborn. *N Engl J Med.* 1997;336(9):605-610.
11. Clark RH, Kueser TJ, Walker MW, et al. Low-dose nitric oxide therapy for persistent pulmonary hypertension of the newborn. *N Engl J Med.* 2000;342(7):469-474.
12. Miller OI, Fong Tang S, Keech A, Pigott NB, Beller E, Celermajer DS. Inhaled nitric oxide and prevention of pulmonary hypertension after congenital heart surgery: a randomised double-blind study. *Lancet.* 2000;356:1464-1469.
13. Gupta VK, Cheifetz IM. Heliox administration in the pediatric intensive care unit: an evidence-based review. *Pediatr Crit Care Med.* 2005;6(2):204-211.
14. The ARDS Definition Task Force. Acute respiratory distress syndrome: the Berlin Definition. *JAMA.* 2012;307(23):2526-2533.
15. The Pediatric Acute Lung Injury Consensus Conference Group. Pediatric acute respiratory distress syndrome: consensus recommendation from the pediatric acute lung injury consensus conference. *Pediatr Crit Care Med.* 2015;16(5):428-439.
16. Zimmerman JJ, Akhtar SR, Caldwell E, Rubenfeld GD. Incidence and outcomes of pediatric acute lung injury. *Pediatrics.* 2009;124(1):87-95.
17. Flori HR, Glidden DV, Rutherford GW, Matthay MA. Pediatric acute lung injury. *Am J Respir Crit Care Med.* 2005;171:995-1001.
18. Erickson S, Schibler A, Numa A, et al. Acute lung injury in pediatric intensive care in Australia and New Zealand: a prospective, multicenter, observational study. *Pediatr Crit Care Med.* 2007;8:317-323.
19. Ben-Abraham R, Weinbroum AA, Augerten A, et al. Acute respiratory distress syndrome in children with malignancy: Can we predict outcome? *J Crit Care.* 2001;16(2):54-58.
20. Lamas A, Otheo E, Ros P, et al. Prognosis of child recipients of hematopoietic stem cell transplantation requiring intensive care. *Intensive Care Med.* 2003;29:91-96.
21. Dahlem P, van Aalderen WMC, Hamaker ME, Dijkgraaf MGW, Bos AP. Incidence and short-term outcome of acute lung injury in mechanically ventilated children. *Eur Respir J.* 2003;22:980-985.
22. Keenan HT, Bratton SL, Martin LD, Crawford SW, Weiss NS. Outcome of children who require mechanical ventilatory support after bone marrow transplantation. *Crit Care Med.* 2000;28(3):830-835.
23. Piastra M, De Luca D, Marzano L, et al. The number of failing organs predicts non-invasive ventilation failure in children with ALI/ARDS. *Intensive Care Med.* 2011;37:1510-1516.
24. Weiss I, Ushay HM, DeBruin W, O'Loughlin J, Rosner I, Notterman D. Respiratory and cardiac function in children after acute hypoxemic respiratory failure. *Crit Care Med.* 1996;24(1):148-154.

25. Golder NDB, Lane R, Tasker RC. Timing of recovery of lung function after severe hypoxemic respiratory failure in children. *Intensive Care Med*. 1998;24:530-533.

26. Fanconi S, Kraemer R, Weber J, Tschaeppeler H, Pfenninger J. Long-term sequelae in children surviving adult respiratory distress syndrome. *J Pediatr*. 1985;106(2):218-222.

27. Effmann EL, Merten DF, Kirks DR, Pratt PC, Spock A. Adult respiratory distress syndrome in children. *Radiology*. 1985;157:69-74.

28. Ben Abraham R, Weinbroum AA, Roizin H, et al. Long-term assessment of pulmonary function tests in pediatric survivors of acute respiratory distress syndrome. *Med Sci Monit*. 2002;8(3):CR153-CR157.

29. Dahlem P, van Aalderen WMC, de Neef M, Dijkgraaf MGW, Bos AP. Randomized controlled trial of aerosolized prostacyclin therapy in children with acute lung injury. *Crit Care Med*. 2004;32:1055-1060.

30. Yanez LJ, Yunge M, Emilfork M. et al. A prospective, randomized, controlled trial of noninvasive ventilation in pediatric acute respiratory failure. *Pediatr Crit Care Med*. 2008;9:484-489.

31. Dreyfuss D, Saumon G. Ventilator-induced lung injury. *Am J Respir Crit Care Med*. 1998;157:294-323.

32. The Acute Respiratory Distress Syndrome Network. Ventilation with lower tidal volumes as compared with traditional tidal volumes for acute lung injury and the acute respiratory distress syndrome. *N Engl J Med*. 2000;342(18):1301-1308.

33. Khemani RG, Conti D, Alonzo TA, Bart RD III, Newth CJL. Effect of tidal volume in children with acute hypoxemic respiratory failure. *Intensive Care Med*. 2009;35:1428-1437.

34. Briel M, Meade M, Mercat A, et al. Higher vs lower positive end-expiratory pressure in patients with acute lung injury and acute respiratory distress syndrome. *JAMA*. 2010;203(9):865-873.

35. Phoenix SJ, Paravastu S, Columb M, Vincent J, Nirmalan M. Does a higher positive end-expiratory pressure decrease mortality in acute respiratory distress syndrome. *Anesthesiology*. 2009;110:1098-1105.

36. Arnold JH, Hanson JH, Toro-Figuero LO, Gutierrez J, Berens RJ, Anglin DL.Prospective, randomized comparison of high-frequency oscillatory ventilation and conventional mechanical ventilation in pediatric respiratory failure. *Crit Care Med*. 1994;22(10):1530-1539.

37. Bollen CW, van Well GTJ, Sherry T, et al. High frequency oscillatory ventilation compared with conventional mechanical ventilation in adult respiratory distress syndrome: a randomized controlled trial. *Critical Care*. 2005;9(4):R430-R439.

38. Hickling KG, Walsh J, Henderson S, Jackson R. Low mortality rate in adult respiratory distress syndrome using low-volume, pressure-limited ventilation with permissive hypercapnia: a prospective study. *Crit Care Med*. 1994;22(10):1568-1578.

39. Milberg JA, Davis DR, Steinberg KP, Hudson LD. Improved survival of patients with acute respiratory distress syndrome (ARDS): 1983–1993. *JAMA*. 1995;273:306-309.

40. Afshari A, Brok J, Moller AM, Wetterslev J. Inhaled nitric oxide for acute respiratory distress syndrome and acute lung injury in adults and children: a systematic review with meta-analysis and trial sequential analysis. *Anesth Analg*. 2011;112:411-421.

41. Tamburro RF, Kneyber MCJ, for the Pediatric Acute Lung Injury Consensus Conference Group. Pulmonary specific ancillary treatment for pediatric acute respiratory distress syndrome: proceedings from the pediatric acute lung injury consensus conference. *Pediatr Crit Care Med*. 2015;16:S61-S72.

42. Willson DF, Thomas NJ, Tamburro R, et al. Pediatric calfactant in acute respiratory distress syndrome trial. *Pediatr Crit Care Med*. 2013;14:657-665.

43. Curley MAQ, Hibberd PL, Fineman LD, et al. Effect of prone positioning on clinical outcomes in children with acute lung injury: a randomized controlled trial. *JAMA*. 2005;294(2):229-237.

44. Guerin C, Reignier J, Richard JC, et al. Prone positioning in severe acute respiratory distress syndrome. *N Engl J Med*. 2013;368(23):2159-2168.

45. Peter JV, John P, Graham PL, Moran JL, George IA, Bersten A. Corticosteroids in the prevention and treatment of acute respiratory distress syndrome (ARDS) in adults: meta-analysis. *BMJ*. 2008;336(7651):1006-1009.

46. Tang BMP, Craig JC, Eslick GD, Seppelt I, McLean AS. Use of corticosteroids in acute lung injury and acute respiratory distress syndrome: a systematic review and meta-analysis. *Crit Care Med*. 2009;37:1594-1603.

47. Valentine SL, Nadkarni VM, Curley MAQ, for the Pediatric Acute Lung Injury Consensus Conference Group. Nonpulmonary treatments for pediatric acute respiratory distress syndrome: proceeding from the pediatric acute lung injury consensus conference. *Crit Care Med*. 2015;16:S73-S85.

48. Smith LS, Badugu S, Hernan LJ. Shock states. In: Fuhrman BP, Zimmerman JJ, eds. *Fuhrman and Zimmerman's Pediatric Critical Care*. 5th ed. Philadelphia, PA: Elsevier; 2017:417-429.

49. Goldstein B, Giroir B, Randolph A; International Consensus Conference On Pediatric Sepsis. International pediatric sepsis consensus conference: definitions for sepsis and organ dysfunction in pediatrics. *Pediatr Crit Care Med*. 2005;6:2-8.

50. Carvalho PR, Feldens L, Seitz EE, et al. Prevalence of systemic inflammatory syndromes at a tertiary pediatric intensive care unit. *J Pediatr (Rio J)*. 2005;81:143-148.

51. Kawasaki T. Update on pediatric sepsis: a review. *J Intensive Care*. 2017;5:47.

52. Schlapbach LJ, Straney L, Bellomo R, et al. Prognostic accuracy of age-adapted SOFA, SIRS, PELOD-2, and qSOFA for in-hospital mortality among children with suspected infection admitted to the intensive care unit. *Intensive Care Med*. 2017; doi:10.1007/s00134-017-5021-8.

53. Zanotti Cavazzoni SL, Dellinger RP. Hemodynamic optimization of sepsis-induced tissue hypoperfusion. *Crit Care*. 2006;10(Suppl 3):S2.

54. Balamuth F, Fitzgerald J, Weiss SL. Shock. In: Shaw KN, Bachur RG, eds. *Fleisher & Ludwig's Textbook of Pediatric Emergency Medicine*. 7th ed. Philadelphia, PA: Lippincott Williams & Wilkins; 2016:55.

55. Zimgarelli B. Shock, ischemia, and reperfusion injury. In: Nichols DG, ed. *Rogers' Textbook of Pediatric Intensive Care*. 5th ed. Philadelphia, PA: Wolters Kluwer; 2016:253.

56. Levraut J, Ciebiera JP, Chave S, et al. Mild hyperlactatemia in stable septic patients is due to impaired lactate clearance rather than overproduction. *Am J Respir Crit Care Med*. 1998;157:1021.

57. Bell LM. Shock. In: Fleisher GR, Ludwig S, Henretig FM, eds. *Textbook of Pediatric Emergency Medicine*. 6th ed. Philadelphia, PA: Lippincott Williams & Wilkins; 2010:46.

58. Rhodes A, Evans LE, Alhazzani W, et al. Surviving sepsis campaign: international guidelines for management of sepsis and septic shock: 2016. *Intensive Care Med*. 2017;43:304-377.

59. Cantle PM, Cotton BA. Balanced resuscitation in trauma management. *Surg Clin North Am*. 2017;97:999-1014.

60. Kalkwarf KJ, Cotton BA. Resuscitation for hypovolemic shock. *Surg Clin North Am*. 2017;97:13071321.

61. Jayaraman AL, Cormican D, Shah P, Ramakrishna H. Cannulation strategies in adult veno-arterial and veno-venous extracorporeal membrane oxygenation: techniques, limitations, and special considerations. *Ann Card Anaesth.* 2017;20:S11-S18.

62. King CS, Roy A, Ryan L, Singh R. Cardiac support: emphasis on venoarterial ECMO. *Crit Care Clin.* 2017;33:777-794.

63. Le Gall A, Follin A, Cholley B, et al. Veno-arterial-ECMO in the intensive care unit: from technical aspects to clinical practice. *Anaesth Crit Care Pain Med.* 2017. doi:10.1016/j.accpm.2017.08.007.

64. Anton-Martin P, Thompson MT, Sheeran PD, et al. Extubation during pediatric extracorporeal membrane oxygenation: a single-center experience. *Pediatr Crit Care Med.* 2014;15:861-869.

65. Stein DR, Ferguson MA. Evaluation and treatment of hypertensive crises in children. *Integr Blood Press Control.* 2016;9:49-58.

66. Johnson NJ, Carlbom DJ, Gaieski DF. Ventilator management and respiratory care after cardiac arrest: oxygenation, ventilation, infection, and injury. *Chest.* 2017. doi:10.1016/j.chest.2017.11.012.

67. Moler FW, Silverstein FS, Holubkov R, et al. Therapeutic hypothermia after in-hospital cardiac arrest in children. *N Engl J Med.* 2017;376:318-329.

68. Ferguson LP, Durward A, Tibby SM. Relationship between arterial partial oxygen pressure after resuscitation from cardiac arrest and mortality in children. *Circulation.* 2012;126:335-342.

69. Sutton RM, Morgan RW, Kilbaugh TJ. Cardiopulmonary resuscitation in pediatric and cardiac intensive care units. *Pediatr Clin North Am.* 2017;64:961-972.

70. Leite HP, Isatugo MK, Sawaki L, Fisberg M. Anthropometric nutritional assessment of critically ill children. *Rev Paul Med.* 1993;111(1):309-313.

71. Singer P, Blaser AR, Berger MM, et al. ESPEN guideline on clinical nutrition in the intensive care unit. *Clin Nutr.* 2019;38:48-79.

72. Taylor BE, McClave SA, Martindale RG, et al. Guidelines for the provision and assessment of nutrition support therapy in the adult critically ill patient: Society Of Critical Care Medicine (SCCM) and American Society for Parenteral and Enteral Nutrition (A.S.P.E.N.). *Crit Care Med.* 2016;44:390-438.

73. Mehta NM, McAleer D, Hamilton S, et al. Challenges to optimal enteral nutrition in a multidisciplinary pediatric intensive care unit. *J Parenter Enteral Nutr.* 2010;34:38-45.

74. American Society of Anesthesiologists: Practice guidelines for preoperative fasting and the use of pharmacologic agents to reduce the risk of pulmonary aspiration: An updated report. *Anesthesiology.* 2011;114:495-511

75. King W, Petrillo T, Pettignano R. Enteral nutrition and cardiovascular medications in the pediatric intensive care unit. *J Parenter Enteral Nutr.* 2004;28:334-338.

76. Casaer MP, Mesotten D, Hermans G, et al. Early versus late parenteral nutrition in critically ill adults. *N Engl J Med.* 2011;365:506-517.

77. Reignier J, Boisrame-Helms J, Brisard L, et al. Enteral versus parenteral early nutrition in ventilated adults with shock: a randomised, controlled, multicentre, open-label, parallel-group study (NUTRIREA-2). *Lancet.* 2017; pii: S0140-6736(17)32146-3.

78. Fivez T, Kerklaan D, Mesotten D, et al. Early versus late parenteral nutrition in critically ill children. *N Engl J Med.* 2016;374:1111-1122.

79. Faraon-Pogaceanu C, Banasiak KJ, Hirshberg EL, Faustino EVS. Comparison of the effectiveness and safety of two insulin infusion protocols in the management of hyperglycemia in critically ill children. *Pediatr Crit Care Med.* 2010;11:741-749.

80. Agus MSD, Steil GM, Wypij D, et al. Tight glycemic control versus standard care after pediatric cardiac surgery. *N Engl J Med.* 2012;357:1208-1219.

81. Agus MSD, Asaro LA, Steil GM, et al. Tight glycemic control after pediatric cardiac surgery in high-risk patient populations. *Circulation.* 2014;129:2297-2304.

82. Macrae D, Grieve R, Allen E, et al. A randomized trial of hyperglycemic control in pediatric intensive care. *N Engl J Med.* 2014;3740:107-118.

83. Basu RK, Kaddourah A, Terrell T, et al. Assessment of worldwide acute kidney injury, renal angina and epidemiology in critically ill children (AWARE): a prospective study to improve diagnostic precision. *J Clin Trials.* 2015;5:222.

84. Akcan-Arikan A, Zappitelli M, Loftis LL, Washburn KK, Jefferson LS, Goldstein SL. Modified RIFLE criteria in critically ill children with acute kidney injury. *Kidney Int.* 2007;71:1028-1035.

85. Kwiatkowski DM, Sutherland SM. Acute kidney injury in pediatric patients. *Best Pract Res Clin Anaesthesiol.* 2017;31:427-439.

86. Bunchman TE, McBryde KD, Mottes TE, et al. Pediatric acute renal failure: outcome by modality and disease. *Pediatr Nephrol.* 2001;16:1067.

87. Sutherland SM, Byrnes JJ, Kothari M, et al. AKI in hospitalized children: comparing the pRIFLE, AKIN and KDIGO definitions. *Clin J Am Soc Nephrol.* 2015;10:554-561.

88. Teo SH, Endre ZH. Biomarkers in acute kidney injury (AKI). *Best Pract Res Clin Anaesthesiol.* 2017;31:331-344.

89. Bellomo R, Ronco C, Kellum JA, Mehta RL, Palevsky P, the ADQI workgroup. Acute renal failure—definition, outcome measures, animal models, fluid therapy and information technology needs: the second international consensus conference of the acute dialysis quality initiative (ADQI) group. *Crit Care.* 2004;8:R204-R212.

90. Bresolin N, Bianchini AP, Haas CA. Pediatric acute kidney injury assessed by pRIFLE as a prognostic factor in the intensive care unit. *Pediatr Nephrol.* 2013;28:485-492.

91. Sutherland SM, Alexander SR. Continuous renal replacement therapy in children. *Pediatr Nephrol.* 2012;27:2007-2016.

92. Gibney N, Hoste E, Burdmann EA, et al. Timing of initiation and discontinuation of renal replacement therapy in AKI: unanswered key questions. *Clin J Am Soc Nephrol.* 2008;3:876.

93. Sutherland SM, Zappitelli M, Alexander SR, et al. Fluid overload and mortality in children receiving continuous renal replacement therapy: the prospective pediatric continuous renal replacement therapy registry. *Am J Kidney Dis.* 2010;55:316.

94. Ricci Z, Ronco C. Dose and efficiency of renal replacement therapy: continuous renal replacement therapy versus intermittent hemodialysis versus slow extended daily dialysis. *Crit Care Med.* 2008;36:S229.

95. Cullis B, Abdelraheem M, Abrahams G, et al. Peritoneal dialysis for acute kidney injury. *Perit Dial Int.* 2014;34:494-517.

96. Bouty A, Faure A, Shaw L, et al. Is peritoneal dialysis feasible after laparotomy in children? A case-control series to compare outcomes. *J Pediatr Urol.* 2017;13:612.

97. Miyata S, Golden J, Lebedevskiy O, et al. The rate of PD catheter complication does not increase with simultaneous abdominal surgery. *J Pediatr Surg.* 2017. Retrieved from https://doi.org/10.1016/j.jpedsurg.2017.11.052.

98. Kwiatkowski DM, Menon S, Krawczeski CD, et al. Improved outcomes with peritoneal dialysis catheter placement after cardiopulmonary bypass in infants. *J Thorac Cardiovasc Surg.* 2015;149:230-236.

99. Bonilla-Felix M. Peritoneal dialysis in the pediatric intensive care unit setting. *Perit Dial Int.* 2009;29(Suppl 2):S183-S185.

100. Fischbach M, Terzic J, Menouer S, et al. Hemodialysis in children: principles and practice. *Semin Nephrol.* 2001;21:470-479.

101. Sakarcan A, Quigley R. Hyperphosphatemia in tumor lysis syndrome: the role of hemodialysis and continuous venovenous hemofiltration. *Pediatr Nephrol.* 1994. 8:351-353.

102. Ricci Z, Goldstein SL. Pediatric continuous renal replacement therapy. *Contrib Nephrol.* 2016;187:121-130.

103. Sutherland SM, Goldstein SL, Alexander SR. The prospective pediatric continuous renal replacement therapy (ppCRRT) registry: a critical appraisal. *Pediatr Nephrol.* 2014;29:2069-2076.

104. Davis TK, Neumayr T, Geile K, et al. Citrate anticoagulation during continuous renal replacement therapy in pediatric critical care. *Pediatr Crit Care Med.* 2014;15:471-485

105. Rodriguez K, Srivaths PR, Tal L, et al. Regional citrate anticoagulation for continuous renal replacement therapy in pediatric patients with liver failure. *PLoS One.* 2017;12:e0182134.

106. Lacroix J, Hebert PC, Hutchison JS, et al. Transfusion strategies for patients in pediatric intensive care units. *N Engl J Med.* 2007;356:1609-1619.

107. de Gast-Bakker DH, de Wilde RBP, Hazekamp MG, et al. Safety and effects of two red blood cell transfusion strategies in pediatric cardiac surgery patients: a randomized controlled trial. *Intensive Care Med.* 2013;39:2011-2019.

108. Cholette JM, Rubenstein JS, Alfieris GM, Powers KS, Eaton M, Lemer NB. Children with single-ventricle physiology do not benefit from higher hemoglobin levels post cavopulmonary connection: Results of a prospective, randomized, controlled trial of a restrictive versus liberal red-cell transfusion strategy. *Pediatr Crit Care Med.* 2011;12:39-45.

109. Doctor A, Cholette JM, Remy KE, et al. Recommendations on RBC transfusion in general critically ill children based on hemoglobin and/or physiologic thresholds from the pediatric critical care transfusion and anemia expertise initiative. *Pediatr Crit Care Med.* 2018;19:S98-S113.

110. Lavoie J. Blood transfusion risks and alternative strategies in pediatric patients. *Pediatr Anesth.* 2011; 21:14-24.

111. Stainsby D, Jones H, Wells AW, Gibson B, Cohen H. Adverse outcomes of blood transfusion in children: analysis of UK reports to the serious hazards of transfusion scheme 1996-2005. *Br J Haematol.* 2008;141:73-79.

112. Vamvakas EC, Blajchman MA. Transfusion-related immunomodulation (TRIM): an update. *Blood Rev.* 2007;21:327-348.

113. Watson RS, Carcillo JA, Linde-Zwirble WT, Clermont G, Lidicker J, Angus DC. The epidemiology of severe sepsis in children in the United States. *Am J Respir Crit Care Med.* 2003;167:695-701.

114. Black RE, Cousens S, Johnson HL, et al. Global, regional, and national causes of child mortality in 2008: a systematic analysis. *Lancet.* 2010;375:1969-1987.

115. Singer M, Deutschman CS, Seymore CW, et al. The third international consensus definitions for sepsis and septic shock (Sepsis-3). *JAMA.* 2016;315(8):801-810.

116. Goldstein B, Giroir B, Randolph A; the Members of the International Consensus Conference on Pediatric Sepsis. International pediatric sepsis consensus conference: Definitions for sepsis and organ dysfunction in pediatrics. *Pediatr Crit Care Med.* 2005;6:2-8.

117. Matics TJ, Sanchez-Pinto LN. Adaptation and validation of a pediatric sequential organ failure assessment score and evaluation of the sepsis-3 definitions in critically ill children. *JAMA Pediatr.* 2017;17(10):e172352. doi:10.1001/jamapediatrics.2017.2352.

118. Ceneviva G, Paschall JA, Maffei F, Carcillo JA. Hemodynamic support in fluid-refractory pediatric septic shock. *Pediatrics.* 1998;102(2):1-6.

119. Rhodes A, Evans LE, Alhazzani W, et al. Surviving sepsis campaign: international guidelines for management of sepsis and septic shock: 2016. *Intensive Care Med.* 2017;43:34-377.

120. Kawasaki T. Update on pediatric sepsis: a review. *J Intensive Care.* 2017;5, 47(2017). doi:10.1186/s40560-017-0240-1.

121. Chugani HT, Phelps ME, Mazziotta JC. Positron emission tomography study of human brain functional development. *Ann Neurol.* 1987;22:487-497.

122. Thurman DJ. The epidemiology of traumatic brain injury in children and youths: a review of research since 1990. *J Child Neurol.* 2016;31:20-27.

123. Teasdale G, Jennett B. Assessment of coma and impaired consciousness. A practical scale. *Lancet.* 1974;2:81-84.

124. Baum J, Entezami P, Shah K, Medhkour A. Predictors of outcomes in traumatic brain injury. *World Neurosurg.* 2016;90:525-529.

125. Seule M, Brunner T, Mack A, et al. Neurosurgical and intensive care management of traumatic brain injury. *Facial Plast Surg.* 2015;31:325-331.

126. Grote S, Bocker W, Mutschler W, et al. Diagnostic value of the Glasgow Coma Scale for traumatic brain injury in 18,002 patients with severe multiple injuries. *J Neurotrauma.* 2011;28:527-534.

127. Fodstad H, Kelly PJ, Buchfelder M. History of the cushing reflex. *Neurosurgery.* 2006;59:1132-1137.

128. Depreitere B, Bruyninckx D, Guiza F. Monitoring of intracranial pressure in meningitis. *Acta Neurochir Suppl.* 2016;122:101-104.

129. Kochanek PM, Carney N, Adelson PD, et al. Indications for intracranial pressure monitoring. In: *Guidelines for the Acute Medical Management of Severe Traumatic Brain Injury in Infants, Children, and Adolescents.* 2nd ed. *Pediatr Crit Care Med.* 2012;S11–S17.

130. Orliaguet GA, Meyer PG, Baugnon T. Management of critically ill children with traumatic brain injury. *Paediatr Anaesth.* 2008;18:455-461.

131. O'Neill BR, Handler MH, Tong S, Chapman KE. Incidence of seizures on continuous EEG monitoring following traumatic brain injury in children. *J Neurosurg Pediatr.* 2015;16:167-176.

132. Ruzas CM, DeWitt PE, Bennett KS, et al. EEG monitoring and antiepileptic drugs in children with severe TBI. *Neurocrit Care.* 2017;26:256-266.

133. Adelson PD, Bratton SL, Carney NA, et al. Guidelines for the acute medical management of severe traumatic brain injury in infants, children, and adolescents. *Pediatr Crit Care Med.* 2003;4:S1-S75.

134. Mazzola CA, Adelson PD. Critical care management of head trauma in children. *Crit Care Med.* 2002;30:S393-S401.

135. Bennett TD, Statler KD, Korgenski EK, Bratton SL. Osmolar therapy in pediatric traumatic brain injury. *Crit Care Med.* 2012;40:208-215.

136. Stocchetti N, Zanaboni C, Colomba A, et al. Refractory intracranial hypertension and "second tier" therapies in traumatic brain injury. *Intensive Care Med.* 2008;34:461-467.

137. Vet NJ, Ista E, de Wildt SN, et al. Optimal sedation in pediatric intensive care patients: a systematic review. *Intensive Care Med.* 2013;39:1524-1534.

138. Schultheis JM, Heath TS, Turner DA. Association between deep sedation from continuous intravenous sedatives and extubation failures in mechanically ventilated patients in the pediatric intensive care unit. *J Pediatr Pharmacol Ther.* 2017;22:106-111.

139. Curley MA, Harris SK, Fraser KA, et al. State behavioral scale: a sedation assessment instrument for infants and young children supported on mechanical ventilation. *Pediatr Crit Care Med.* 2006;7:107-114.

140. Curley MA, Wypij D, Watson RS, et al. Protocolized sedation vs usual care in pediatric patients mechanically ventilated for acute respiratory failure: a randomized clinical trial. *JAMA.* 2015;313:379-389.

141. Van Tuijl SG, Van Cauteren YJ, Pkhard T et al. Management of pediatric delirium in critical illness: a practical update. *Minerva Anestesiol.* 2015 Mar;81(3):333-341.

142. Traube C, Silver G, Kearney J, et al. Cornell assessment of pediatric delirium: a valid, rapid, observational tool for screening delirium in the PICU. *Crit Care Med.* 2014;42:656-663.

143. Turkel SB, Hanft A. The pharmacologic management of delirium in children and adolescents. *Paediatr Drugs.* 2014;16:267-274.

144. Ramjee V, Abella BS. The neuroprognostic challenge of post-arrest care. *Resuscitation.* 2013;84:537-538.

145. Girotra S, Chan PS, Bradley SM. Post-resuscitation care following out-of-hospital and in-hospital cardiac arrest. *Heart.* 2015;101:1943-1949.

146. Singh-Nas N, Sprague BM, Patel KM, Pollack MM. Risk factors for nosocomial infection in critically ill children: a prospective cohort study. *Crit Care Med.* 1996;24(5):875-878.

147. Dudeck MA, Edwards JR, Allen-Bridson K, et al. National Healthcare Safety Network Report, data summary for 2013: Device-associated module. *Am J Infect Control.* 2015;43:206-221.

148. Ortega HW, Cutler G, Dreyfus J, Flood A, Kharbanda A. Hospital-acquired pneumonia among pediatric trauma treated at national trauma centers. *J Trauma Acute Care Surg.* 2015;78:1149-1154.

149. Horan TC, Andrus M, Dudeck MA. CDC/NHSN surveillance definition of health care-associated infection and criteria for specific types of infections in the acute care setting. *Am J Infect Control.* 2008;36(5):309-332.

150. Hooton TM, Bradley SF, Cardenas DD, et al. Diagnosis, prevention, and treatment of catheter-associated urinary tract infection in adults: 2009 international practice guidelines from the Infectious Disease Society of America. *Clin Infect Dis.* 2010;50(5):625-663.

151. Merrer J, De Jonghe B, Golliot F, et al. Complications of femoral and subclavian venous catheterization in critically ill patients. *JAMA.* 2001;286:700-707.

152. Parienti JJ, Mongardon N, Megarbane B, et al. Intravascular complications of central venous catheterization by insertion site. *N Engl J Med.* 2015;373(13):1220-1229.

153. Reyes JA, Habash ML, Taylor RP. Femoral central venous catheters are not associated with higher rates of infection in the pediatric critical care population. *Am J Infect Control.* 2012;40:43-47.

154. Nahum E, Levy I, Katz J, et al. Efficacy of subcutaneous tunneling for prevention of bacterial colonization of femoral central venous catheters in critically ill children. *Pediatr Infect Dis J.* 2002;21:1000-1004.

155. Jumani K, Advani S, Reich NG, Gosey L, Milstone AM. Risk factors for peripherally inserted central venous catheter complications in children. *JAMA Pediatr.* 2013;167(5):429-435.

156. Mermel LA, Allon M, Bouza E, et al. Clinical practice guidelines for the diagnosis and management of intravascular catheter-related infection: 2009 update by the Infectious Diseases Society of America. *Clin Infect Dis.* 2009;49:1-45.

157. Guidelines for the prevention of intravascular catheter-related infections (2011). Centers for Disease Control and Prevention. Retrieved from https://www.cdc.gov/infection-control/guidelines/bsi/. Accessed December 19, 2017.

158. Andrew M, David M, Adams M, et al. Venous thromboembolic complications (VTE) in children: first analyses of the Canadian Registry of VTE. *Blood.* 1994;83(5):1251-1257.

159. Raffini L, Trimarchia T, Beliveau J, Davis D. Thromboprophylaxis in a pediatric hospital: a patient-safety and quality-improvement initiative. *Pediatrics.* 2011;127:E1326-E1332.

160. Barbar S, Noventa F, Rossetto V, et al. A risk assessment model for the identification of hospitalized medical patients at risk for venous thromboembolism: the Padua Prediction Score. *J Thromb Haemost.* 2010;8:2450-2457.

161. Reveiz L, Guerrero-Lozano R, Camacho A, Yara L, Mosquera PA. Stress ulcer, gastritis, and gastrointestinal bleeding prophylaxis in critically ill pediatric patients: a systematic review. *Pediatr Crit Care Med.* 2010;11:124-132.

162. Gautam A, Ganu SS, Tegg OJ, Andresen DN, Wilkins BH, Schell DN. Ventilator-associated pneumonia in a tertiary paediatric intensive care unit: a 1-year prospective observational study. *Crit Care Resusc.* 2012;14(4):283-289.

163. Grindlinger GA, Cairo SB, Duperre CB. Pneumonia prevention in intubated patients given sucralfate versus proton-pump inhibitors and/or histamine II receptor blockers. *J Surg Res.* 2016;206:398-404.

164. Raff T, Germann G, Hartmann B. The value of early enteral nutrition in the prophylaxis of stress ulceration in the severely burned patient. *Burns.* 1997;23(4):313-318.

165. Plotz FB, Bouma AB, van Wijk JA, Kneyber MC, Bokenkamp A. Pediatric acute kidney injury in the ICU: an independent evaluation of pRIFLE criteria. *Intensive Care Med.* 2008;34:1713-1717.

Cardiopulmonary Resuscitation

Shilpa Narayan and Chelsea Willie

39

HISTORY OF CPR AND EPIDEMIOLOGY

Perioperative cardiac arrest is rare and the incidence in children can be difficult to define as the time frame for anesthesia-related cardiac arrest can range from intraoperative up to 30 days postoperatively.[1] There is a discrepancy in whether studies include events during cardiac surgery or noncardiac cases. It is estimated that in-hospital pediatric cardiac arrest involves 5000 to 10,000 children per year in the United States.[2,3] Pediatric perioperative cardiac arrests excluding cardiac surgery have been found to occur in 2.9 to 7.4 per 10,000 procedures.[4,5] The incidence of specific anesthesia-related cardiac arrests when cardiac surgery is included ranges from 0.8 to 4.6 per 10,000 procedures with the highest incidence of 79 to 127 per 10,000 procedures in cardiac surgery.[4,6]

Beyond those having cardiac surgery, the highest risk patients include infants under 1 year of age (greatest in neonate) and those with an ASA physical status of 3 or higher.[4,5,7] The etiology of cardiac arrest can be divided into four broad categories to include medication-related (anesthesia overdose), cardiovascular (hypovolemia), respiratory, and equipment-related causes.[8] Within these categories the most common causes associated with perioperative pediatric arrest include hypovolemia, hyperkalemia, laryngospasm, inhaled induction, central-line complications, venous air embolism, and hypoxia.[9] Cardiovascular (CV) etiologies make up 40% of anesthesia-related cardiac arrests with decreased intravascular volume being the most common culprit. Hypovolemia due to unrecognized ongoing hemorrhage is the most common cause of intraoperative hypovolemia and is worsened by the lack of vital sign variations (e.g., lack of heart rate increase) and inadequate IV access for appropriate resuscitation.[4,7,9]

Following CV causes, respiratory etiologies make up about 31% of cardiac arrest related to anesthesia in children and involve inadequate ventilation, inadequate oxygenation, and the "loss of airway" in the form of laryngospasm, bronchospasm, and airway difficulty.[4,7]

Determining the outcome for pediatric patients after a cardiac arrest varies depending on whether events are defined as "anesthesia-related" versus "perioperative" in nature. "Anesthesia-related" mortality is estimated to be 0.1 to 1.6 per 10,000 procedures, whereas perioperative cardiac arrest (including anesthesia, surgical, and patient disease) mortality is higher at 3.8 to 13.4 per 10,000 procedures.[1,4,8,10] Overall the quality of survival is more favorable after cardiac arrest from an anesthesia-related cause compared to a nonanesthesia cause in that patients have a 62% chance of surviving and survivors have a 92% chance of having a positive neurological outcome after an anesthesia-related cause. Survival rates are only estimated to be 36% with 22% of survivors returning to their neurological status when all perioperative cardiac arrest causes are assessed.[8] It is difficult to pinpoint factors that may lead to improved outcomes after anesthesia-related causes but may include reversible causes of operating room cardiac arrest, continuous hemodynamic and respiratory monitoring during anesthesia, and the advanced preparation paired with the resuscitation skills of the anesthesiologist.[8]

RECOGNIZING ARREST

In hospital pediatric cardiac arrest most commonly occurs in the pediatric ICU due to progression of respiratory failure and/or circulatory shock.[11] One study using a multicenter registry of adverse events in pediatric anesthesia demonstrated the incidence of cardiac arrest in the perioperative period to be 5.3 per 10,000 anesthetic cases.[12] There are four recognized phases of cardiac arrest: prearrest, no flow (untreated cardiac arrest), low flow (CPR), and postresuscitation. The goals of care during each phase are vastly different; however, early recognition of the early phase gives the greatest chance of changing patient outcomes by potentially preventing the subsequent phases. Delay in starting CPR and prolonged periods of no flow are all associated with worse outcomes.[11] Thus, recognizing that a patient has progressive respiratory or circulatory failure is important for preventing progression or time spent in the no-flow phase of cardiac arrest and for prompt management with rapid initiation of basic life support (BLS) or pediatric advanced life support (PALS) once in the no-flow phase. The postresuscitative phase will be discussed later in this chapter.

MECHANICS OF CPR

The goal of CPR is to maintain coronary perfusion pressure, which is the primary factor of myocardial blood flow. Maintaining appropriate diastolic blood pressure (DBP) and thus coronary perfusion pressure is associated with increased likelihood of survival to discharge and favorable neurological outcomes after in-hospital cardiac arrest (IHCA).[13] It is important to recognize that CPR has limitations, providing only about 10% to 30% of normal blood flow to the heart and 30% to 40% of normal blood flow to the brain.[14] Being well-versed in the mechanics of BLS during pediatric CPR and resuscitation is vital to pediatric providers in order to provide optimal support during cardiac arrest.

To minimize the time to first compressions and to better align with the adult BLS recommendations that emphasize chest compressions to ventilations,[15] in 2015, the American Heart Association (AHA) adopted a major change to the sequence of chest compressions and ventilation from Airway-Breathing-Circulation (ABC) to Circulation-Airway-Breathing (CAB).[16,17] Recognizing that asphyxia and other respiratory etiologies are more common in pediatric cardiac arrest, the AHA acknowledges that ventilation may be more important in pediatric resuscitation; however, simulation studies suggest a greater delay in first compressions in the ABC approach than delay in initiation of ventilation in the CAB approach.[17-19] For in-hospital cardiac arrest, the first rescuer should begin immediate chest compressions and call for further assistance, while the second rescuer to arrive should focus on the airway and breathing components.[20]

▶ Depth and Recoil

The AHA guidelines for pediatric cardiac arrest recognize that there is limited evidence supporting the targeted depth for compression in pediatric patients. The consensus recommendations are that pediatric patients require compression of the chest by at least one-third of the anterior-posterior diameter. In infants, this is approximately 1.5 in., while in children this is 2 in. or greater. Of note, overly deep compressions have been associated with potentially worse patient outcomes.[15]

Allowing for complete chest recoil between compressions is a key element often missed in high-quality CPR. Incomplete chest recoil can lead to higher intrathoracic pressures, decreased venous return, decreased coronary perfusion and blood flow, and decreased cerebral perfusion.[17,21]

▶ Focal Versus Circumferential Compressions in Infants

Due to children's size and chest wall compliance, the use of focal versus circumferential compressions is debated. Focal compressions utilize two fingers placed over the infant's sternum to administer compressions, while circumferential compressions are administered by encircling the chest with two hands and placing the rescuer's thumbs to depress the sternum.[17,20] The AHA endorses the use of two fingers or focal technique in pediatric resuscitation; however, several animal and simulation studies have supported the use of the two hands or circumferential technique.[17] The latter method in these studies resulted in higher mean arterial, systolic, and diastolic blood pressures.[22,23] The AHA recommendations suggest either technique can be utilized, as long as adequate depth and recoil can be achieved.[17]

Ratios and Rate

During cardiac arrest, the ratio of compressions to ventilations depends on the presence of an advanced airway and the number of rescuers. This ratio is based on achieving a balance that optimizes oxygen delivery to the vital organs, which requires compressions and minute ventilation. Rescuers must also recognize the positive pressure ventilation (PPV) benefits, but know that PPV can be detrimental if it is used too aggressively due to the impedance to forward flow PPV may cause.[20] At the writing of this text, the most updated AHA recommendations for compression to ventilation ratios come from their 2010 consensus.[24]

Single Rescuer

In a study on out-of-hospital cardiac arrests (OHCA) comparing favorable neurological outcomes for children receiving standard bystander CPR (compressions with rescue breaths) versus compression only, CPR showed that children with noncardiac etiology of their cardiac arrest had more favorable neurological outcomes with standard bystander CPR.[25] Several animal studies also support this finding as well, which is why the AHA continues to recommend a compression to ventilation of 30 compressions to 2 rescue breaths for infants and children (same recommendation for adults).[24]

Two Rescuers; No Advanced Airway in Place

For most IHCAs, there will likely and fortunately be more than one provider available. If there is no advanced airway present, the compression-to-ventilation ratio should be 15 compressions for every 2 breaths, provided by bag-mask ventilation.[24] Efforts should be made to obtain a secure, advanced airway as soon as possible, while minimizing interruptions to chest compressions when in a hospital setting.

Two Rescuers; Advanced Airway in Place

Once an advanced airway has been established, compressions should be performed continuously with no pauses.[20,24] A rapid ventilation rate should be avoided during CPR. A CPR study on a pig model revealed that excessive ventilation led to significantly decreased coronary perfusion pressure, increased intrathoracic pressure, and decreased survival rates.[26,27] The AHA does not provide a suggested rate for ventilation during pediatric cardiac arrest, but merely recommends avoidance of excessive ventilation.[24] A generally accepted rate is 8 to 12 breaths per minute during cardiac arrest. This should be titrated by the provider based on end-tidal CO_2 or signs of increased intrathoracic pressure.

SPECIAL CONSIDERATIONS FOR INTRAOPERATIVE CPR

Surgical procedures require an array of positions including the prone and sitting positions that may expose pediatric patients to a higher risk of both cardiac arrest and delay in CPR. Patients are also exposed to multiple drugs that are necessary for the anesthetic, which might predispose the child to toxicity that may lead to cardiac arrest. Open-chest CPR is a viable option in postoperative cardiac patients or abdominal surgeries during which the chest or abdomen are left open. Studies show that open-chest CPR can achieve near-normal blood flow and increase cardiac output two to three times above conventional closed-chest CPR.[28,29]

Spine surgeries and posterior cranial surgeries may delay conventional supine CPR due to the stage of the surgery requiring surgical stabilization and preparation for repositioning. To prevent delay of life-saving therapies, CPR should be initiated in the prone position. One method to deliver prone compressions involves one hand over each scapula while counterpressure is provided by a second rescuer's hand/fist or sandbag on the sternum. The second method is identical except the compressions are done with the heel of one hand on the spine with the second hand on top, similar to that of conventional sternum compressions and can be done when surgical exposure does not include the midline spine.[30,31] Prone compressions have been shown to achieve an effective depth 75% of the time when compared to supine compressions using a high-fidelity simulation model.[32] The efficacy of prone compressions was noted in a clinical study that showed six adults in an ICU had better hemodynamics when CPR was done in the prone position versus the supine position.[33]

Not only does alternative positioning lead to limitations to CPR, but procedures in which large open blood vessels are above the level of the heart can place the patient at higher risk for a venous air embolus (VAE). Craniofacial, other neurosurgical procedures, and spine surgeries are common culprits for this complication as they also may be associated with hypovolemia that can lower the CVP and worsen entrainment of air.[9] A VAE is typically recognized as an abrupt decrease in blood pressure and ETCO2, which can be further verified by end-tidal nitrogen, transesophageal echocardiography, or audible doppler bubbles.[8] Initial steps should involve lowering the operative site below the heart, flooding the site with fluid, and if possible positioning the patient in the left lateral decubitus position to prevent air entry into the pulmonary artery which could cause further obstruction to left heart flow.

Inhalational induction exposes patients to rapid physiological changes such as vasodilation and a hyperstimulating state that can lead to significant hemodynamic changes and respiratory compromise in an unsecured airway. It is estimated that 25% of perioperative cardiac arrests occur during induction due to hypotension and laryngospasm.[7] Hypotension may be significant when the vasodilation from volatile anesthetics is paired with the relative hypovolemic patient from causes such as NPO requirements, bowel preparations, and shock. Treatment should involve decreasing the inhalational agent and administering fluid or blood with possible temporization with vasoactive medications. If laryngospasm occurs, positive pressure with deepening of the anesthetic should be initiated. Depending on vascular access, a muscle relaxant (such as succinylcholine) should be administered via the IV or IM route. Careful induction and vigilant awareness with appropriate response to cardiovascular and respiratory changes can improve the safety profile during an inhalational induction.

The risk for intraoperative cardiac arrest from hyperkalemia in children is high when rapid infusion of blood occurs and increases proportionately with the age of the blood transfused.[7] Hemodynamic signs of hyperkalemia include peaked T waves, arrhythmias (VT or VF), and widening QRS complexes which should be immediately treated with discontinuation of the blood transfusion, alkalosis (hyperventilation and bicarbonate), and stabilization of the cardiac membrane with calcium. Potassium can be further driven intracellularly with insulin/glucose and beta-agonists.

Medication-related intraoperative cardiac arrest is commonly associated with local anesthetic toxicity and anaphylaxis. Regional anesthesia is typically performed when children are already under general anesthesia, so early signs of toxicity (neurological changes) are not present in prevention of the later effects of conduction abnormalities and cardiovascular collapse. Cardiac arrest caused by local anesthetic toxicity is unique in that hemodynamic support is accomplished with lower doses of epinephrine (less than 1 mcg/kg per bolus) and drugs that could further compromise cardiac function (vasopressin, calcium channel blockers, beta blockers, and lidocaine) should be avoided. The mainstay treatment is lipid emulsion 20% 1.5 mL/kg (maximum dose 12 mL/kg) followed by an infusion 0.25 mL/kg/min. If hemodynamic stability cannot be accomplished medically, extracorporeal life support should be an early consideration.[34] Another medication-associated etiology for sudden cardiovascular collapse is anaphylaxis which is most commonly related to the administration of antibiotics or neuromuscular blockers. Anaphylaxis may be exhibited by tachycardia, bronchospasm, angioedema, and rash. Treatment includes 100% oxygen, epinephrine IV or IM, corticosteroids, antihistamines, and supportive care with albuterol and H1 blockers. CPR should commence as indicated by the AHA guidelines for PALS if anaphylaxis progresses to shock.[8]

VENTRICULAR FIBRILLATION/TACHYCARDIA

Ventricular fibrillation is an uncommon yet fatal arrhythmia. Children with a sudden, witnessed collapse in an out-of-hospital situation should arouse a strong suspicion for ventricular fibrillation (VF) or ventricular tachycardia (VT).[17] In a large, multicenter study, it was found that 27% of pediatric patients who had an IHCA had VF or VT at some point during their arrest. In 10% of the patients, it was the initial pulseless rhythm. Notably, this study found that in patients whose initial rhythm was not VT/VF but subsequently deteriorated into VT/VF during their resuscitation had worse outcomes than those patients who were in VF/VT as their initial rhythm.[35]

Causes

Underlying cardiac disease is one of the most common causes of IHCA from VF/VT, with up to 40% of in-hospital cases occurring in pediatric cardiac patients.[36] Other common causes include tricyclic antidepressant overdose, hyperkalemia, cardiomyopathy, prolonged QT syndromes, and asphyxiation.[20]

Treatment

A study of witnessed OHCA in adults showed that rapid defibrillation of VF led to a long-term survival of >70% when defibrillation was administered in less than 3 minutes.[37] Although mortality increases by as much as 7% to 10% with each minute of delay of defibrillation, earlier electrical treatment increases the success rate of returning to an organized rhythm.[20] Thus, it is imperative to both recognize and aggressively treat VT/VF when present during a cardiac arrest.

For IHCA, manual defibrillation should be administered by trained healthcare providers. The evidence supporting the dosing of defibrillation is limited in pediatrics and extrapolated from adult data. The initial recommended dose for pediatric VT/VF is 2 J/kg. Subsequent doses should be increased by 2 J/kg to a maximum of 10 J/kg or maximum adult dose.[20] In between delivered shocks, efforts should be made to minimize interruptions of chest compressions, with resumption immediately upon delivery of the shock and analyzed rhythm after 2 minutes of effective CPR.[17]

CARDIOPULMONARY RESUSCITATION MEDICATIONS (TABLE 39-1)

Epinephrine

Epinephrine has long been proven to increase diastolic pressure and systemic vascular resistance, thereby becoming the mainstay medication for CPR as it directly improves coronary perfusion which increases the chances for a successful resuscitation.[38] The alpha-agonist action of epinephrine is probably the most important in increasing coronary blood flow to maintain myocardial blood flow and in providing cerebral blood flow with peripheral vasoconstriction.[39] Although the beta-adrenergic stimulation may increase the "vigor" of VF to help in defibrillation, it increases myocardial oxygen demand which can increase the risk of ischemic injury.[40] There is varying evidence about the use of high-dose epinephrine (0.1 mg/kg) versus standard dose epinephrine (0.01 mg/kg). Some studies have found that cerebral and coronary blood flow may be increased, but other studies have noted that this may result in detrimental increase in myocardial oxygen consumption which may lead to postresuscitation adverse effects with no benefits in return of spontaneous circulation (ROSC), neurological outcome, or survival to hospital discharge.[41] A randomized, prospective study by Perondi et al revealed that there was no difference in survival in children given high-dose versus standard-dose epinephrine in witnessed in-hospital cardiac arrest and patients with asphyxia-related cardiac arrest did worse.[42] The situations in which high-dose epinephrine may be helpful are beta-blocker or calcium channel–blocker overdose, severe anaphylaxis, or septic shock.[24] In summary, the 2015 AHA guidelines recommend standard dose epinephrine for serial doses in pulseless cardiac arrest.[18]

Vasopressin

Vasopressin tends to be compared in efficacy to epinephrine in that it provides vasoconstriction (V1 receptors) and causes water reabsorption by binding to renal tubule receptors (V2 receptors) without the adrenergic effects that cause increased myocardial demand. The use of vasopressin in pediatric cardiac arrest is not well studied and in one multivariate analysis from October 1999 to November 2004 it was noted that vasopressin was associated with worse ROSC, but without any difference in discharge survival.[43] The AHA guidelines do not provide recommendations for vasopressin in pediatric patients, but in adults with refractory VF it is recommended to use 40 units of vasopressin. In one retrospective case series of four children undergoing prolonged CPR (> 60 minutes) there was ROSC in three of the four patients following vasopressin (0.4 U/kg) administration, so this may warrant further study about the use of vasopressin in prolonged pediatric cardiac arrest.[44]

Atropine

Atropine is a parasympatholytic drug that increases heart rate by its effects on the sinus node, shortening of AV conduction, and activating latent ectopic pacemakers.[45] It is especially useful for bradycardia as a result of increased parasympathetic tone. Atropine should be considered in second-and third-degree AV blocks, and bradycardia with associated hypotension.[46] In pediatric patients, atropine is occasionally given before intubation to prevent the parasympathetic response that might result from airway manipulation in a neonate.

Adenosine

Adenosine is a purine nucleoside that binds to adenosine receptors in the myocardium and peripheral vasculature to cause slower conduction through the AV node by prolonging the AV-node refractory period. Adenosine is used to treat supraventricular tachycardia by terminating the reentrant circuit.[47] It must be given very rapidly (typically in a stopcock followed by a 10-mL flush) due to its very rapid metabolism by adenosine deaminase on red blood cells, which clears it within 30 seconds.[48]

Amiodarone

Amiodarone is an antiarrhythmic drug that is classified as a class III antiarrhythmic (increases action potential and refractory period), but spans over all the classes in its effect as potassium channel blocker, sodium influx blocker, noncompetitive beta-blocker, and calcium channel blocker.[49] The effect of amiodarone is directly associated with the route of administration. Oral administration leads to a mostly class III effect, but the IV loading dose most commonly used in an emergency results in a class II effect with increased AV node refraction and AV node conduction.[50] The alpha-adrenergic blockade effect of amiodarone leads to coronary and systemic vasodilation, so while enhancing heart perfusion it may lead to overall hypotension.[51] With its wide pharmacological profile, amiodarone has become one of the recommended drugs (along with lidocaine) for shock refractory VF and pulseless VT (pVT).[18]

Lidocaine

Lidocaine is a class 1B antiarrhythmic that acts on the sodium channels to increase the refractory period and decrease the action potential to stop reentrant ventricular arrhythmias. As there is no effect on AV conduction time, lidocaine does not have an effect on atrial or junctional arrhythmias, but is useful in decreasing the ventricular accelerated ectopic foci.[52] Lidocaine is used for ventricular tachyarrhythmias and can be used interchangeably with amiodarone for shock-refractory VF or pVT.[18]

Magnesium

Hypomagnesemia may occur in critically ill children and with coming off cardiopulmonary bypass, which may increase the risk of arrhythmias. Administering magnesium emergently (during CPR) is only indicated for hypomagnesemia and torsades de pointes VT. If magnesium is given rapidly it can lead to hypotension due to a decrease in systemic vascular resistance, so the infusion rate may be limited by this adverse effect.[8]

Calcium

Calcium directly affects contractility and ventricular automaticity, but despite its essential role in cardiac contractility it has been found to be associated with poor survival and neurological outcomes in pediatric patients when used during CPR.[53] This negative effect may be due to the role of calcium in cell death of many organs. The only indications for calcium during cardiopulmonary resuscitation are suspected hypocalcemia, hyperkalemia, hypermagnesemia, and calcium channel blocker overdose.[52] Giving calcium during an intraoperative cardiac arrest may be warranted as there is a higher potential for hypocalcemia and hyperkalemia with rapid blood product administration.[54] As electrolyte imbalance was noted to be associated with 5% of pediatric perioperative arrests in the Pediatric Perioperative Cardiac Arrest Registry, intraoperative CPR is a special situation during which calcium administration should likely occur.[7] Calcium administration should be carried out with care as it can lead to bradycardia, heart block, and ventricular standstill.[7]

Sodium Bicarbonate

Sodium bicarbonate administration during cardiopulmonary arrest remains very controversial. The use of sodium bicarbonate is beneficial in correcting the metabolic acidosis that can lead to depressed myocardial function and decreased response to catecholamines. It may also treat the acidosis that leads to systemic vasodilation and increased pulmonary vascular resistance.[8,55] The worrisome effects of bicarbonate administration include metabolic alkalosis that can impair oxygen delivery to tissues (shift the oxyhemoglobin dissociation curve to the left), hypernatremia, hypercapnia, and hyperosmolarity which all may be associated with increased mortality.[56,57] This leaves the use of sodium bicarbonate limited to hyperkalemic arrest, hypermagnesemia, long CPR time, tricyclic antidepressant overdose, and overdose from sodium-blocking drugs (cocaine, beta-blockers, and diphenhydramine).[8,51]

QUALITY CPR

While survival outcomes have continued to improve over the years, the degree of mortality and morbidity remains quite high even among IHCA patients.[2,58] With this knowledge, there has been a growing focus on identifying methods to monitor the quality of CPR efforts being provided by healthcare providers, particularly in the inpatient setting (ICU or OR) where patients often already have advanced airways and invasive monitoring. The AHA recommends the use of arterial line waveforms and in-line capnography as guidance for the quality of compressions being provided.

Capnography

Capnography should be used to verify tracheal tube placement during perfusing rhythms and assess cardiac output by chest compressions during cardiac arrest. If $ETCO_2$ is not detected during cardiac arrest, the position of the tracheal tube should be confirmed by direct laryngoscopy, taking care to minimize interruptions to compressions.

The AHA previously recommended a target $ETCO_2$ of 15 mm Hg or higher, as animal studies supported a direct association between $ETCO_2$ and ROSC. Adjustments to the quality of compressions should occur if this target is not being met by optimizing the depth, rate, and recoil. An effort to ensure the patient is not being ventilated excessively should also be made. A rapid rise in $ETCO_2$ can also be a visual indicator of ROSC, which is another significant utility of capnography monitoring during cardiac arrest.

In cases of low pulmonary blood flow, such as pulmonary embolism or obstructed caval shunts, $ETCO_2$ may not be detectable regardless of adequacy of compressions. In cases of severe airway obstruction, such as status asthmaticus or pulmonary edema, the $ETCO_2$ may be undetectably high.

Invasive Hemodynamic Monitoring

If a patient has an invasive arterial catheter during cardiac arrest, the waveform can be used to optimize the delivery of chest compressions. Animal studies showed an increased likelihood of ROSC when invasive monitoring is used to guide CPR. At this time, there are no evidence-based guidelines for goal systolic or diastolic blood pressures.[18]

POSTRESUSCITATION CONSIDERATIONS

In the postresuscitative phase, after achieving ROSC, the goals of management focus on preserving neurological function and preventing further secondary organ damage. During this phase, the patient is at the highest risk for brain injury, ventricular arrhythmias, and reperfusion injury. After stabilization, the goal should be to diagnose the underlying etiology of the arrest and provide appropriate interventions, otherwise the patient remains at risk for additional events.

Myocardial Function

Myocardial stunning is common after cardiac arrest and usually involves global, biventricular systolic and diastolic dysfunction. The severity of myocardial dysfunction increases with prolonged untreated cardiac arrest time, prolonged CPR, and after administration of multiple shocks of higher energy for defibrillation. Myocardial stunning will often lead to hypotensive shock, further exacerbating secondary organ damage.[11] Several pediatric studies demonstrated that post-ROSC hypotension was associated with worse survival to discharge and less

Table 39-1. Resuscitation Drug Guide

Drug	Dose/Route	Indication	Action
Epinephrine (1:10,000 IV/IO) (1:1,000 ETT)	IV/IO (1:10K): 0.01 mg/kg (0.1 mL/kg) (max 1 mg) ETT (1:1K): 0.1 mg/kg IM/SQ (1:1K): 0.01 mg/kg (anaphylaxis)	• Bradycardia • Pulseless arrest • Anaphylaxis	• Alpha-adrenergic • Beta-adrenergic
Vasopressin	IV/IO: 0.4 U/kg (max 40 U)	• Refractory VF	• V1 (vasoconstriction) • V2 (renal water reabsorption)
Atropine	IV/IO/IM: 0.02 mg/kg (max 1 mg) ETT: 0.03–0.05 mg/kg	• Bradycardia • AV node block •	• Blocks cholinergic stimulation
Adenosine	IV/IO: 0.1 mg/kg (first dose; max 6 mg) 0.2 mg/kg (second dose; max 12 mg)	• SVT	• Prolongs AV-node refractory period • Slows conduction •
Amiodarone	IV/IO: 5 mg/kg (pulseless) over 20–60 minutes (if perfusing rhythm) (max 20 mg/kg/day)	• VF, VT and SVT	• Alpha-adrenergic blockade • Beta-adrenergic blockade • Ca channel blockade • Action potential prolongation
Lidocaine	IV/IO: 1 mg/kg (max 100 mg) ETT: 1.5–2.5 mg/kg	• Ventricular • arrhythmias	• Deceases automaticity of ventricular ectopic foci
Magnesium	IV/IO: 25–50 mg/kg (max 2 g)	• Torsades de pointes • Hypomagnesemia	• In enzymatic reactions as intracellular cation
Calcium	IV/IO: 20 mg/kg ($CaCl_2$) 60 mg/kg (CaGlc) (max 2 g)	• Hypocalcemia • Hyperkalemia • Hypermagnesemia • Calcium channel blocker overdose	• Myocardial excitation-contraction coupling • Myocardial contractility
Sodium Bicarbonate	IV/IO: 1 meq/kg or calculate base deficit	• Metabolic acidosis • Hyperkalemia • Long CPR time	• Buffers excess H^+ thus increasing the pH

likelihood of discharge with favorable neurological outcomes.[59] Specific treatment for this phenomenon has not been well-described in pediatric patients; however, the use of fluid resuscitation followed by continuous infusions of vasoactive agents with inotropic properties is recommended to maintain a systolic blood pressure greater than the 5th percentile for age.[18] Care should be taken not to increase the afterload to the left ventricle through aggressive use of vasoactive agents leading to hypertension in the postarrest phase of care, which may cause further myocardial dysfunction.[20]

Targeted Temperature Management

Hyperthermia is known to lead to worse outcomes and is common in postarrest children.[20,60] Fevers should be treated aggressively, with the goal to achieve normothermia. Trials in adults have shown induced hypothermia to be neuroprotective postcardiac arrest; however, this was not replicated in a pediatric study.[61] At this time, there is inadequate evidence to support cooling after IHCA for pediatric patients, thus the mainstay of treatment should be avoidance of hyperthermia.[18]

Oxygenation

Hyperoxemia after cardiac arrest was shown to increase oxidative stress in animal studies. There is limited evidence in the pediatric population about the effect of hyperoxemia on outcomes, though one large observational study showed improved survival to ICU discharge in patients with normoxemia when compared to those with hypoxemia (PaO_2 < 60 mm Hg) or hyperoxemia (PaO_2 > 300 mm Hg).[62] Thus, it is suggested to target normoxemia in pediatric patients in the postresuscitative phase.

Extracorporeal Life Support (ECLS)

Initiating CPR is the gold standard for the low-flow and no-flow states during a cardiopulmonary arrest, but early activation of ECLS should be considered in cardiac arrest with reversible causes that are refractory to standard resuscitation measures.[18] ECLS is now part of the 2015 AHA PALS guidelines and is recommended for in-house cardiac arrest and has been especially useful in patients with congenital heart disease, as several studies have found that ECLS in this patient cohort has higher survival rates.[36,63,64] The use of ECLS in the operating room is important as typically this is an environment in which cardiac arrest is recognized very quickly by personnel highly trained in resuscitation and many times the surgeon is readily available to initiate ECMO. ECLS should be considered in reversible causes that include hyperkalemia, local anesthetic toxicity, general anesthetic overdose, and airway emergency. Patients with bleeding issues may be a challenge on ECMO, but the only contraindications to ECMO are patients with irreversible pathology or disability that would prevent an acceptable quality of life after conclusion of ECMO.[8]

REFERENCES

1. van der Griend BF, Lister NA, McKenzie IM, et al. Postoperative mortality in children after 101,885 anesthetics at a tertiary pediatric hospital. *Anesth Analg.* 2011;112(6):1440-1447.
2. Sutton RM, Morgan RW, Kilbaugh TJ, Nadkarni VM, Berg RA. Cardiopulmonary resuscitation in pediatric and cardiac intensive care units. *Pediatr Clin North Am.* 2017;64(5):961-972.
3. Knudson JD, Neish SR, Cabrera AG, et al. Prevalence and outcomes of pediatric in-hospital cardiopulmonary resuscitation in the United States: an analysis of the Kids' Inpatient Database. *Crit Care Med.* 2012;40(11):2940-2944.
4. Flick RP, Sprung J, Harrison TE, et al. Perioperative cardiac arrests in children between 1988 and 2005 at a tertiary referral center: a study of 92,881 patients. *Anesthesiology.* 2007;106(4):226-237; quiz 413-224.
5. Bharti N, Batra YK, Kaur H. Paediatric perioperative cardiac arrest and its mortality: database of a 60-month period from a tertiary care paediatric centre. *Eur J Anaesthesiol.* 2009;26(6):490-495.
6. Odegard KC, DiNardo JA, Kussman BD, et al. The frequency of anesthesia-related cardiac arrests in patients with congenital heart disease undergoing cardiac surgery. *Anesth Analg.* 2007;105(2):335-343.
7. Bhananker SM, Ramamoorthy C, Geiduschek JM, et al. Anesthesia-related cardiac arrest in children: update from the Pediatric Perioperative Cardiac Arrest Registry. *Anesth Analg.* 2007;105(2):344-350.
8. Cladis FP. *Smith's Anesthesia for Infants and Children.* 9th ed. Philadelphia, PA: Elsevier; 2016.
9. Shaffner DH, Heitmiller ES, Deshpande JK. Pediatric perioperative life support. *Anesth Analg.* 2013;117(4):960-979.
10. Morray JP, Geiduschek JM, Ramamoorthy C, et al. Anesthesia-related cardiac arrest in children: initial findings of the Pediatric Perioperative Cardiac Arrest (POCA) Registry. *Anesthesiology.* 2000;93(1):6-14.
11. Topjian AA, Berg RA, Nadkarni VM. Advances in recognition, resuscitation, and stabilization of the critically ill child. *Pediatr Clin North Am.* 2013;60(3):605-620.
12. Christensen RE, Lee AC, Gowen MS, Rettiganti MR, Deshpande JK, Morray JP. Pediatric Perioperative Cardiac Arrest, Death in the Off Hours: a report from Wake Up Safe, the Pediatric Quality Improvement Initiative. *Anesth Analg.* 2018;127(2):472-477.
13. Atkins DL, de Caen AR, Berger S, et al. 2017 American Heart Association Focused Update on Pediatric Basic Life Support and Cardiopulmonary Resuscitation Quality: An update to the American Heart Association Guidelines for Cardiopulmonary Resuscitation and Emergency Cardiovascular Care. *Circulation.* 2018;137(1):e1-e6.
14. Marino BS, Tabbutt S, MacLaren G, et al. Cardiopulmonary resuscitation in infants and children with cardiac disease: a scientific statement from the American Heart Association. *Circulation.* 2018;137(22):e691-e782.
15. de Caen AR, Maconochie IK, Aickin R, et al. Part 6: Pediatric basic life support and pediatric advanced life support: 2015 International Consensus on Cardiopulmonary Resuscitation and Emergency Cardiovascular Care Science with Treatment Recommendations (Reprint). *Pediatrics.* 2015;136(suppl 2):S88-S119.
16. Berg MD, Schexnayder SM, Chameides L, et al. Part 13: Pediatric basic life support: 2010 American Heart Association Guidelines for Cardiopulmonary Resuscitation and Emergency Cardiovascular Care. *Circulation.* 2010;122(18 Suppl 3):S862-S875.
17. Atkins DL, Berger S, Duff JP, et al. Part 11: Pediatric basic life support and cardiopulmonary resuscitation quality: 2015 American Heart Association Guidelines Update for Cardiopulmonary Resuscitation and Emergency Cardiovascular Care. *Circulation.* 2015;132(18 Suppl 2):S519-S525.
18. de Caen AR, Berg MD, Chameides L, et al. Part 12: Pediatric advanced life support: 2015 American Heart Association Guidelines Update for Cardiopulmonary Resuscitation and Emergency Cardiovascular Care. *Circulation.* 2015;132(18 Suppl 2):S526-S542.
19. Marsch S, Tschan F, Semmer NK, Zobrist R, Hunziker PR, Hunziker S. ABC versus CAB for cardiopulmonary resuscitation: a prospective, randomized simulator-based trial. *Swiss Med Weekly.* 2013;143:w13856.
20. Nichols DG, Shaffner DH. *Rogers' Textbook of Pediatric Intensive Care.* 5th ed. Philadelphia, PA: Wolters Kluwer; 2016.
21. Zuercher M, Hilwig RW, Ranger-Moore J, et al. Leaning during chest compressions impairs cardiac output and left ventricular myocardial blood flow in piglet cardiac arrest. *Crit Care Med.* 2010;38(4):1141-1146.
22. Houri PK, Frank LR, Menegazzi JJ, Taylor R. A randomized, controlled trial of two-thumb vs two-finger chest compression in a swine infant model of cardiac arrest [see comment]. *Prehosp Emerg Care.* 1997;1(2):65-67.
23. Dorfsman ML, Menegazzi JJ, Wadas RJ, Auble TE. Two-thumb vs. two-finger chest compression in an infant model of prolonged cardiopulmonary resuscitation. *Acad Emerg Med.* 2000;7(10):1077-1082.
24. Kleinman ME, de Caen AR, Chameides L, et al. Part 10: Pediatric basic and advanced life support: 2010 International Consensus on Cardiopulmonary Resuscitation and Emergency Cardiovascular Care Science With Treatment Recommendations. *Circulation.* 2010;122(16 Suppl 2):S466-S515.

25. Kitamura T, Iwami T, Kawamura T, et al. Conventional and chest-compression-only cardiopulmonary resuscitation by bystanders for children who have out-of-hospital cardiac arrests: a prospective, nationwide, population-based cohort study. *Lancet (London, UK)*. 2010;375(9723):1347-1354.

26. Aufderheide TP, Sigurdsson G, Pirrallo RG, et al. Hyperventilation-induced hypotension during cardiopulmonary resuscitation. *Circulation*. 2004;109(16):1960-1965.

27. Aufderheide TP, Lurie KG. Death by hyperventilation: a common and life-threatening problem during cardiopulmonary resuscitation. *Crit Care Med*. 2004;32(9 Suppl):S345-S351.

28. Weiser FM, Adler LN, Kuhn LA. Hemodynamic effects of closed and open chest cardiac resuscitation in normal dogs and those with acute myocardial infarction. *Am J Cardiol*. 1962;10:555-561.

29. Bircher N, Safar P. Comparison of standard and "new" closed-chest CPR and open-chest CPR in dogs. *Crit Care Med*. 1981;9(5):384-385.

30. Sun WZ, Huang FY, Kung KL, Fan SZ, Chen TL. Successful cardiopulmonary resuscitation of two patients in the prone position using reversed precordial compression. *Anesthesiology*. 1992;77(1):202-204.

31. Tobias JD, Mencio GA, Atwood R, Gurwitz GS. Intraoperative cardiopulmonary resuscitation in the prone position. *J Pediatr Surg*. 1994;29(12):1537-1538.

32. Atkinson MC. The efficacy of cardiopulmonary resuscitation in the prone position. *Crit Care Resuscitat*. 2000;2(3):188-190.

33. Mazer SP, Weisfeldt M, Bai D, et al. Reverse CPR: a pilot study of CPR in the prone position. *Resuscitation*. 2003;57(3):279-285.

34. Neal JM, Woodward CM, Harrison TK. The American Society of Regional Anesthesia and Pain Medicine Checklist for Managing Local Anesthetic Systemic Toxicity: 2017 version. *Reg Anesth Pain Med*. 2018;43(2):150-153.

35. Samson RA, Nadkarni VM, Meaney PA, Carey SM, Berg MD, Berg RA. Outcomes of in-hospital ventricular fibrillation in children. *New Engl J Med*. 2006;354(22):2328-2339.

36. Ortmann L, Prodhan P, Gossett J, et al. Outcomes after in-hospital cardiac arrest in children with cardiac disease: a report from Get With the Guidelines—Resuscitation. *Circulation*. 2011;124(21):2329-2337.

37. Valenzuela TD, Roe DJ, Nichol G, Clark LL, Spaite DW, Hardman RG. Outcomes of rapid defibrillation by security officers after cardiac arrest in casinos. *New Engl J Med*. 2000;343(17):1206-1209.

38. Pearson JW, Redding JS. Peripheral vascular tone on cardiac resuscitation. *Anesth Analg*. 1965;44(6):746-752.

39. Michael JR, Guerci AD, Koehler RC, et al. Mechanisms by which epinephrine augments cerebral and myocardial perfusion during cardiopulmonary resuscitation in dogs. *Circulation*. 1984;69(4):822-835.

40. Livesay JJ, Follette DM, Fey KH, et al. Optimizing myocardial supply/demand balance with alpha-adrenergic drugs during cardiopulmonary resuscitation. *J Thorac Cardiovasc Surg*. 1978;76(2):244-251.

41. Brown CG, Martin DR, Pepe PE, et al. A comparison of standard-dose and high-dose epinephrine in cardiac arrest outside the hospital. The Multicenter High-Dose Epinephrine Study Group. *New Engl J Med*. 1992;327(15):1051-1055.

42. Perondi MB, Reis AG, Paiva EF, Nadkarni VM, Berg RA. A comparison of high-dose and standard-dose epinephrine in children with cardiac arrest. *New Engl J Med*. 2004;350(17):1722-1730.

43. Duncan JM, Meaney P, Simpson P, Berg RA, Nadkarni V, Schexnayder S. Vasopressin for in-hospital pediatric cardiac arrest: results from the American Heart Association National Registry of Cardiopulmonary Resuscitation. *Pediatr Crit Care Med*. 2009;10(2):191-195.

44. Mann K, Berg RA, Nadkarni V. Beneficial effects of vasopressin in prolonged pediatric cardiac arrest: a case series. *Resuscitation*. 2002;52(2):149-156.

45. Goodman LS, Gilman A, Brunton LL, Chabner BA, Knollmann BC. *Goodman & Gilman's The Pharmacological Basis of Therapeutics*. New York: McGraw-Hill Medical; 2011.

46. Neumar RW, Otto CW, Link MS, et al. Part 8: Adult advanced cardiovascular life support: 2010 American Heart Association Guidelines for Cardiopulmonary Resuscitation and Emergency Cardiovascular Care. *Circulation*. 2010;122(18 Suppl 3):S729-S767.

47. Crosson JE, Etheridge SP, Milstein S, Hesslein PS, Dunnigan A. Therapeutic and diagnostic utility of adenosine during tachycardia evaluation in children. *Am J Cardiol*. 1994;74(2):155-160.

48. Losek JD, Endom E, Dietrich A, Stewart G, Zempsky W, Smith K. Adenosine and pediatric supraventricular tachycardia in the emergency department: multicenter study and review. *Ann Emerg Med*. 1999;33(2):185-191.

49. Singh BN, Venkatesh N, Nademanee K, Josephson MA, Kannan R. The historical development, cellular electrophysiology and pharmacology of amiodarone. *Prog Cardiovasc Dis*. 1989;31(4):249-280.

50. Nattel S. Comparative mechanisms of action of antiarrhythmic drugs. *Am J Cardiol*. 1993;72(16):13f-17f.

51. Cote P, Bourassa MG, Delaye J, Janin A, Froment R, David P. Effects of amiodarone on cardiac and coronary hemodynamics and on myocardial metabolism in patients with coronary artery disease. *Circulation*. 1979;59(6):1165-1172.

52. CotÈ CJ, Lerman J, Anderson BJ. *A Practice of Anesthesia for Infants and Children, 6th ed*. Philadelphia, PA: Elsevier; 2019.

53. de Mos N, van Litsenburg RR, McCrindle B, Bohn DJ, Parshuram CS. Pediatric in-intensive-care-unit cardiac arrest: incidence, survival, and predictive factors. *Crit Care Med*. 2006;34(4):1209-1215.

54. Denlinger JK, Nahrwold ML, Gibbs PS, Lecky JH. Hypocalcaemia during rapid blood transfusion in anaesthetized man. *Br J Anaesth*. 1976;48(10):995-1000.

55. Wood WB, Manley ESJr, Woodbury RA. The effects of CO_2-induced respiratory acidosis on the depressor and pressor components of the dog's blood pressure response to epinephrine. *J Pharmacol Experiment Therapeut*. 1963;139:238-247.

56. Mattar JA, Weil MH, Shubin H, Stein L. Cardiac arrest in the critically ill. II. Hyperosmolal states following cardiac arrest. *Am J Med*. 1974;56(2):162-168.

57. Bishop RL, Weisfeldt ML. Sodium bicarbonate administration during cardiac arrest. Effect on arterial pH PCO2, and osmolality. *JAMA*. 1976;235(5):506-509.

58. Berg RA, Nadkarni VM, Clark AE, et al. Incidence and outcomes of cardiopulmonary resuscitation in PICUs. *Crit Care Med*. 2016;44(4):798-808.

59. Topjian AA, French B, Sutton RM, et al. Early postresuscitation hypotension is associated with increased mortality following pediatric cardiac arrest. *Crit Care Med*. 2014;42(6):1518-1523.

60. Zeiner A, Holzer M, Sterz F, et al. Hyperthermia after cardiac arrest is associated with an unfavorable neurologic outcome. *Arch Int Med*. 2001;161(16):2007-2012.

61. Moler FW, Silverstein FS, Holubkov R, et al. Therapeutic hypothermia after in-hospital cardiac arrest in children. *New Engl J Med.* 2017;376(4):318-329.

62. Ferguson LP, Durward A, Tibby SM. Relationship between arterial partial oxygen pressure after resuscitation from cardiac arrest and mortality in children. *Circulation.* 2012;126(3):335-342.

63. Morris MC, Wernovsky G, Nadkarni VM. Survival outcomes after extracorporeal cardiopulmonary resuscitation instituted during active chest compressions following refractory in-hospital pediatric cardiac arrest. *Pediatr Crit Care Med.* 2004;5(5):440-446.

64. Raymond TT, Cunnyngham CB, Thompson MT, Thomas JA, Dalton HJ, Nadkarni VM. Outcomes among neonates, infants, and children after extracorporeal cardiopulmonary resuscitation for refractory inhospital pediatric cardiac arrest: a report from the National Registry of Cardiopulmonary Resuscitation. *Pediatr Crit Care Med.* 2010;11(3):362-371.

Syndromes

Laura Rhee

FOCUS POINTS

1. Trisomy 21 (Down syndrome): Congenital heart disease, sleep apnea, and subglottic stenosis.
2. Trisomy 13 and 18: High infant mortality rate, apnea, and airway challenges.
3. Turner syndrome: Cardiac evaluation, webbed neck with limited mobility, and difficult IV access.
4. VACTERL: Three defining features for diagnosis, cardiac evaluation, and spontaneous ventilation for TEF.
5. CHARGE: Major features include choanal atresia, coloboma, cranial nerve dysfunction, and characteristic ear anomalies.
6. 22q11 deletion syndrome: Cardiac abnormalities, abnormal facies, thymic hypoplasia, cleft palate, hypocalcemia.
7. Muscular dystrophy does not increase the risk of malignant hyperthermia (MH).
8. Williams syndrome: "Cocktail-party" personality, supravalvar aortic stenosis at high risk for perioperative myocardial ischemia.

INTRODUCTION

With advances in the field of molecular cytogenetics, more genetic syndromes are being formally diagnosed than ever before. Likewise, further innovations in medical care have fostered the survival of children with multiple congenital malformations further into adulthood. Children with a chronic underlying disorder of genetic origin account for over two-thirds of hospital admissions[1]—and are consequently quite likely to require (anesthesia for) diagnostic imaging or procedures. While syndromes do not account for all "disorders of genetic origin," they are collectively common (albeit individually rare) and likely to be encountered with regularity by the anesthesiologist caring for pediatric patients.

Children with genetic dysmorphic conditions are at greater risk for perioperative morbidity and mortality with multiple organ systems often affected.[1] While neurologic and developmental abnormalities are frequent and can impact perioperative care, many are also associated with cardiovascular disease, and various craniofacial abnormalities that may affect airway management. To successfully anticipate perioperative challenges and provide safe and effective care, it is imperative that pediatric anesthesiologists are aware of potential congenital anomalies and their associated anatomic and physiologic disturbances. This chapter reviews the major features and perioperative implications of common syndromes that are pertinent to the pediatric anesthesiologist.

TRISOMY 21 (DOWN SYNDROME)

Trisomy 21 or down syndrome (DS) (see Figure 40-1), which is caused by an extra 21st chromosome, is the most common autosomal chromosomal disorder in humans, with an incidence of 1:700 live births.[2,3] The characteristic phenotypic features of these patients include brachycephaly, oblique palpebral fissures, epicanthal folds, small low-set ears, midfacial and mild mandibular hypoplasia, and a short neck.[3] Individuals with DS may have multiple reasons of airway obstruction such as protruding tongue and adenotonsillar hypertrophy, in combination with pharyngeal hypotonia, which frequently contribute to upper airway obstructive symptoms and obstructive sleep apnea (OSA). Subglottic stenosis, cleft palate, and choanal atresia are also more frequently seen in DS. There is a high rate (40% to 50%) of congenital heart disease, particularly endocardial cushion defects, such as ASD, vertebral artery.[6] Both clinical and radiologic assessments of cervical spine instability (CSI) are challenging in this patient population. While the frequency of atlanto-occipital and atlanto-axial instability is estimated at 15%, only 1% to 2% of individuals will present with overt symptoms.[4] Radiologic assessment is typically measured by the atlanto-dens interval on plain cervical spine radiographs, which changes with neck position. Prior guidelines from the American Academy of Pediatrics recommended obtaining cervical spine films to assess for CSI in all patients 3 to 5 years of age with DS but more recent evidence suggests no routine radiographs in asymptomatic children: "Plain radiographs do not predict well which children are at increased risk of developing spine problems, and normal radiographs do not provide assurance that a child will not develop spine problems later."[6]

A variety of neuropsychiatric features are common in individuals with DS. Intellectual disability of varying degrees and developmental delay are ubiquitous; achievement of all developmental milestones in the early years lags behind that of their unaffected peers. Individuals with DS are frequently affected by autism spectrum disorders, behavioral disorders, depression and early-onset Alzheimer's disease.[5]

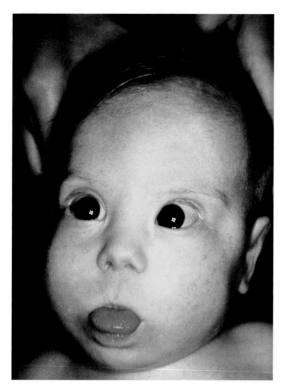

▲ **Figure 40-1.** Trisomy 21 features. (Reproduced with permission, from Bissonnette B, Luginbuehl I, Marciniak B, et al., eds. *Syndromes: Rapid Recognition and Perioperative Implications.* 2006. https://accessanesthesiology.mhmedical.com. Copyright © McGraw Hill LLC. All rights reserved.)

VSD, and atrioventricular canal defects (though PDA and TOF are also common).[3] There is a higher incidence of pulmonary hypertension in children with DS; coexisting congenital heart disease, higher rates of persistent pulmonary hypertension of the newborn, and predisposition to upper airway obstruction (leading to chronic hypoxemia) may all contribute.[4] GI malformations detected in the neonatal period (duodenal atresia, annular pancreas, tracheo-esophageal fistula, Hirschsprung disease, imperforate anus) are common as well.[4] Growth delay, obesity, and thyroid disease frequently occur in patients with DS and 1% of individuals with DS are diagnosed with leukemia.[5] Musculoskeletal abnormalities may include polydactyly, recurrent joint dislocation, and extreme joint laxity, in addition to generalized hypotonia.[5]

Because of ligamentous laxity and bony anomalies in the cervical vertebrae, patients with DS are prone to atlanto-occipital (occiput-C1) and (more commonly) atlanto-axial (C1-C2) instability.

Anterior subluxation of C1-C2 may lead to spinal cord compression and rotary subluxation of C1-C2 may lead to neck pain, immobility, and kinking of the ipsilateral

Perioperative Implications

Particular care should be given to the maintenance of airway patency and airway management in patients with DS. Their high risk for airway obstruction (subglottic stenosis, narrowed nasopharynx, upper airway obstruction secondary to macroglossia, and adenotonsillar hypertrophy) and for OSA render them a higher risk perioperatively thus requiring closer monitoring. Endotracheal tubes should be downsized given the likelihood of subglottic narrowing. Discretion should be used with placement of nasal endotracheal tubes, especially if there is a history of choanal atresia or stenosis. Because of the risk of cervical spine instability, a thorough preoperative history and physical should be performed to elicit any signs or symptoms of cord compression. As clinical assessment is still somewhat unreliable, even asymptomatic children should be considered at risk of acute dislocation and special attention should be given to positioning during intubation and surgery to maintain a neutral cervical spine position (consider avoiding the typical headrest).

Patients with congenital heart disease and/or pulmonary hypertension may require a cardiac evaluation (depending on severity of lesion and status of the repair). Caution should be used during inhaled induction as individuals with DS are known to have a higher prevalence and degree of bradycardia during sevoflurane induction.[7] Given the high incidence of hypothyroidism in this patient population, recent thyroid function testing should be reviewed prior to major procedures. Lastly, due to obesity, obtaining vascular access (venous and arterial) in these children can be challenging.[8]

TRISOMY 13 (PATAU SYNDROME) AND TRISOMY 18 (EDWARD SYNDROME)

Trisomy 13 (Patau syndrome) is caused by an additional 13th chromosome. The incidence of trisomy 13 is approximately 1:5000 births and it is associated with a high infant mortality rate (over 90% of patients die by one year of age).[9] Common features include microcephaly, cleft lip and/or palate, ocular hypertelorism, microphthalmia, low-set ears, and polydactyly. CNS defects may include holo-prosencephaly (most common), seizures, deafness, and significant neurodevelopmental delay. Cardiac malformations are frequent as are visceral and genital anomalies.[10,11]

Trisomy 18 (Edward syndrome) is caused by an additional 18th chromosome. The incidence of trisomy 18 is approximately 1:6–8000 live births, with a predisposition toward females.[12,13] Prognosis is similar to that of trisomy 13. Children with trisomy 18 commonly have microcephaly with a prominent occiput, a small mouth, microretrognathia, short sternum, and positional foot deformities. Clenched fists with overlapping digits are a distinctive feature of this syndrome. CNS abnormalities include cerebellar hypoplasia, agenesis of corpus callosum, polymicrogyria, hydrocephalus, seizures, and myelomeningocele.[13] Cardiac malformations occur in over 95% of patients.[14] Renal anomalies are quite common. Like patients with trisomy 13, these patients also suffer intellectual disability and neurodevelopmental delay.[13]

Perioperative Implications for Trisomy 13 and Trisomy 18

While the prognosis for these two disorders is very poor, those children that do survive often require many hospitalizations, interventions, and surgical procedures. Preoperative assessment should include a discussion with parents to discern the best interests of the patient and quality of life that is desired.[14] Consideration should be given to the fact that the child may not survive long enough to benefit from a particular procedure. Once the surgical procedure is deemed necessary or beneficial, the anesthesia provider should anticipate potential difficulties with direct laryngoscopy (especially due to a small mouth opening and micrognathia in trisomy 18). For those patients with congenital heart disease, cardiac evaluation is important. Children with both syndromes are prone to apnea and this should be taken into consideration during the perioperative period.

TURNER SYNDROME

Turner syndrome (TS) is caused by the absence of all or part of a normal second sex chromosome (46, XO). While it is the single most common chromosomal abnormality, the incidence is only approximately 1:3000 live (female)

births due to a high rate of spontaneous abortion.[14] The syndrome is characterized by a constellation of physical findings that includes congenital lymphedema, short stature, and gonadal dysgenesis. Approximately 20% to 30% of TS cases are diagnosed in the newborn period (with findings of congenital lymphedema), 30% in mid childhood (presenting with growth delay), and the remainder of cases in adolescence or adulthood (failure to enter puberty or inability to conceive).[15]

These patients can be identified by their short stature, broad chest, low-set ears, and short, webbed neck (often with limited range of motion). Airway exam may reveal micrognathia and a high arched palate.[16,17] Cardiovascular anomalies are present in a large percentage (17% to 45%) of patients. The most frequent cardiovascular anomalies include aortic coarctation and bicuspid aortic valve; however, hypertension, mitral valve prolapse, and conduction defects (including QTc prolongation) can also occur.[16,18] In addition, 15% to 30% of girls and women with TS have ascending aortic dilation and there are numerous case reports that describe spontaneous aortic dissection.[19] The tracheal bifurcation has been reported to be higher than the general population, which can increase the risk of mainstem intubation.[18] Structural renal malformations are relatively common (up to 40%), as are skeletal deformities (such as scoliosis). Because patients with TS have impaired growth, the administration of recombinant human growth hormone is now standard. Due to gonadal dysgenesis, most patients require hormone replacement therapy to enter puberty and continue appropriate growth. While most patients with TS will have normal intelligence, learning disabilities are quite prevalent. Hypothyroidism is more prevalent in adults with TS but also does occur in a small percentage of patients before puberty.[16]

Perioperative Implications

Due to possible micrognathia, a high arched palate, and short neck with limited mobility, tracheal intubation may be difficult in individuals with TS. A supraglottic airway and a difficult airway cart (i.e., video laryngoscope and fiberoptic scope) should be readily available. A short neck and higher tracheal bifurcation can easily lead to endobronchial intubation. A cardiac workup in these patients is mandatory and an echocardiogram and baseline ECG should be obtained preoperatively. Renal function should be evaluated (electrolytes, BUN/Cr) if renal anomalies are suspected or known. *One should confirm the presence of a euthyroid state if the patient is being treated for hypothyroidism.* If congenital lymphedema is present, peripheral vascular access may be difficult to obtain.

VACTERL ASSOCIATION

VACTERL association was originally described in 1972 as VATER association—**V**ertebral defects, **A**nal atresia,

TE fistula, and **R**enal & **R**adial dysplasia—but has since been broadened to include **V**ascular anomalies, **C**ardiac malformations, and **L**imb anomalies (not limited to radial dysplasia). VACTERL association is a clinical definition, as a distinct pattern or mode of inheritance has not yet been identified (though several signaling pathways and genes have been implicated, such as the Sonic hedgehog signaling pathway, WNT signaling, and the HOX gene clusters). The incidence of VACTERL is estimated to be around 1:10,000–40,000 live births.[19]

While the phenotypic spectrum varies and is broad, the diagnosis of VACTERL typically requires three of the following defining features to be present.

Vertebral anomalies (which affect 60% to 90%) may include segmentation defects (such as dysplastic or fused vertebrae) affecting one or more levels, sacral agenesis/dysgenesis, or rib anomalies.

Abnormal spinal curvatures (causing lordosis, kyphosis, or scoliosis) secondary to these vertebral anomalies may occur. Tethered spinal cord is another finding that may be present.[20]

Anal atresia (anorectal malformations) which occur in 55% to 90% of patients include imperforate anus or anal atresia, perineal and/or gastrocutaneous fistulas. Patients with such anomalies often also have accompanying genitourinary malformations (such as hypospadias, cryptorchidism, and cloacal malformations).[21]

Cardiac malformations affect 40% to 80% of individuals and may vary in complexity from a minor anatomic defect to complex congenital heart disease.[21] Vascular anomalies may be cardiac (such as a right-sided aortic arch, anomalous SVC, or vascular rings) or extracardiac (such as a single umbilical artery, which may be the first clue to a diagnosis antenatally).[21]

Tracheo-**E**sophageal fistula with or without esophageal atresia may be diagnosed if neonates demonstrate difficulty with oral secretions or feeds or when a gastric feeding tube cannot be passed. These anomalies affect 50% to 80% of individuals and will require surgical repair.[21] **R**enal abnormalities such as horseshoe kidney, renal agenesis, or cystic and/or dysplastic kidneys affect 50% to 80% of individuals and may be accompanied by ureteral and genitourinary anomalies.

Limb anomalies, while initially thought isolated to the radius, may affect any limb and are found in 40% to 55% of individuals. Polydactyly, limb length discrepancy, or limb hypoplasia may be present.[21]

▶ Perioperative Implications

If VACTERL association is suspected, a cardiac evaluation (with echocardiogram) should be performed prior to any surgical intervention. It is important to obtain imaging studies to evaluate for spinal deformities if neuraxial anesthetic is planned. If significant scoliosis is present, tracheal intubation may be challenging and restrictive lung disease (if severe) may affect oxygenation and ventilation. Special considerations for TEF, if present and unrepaired, apply: beware of the propensity of these patients to aspirate and maintain spontaneous ventilation until fistula ligation is confirmed (or endotracheal tube has been placed beyond fistula). If renal anomalies exist, dosing of renally excreted drugs and fluid management should be tailored accordingly. Obtaining vascular access may be challenging if significant limb anomalies are present.

CHARGE SYNDROME

This syndrome, first described in 1979, was given the acronym CHARGE (**C**oloboma, **H**eart defect, **A**tresia choanae, **R**etarded growth/development, **G**enital hypoplasia, **E**ar anomalies/deafness) shortly thereafter, which described an association of various anomalies.[22] CHARGE is now recognized as a syndrome, and a (de novo) mutation of the *CHD7* gene is thought to be responsible for the majority of cases.[23] Its incidence is estimated at 1:8500–10,000 live births.[24] While the clinical phenotype may be quite heterogeneous, a set of diagnostic criteria have been outlined to aid in diagnosis. The presence of any major feature in a neonate should trigger suspicion and investigation into a diagnosis of CHARGE. A diagnosis of CHARGE is highly likely if an individual has either four of the major characteristics or three major and three minor characteristics. **Major features** (4 C's) of CHARGE are as follows: Choanal atresia, Coloboma, Cranial nerve dysfunction, and Characteristic ear anomalies. **Minor features** are as follows: Cardiovascular malformations, Genital hypoplasia, Cleft lip/palate, TE fistula, Distinctive CHARGE facies, Growth deficiency, and Developmental delay.[23]

Eye malformations, which may range from **colobomas** to microphthalmia to anophthalmos, affect up to 80% of patients.[23] Congenital **heart defects** affect 75% to 80% of patients, the most common types of large-level defects being conotruncal defects, septal defects, and atrioventricular septal defects.[25] Tetralogy of Fallot (a conotruncal defect) is the most frequent (33%). **Choanal atresia** may be bilateral or unilateral, membranous or bony, and is associated with polyhydramnios antenatally on ultrasound. Because neonates are obligate nose breathers, those with bilateral choanal atresia must undergo surgical correction. **Growth retardation** may be secondary to respiratory or cardiac comorbidities, growth hormone deficiency, or feeding difficulties. While most neonates with CHARGE have normal birth weights, by school age these children are often underweight. Developmental delays may include motor and language and/or intellectual disability that can range from mild to profound. Autism spectrum disorder may also be present. **Genital hypoplasia** is easier to recognize and more common in males. Occasionally renal anomalies may also occur. **Ear anomalies,** which affect 80% to 100% of individuals, include abnormally shaped ears as well as sensorineural hearing loss often accompanied by facial nerve palsies.[23]

Cranial nerve anomalies are evident in over 75%[26] and may cause anosmia (CN I), facial nerve palsy (CN VII), and swallowing problems and/or aspiration (CN IX/X/XI) which cause feeding difficulties and/or recurrent respiratory infections. Multiple cranial neuropathies may be present and in general are often asymmetric.[23,27]

While not described in the acronym, there is a higher documented incidence of upper airway abnormalities in patients with CHARGE syndrome.[27] In addition to cleft lip and palate, individuals may have a short neck, micrognathia, and laryngomalacia,[28] all of which may contribute to upper airway obstruction or difficult tracheal intubation. Many patients will require tracheostomy placement secondary to upper airway obstruction.[27]

Perioperative Implications

Individuals with special needs may require premedication and/or child behavioral support perioperatively. Many are affected by intellectual disability or autism spectrum disorder and 80% to 90% have at least mild *dual* sensory loss (deafblindness)[28] which can impair perioperative communication. Cardiac evaluation should be performed to identify any congenital heart defects. The presence of choanal atresia or stenosis precludes placement of nasogastric tube or nasal airway. Mask ventilation on induction may require CPAP if laryngomalacia is present and tracheal intubation may be challenging if anatomic airway abnormalities (cleft lip/palate, micrognathia, short neck) are present. Laryngeal discoordination from cranial nerve palsies may contribute to pooling of oral secretions, aspiration, and airway obstruction. As these patients are at higher risk of postoperative airway events (airway obstruction and need for reintubation),[29] intensive care unit monitoring with or without postoperative ventilation should be considered.

22Q11 DELETION SYNDROME (22Q11DS)

This syndrome is a major cause of developmental delay and major congenital heart disease second only to trisomy 21. 22q11DS occurs in approximately 1:4,000 births (Bassett).[30] The most common cause is a deletion of a segment of 35 genes on chromosome 22 (though this is usually a de novo event, this mutation can be inherited in an autosomal dominant fashion).[31] The constellation of clinical findings are the result of aberrant migration of neural crest cells during embryonic development which leads to abnormal development of the pharyngeal arches (which form the aortic arch and its branches, cardiac outflow tract, the thymus, the parathyroid, parts of the palate, pharynx, and face).[32] There is significant variability in the severity and extent of phenotypic expression. 22q11DS encompasses three syndromes with overlapping phenotypic features:

DiGeorge syndrome, velocardiofacial syndrome, and conotruncal anomaly face syndrome (historically these were described as three separate entities but it is now known that most cases of these syndromes are caused by the 22q11 deletion).[31] Some of the more prominent clinical features of 22q11DS may be recalled using the "**CATCH-22**" mnemonic: **C**ardiac abnormalities, **A**bnormal facies, **T**hymic hypoplasia, **C**left palate, **H**ypocalcemia.

Cardiac anomalies are present in approximately 75% of patients, with conotruncal defects being the most prevalent: tetralogy of Fallot, truncus arteriosus, interrupted aortic arch, and pulmonary atresia with VSD.[32,33] Aberrant vascular anomalies, such as vascular rings or medial carotid arteries, are often identified in these patients.[33,34] Characteristics that contribute to the **dysmorphic facial features** in this syndrome include a long face, ocular hypertelorism, narrow palpebral fissures, a squared nasal root, narrow nares, low-set ears, small mouth, and retrognathia. A small percentage (11% to 17%) of patients have Pierre Robin sequence.[35] While the original description by DiGeorge included an absent thymus, **thymic aplasia** and hypoplasia are far less common than low T-cell counts which affect 75% to 80% of infants (<1% have no T cells). Impaired immunity may lead to recurrent infections (especially upper respiratory infections) in affected patients. **Abnormalities of the palate**, pharynx, and trachea affect three-fourths of patients: bifid uvula, cleft palate, tracheo- and laryngomalacia, and laryngeal webs may be present.[32,35] A short trachea has also been reported in these patients.[35] Velopharyngeal insufficiency (present in 70%) quite commonly contributes to feeding difficulties and speech delays.[35] **Hypocalcemia** secondary to hypoparathyroidism is common, and although it tends to resolve with age, hypocalcemia may recur during periods of increased metabolic demand.[36] Approximately ⅓ of patients have a structural genitourinary tract abnormality but generally these require no intervention.[32] Scoliosis affects nearly half of individuals with 22q11DS and may require surgical intervention. Learning disabilities affect over 90% of patients and approximately 35% of patients have cognitive delays. Behavioral and psychiatric disorders are also very common, both in children and adults.[31]

Perioperative Implications

Palatal defects, micrognathia, and a small mouth opening can make direct laryngoscopy and tracheal intubation difficult (especially if Pierre Robin sequence is present). Beyond direct visualization of the glottic opening, the potential for a shorter trachea, laryngeal web, and/or vascular rings may hinder endotracheal tube advancement. Evaluation for potential congenital heart disease should be performed to determine the severity of a lesion and status of a repair if present. Anatomy of vascular structures (carotid and subclavian arteries) should be confirmed prior to central line insertion (or velopharyngoplasty) given the potential presence of major arterial malformations. In case of impaired immune function, administration of irradiated blood may be necessary and strict aseptic technique should be followed during placement of lines or other invasive monitors or regional anesthetic technique. Symptomatic hypocalcemia, which can be aggravated by hyperventilation (alkalosis) and citrate-containing blood products, should be monitored and corrected perioperatively.

BECKWITH–WIEDEMANN SYNDROME

Beckwith–Wiedemann syndrome (BWS) is an overgrowth syndrome, characterized by pre- and post-natal macrosomia, various malformations, and an elevated risk of embryonal tumors.[37] It is caused by an alteration in chromosome 11p15, which is usually sporadic but can be inherited.[38] It occurs at a rate of approximately 1:13,700 births and its clinical picture is extremely variable.[39]

While patients with BWS often exhibit macrosomia and are large for gestational age, the syndrome is also frequently associated with prematurity (and its associated comorbidities).[40]

Macroglossia, which may contribute to chronic upper airway obstruction, is one of the more distinguishing features of this syndrome. Occasionally the obstruction may become so severe leading to alveolar hypoventilation and cor pulmonale; some patients may require tracheostomy or partial glossectomy.[41,42] Hemihypertrophy and visceromegaly (disproportionately oversized organs—adrenals, kidneys, pancreas, gonads) are major findings as are abdominal wall defects (omphalocele and umbilical hernia).[39] Cardiac anomalies (particularly cardiomegaly, which usually spontaneously regresses) have been reported in some children.[42] Children with BWS are at much greater risk of developing childhood malignancies, particularly Wilms tumor, hepatoblastoma, neuroblastoma, rhabdomyosarcoma, as well as some benign tumors.[38,39] Severe neonatal hypoglycemia (related to pancreatic islet cell hypertrophy) may occur, though hypoglycemic episodes usually spontaneously resolve with growth.[42]

Perioperative Implications

Macroglossia usually regresses as the patient grows (as facial bones grow more, room is available in the oral cavity). In the neonatal period, macroglossia can be a source of significant upper airway obstruction and cause difficulty visualizing the glottis during direct laryngoscopy. Preoperative sedation is best avoided. Awake direct laryngoscopy can aid in detecting visualization of the glottis.[42] Fiberoptic intubation may be necessary. Intubation via video laryngoscopy and placement of supraglottic devices have both been successful in these patients.[43] A preoperative echocardiogram may be indicated. Close monitoring of blood glucose in the neonatal period is warranted and may necessitate a bolus and infusion of dextrose.

MUSCULAR DYSTROPHINOPATHIES

Duchenne and Becker muscular dystrophy (together) are the most common forms of muscular dystrophy found in children,[44] with an incidence of approximately 1:3500 live male births. Both are the result of X-linked recessive mutations in the dystrophin gene; a mutation resulting in a partially functional dystrophin protein causes Becker muscular dystrophy (BMD), while a mutation resulting in complete absence of dystrophin causes Duchenne muscular dystrophy (DMD).[45]

Both DMD and BMD are characterized by progressive (skeletal and cardiac) muscle degeneration and weakness, though BMD is less severe and progression of the disease is much slower than DMD. Due to such severe muscle breakdown, serum CK in DMD may be 50 to 100 times normal.[46]

Individuals with DMD are asymptomatic in infancy, but generally begin walking later than their peers and have a waddling gait with toe-walking. Pseudohypertrophy, especially of the calf muscles, is characteristic and because of proximal muscle (pelvic muscle) weakness, individuals may exhibit the Gower maneuver (see Figure 40-2). As lower extremity muscles deteriorate before upper

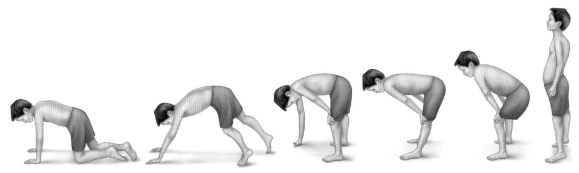

▲ **Figure 40-2.** Gower sign. (Reproduced with permission, from Kline MW. eds. *Rudolph's Pediatrics*. 23rd ed. 2018. https://accesspediatrics.mhmedical.com. Copyright © McGraw Hill LLC. All rights reserved.)

extremity muscles, the ability to ambulate is generally lost around age 10,[47] after which nearly all boys will rapidly develop scoliosis.

Initially boys have increased chest wall compliance and increased forced vital capacity (FVC) for their age. Deterioration of pulmonary function and decreased compliance begin at around 10 years of age, with a gradual decline in FVC[47] and the development of restrictive lung disease.

The ability to cough and clear secretions likewise worsens, and pneumonia is frequent in these patients. Nocturnal hypoventilation may require assisted ventilation by the late teenage years.

Cardiomyopathy presents on echocardiography earlier in life, and is often asymptomatic until the early teenage years.[48] Left ventricular hypertrophy is commonly found on electrocardiograms of younger patients. A progressive decline in LV ejection fraction leads to LV failure and the development of a dilated cardiomyopathy. Resting sinus tachycardia is common and may be present prior to the development of impaired systolic function;[49] the incidence of arrhythmias, however, has been shown to correlate with a decrease in ejection fraction.[49]

Glucocorticoid administration has been shown to delay the overall progression of muscle weakness in DMD and advances have been made in management of the respiratory component of this disease. As such, the longevity of these patients has improved into the third and fourth decades and cardiomyopathy has emerged as the major cause of morbidity and mortality.[50]

Perioperative Implications

Patients with BMD and DMD often present for procedures such as scoliosis surgery, and release of contractures, gastric tube placement, or tracheostomy. A thorough preoperative evaluation should take place prior to any surgical procedure. Cardiology consultation is a must prior to any major procedure (i.e., scoliosis) and a baseline ECG, and either echocardiogram or cardiac MRI should be reviewed. Dobutamine stress echocardiogram or Holter monitor may be warranted (upon evaluation by the child's cardiologist).[49] Consultation with pulmonologist should occur to assess the degree of respiratory insufficiency. A decline in FVC may predict moderate (FVC <50% predicted) or high (FVC <30% predicted) risk of respiratory complications perioperatively.[48]

Caution should be exercised with administration of preoperative anxiolysis or sedation which can further compromise existing respiratory insufficiency. Potential airway involvement should be considered: fibrosis of masseter muscles may lead to limited mouth opening and involvement of neck muscles may restrict cervical range of motion. These factors combined with tongue hypertrophy and high rates of obesity may contribute to difficulty with direct laryngoscopy, the incidence of which has been higher in DMD, especially in older patients.[50] Nondepolarizing neuromuscular blocking agents (such as rocuronium) may be safely used in muscular dystrophy, though prolongation of time to peak blockade and recovery should be expected.[49,51]

If cardiomyopathy exists, abrupt changes to CO may occur with patient position (supine to prone), institution of positive pressure ventilation, or abdominal insufflation during laparoscopy.[49] Likewise, the presence of cardiomyopathy should guide fluid management perioperatively (in any type of procedure) to avoid fluid shifts that may promote heart failure.[48] The presence of contractures in the extremities may make peripheral arterial or venous cannulation challenging and also impact positioning.

Significantly higher amounts of blood loss and "impaired hemostatic function" have been documented in patients with DMD undergoing spinal surgery; preoperative planning should focus on ways to minimize homologous transfusion but also avoid hypovolemia in the setting of potential cardiovascular impairment (use of antifibrinolytics or cell salvage with intraoperative autotransfusion).[49,51]

Patients with DMD are at increased risk of acute rhabdomyolysis and subsequent hyperkalemic cardiac arrest. Succinylcholine is a known trigger for this reaction and should be avoided; however, volatile anesthetics are also associated with this reaction, and their use in this patient population is controversial. Many advocate for a nontriggering anesthetic technique (total intravenous anesthetic, or TIVA) to avoid rhabdomyolysis, though reactions have been reported with nontriggering anesthetic agents as well. Acute rhabdomyolysis from triggering agents may cause a hypermetabolic state that can mimic malignant hyperthermia (MH), but it is not caused by MH nor does muscular dystrophy increase the risk of MH.[46]

Postoperatively, patients may require extubation to noninvasive PPV (especially if required at baseline).[49] Prolonged intubation and mechanical ventilatory support may be required after more extensive procedures (such as posterior spine fusion).

SYNDROMES WITH SPECIFIC CARDIAC CONSIDERATIONS

In addition to Down syndrome, 22q11 deletion syndrome, Turner syndrome, CHARGE syndrome, and VACTERL association, the following syndromes merit special attention because of their high incidence of cardiac involvement and its impact on perioperative planning.

Noonan syndrome is an autosomal dominant genetic disorder with an incidence of approximately 1:1000–2500 live births.[51] A mutation in the RAS/MAPK signaling pathway can be identified in many but not all patients with Noonan syndrome. Many phenotypic features may overlap with those of Turner syndrome, including short stature, webbed neck, broad chest with wide spaced nipples, lymphatic issues, and renal malformations. Cardiac anomalies affect 80% of individuals with pulmonary stenosis (valvar or supravalvar) being the most common defect.

Other frequent anomalies include ASD, partial atrioventricular canal defect, and hypertrophic cardiomyopathy. Bleeding diatheses have been reported in a large proportion of individuals, and may be secondary to platelet dysfunction, thrombocytopenia, or factor deficiencies.[52] Spinal anomalies such as scoliosis, kyphosis, spina bifida, and vertebral or rib abnormalities may be present.[52]

Perioperative Implications

An airway evaluation should be performed preoperatively; like individuals with Turner syndrome, those with Noonan may have a high arched palate and micrognathia. This facial feature combined with a short neck and limited extension may contribute to difficulty with direct laryngoscopy and tracheal intubation. Preoperative assessment should include echocardiography; imaging should be included to evaluate for spinal deformities if neuraxial anesthetic is planned. Coagulation studies and platelet function tests should be performed prior to procedures with potential for significant blood loss.

Williams syndrome (WS) (or Williams–Beuren syndrome) is caused by a contiguous gene deletion on chromosome 7 (usually sporadic but it may be inherited in an autosomal dominant fashion).[53] Its incidence is estimated at 1:20,000 live births.[54] Of primary concern for the anesthesiologist is the potential for cardiovascular disease, but this syndrome like others has a multisystem involvement. Patients may be distinguished by characteristic facies such as midfacial flattening, mandibular hypoplasia, and dental malocclusion, all contributing to difficulty with tracheal intubation.[54] Intellectual disability and developmental delay are also typical. While individuals with WS are known for their unique outgoing "cocktail party" personality, anxiety and ADHD are common.[54,55] Endocrine disease may include hypercalcemia (primarily affecting infants and resolved by age 4 years), hypercalciuria, hypothyroidism, and early puberty. Failure to thrive with feeding difficulties commonly affects infants with WS.[54] Renal or genitourinary involvement incorporates anatomic renal abnormalities, nephrocalcinosis, or bladder diverticuli.[55] Because part of the region of deleted genes on chromosome 7 includes the elastin gene, connective tissue abnormalities may be present, and may manifest as joint laxity or more importantly, as elastin arteriopathy, the cause of cardiovascular pathology in these individuals.[55]

Cardiovascular disease affects 80% of individuals, with most diagnosed by one year of age.[54] Supravalvar aortic stenosis (SVAS) is the most common lesion, present in 45% to 75% of individuals.[54,55] Pulmonary artery stenosis is also quite common and peripheral stenosis is more frequently encountered than central;[54] these lesions typically improve as children age.[56] Coronary anomalies are frequently encountered resulting in coronary artery disease in 5% to 9% of patients. Left or right ventricular hypertrophy caused by outflow obstructive lesions may be present. Hypertension affects over half of individuals with WS and may be secondary to renal artery stenosis; vascular stenoses secondary to elastin arteriopathy are common and may be seen at the thoracic aorta (causing middle aortic syndrome), or mesenteric, carotid, or peripheral arteries. Prolonged QTc has also been observed in WS.[54]

Perioperative Implications

Individuals with WS are at a high risk of sudden cardiac death, and the literature abounds with case reports of anesthesia-related cardiac arrest.[57] Most are secondary to myocardial ischemia. Therefore, a very thorough preoperative evaluation should precede sedation or general anesthesia for any type of diagnostic imaging or surgical procedure. The necessity of the procedure should be determined (given the high risk in the perioperative setting) as should the location—ideally any elective procedure should occur at a tertiary care facility where a pediatric anesthesia team can be involved, and where ECMO is readily available.[57] A cardiologist should be consulted preoperatively and the patient's most recent ECG, ECHO, and cardiac catheterization (if applicable) should be reviewed. Screening for hypercalcemia and hypothyroidism should occur in frequent intervals and calcium/creatinine ratio annually.[56] An airway exam should be performed to assess for potential indicators of difficult airway.

Since anxiety is common in patients with WS, the perioperative hospital setting may exacerbate such behavior; premedication may aid in a smoother induction. Preoperative hydration should be stressed to maintain adequate preload, and scheduling should attempt to minimize prolonged NPO times. Intraoperatively, a five-lead ECG should be utilized to monitor for ischemia, and a lower threshold should exist for placing invasive monitors. According to Burch, "All patients with SVAS should be considered at risk for myocardial ischemia."[57] Anesthetic goals should reflect this and should include maintenance of an age-appropriate heart rate and sinus rhythm, maintenance of preload, contractility and SVR (with vasopressors if needed), and avoidance of increased PVR.[57] Attempts to stratify perioperative risk in individuals with WS indicate that children with biventricular outflow tract obstruction and age <3 years are at highest risk of cardiac arrest,[57] although the potential for perioperative cardiac complications should not be underestimated in any child with WS.

SYNDROMES WITH AIRWAY MANAGEMENT CONCERNS

Several syndromes are of interest to the pediatric anesthesiologist because of potential difficulty with ventilation

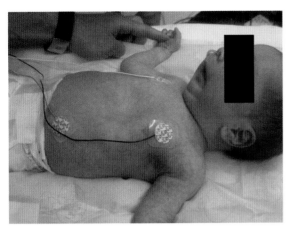

▲ **Figure 40-3.** Pierre Robin neonate. Note the micrognathia and resultant sternal retraction. (Reproduced with permission, from Hung OR, Murphy MF. eds. *Hung's Difficult and Failed Airway Management*. 3rd ed. 2018. https://accessanesthesiology.mhmedical. com. Copyright © McGraw Hill LLC. All rights reserved.)

or tracheal intubation. Airway concerns for the following syndromes are outlined below.

Micrognathia or Mandibular Hypoplasia

Pierre Robin Sequence (PRS) is defined by the triad of micrognathia, glossoptosis, and airway obstruction (see Figure 40-3). An underlying genetic abnormality has not been identified and PRS may occur in isolation or in association with a syndrome (commonly Stickler syndrome, 22q11DS, fetal alcohol syndrome, and Treacher–Collins syndrome). Its incidence ranges from 1:5000 to 1:85,000.[58] In non-syndromic PRS, jaw size may increase (and airway difficulty may improve) with age.[43,59] Symptoms in PRS may range from mild to severe, with severe airway obstruction causing respiratory distress and failure to thrive. Affected infants may require various interventions to relieve airway obstruction, including prone positioning, nasopharyngeal airway placement, tongue lip adhesion, mandibular distraction osteogenesis, and/or tracheostomy. Cleft palate is common among individuals with PRS. Due to severe micrognathia and airway obstruction, airway management may be quite challenging. Maintenance of spontaneous ventilation should be emphasized and specialized airway equipment (fiberoptic bronchoscopy, video laryngoscopy) and adjuncts (nasopharyngeal and oropharyngeal airways) should be available. Awake supraglottic device placement (with subsequent fiberoptic intubation) is a well-known successful technique in patients with severe airway obstruction.[60]

Treacher-Collins syndrome (or mandibulofacial dysostosis) is caused by a mutation of the *TCOF1* gene and is inherited in an autosomal dominant manner (though 60% arise from new mutations). Its incidence is estimated at 1:50,000 live births. Craniofacial features affecting the airway include maxillary, zygomatic, and mandibular hypoplasia combined with small mouth opening, high arched palate, and temporomandibular joint abnormalities. These features may contribute to airway obstruction hindering bag mask ventilation and difficult direct laryngoscopy and intubation.[60] Unlike individuals with PRS, airway management in Treacher-Collins may increase in difficulty with patient age.[43,61] Airway devices such as nasopharyngeal airways and supraglottic devices should be readily available as should specialized intubating equipment (fiberoptic bronchoscopy, video laryngoscopy) as conventional direct laryngoscopy is often insufficient in these patients.

Craniofacial Microsomia

Hemifacial microsomia is caused by a derangement in the development of the first and second pharyngeal arches during embryogenesis; its cause is unknown, but is thought to be multifactorial (most cases are sporadic, with few inherited; maternal exposure and environmental factors may play a role).[61] Its incidence ranges from 1: 3500 to 1: 27,000 live births.[62] This malformation results in unilateral cranial bone abnormalities, microtia/anotia with preauricular skin tags/pits, microphthalmia, and, most significantly, mandibular hypoplasia which may cause difficulties in direct laryngoscopy and intubation (bilateral microsomia does occur in approximately 20% and may resemble Treacher–Collins syndrome in both clinical phenotype and level of airway difficulty).[63]

Goldenhar syndrome is considered a variant of hemifacial microsomia that, in addition to unilateral cranial and soft tissue deformities, also includes vertebral anomalies and epibulbar dermoids (benign eye cysts).[63] Vertebral anomalies may include fused or hemivertebrae which may limit neck flexion and extension and worsen intubating conditions.[43]

Limited Cervical Mobility

Klippel-Feil syndrome occurs in 1:42,000 births and its etiology is yet unknown. Individuals with Klippel–Feil syndrome have a short neck, low posterior hairline and severe limitation in cervical motion. The *limitation in cervical motion* is caused by congenital fusion of two or more cervical vertebrae (and may be classified into Types I to III based on degree of fusion on radiographic examination). Cervical fusion typically worsens with age.[64] Bag mask ventilation is not typically difficult,[43] but severe restriction of range of cervical motion may make direct laryngoscopy very difficult, and fiberoptic intubation or supraglottic airway device is often the preferred route of airway instrumentation. In addition, individuals with Klippel–Feil syndrome are more likely to have additional skeletal abnormalities, such as atlanto-occipital abnormalities, spinal canal stenosis, and scoliosis.[65] As such, caution with head and neck positioning is advised to avoid neurologic injury during airway manipulation.

Turner, **Noonan**, and **Goldenhar** syndromes are also known for limited cervical mobility, which can hinder tracheal intubation by direct laryngoscopy.

Craniofacial Synostosis

Apert syndrome (AS), **Crouzon syndrome** (CS), and **Pfeiffer syndrome** (PS) are three of several common genetic syndromes associated with craniosynostosis. All are caused by (usually) de novo mutations in the *FGFR1-3* genes, though these can be inherited in an autosomal dominant fashion. Their incidence ranges from 1:100,000 (Pfeiffer syndrome) to 6–16:1,000,000 (Apert and Crouzon syndromes). In addition to craniosynostosis, all have flat foreheads, proptosis, and midfacial hypoplasia with narrowed nasopharynx or choanal atresia. Individuals with **Apert syndrome** frequently have bilateral symmetrical syndactyly of upper and lower extremities, cleft palate, and fusion of the cervical spine at C5-6.[65,66] **Pfeiffer syndrome** can be differentiated by the presence of broad, radially deviated thumbs or big toes and occasional partial syndactyly. Patients with **Crouzon syndrome** typically have normal hands and feet and may have fusion of the cervical spine at C2-3.[66,67] Learning disability or delayed development are common in AS and PS but individuals with CS usually have normal intelligence.[68]

These individuals are often prone to upper airway obstruction because of midfacial hypoplasia, and many develop OSA. Those with severe respiratory distress often require tracheostomy. Bag mask ventilation may be challenging not only because of upper airway obstruction but also because of insufficient mask fit secondary to midfacial hypoplasia and proptosis. Direct laryngoscopy, however, is not typically difficult unless cervical spine abnormalities are present.[43]

Tracheal cartilaginous sleeve is associated with syndromic craniosynostosis; lower airway stenosis may result and a smaller endotracheal tube than expected may be necessary.[68]

Mucopolysaccharidoses

The mucopolysaccharidoses are a group of hereditary multisystem disorders that lead to cognitive impairment, organ failure, and shortened lifespan.[69] Except MPS II (Hunter syndrome; X-linked recessive) inheritance is autosomal recessive; their incidence ranges from 1:100,000 (MPS I) to 1: 2,000,000 (MPS VI).[70] They are caused by deficiencies of different lysosomal storage enzymes creating progressive buildup of glycosaminoglycans (GAGs) in various tissues throughout the body. These diseases are heterogenous and the severity of phenotype varies.

MPS I (**Hurler syndrome**) and MPS II (**Hunter syndrome**) have very similar clinical features, which include progressive development of coarse facial features, corneal clouding, hearing loss, short stature, hepatomegaly and splenomegaly, communicating hydrocephalus, and spinal cord compression with cognitive impairment.[70]

Clinical features of individuals with MPS IV (**Morquio syndrome**) include those for MPS I and II, but these individuals also exhibit skeletal dysplasia, ligamentous laxity and joint hypermobility (rather than stiff joints with decreased mobility in MPS I/II), and odontoid hypoplasia leading to potential cervical spine instability.[70] Individuals also may develop kyphoscoliosis with subsequent restrictive pulmonary defects. Tracheal collapse has also been reported with flexion of the head (which causes buckling of the posterior tracheal wall).[71] In contrast to MPS I and II, these patients typically do not have cognitive impairment.

Airway management is a primary concern in patients with MPS. Submucosal GAG deposition in the tongue, nasopharynx, oropharynx, and larynx leads to progressive upper airway obstruction;[72] mask ventilation can be very challenging or impossible. Additionally, a short neck with limited range of motion and limited mobility of the temporomandibular joint (combined with narrowed and rigid airway anatomy) contribute to difficult direct laryngoscopy and intubation.[71] Incidence of difficult airway in MPS patients has been reported at around 25%;[73] preoperative airway examination is critical as is careful preparation for airway instrumentation. Fiberoptic intubation or video laryngoscopy is often needed and a supraglottic device should be available as a rescue device. As would be expected with progressive GAG buildup, airway difficulty worsens with age.

Secondarily, GAG deposition in the heart can lead to valve thickening and subsequent dysfunction (insufficiency more commonly than stenosis). Generally mitral and aortic valves are affected more frequently; valvular disease can progress to LV volume overload, LVH, or dilation, followed by ventricular dysfunction. Coronary artery narrowing secondary to GAG deposition has also been described.[74]

Enzyme replacement therapy and hematopoetic stem cell transplant are therapies that have been instituted and if initiated early on, they may alter progression of the disease.

REFERENCES

1. Galinkin JL, Demmer L, Yaster M. Genetics for the pediatric anesthesiologist. *Anesth Analg.* 2010;111(5):1264-1274.
2. Borland LM, Colligan J, Brandom BW. Frequency of anesthesia- related complications in children with down syndrome under general anesthesia for noncardiac procedures. *Pediatr Anesth.* 2004;14(9):733-738.
3. Lewanda AF, Matisoff A, Revenis M, et al. Preoperative evaluation and comprehensive risk assessment for children with Down syndrome. *Pediatr Anesth.* 2016;26(4): 356-362.

4. Kliegman RM, St Geme III JW, Blum NJ, et al. *Cytogenetics: Nelson Textbook of Pediatrics, 2-Volume Set.* 21st ed. Elsevier; 2016:chap. 98.

5. Bull MJ; the Committee on Genetics. Health supervision for children with Down syndrome. *Pediatrics.* 2011;128(2): 393-406.

6. Hata T, Todd MM. Cervical spine considerations when anesthetizing patients with Down syndrome. *Anesthesiology.* 2005;102(3):680-685.

7. Bai W, Voepel-Lewis T, Malviya S. Hemodynamic changes in children with Down syndrome during and following inhalation induction of anesthesia with sevoflurane. *J Clin Anesth.* 2010;22(8):592-597.

8. Sulemanji DS, et al. Vascular catheterization is difficult in infants with Down syndrome. *Acta Anaesthesiol Scand.* 2009;53(1):98-100.

9. Rios A, et al. Recognizing the clinical features of trisomy 13 syndrome. *Adv Neonat Care.* 2004;4(6):332-343.

10. Pollard RC, Beasley JM. Anaesthesia for patients with trisomy 13 (Patau's syndrome). *Pediatr Anesth.* 1996;6(2): 151-153.

11. Martlew RA, Sharples A. Anaesthesia in a child with Patau's syndrome. *Anaesthesia.* 1995;50(11):980-982.

12. Cereda A, Carey JC. The trisomy 18 syndrome. *Orphanet J Rare Dis.* 2012;7(1):81.

13. Courreges P, Nieuviarts R, Lecoutre D. Anaesthetic management for Edward's syndrome. *Pediatr Anesth.* 2003;13(3):267-269.

14. Mashour GA, Sunder N, Acquadro MA. Anesthetic management of Turner syndrome: A systematic approach. *J Clin Anesth.* 2005;17(2):128-130.

15. Sybert VP, McCauley E. Turner's syndrome. *New Engl J Med.* 2004;351(12):1227-1238.

16. Maranhão, Marcius VM. Turner syndrome and anesthesia. *Rev. Bras. Anestesiol.* 2008;58(1):84-89.

17. Divekar VM, Kothari MD, Kamdar BM. Anaesthesia in Turner's syndrome. *Can Anaesth Soc J.* 1983;30(4): 417-418.

18. Bondy CA. Congenital cardiovascular disease in Turner syndrome. *Congenit Heart Dis.* 2008;3(1):2-15.

19. Solomon BD, et al. Clinical geneticists' views of VACTERL/VATER association. *Am J Med Genet A.* 2012;158(12):3087-3100.

20. Solomon BD, et al. An approach to the identification of anomalies and etiologies in neonates with identified or suspected VACTERL (vertebral defects, anal atresia, tracheoesophageal fistula with esophageal atresia, cardiac anomalies, renal anomalies, and limb anomalies) association. *J Pediatr.* 2014;164(3):451-451.

21. Solomon BD. VACTERL/VATER association. *Orphanet J Rare Dis.* 2011;6(1):56.

22. Blake KD, Prasad C. CHARGE syndrome. *Orphanet J Rare Dis.* 2006;1(1):34-38.

23. Jongmans MCJ. CHARGE syndrome: the phenotypic spectrum of mutations in the CHD7 gene. *J Med Genet.* 2005;43(4):306-314.

24. Jyonouchi S, McDonald-McGinn DM, Bale S, Zackai EH, Sullivan KE. CHARGE (Coloboma, Heart Defect, Atresia Choanae, Retarded Growth and Development, Genital Hypoplasia, Ear Anomalies/Deafness) syndrome and chromosome 22q11.2 deletion syndrome: a comparison of immunologic and nonimmunologic phenotypic features. *Pediatrics.* 2009;123(5):e871-e877.

25. Corsten-Janssen N, et al. The cardiac phenotype in patients with a CHD7 mutation. *Circ Cardiovasc Genet.* 2013;6(3):248-254.

26. White DR, et al. Aspiration in children with CHARGE syndrome. *Int J Pediatr Otorhinolaryngol.* 2005;69(9): 1205-1209.

27. Stack CG, Wyse RK. Incidence and management of airway problems in the CHARGE association. *Anaesthesia.* 1991;46(7):582-585.

28. Hartshorne TS, Hefner MA, Davenport SLH. Behavior in CHARGE syndrome: Introduction to the special topic. *Am J Med Genet A.* 2005;133(3):228-231.

29. Blake K, et al. Postoperative airway events of individuals with CHARGE syndrome. *Int J Pediatr Otorhinolaryngol.* 2009;73(2):219-226.

30. Bassett AS, et al. Practical guidelines for managing patients with 22q11.2 deletion syndrome. *J Pediatr.* 2011;159(2):332-339.e1.

31. Kobrynski LJ, Sullivan KE. Velocardiofacial syndrome, DiGeorge syndrome: the chromosome 22q11.2 deletion syndromes. *Lancet.* 2007;370(9596):1443-1452.

32. Momma K. Cardiovascular anomalies associated with chromosome 22q11.2 deletion syndrome. *Am J Cardiol.* 2010;105(11):1617-1624.

33. Yeoh TY, et al. Perioperative management of patients with DiGeorge syndrome undergoing cardiac surgery. *J Cardiothorac Vasc Anesth.* 2014;28(4):983-989.

34. Yotsui-Tsuchimochi H, et al. Anesthetic management of a child with chromosome 22q11 deletion syndrome. *Pediatr Anesth.* 2006;16(4):454-457.

35. Cuneo BF. 22q11.2 deletion syndrome: DiGeorge, velocardiofacial, and conotruncal anomaly face syndromes. *Curr Opin Pediatr.* 2001;13(5):465-472.

36. Weinzimer SA. Endocrine aspects of the 22q11.2 deletion syndrome. *Genet Med.* 2001;3(1):19-22.

37. Li M, Squire JA, Weksberg R. Molecular genetics of Wiedemann-Beckwith syndrome. *Am J Med Genet A.* 1998;79(4):253-259.

38. Shuman C, Beckwith JB, Weksberg R. Beckwith-Wiedemann syndrome. 2000 March 3 [Updated 2016 August 11]. In: Pagon RA, Adam MP, Ardinger HH, et al., eds. *GeneReviews*® [Internet]. Seattle, WA: University of Washington, Seattle; 1993-2016. Available at https://www.ncbi.nlm.nih.gov/books/NBK1394/. Accessed July 31, 2020.

39. Celiker V, Basgul E, Karagoz AH. Anesthesia in Beckwith-Wiedemann syndrome. *Pediatr Anesth* 2004;14(9):778-780.

40. Tobias JD, Lowe S, Holcomb GW. Anesthetic considerations of an infant with Beckwith-Wiedemann syndrome. *J Clin Anesth.* 1992;4(6):484-486.

41. Suan C, et al. Anaesthesia and the Beckwith-Wiedemann syndrome. *Pediatr Anesth.* 1996;6(3):231-233.

42. Nargozian C. The airway in patients with craniofacial abnormalities. *Pediatr Anesth.* 2004;14(1):53-59.

43. Eaton J, Atiles R, Tuchman JB. GlideScope for management of the difficult airway in a child with Beckwith-Wiedemann syndrome. *Pediatr Anesth.* 2009;19(7):696-698.

44. Roland EH. Muscular dystrophy. *Pediatr Rev.* 2000;21(7): 233-237-quiz 238.

45. Segura LG, et al. Anesthesia and Duchenne or Becker muscular dystrophy: Review of 117 anesthetic exposures. *Pediatr Anesth.* 2013;23(9):855-864.

46. Biggar WD. Duchenne Muscular dystrophy. *Pediatr Rev.* 2006;27(3):83-88.

47. Blatter JA, Finder JD. Perioperative respiratory management of pediatric patients with neuromuscular disease. *Pediatr Anesth.* 2013;23(9):770-776.

48. Cripe LH, Tobias JD. Cardiac considerations in the operative management of the patient with Duchenne or

Becker muscular dystrophy. *Pediatr Anesth.* 2013;23(9): 777-784.

49. Chiang DY, et al. Relation of cardiac dysfunction to rhythm abnormalities in patients with Duchenne or Becker muscular dystrophies. *Am J Cardiol.* 2016;117(8):1349-1354.

50. Muenster T, et al. Anaesthetic management in patients with duchenne muscular dystrophy undergoing orthopaedic surgery. *Eur J Anaesthesiol.* 2012;29(10):489-494.

51. Romano AA, et al. Noonan syndrome: Clinical features, diagnosis, and management guidelines. *Pediatrics.* 2010;126(4):746-759.

52. Artoni A, et al. Hemostatic abnormalities in Noonan syndrome. *Pediatrics.* 2014;133(5):e1299-e1304.

53. Matisoff AJ, et al. Risk assessment and anesthetic management of patients with Williams syndrome: A comprehensive review. *Pediatr Anesth.* 2015;25(12):1207-1215.

54. Medley J, Russo P, Tobias JD. Perioperative care of the patient with Williams syndrome. *Pediatr Anesth.* 2005;15(3):243-247.

55. Morris CA. Williams syndrome. 1999 April 9 [Updated 2013 June 13]. In: Pagon RA, Adam MP, Ardinger HH, et al., eds. *GeneReviews* [Internet]. Seattle, WA: University of Washington, Seattle; 1993-2016. Available at https://www.ncbi.nlm.nih.gov/books/NBK1249/. Accessed July 31, 2020.

56. Burch TM, et al. Congenital supravalvular aortic stenosis and sudden death associated with anesthesia: What's the mystery? *Anesth Analg.* 2008;107(6):1848-1854.

57. Latham GJ, et al. Perioperative morbidity in children with elastin arteriopathy. *Pediatr Anesth.* 2016;26(9):926-935.

58. Cladis F, et al. Pierre Robin sequence. *Anesth Analg.* 2014;119(2):400-412.

59. Sims C, von Ungern-Sternberg BS. The normal and the challenging pediatric airway. *Pediatr Anesth.* 2012;22(6):521-526.

60. Hosking J, et al. Anesthesia for Treacher-Collins syndrome: A review of airway management in 240 pediatric cases. *Pediatr Anesth.* 2012;22(8):752-758.

61. Heike CL, Luquetti DV, Hing AV. Craniofacial microsomia overview. 2009 March 19 [Updated 2014 Oct 9]. In: Pagon RA, Adam MP, Ardinger HH, et al., eds. *GeneReviews* [Internet]. Seattle, WA: University of Washington, Seattle; 1993-2016. Available at https://www.ncbi.nlm.nih.gov/books/NBK5199/. Accessed July 31, 2020.

62. Nargozian C. Hemifacial microsomia: Anatomical prediction of difficult intubation. *Pediatr Anesth.* 1999;9(5):393-398.

63. Tuin J, et al. Distinguishing Goldenhar syndrome from craniofacial microsomia. *J Craniofacial Surg.* 2015;26(6):1887-1892.

64. Stallmer ML, Vanaharam V, Mashour GA. Congenital cervical spine fusion and airway management: A case series of Klippel-Feil syndrome. *J Clin Anesth.* 2008;20(6):447-451.

65. Barnett S, Moloney C, Bingham R. Perioperative complications in children with apert syndrome: A review of 509 anesthetics. *Pediatr Anesth.* 2010;21(1):72-77.

66. Johnson D, Wilkie AOM. Craniosynostosis. *Eur J Human Genet.* 2011;19(4):369-376.

67. Ko JM. Genetic syndromes associated with craniosynostosis. *J Korean Neurosurg Soc.* 2016;59(3):187-191.

68. Wenger TL, et al. Tracheal cartilaginous sleeves in children with syndromic craniosynostosis. *Genet Med.* May 26, 2016.

69. Muenzer J. Overview of the mucopolysaccharidoses. *Rheumatology.* 2011;50(5):v4-v12.

70. Frawley G, et al. A retrospective audit of anesthetic techniques and complications in children with mucopolysaccharidoses. *Pediatr Anesth.* 2012;22(8):737-744.

71. Theroux MC, et al. Anesthetic care and perioperative complications of children with morquio syndrome. *Pediatr Anesth.* 2012;22(9):901-907.

72. Megens JHAM, et al. Perioperative complications in patients diagnosed with mucopolysaccharidosis and the impact of enzyme replacement therapy followed by hematopoietic stem cell transplantation at early age. *Pediatr Anesth.* 2014;24(5):521-527.

73. Kirkpatrick K, Ellwood J, Walker RWM. Mucopolysaccharidosis type I (Hurler syndrome) and anesthesia: The impact of bone marrow transplantation, enzyme replacement therapy, and fiberoptic intubation on airway management. *Pediatr Anesth.* 2012;22(8):745-751.

74. Braunlin EA, et al. Cardiac disease in patients with mucopolysaccharidosis: Presentation, diagnosis and management. *J Inherit Metab Dis.* 2011;34(6):1183-1197.

Index

Note: Page numbers followed by "*f*" are to figures; page numbers followed by "*t*" are to tables; page numbers followed by "*b*" are to boxes.